Examination and Diagnosis
of Musculoskeletal Disorders

Examination and Diagnosis of Musculoskeletal Disorders

Clinical Examination · Imaging Modalities

William H. M. Castro, M.D.
Professor and Supervising Physician
Münster Orthopedic Research Institute
Formerly Supervising Physician
for the Academy for Manual Medicine
Westfälische Wilhelms University
Münster
Germany

Jörg Jerosch, M.D.
Professor and Director
Clinic for Orthopedic Surgery
Johanna-Etienne-Krankenhaus
Neuss
Germany

Thomas W. Grossman, Jr., M.D., F.A.C.S.
Adjunct Assistant Professor of Surgery
Uniformed Services University of the Health Sciences
Bethesda, Maryland
Orthopedics, Aurora Medical Group
Burlington and Elkhorn, Wisconsin
USA

With contributions by

Josef Assheuer, Henry Halm, Susanne Fuchs, Ulf Liljenqvist, Ulrich Plewka, Horst Rieger, Thomas Schneider, Michael Schröder, Ludwig Schwering, Joachim Scuik, and Jörn Steinbeck

1166 illustrations

Thieme
Stuttgart · New York 2001

Library of Congress Cataloging-in-Publication Data is available from the publisher.

Translated by John Grossman, Berlin, Germany

This book is an authorized, revised translation of the German editions published and copyrighted 1995 and 1996 by Ferdinand Enke Verlag, Stuttgart, Germany. Title of the German editions: Orthopädisch-traumatologische Gelenkdiagnostik and Orthopädisch-traumatologische Wirbelsäulen- und Beckendiagnostik.

© 2001 Georg Thieme Verlag,
Rüdigerstraße 14, D-70469 Stuttgart, Germany
Thieme New York, 333 Seventh Avenue,
New York, N.Y. 10001 U.S.A.

Typesetting by Mitterweger & Partner,
D-68723 Plankstadt

Printed in Germany by Grammlich, Pliezhausen

ISBN 3-13-111031-7 (GTV)
ISBN 1-58890-032-0 (TNY)   1 2 3 4 5

Foreword

William Castro and his co-authors have provided us with an important as well as timely addition to the reference works that should be part of every orthopedic surgeon's library. Their techniques produce the most exact and enduring picture that we can obtain of a patient. Beginning with the patient and his/her complaint, we are shown how to help the patient flesh out the details of the history and subsequently how to perform the examination. This is almost all the information that we actually have on our patient.

Diagnostic entities, while essential to the treatment, are frequently shown to be incomplete concepts by rapid progress in medicine. Recently touted diagnostic tests have been demonstrated to show lesions in asymptomatic patients that could lead to misdiagnosis if not interpreted in the light of a proper history and physical examination. On the other hand, at least one recent study has shown strong variations in the manner in which some stages of the physical examination are performed.

While our mental picture of diseases may change, we, the patient, and his/her complaint remain the only constant. The patient deserves a proper work-up. Herein lies the value of this text as an essential reference for all orthopedic surgeons and residents.

Christopher M. Jobe, M.D.
Professor and Program Director
Loma Linda University Medical Center
Department of Orthopedic Surgery
Loma Linda, California

Contributors' Addresses

Josef Assheuer, M.D.
Attending Physician
Department of Neuroanatomy
University of Düsseldorf
Düsseldorf, Germany

Henry Halm, M.D.
Director
Clinic for Spinal Surgery/Center for
Scoliosis/Center for Thorax Deformities
Neustadt Clinic
Neustadt, Germany

Susanne Fuchs, M.D.
Associate Professor and Supervising Physician
Clinic for Orthopedic Surgery
Westfälische-Wilhelms University
Münster, Germany

Ulf Liljenqvist, M.D.
Supervising Physician
Clinic for Orthopedic Surgery
Westfälische-Wilhelms University
Münster, Germany

Ulrich Plewka, M.D.
Medical Consultant for the German
National Health Service

Horst Rieger, M.D.
Professor and Director
Clinic for Trauma, Hand, and Reconstructive Surgery
Clemens Hospital
Münster, Germany

Thomas Schneider, M.D.
Director
Clinic for Orthopedic and Trauma
Dreifaltigkeits Hospital
Cologne, Germany

Michael Schröder, M.D.
Private Practice in Orthopedic Surgery
Krefeld, Germany

Ludwig Schwering, M.D.
Supervising Physician
Seepark Hospital
Langen, Germany

Joachim Scuik, M.D.
Professor and Supervising Physician
Clinic for Nuclear Medicine
Westfälische-Wilhelms University
Münster, Germany

Jörn Steinbecks, M.D.
Associate Professor and Supervising Physician
Clinic for Orthopedic Surgery
Westfälische-Wilhelms University
Münster, Germany

Contents

2 Elbow

3 Hand

4 Hip

5 Knee

9   Pelvis

1 Shoulder

1.1 Introduction

Acute shoulder injuries and chronic shoulder symptoms have become an increasing problem in recent years. Degenerative shoulder symptoms are exceeded only by degenerative back and knee disorders. Causes include sports, leisure activities, and occupational stresses overlaid on age-related degeneration. Decades of repetitive overhead movements in occupational, leisure, or domestic activities can cause stress syndromes. With increasing age, the incidence of degenerative changes of the shoulder approaches 100%.

Occupational shoulder complaints are not a new phenomenon. The galley slaves of ancient times were well acquainted with the effects of asymmetric stress from rowing. The modern physiologic equivalents of these galley slaves are world-class tennis players. Here, asymmetric stress and adaptation result in complex changes in the muscles, tendons, and bones referred to as "tennis shoulder." While the shoulder complex is crucial to the coordinated movements of most sports, the force, flexibility, and endurance requirements of athletic activity often exceed physiologic limits. Repetitive overhead movements can induce attritional mechanisms with resulting pathologic changes to the rotator cuff. In the throwing athlete, forceful windup, cocking, and acceleration motions can produce anterior instability. Deceleration on follow-through can produce posterior instability. Eccentric loads can cause tenosynovitis. The adolescent athlete is faced with age-specific problems in the form of incomplete epiphyseal fusion, just as the older athlete must contend with degenerative changes to the tendon of the supraspinatus muscle.

1.2 Clinical Examination

Standard Examination

The patient is observed from the front. The sternoclavicular joint, clavicle, acromioclavicular joint, and the pectoralis major and biceps are evaluated. Posterior observation to evaluate for atrophy in the infraspinatus and supraspinatus follows. For the rest of the examination, stand behind the patient. After a preliminary examination of the cervical spine, palpate the sternoclavicular joint, clavicle, acromioclavicular joint, coracoid process, the long tendon of the biceps, and the supraspinatus tendon in internal rotation. Range-of-motion tests are then performed using the neutral-0 method (flexion/extension, abduction/adduction, external rotation/internal rotation in a neutral position and abduction). The painful arc of motion can be assessed. Horizontal adduction may also reveal pain with cross-body compression. The apprehension test is also performed standing behind the patient, as is evaluation of the sulcus sign. Move to the front of the patient to conduct the Jobe test and to assess the strength and sensation of the upper extremities.

Depending on the working diagnosis, this standard examination is supplemented by various specific tests discussed in the following section.

Patient History

As in any medical encounter, the examination of the shoulder begins with taking the patient's history. This forms the basis for the working diagnosis. The various disorders of the shoulder can be caused by acute trauma, repetitive microtrauma, age-related degeneration, or systemic disorders. In patients with acute injuries, the manner in which the accident occurred and observation of the cardinal symptoms (redness, warmth, swelling, loss of function, etc.) can provide sufficient information for a diagnosis. Chronic complaints require an extensive history. This requires a good memory on the part of the patient, an extensive review of medical records, and no small amount of detective work on the part of the physician to make the diagnosis and identify the cause.

Many of the systemic disorders that affect the shoulder are hereditary. If a hereditary disorder is suspected, a detailed family history must be explored.

The age of the patient is a critical factor in the overall evaluation of symptoms. Many disorders of the shoulder girdle occur more frequently within certain age-groups. For example, clavicular fractures and torticollis frequently occur in newborns and infants. Congenital deformities such as Sprengel deformity, Klippel–Feil syndrome, or cleidocranial dysostosis are first observed at this age. Septic arthritides or osteomyelitis can be the cause of fevers in infants (Table 1.1). Acute injuries predominate in adolescents and young adults. These include dislocated shoulders, injuries to the acromioclavicular joint, and clavicular

Table 1.**1**   Typical shoulder disorders in various age-groups

Newborn/infant	Adolescent/young adult	Older adult
Clavicular fracture	Traumatic instability	Partial tear of the rotator cuff
Torticollis	Acromioclavicular-joint separation	Complete tear of the rotator cuff
Septic arthritis	Clavicular fracture	Arthritis of the acromioclavicular joint
Osteomyelitis	Dislocation of the sternoclavicular joint	Fracture of the proximal humerus
Sprengel deformity	Tenosynovitis	Calcific tendinitis
Klippel–Feil syndrome	Atraumatic instability	Subacromial bursitis
Cleidocranial dysostosis	Subacromial bursitis	

fractures. After the age of 30, degenerative symptoms tend to predominate, primarily impingement syndrome, tears in the rotator cuff, and degenerative changes in the acromioclavicular joint. Impingement syndromes can occur in athletes, even at a young age. In this case, primary impingement syndrome must be carefully distinguished from impingement of instability. In the older population, degenerative changes in the rotator cuff and glenohumeral joint predominate.

Inquiring about **occupational** and **athletic activity** provides important information. Occupations that involve overhead work (such as painting) and sports that make similar demands (such as basketball, baseball, tennis, swimming, and volleyball) often lead to symptoms in the subacromial area. Degenerative changes may occur in the acromioclavicular joint. For possible occupational causes, carefully evaluate information on force, repetition, posture, duration of exposure, contact stress, vibration exposure, and low-temperature exposure. Confirm information provided by the patient with material such as formal position descriptions, workplace videos, or job-site analysis provided by a third party. Making a diagnosis of an occupational injury can have a profound negative response to treatment, as it appears that success rates in worker's compensation situations is less than in other settings.

With athletes, taking a history requires knowledge of the specific sport. Only in this manner can characteristic patterns of injury for specific sports be identified. Often these patients do not suffer acute trauma, but repetitive microtrauma can occur with hyperextension at maximum abduction and external rotation in "overhead" sports. This can lead to instability of the shoulder. Often these patients will pre-

sent with symptoms resembling impingement. Instability problems are less prominent in bodybuilders or competitive weight lifters. Be alert for degenerative changes in the acromioclavicular joint and rotator cuff.

With precise knowledge of a particular sport, important information can be obtained by inquiring specifically when pain occurs. A baseball player whose primary symptoms occur during the early cocking phase (abduction and external rotation) may suffer from anterior instability as a result of chronic overloading of the anterior stabilizers of the joint. If complaints occur primarily during the follow-through phase of throwing motion (flexion and internal rotation), then the disorder could involve either posterior instability or tendonopathy. Other related activities exist that can cause symptoms if instability is present. These include reaching high overhead while rebounding in basketball, a running spike in volleyball with the shoulder hyperextended, or a hard stroke in tennis with the arm extended overhead.

Taking a detailed history can also provide important information about degenerative disorders or repetitive microtrauma. For example, a tennis player with supraspinatus tendinitis may complain of sharp pain during a backhand stroke, while a forehand stroke presents no problem at all. The same applies to the serve. A tennis player with supraspinatus tendinitis can have discomfort when the tendon is compressed between the greater tuberosity of the humerus and the acromion in the final phase of an overhead serve when there is maximum internal rotation on the follow-through. This internal rotation is avoided in a forehand serve that can be performed without any pain.

When the history reveals dysfunction following prior trauma, it is important to reconstruct the mechanism of injury as precisely as possible. The magnitude, direction, and point of impact of the forces acting on the joint are important in establishing whether a direct or indirect mechanism of injury was involved. This inquiry yields important diagnostic information about the type and extent of injury. Acute trauma with the arm abducted and externally rotated generally results in an anteroinferior dislocation of the shoulder. A typical example is the quarterback who is sacked by the defensive lineman in the midst of throwing. Internal rotation and adduction often

Table 1.**2**   Occupational and athletic activities associated with increased shoulder stress. (The role of occupational stress is less well studied than the role of athletic exposure.)

Occupation	Sport
Painting	Throwing sports
Drywalling	Tennis
Plastering	Weight lifting
Air-hammer operation	Racquetball
	Swimming

Table 1.**3**   Associations between sports and shoulder complaints

Known association with shoulder complaints	Possible association with shoulder complaints	Rare association with shoulder complaints
Handball	Windsurfing	Cross-country skiing
Volleyball	Rowing	Cycling
Tennis	Waterskiing	Riding
Basketball	Dancing	Hockey
Squash	Ballet	Soccer
Swimming	Swimming	Roller skating
Butterfly, backstroke, crawl	Breaststroke	Ice skating
Badminton	Ice hockey	
Weight lifting	Archery	
Fencing		
Boxing		
Throwing sports		
Baseball, shot put, javelin, discus, hammer		
Martial arts		
Judo, aikido, karate, teakwondo		
Gymnastics		
Floor exercises, horizontal bar, parallel bars, uneven parallel bars, beam		

causes posterior dislocation of the shoulder. A fall with the arm extended can cause dislocation if the player fails to tense his or her muscles in anticipation of the fall. A direct blow to the lateral aspect of the shoulder suggests acromioclavicular joint separation. A direct blow to the clavicle or a fall on the extended arm can cause a clavicular fracture. If the patient has a history of shoulder instability, then the question of whether the instability was triggered by acute trauma or a unique motion is important. It is also important to ask if reduction was necessary. Did reduction occur spontaneously, or did the patient position the arm to obtain reduction? Was reduction only possible in an emergency-room setting or only under anesthesia? Was reduction painful? In the case of recurrent instability, documenting the initial event is particularly important. Did trauma precede this dislocation? How old was the patient when the first dislocation occurred? All these questions are crucial for classifying the instability and determining appropriate therapy (Table 1.**4a, b**)

However, acute trauma is not always the cause of acute symptoms. In patients with previous tendon degeneration, even normal motion can lead to rupture of the supraspinatus tendon. For example, if a 40-year-old tennis player with a 4-year history of shoulder discomfort complains of a sudden stabbing pain during a serve, this would suggest a rotator-cuff tear. On the other hand, sudden pain during a tennis serve in a 20-year-old tennis player is more likely to be a sign of shoulder subluxation (dead-arm syndrome).

Table 1.**4a**   Classification of shoulder instability for purposes of therapy

Timing	Cause	Direction	Degree
Acute	Traumatic	Anterior	Subluxation
Recurrent	Repetitive microtrauma	Posterior	Dislocation
Chronic	Atraumatic	Inferior	
		Multidirectional	

Table 1.**4b**   Classification of glenohumeral instability. Instability of the shoulder is differentiated as follows:

Timing	Cause	Direction	Degree	Volition
Acute	Traumatic	Anterior	Dislocation	Involuntary
Primary	Atraumatic	Posterior	Subluxation	Voluntary
Recurrent	Repetitive micro-	Inferior		— Positional
Chronic	trauma (overuse)	Bidirectional		— Muscular
		— Anterior inferior		— Psychological disorder
		— Posterior inferior		
		Multidirectional		

In the presence of chronic complaints, the type of pain should be quantified:

— When did the pain first occur?
— How long does the pain usually last?
— What type of pain is it, diffuse or stabbing?
— Where is the pain localized?
— Into which parts of the body does the pain radiate?
— Are there specific movements that provoke the pain?
— Does the pain occur before, during, or after exercise?
— Does the pain occur at night?
— Is the night pain intense enough to wake the patient?

The type of pain can suggest probable diagnoses to the experienced examiner. For example, the diffuse deep pain that occurs in disorders of the rotator cuff can be clearly differentiated by the patient's history from the sharp localized pain of acute calcific bursitis. Even in degenerative shoulder disorders, the motion triggering the pain is a crucial piece of diagnostic information. Supraspinatus disorders often produce symptoms from 40° to 120° of abduction; a degenerative acromioclavicular joint will cause problems at the end of range of motion in abduction and when grasping the contralateral shoulder. Frequently, pain will manifest itself in two phases. For example, adhesive capsulitis can be divided into an initial painful phase (freezing phase), in which mobility still exists, and a second painless phase (frozen phase), in which the joint is immobile. The acute pain of a degenerative rotator-cuff tear is almost always preceded by an extended episode of diffuse shoulder pain, pain at night, and pain with the arms extended overhead.

Sometimes a patient will complain of weakness; he or she is no longer able to make certain movements or may notice changes in muscle contour. Atrophy of the supraspinatus or infraspinatus musculature is noticed far more than the conspicuous and typical changes in the contour of the upper arm after a tear in the long biceps tendon. The patient's spouse, parents, coach, or tennis partner are more likely to notice compensatory movements than the patient.

Aside from the specific questions focusing primarily on the shoulder girdle, inquire about systematic diseases and other disease processes (Table 1.5). For example, angina often radiates into the shoulder and arm; the radiating pain does not always occur on the left side. Depending on variations in myocardial

vascular anatomy, pain can radiate into the right upper extremity. Gallbladder and liver disorders can also produce pain in the right shoulder. The patient's neurologic and endocrine status should be explored. Both rheumatoid arthritis and hyperuricemia manifest themselves in the shoulder. Patients with diabetes mellitus experience an above-average incidence of shoulder complaints.

Even in young patients the possibility of a neoplastic process cannot be ignored, particularly when the history is inconsistent with known primary shoulder disorders. One of the most frequent neoplastic causes for shoulder pain is a Pancoast tumor with a typical Horner syndrome. Other causes include primary osteogenic tumors in younger patients, and metastatic disease in older patients. A history of cold or numb fingers suggests a compressive neuropathy or vascular compromise.

To complete the history, document previous interventions. Inquire specifically about the number, type, and site of previous injections. It is also essential to elicit a history of other medications. Any indication of treatment with anabolic steroids is important, particularly in athletes, because these drugs significantly decrease the ability of muscle-tendon units to respond to exertion. Tears can occur in these weakened structures.

As in any physical examination, a systemic approach is the key to clinical examination of the shoulder. Such an approach can help to prevent important findings from being overlooked and can reduce the risk of inadequate documentation.

Every clinical examination consists of three parts: observation, palpation, and tests.

Observation

Observing the patient provides an initial insight into the diagnosis. This begins the moment the patient's name is called in the waiting room. Note how the patient arises from the chair, his/her gait, and the motion of the contralateral upper extremity. Does the patient undress smoothly and symmetrically? A patient with a frozen shoulder will avoid any shoulder rotation and movements above horizontal when undressing. If acute calcific bursitis is present, the intense pain will cause the patient to anxiously hold the affected arm fixed to the side; often the patient will hold the affected arm with the other hand. Patients with a tear in the rotator cuff will often ask for help when undressing because they lack the

Table 1.5   Non-shoulder–related disorders that have components of shoulder complaints

Angina	Rheumatoid arthritis	Primary neoplasms
Myocardial infarcts	Hyperuricemia	Secondary neoplasms
Biliary disease	Hematologic disease (hemophilia, sickle cell)	Pancoast tumor
Liver diseases	Cervical spine syndrome	Neurovascular entrapment
Irritation of the diaphragm	Epicondylitis	

Fig. 1.**1** Typical appearance of Erb palsy with the arm adducted and in internal rotation.

Fig. 1.**3** Proximal tear of the long head of the biceps showing distal migration of the muscular belly.

Fig. 1.**2** Separation of the acromioclavicular joint showing the superiorly protruding lateral clavicle.

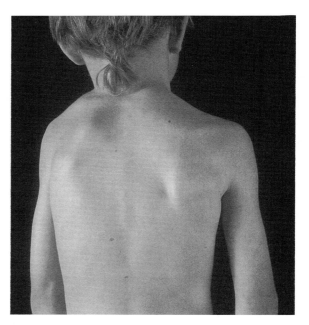

Fig. 1.**4** Sprengel deformity showing the superiorly protruding scapula.

strength to abduct the arm. An arm adducted and held in internal rotation (in the "porter's tip" position) suggests Erb palsy (Fig. 1.**1**).

Always uncover both shoulders for the examination. Examination gowns that leave the shoulder girdle exposed may be helpful with female patients. Inspection begins anteriorly and proceeds posteriorly. Note any blisters, hematomas, scrapes, or other pathologic skin changes. Asymmetry, especially muscular atrophy, is best revealed by comparing one side with the other. A lateral tangential view is better for comparing the sides. This view will reveal minor differences between the sides in the sternoclavicular joints. These may be caused by subluxation or dislocation, or by degenerative changes in the joint. When observing

and comparing the acromioclavicular joint from both sides, be alert to swelling or step-off resulting from acromioclavicular joint separation. The superiorly protruding clavicle with a "piano key" phenomenon is a diagnosis from observation (Fig. 1.**2**) like a tear of the long head of the biceps tendon with distal migration of the muscular belly (Fig. 1.**3**). The same applies to many congenital disorders such as Sprengel deformity (Fig. 1.**4**), Klippel–Feil syndrome, congenital torticollis, or a clavicular fracture frequently occurring in newborns and infants.

Isolated atrophy of the supraspinatus muscle suggests a tear in this tendon. Atrophy of the supraspinatus and infraspinatus muscles can be due to a tear in the rotator cuff or a scapular notch syndrome.

Fig. 1.**5**   Winged scapula, a sequela of a long thoracic nerve injury.

Isolated atrophy of the infraspinatus muscle can be caused by entrapment of the infraspinatus branch of the suprascapular nerve.

If there is one-sided atrophy of the trapezius muscle, possibly in conjunction with scarring after lymph-node dissection, this may imply a lesion of the accessory nerve.

Is the patient a muscular athletic type or an asthenic type? Several injuries and disorders can be detected by observation. An interrupted shoulder contour with the arm slightly abducted and in slight internal rotation is a sign of anterior dislocation. This contrasts with posterior dislocation, in which the arm is more frequently held in internal rotation and adduction.

The drooping dominant shoulder in a tennis player is a frequently seen posture, as is an internally rotated posture with hypertrophy of the pectoralis muscle. The drooping shoulder can result in a secondary thoracic outlet syndrome and secondary impingement syndrome. Scoliotic changes in the spine can also develop. An obvious hematoma in the middle third of the clavicle is a sure sign of a clavicular frac-

Table 1.**6**   Typical diagnoses of disorders made by observation

- Tear of the long head of the biceps
- Chronic tear of the rotator cuff
- Acute anterior shoulder dislocation
- Separation of the acromioclavicular joint
- Erb palsy
- Winged scapula
- Sprengel deformity
- Torticollis

ture. Conspicuous protrusion of the scapula (winged scapula) is often the result of paralysis of the muscles by which it is fixed (serratus anterior and trapezius; Fig. 1.**5**).

Preliminary Examination of the Cervical Spine and Arm

Every examination of the shoulder girdle also includes an examination of the cervical spine (see p. 289). Often, the cause of shoulder symptoms may be found in the cervical spine and vice versa. The examination includes evaluating mobility in flexion and extension, right and left lateral bending, and right and left rotation in neutral head position and with the head flexed and extended. Next, palpate the bony structures, such as the transverse and spinous processes. Often, muscle tension in the paravertebral musculature and the trapezius will cause pain in the shoulder and the back of the neck. The pain is often localized in the descending part of the trapezius muscle. Finally, seek enlarged lymph nodes in the shoulder and neck area.

Look for tenderness to palpation about the elbow that may include medial or lateral epicondylitis. Pain in typical sensory nerve distribution may provide clues about compression neuropathies (cubital tunnel syndrome, carpal tunnel syndrome, or radial tunnel syndrome).

Palpation

The next step involves systematic palpation of the shoulder girdle. This is performed with the patient sitting or standing.

Sternoclavicular joint. Stand behind the patient and begin by examining the sternoclavicular joint. Grasp the clavicle between the thumb and forefinger and move it back and forth to evaluate instability. Tenderness to palpation without instability is a sign of joint irritation. Move laterally along the clavicle from the sternoclavicular joint to the acromioclavicular joint. Any irregularities from an old clavicular fracture will be palpable.

Acromioclavicular joint. The joint space is easily palpable when approached from the medial aspect of the clavicle. Particularly in athletes, whose sport involves overhead movements, and in weight lifters or body builders, the joint will often be tender to palpation, indicating irritation of the joint or the onset of degenerative changes. Instability or a loose acromioclavicular joint can be detected by grasping the clavicle between the thumb and forefinger and moving it back and forth. If the lateral end of the clavicle protrudes as the result of acromioclavicular joint separation, it can be reduced by applying vertical pressure. When the pressure is released, it will spring back into the original position ("piano key" phenomenon).

Fig. 1.**6**   The long tendon of the biceps is palpated in the bicipital groove with the arm in external rotation.

Fig. 1.**7**   The supraspinatus tendon and the subacromial bursa are palpated with the arm in extension.

Coracoid process. Next move the finger approximately one to two finger breadths medially and inferiorly to palpate the coracoid process. If the short head of the biceps or the coracobrachialis is overloaded, the area will be tender to palpation. In rare cases of coracoid impingement there may be local symptoms at this bony prominence.

Bicipital groove. The proximal part of the long tendon of the biceps lies in the subacromial space and courses through the narrow bicipital groove. This groove can be palpated deep in the anterior deltoid region. With the patient's arm flexed at the elbow, passively rotating the arm internally and externally presents the lesser tuberosity, bicipital groove, and greater tuberosity in a more exposed position (Fig. 1.**6**). If pathology is present, this examination will cause the patient discomfort. If the tendon has a tendency to sublux or dislocate, this test can be used to trigger instability for diagnostic purposes.

Subscapularis tendon. Irritation of the subscapularis tendon in athletes is often the result of overuse in throwing sports. With the arm in external rotation, the tendinous insertion can be palpated near the lesser tuberosity.

Anterior joint capsule. With the arm in external rotation, the anterior joint capsule and labrum complex can be palpated between the coracoid process

and the lesser tuberosity. Localized pain in this area due to irritation and lesions of the anterior passive stabilizers, is a sign of anterior instability.

Pectoralis major. The tendinous insertion of the pectoralis major is located distal to the lesser tuberosity. Changes in this muscle will often be found in weight lifters. If the history reveals use of anabolic steroids, a steroid-induced pectoralis tear can occur.

Subacromial space. With the shoulder in a neutral position, neither the subacromial bursa nor the supraspinatus tendon are accessible for palpation. Passively extending the shoulder rotates the structures underneath the acromion outward, allowing palpation of the anterior part of the supraspinatus tendon (Fig. 1.**7**). The parts located further posteriorly are exposed by flexing the arm and palpating immediately behind the posterior margin of the acromion.

Infraspinatus tendon. The infraspinatus tendon in the posterior and lateral portion of the humeral head is accessible with the shoulder in a neutral position. Degenerative changes or overuse injuries are less frequent than in the supraspinatus tendon. Pathologic findings, however, may be present, particularly in athletes with hypermobile or unstable joints as a

Fig. 1.**8**   Complex movements such as the Apley "scratch" test where the patient touches the superior medial angle of the contralateral scapula are used for testing combined external rotation and abduction.

Fig. 1.**9**   To test internal rotation and adduction, the patient touches the anterior aspect of the contralateral shoulder.

Fig. 1.**10**   To test internal rotation and adduction, the patient touches the inferior angle of the contralateral scapula.

result of repetitive eccentric stress from the external rotators.

Systematic and orderly palpation paves the way for further investigation. Despite the important information that can be acquired by physical examination, it may not be sufficient for positive differentiation of bursal-sided, intratendinous, or inferior tears in the rotator cuff. Since this differentiation is crucial in determining treatment, a tentative diagnosis should be confirmed by additional studies.

Assessing Range of Motion

Active range of motion. Several tests utilizing complex motions are suitable for initial evaluation of the patient's active range of motion. These complex motions themselves comprise several separate component motions. One such test is the Apley "scratch" test. To test abduction and external rotation, ask the patient to reach behind his or her head and touch the superior medial angle of the contralateral scapula (Fig. 1.**8**) Internal rotation and adduction are tested by having the patient grasp the contralateral acromion (Fig. 1.**9**). Internal rotation and adduction can also be demonstrated by instructing the patient to touch the inferior angle of the contralateral scapula behind his or her back (Fig. 1.**10**). To test full bilateral abduction, instruct the patient to abduct both arms with the elbows extended and the palms in supination. The patient should be able to touch both hands together in the midline above his or her head (Fig. 1.**11**). The advantage of these tests is that they quickly demonstrate the patient's range of motion for both sides simultaneously. Symmetry of motion and even slight limitations on the affected side are easily detected. In the range-of-motion examination, the patient first demonstrates the active range-of-motion of the unaffected side. Then he or she performs the same motions with the affected extremity.

Passive range of motion. These tests are best performed standing behind the patient. The patient may sit or stand. Holding the patient's arm above the flexed elbow, place the other hand on the shoulder. The hand on the upper arm guides the patient's arm through the arc of motion as the hand on the shoulder monitors the movements of the scapula and the

Fig. 1.**12**   The pendulum test for passive forward motion of the shoulder relieves tension on the subacromial space.

Fig. 1.**11**   To evaluate full bilateral abduction, the patient abducts both arms with the elbows extended and the palms in supination.

Fig. 1.**13**   To evaluate laxity in the joint, stabilize the scapula with one hand; with the other hand grasp the humeral head between the thumb and fingers and apply anterior and posterior forces.

humeral head. This permits detection of spasm. If motion is limited due to pain, the pendulum test can be used to document passive range of motion while eliminating the need to use rotator cuff muscles and avoiding stress on the subacromial space. To perform this test, instruct the patient to bend forward and allow the arms to hang down loosely from the body.

This test can be useful to document inconsistencies between reported symptoms and physical examination findings (Fig. 1.**12**).

Limited range of motion after soft-tissue injuries may present as a frozen shoulder syndrome (adhesive capsulitis). Immobilization of the joint in adduction for several weeks can result in shortening of the adductors, which is identifiable by limited abduction and external rotation. Scars in the axilla can contribute to limited motion, as can radiation therapy. Palpable crepitus with audible snapping and grating, particularly during rotation, may have several causes. Crepitus during passive motion is frequently a sign of changes in the subacromial space. These changes may include thickening and irregularities in the subacromial bursa and the rotator cuff, or changes in the greater tuberosity. Crepitus during active motion is suggestive of instability and may indicate a labral lesion. Palpable snapping, particularly with horizontal adduction and abduction, is encountered with acromioclavicular joint pathology. Crepitus with external or internal rotation in abduction may point to instability of the long head of the biceps.

Normal and abnormal range of motion of the joint must be documented. Abnormal motion may be due to labral or capsular pathology or to weakness in the muscles used to actively stabilize the shoulder. Grasp the humeral head between the thumb and fingers and translate it anteriorly and posteriorly with the shoulder muscles relaxed (Fig. 1.**13**). This will demonstrate laxity in the joint. Excess laxity may be a part of shoulder instability.

Fig. 1.**14** Horizontal stretch. Reduction in cross-body adduction indicates posterior capsular contracture.

Reduced horizontal adduction is a sign of shortening of the posterior joint capsule (Fig. 1.**14**).

The active and passive **ranges of motion** are measured and documented using the neutral-0 method. The following ranges of motion are regarded by some physicians as normal:

— Adduction and abduction: 75°–0°–180°
— Extension and flexion: 60°–0°–180°
— Horizontal extension and flexion: 45°–0°–135°
— Internal and external rotation
    in adduction: 80°–0°–65°
— Internal and external rotation
    at 90° adduction: 70°–0°–90°

These values are not always standardized. Note that any abduction past 90° indicates scapulothoracic, rather than glenohumeral, motion.

Although the neutral-0 method is used for all measurements of abduction and adduction, flexion and extension, and internal rotation, the extent of internal rotation is also frequently documented as the part of the body that the patient can reach with the thumb (for example, the greater trochanter, sacroiliac joint, lumbar spinous process, or thoracic spinous process). Both the active and passive ranges of motion are documented. Concentric limitation of motion is a sign of adhesive capsulitis. If external rotation, in particular, is limited, then the differential diagnosis must include chronic posterior dislocation or severe osteoarthritis of the shoulder. Concentric limitations of motion with relatively good external rotation while supine is suggestive of a chronic tear in the rotator cuff.

Scapulohumeral rhythm. Irregularities in the scapulohumeral rhythm are best observed from behind the patient. A frozen shoulder, degenerative glenohume-

ral arthritis, or rheumatoid arthritis of the shoulder will not permit uniform motion. In these conditions, the motion will be segmented and irregular; abduction of more than 90° is rarely possible. Abduction is achieved by scapulothoracic motion rather than by glenohumeral motion. A complete tear of the rotator cuff leads to an even more severe limitation; generally only a few degrees of abduction can be achieved. Again, most abduction will occur as a result of the scapulothoracic motion. With smaller tears, limited abduction will not be so severe; complete physiologic abduction can occasionally be achieved, albeit painfully. Minimally limited abduction may be seen with longitudinal tears. Any weakness detected in abduction is an indication for further diagnostic studies.

Scapula slide test. Physiologic coordinated motion between the scapula and the arm follows certain regular patterns. Abduction of the arm produces a regular lateral sliding motion of the scapula. Observe whether the coordinated motion of the scapula is symmetric. More than 1 cm of asymmetry is regarded as pathologic. For purposes of objective measurement, the distance between the inferior angle of the scapula and the spinous process of the seventh thoracic vertebra is used.

Nerve injuries can produce uncoordinated scapulothoracic motion. Coordinated motion requires stabilizing the scapula on the chest wall. If the stabilizing muscles are weakened or paralyzed, uncoordinated motion results. The main stabilizing muscles are the trapezius and serratus anterior. With neurologic injuries, a winged scapula can be present.

Paralysis of the serratus anterior is encountered most frequently. If this muscle is completely denervated, the diagnosis is made by inspection. Muscular imbalance causes the scapula to protrude, and the inferior angle migrates medially. Maximum scapular winging is demonstrated when the patient elevates his or her arms and presses against a wall (Figs. 1.**15a–c**). This test will clearly demonstrate slight weakness that will not cause noticeable changes at rest. Paralysis of the trapezius causes an identifiable change in the position of the scapula while the scapula is pulled inferiorly, and the inferior angle migrates laterally and inferiorly from the midline.

A lesion of the long thoracic nerve will cause winged scapula similar to a trapezius lesion and is seen in the setting of shoulder complaints that follow a lymph node biopsy. In such situations, the posterior triangle of the neck should be carefully inspected.

A compressive neuropathy of the suprascapular nerve will produce atrophy of the supraspinatus and infraspinatus muscles. If the syndrome involves only the infraspinatus branch, then only that muscle will be affected.

Dislocation of the shoulder can result in damage to the axillary nerve, producing paresis of the deltoid

Fig. 1.**16** Local anesthesia test for differentiating subacromial pain syndromes (Neer impingement test).

Figs. 1.**15a–c** Different forms of winged scapula. (**a**) Normal position of the scapula. (**b**) Paralysis of the serratus anterior; the scapula migrates superiorly and medially. (**c**) Paralysis of the trapezius; the scapula migrates inferiorly and laterally.

and an area of sensory deficit on the lateral aspect of the shoulder.

Paralysis of the deltoid muscle severely limits abduction. The first 45° of motion is largely unchanged; motion beyond this point can only be achieved with difficulty and requires rotation of the scapula and the use of accessory muscles, specifically

the descending part of the trapezius, the serratus anterior, levator scapulae, supraspinatus, and infraspinatus.

Specific Tests (see Table 1.**7**)

Painful arc. This is a painful segment of passive or active motion. It should be described in flexion, abduction, or external rotation. It is generally accepted to demonstrate subacromial pathology.

Acromioclavicular compression test (cross-body compression). With the patient's shoulder flexed 90°, maximum internal rotation, and the elbow flexed 90°, press against the patient's olecranon from lateral to medial. Pain projected into the acromioclavicular joint is a sign of involvement of this joint.

Neer impingement test. Stand behind the patient, immobilizing the scapula with one hand and briskly flexing the patient's arm with the other (Fig. 1.**16**). This will cause the greater tuberosity to decrease the volume of the subacromial space. Pain and weakness may indicate an impingement syndrome. To distinguish between rotator cuff pathology and impingement of instability, repeat the test after infiltrating the subacromial space with local anesthetic. If painless weakness persists after infiltration, consider the possibility of a rotator cuff tear.

Differential anesthetic injection in the shoulder examination. Occasionally it is difficult to differentiate between pain due to degenerative changes in the acromioclavicular joint and subacromial impingement on the basis of the history and physical examination. If there is coexisting radiographic evidence of acromioclavicular and subacromial degenerative changes, the diagnostic dilemma is even greater.

In settings such as this, an extension of the Neer impingement test (using local anesthetic injection to

Table 1.**7**   Overview of specific tests for various clinical syndromes

Rotator cuff	Acromioclavicular joint	Biceps tendon	Instability	Other
Subacromial painful arc	Painful arc at end of range of motion	Speed test	Anterior apprehension	Allen (vascular compression)
Pseudoparalysis		Yergason test	Posterior apprehension	Adson (vascular compression)
Nabot sign	Cross-body compression	Ludington test		
Spontaneous internal rotation		Heuter test	Dead-arm sign	
		Lippman test	Passive drawer	
Impingement test (Neer)		De Anquin test	Active drawer	
Impingement test (Jobe)		Gilcrest test	Sulcus sign	
Impingement test (Hawkins and Kennedy)		Beru sign	Inferior apprehension	
		Stretch test		
Drop-arm test		Compression test	Relocation test	
Jobe test		O'Brien test		
Lift-off test		Clunk test		

isolate the pain generator) is helpful. These techniques are most useful when the possibility of a rotator cuff tear has been eliminated by history, physical examination, or imaging studies.

After obtaining informed consent, prepare and drape the appropriate shoulder. Verify that the patient is not allergic to the anesthetic you propose to use. It may be helpful to have the patient supine in case of a post-injection vasovagal event.

Palpate the acromioclavicular joint. Using a small gauge needle, inject this joint from an anterior or superior approach with a small amount (2–3 mL) of local anesthetic. Injection will be difficult and may require significant force on the plunger of the syringe. Take care not to inject the subacromial space at this point. Allow the anesthetic to take effect and repeat the physical examination, noting any changes in active range of motion and the degree of pain relief. If the needle placement was accurate and only the acromioclavicular joint was infiltrated, changes in motion and pain can be attributed to the acromioclavicular joint. Marked pain relief after isolated acromioclavicular joint injection is predictive of pain relief after acromioclavicular joint decompression.

If acromioclavicular joint injection provides neither pain relief nor a change in active range of motion, or only partial pain relief and minimal change in range of motion, proceed to subacromial injection at the same sitting. At this point the subacromial injection is performed as in the Neer impingement test.

Again, prepare and drape the appropriate shoulder. From an anterior or lateral approach, palpate the edge of the acromion and the subacromial space. Using a small-gauge needle of sufficient length (1.5 or 2 in), advance the tip into the subacromial space. If the needle tip clears the tip of the acromion, and the barrel of the syringe is perpendicular to the floor, the needle tip is almost certainly in the subacromial space. Make sure that the needle tip is not in the rotator cuff by instructing the patient to gently internally and externally rotate the shoulder. If the needle tip is in the subacromial space, the barrel of the syringe should not move significantly with internal or exter-

nal rotation. Inject approximately 10 mL of local anesthetic. The injection should require little effort. Wait for the anesthetic to take effect, then re-examine the shoulder. Note any change in active range of motion and pain relief. Significant pain relief and increased motion is predictive of a good response to subacromial decompression.

A partial response to acromioclavicular joint injection with improvement after subacromial joint injection suggests that both areas are pain generators and therefore must be addressed when surgery is performed. If there is residual pain and restricted motion after injection of both the acromioclavicular and subacromial spaces, this should arouse suspicion of glenohumeral joint pathology.

The glenohumeral joint may be injected from an anterior or posterior approach. If the patient is supine, the anterior approach is easier. Prepare and drape the appropriate shoulder. Palpate the coracoid process. The glenohumeral joint is lateral and inferior to the coracoid, approximately two finger-breadths lateral and one finger-breadth inferior. Use a small-gauge needle of sufficient length; sometimes a short spinal needle is useful. Advance the needle, and if bony resistance is encountered ensure you are not on the humeral head or the glenoid. Inject 10 mL. The injection should require little force. Again, re-examine the shoulder noting any changes in pain and range of motion. If there is residual pain after acromioclavicular joint, subacromial space, and glenohumeral joint injection, consider a referred-pain syndrome.

Vasovagal events can occur after injection. Be prepared to allow the patient to lie down for a few minutes.

Jobe impingement test. Jobe introduced a modification of the impingement test in which the arm is rotated internally in abduction. This is more likely to compress the posterior parts of the supraspinatus tendon in the subacromial space (Fig. 1.**17**).

Hawkins and Kennedy impingement test. The Hawkins and Kennedy impingement test represents a fur-

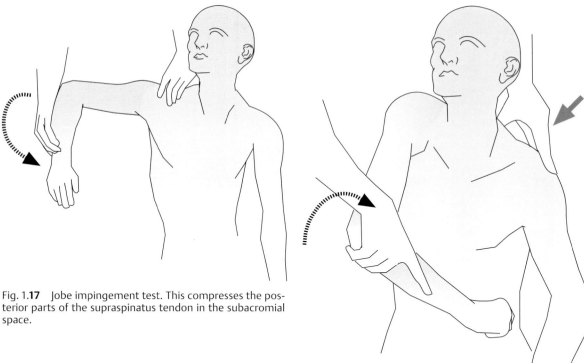

Fig. 1.**17**   Jobe impingement test. This compresses the posterior parts of the supraspinatus tendon in the subacromial space.

ther modification. Here, 90° of shoulder flexion is coupled with simultaneous forced internal rotation (Fig. 1.**18**). A positive test suggests the presence of a subcoracoid impingement syndrome.

Drop-arm test. This test can be used to diagnose larger tears in the rotator cuff. First instruct the patient to fully abduct the arm. The patient may be able to do this using compensatory motions. However, when the arm is lowered from about 90° abduction, any tear that interrupts the continuity of the tendons will make it impossible to actively hold the arm, which will drop to the side. Occasionally the

Fig. 1.**18**   Hawkins and Kennedy impingement test with horizontal flexion and internal rotation suggests the presence of a subcoracoid compression syndrome.

patient can maintain 90° abduction with great effort, but a mere light tap on the forearm will be enough to cause the arm to drop. If active abduction is not possible, passively abduct the arm to 90°. When the supporting hand is removed, the patient will be unable to maintain this position (Figs. 1.**19a, b**).

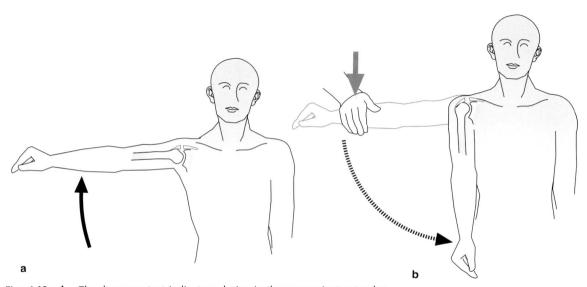

a

b

Figs. 1.**19a, b**   The drop-arm test indicates a lesion in the supraspinatus tendon.

Fig. 1.**20**   Nabot sign with pain in the subacromial space on compression and rotation.

Fig. 1.**22**   Jobe test for the holding function of the supraspinatus tendon.

Fig. 1.**21**   Evaluating the abduction initiation role of the supraspinatus.

abduction is now significantly less painful, this suggests that the bursa is the main cause.

Clinical Signs and Specific Tests for Differentiating Pathology of the Rotator Cuff

Provocative test (isometric rotator tests). If pseudoparalysis is present, further evaluation is needed to precisely determine which component of the rotator cuff is involved. Provocative tests can be very helpful. These evaluate external and internal rotation against resistance with the shoulder in various positions. Weakness is usually attributable to a functional deficit, whereas pain with normal strength is usually attributable to tendinitis or bursitis. Selective testing can evaluate various components of the rotator cuff.

● **Supraspinatus**
Zero-degree abduction test. Abduction of the arm is initiated by the supraspinatus and deltoid muscles. The 0° abduction test is used to evaluate the abduction initiation role of the supraspinatus. The patient attempts to abduct the hanging arm against resistance (Fig. 1.**21**).

Jobe test. The 90° supraspinatus test evaluates the holding function of the supraspinatus muscle. In this test, described in the literature as the Jobe test, the patient holds the arms in 90° abduction with the

Pseudoparalysis. In the presence of pseudoparalysis, the patient will be unable to raise the affected arm. Occasionally, the patient will have learned to abduct the arm using compensatory or swinging motions. This sign suggests the presence of damage to the rotator cuff.

Nabot sign. Press the arm against the acromion along the longitudinal axis of the humerus while rotating it. Crepitus will often be discernible in the presence of rotator cuff pathology (Fig. 1.**20**).

Active abduction while relieving stress on the subacromial space. Pain during abduction from neutral can be caused by irritation of the supraspinatus tendon or by subacromial bursitis. To differentiate between the two, the attempt to decompress the subacromial space by applying traction along the longitudinal axis of the humerus with the arm at the patient's side. This relieves tension on the bursa. If pain persists when the patient now attempts active abduction, this suggests supraspinatus pathology. If

Fig. 1.**23** Full-can test. Optimal manual muscle-testing position for the isolation of the supraspinatus muscle: elevation at 90° of scapular elevation and 45° of external rotation (full-can position).

Fig. 1.**25** Infraspinatus test. Optimal manual muscle-testing position for the isolation of the infraspinatus muscle: 0° of scapular elevation and 45° of internal rotation.

elbows extended. The arms are flexed 30° horizontally in relation to the scapular plane and internally rotated (with the thumbs pointing to the floor). The patient attempts to open the arms further, against resistance (Fig. 1.**22**). The anterior portions of the rotator cuff are tested with the upper arms in the same position but in external rotation.

Fig. 1.**24** Spontaneous internal rotation is a sign of a tear in the infraspinatus and supraspinatus tendon.

Full-can test. This test can also be used to evaluate the supraspinatus muscle in isolation. The arm is abducted 90° in the scapular plane and externally rotated 45°. Attempt to press the arm down ("full-can" position) against the patient's active resistance (Fig. 1.**23**).

- **Supraspinatus and infraspinatus muscles**
Spontaneous internal rotation. The patient stands shirtless or appropriately gowned and as relaxed as possible. Instruct the patient to let the arms hang down at the sides. A tear in the rotator cuff, particularly in the superior and posterior portion, will cause spontaneous internal rotation of the affected arm. This is due to the uncompensated action of the intact internal rotators (Fig. 1.**24**).

To evaluate the infraspinatus and teres minor muscles, the patient's arm is adducted, internally rotated 45°, and flexed 90° at the elbow. With the arm in this position, the patient attempts to externally rotate the arm against resistance (Fig. 1.**25**). To eliminate the deltoid muscle contribution in external rotation, the external rotation can be performed at 90° abduction and 30° flexion. Failure of active external rotation with the arm abducted is indicative of a clinically relevant tear of the infraspinatus tendon (Fig. 1.**26**).

- **Subscapularis**
Increased painless passive external rotation with the patient supine and loss of active internal rotation is a sign of a subscapularis tear.

The internal rotators (subscapularis and pectoralis major) are also tested with the arm adducted and flexed at the elbow, this time with resistance against internal rotation (Fig. 1.**27**). The arm is not placed at

Fig. 1.**26**   Testing the external rotators while eliminating the effect of the deltoid muscle.

Fig. 1.**28**   Lift-off test as the sign of a subscapularis tear.

the side but held in flexion to eliminate contribution of the deltoid muscle. Painful external rotation against resistance in this position is a sign of involvement of the infraspinatus tendon.

Fig. 1.**27**   Testing the internal rotators.

Lift-off test. This test can demonstrate tears in the subscapularis muscle. With the arm in internal rotation, the back of the patient's hand is placed on his or her back at the belt line, and the patient attempts to lift the hand off the back (Fig. 1.**28**). A patient with a tear in the subscapularis will be unable to perform this test.

Modified lift-off test. If internal rotation is limited, the patient might not be able to place his or her hand on the back. In such cases the modified lift-off test can be used. The patient places his or her hand flat on the anterior abdomen and attempts to press with force against the abdominal wall. Inability to do so is a sign of a tear in the subscapularis tendon.

Compression and rotation test. This test is suitable for revealing degenerative changes in the glenohumeral joint. The patient lies on the unaffected side. The arm to be examined is flexed and placed at the side. Press on the humeral head from lateral to medial to produce glenohumeral compression, while the patient rotates the arm internally and externally. Cartilaginous lesions will cause audible and palpable crepitus, and the patient will experience subjective symptoms. To exclude possible accompanying subacromial pathology, inject the subacromial bursa with local anesthetic prior to the test (Fig. 1.**29**).

Specific Tests for the Long Head of the Biceps

Yergason test. This test demonstrates lesions of the long head of the biceps in the bicipital groove, its tendon sheath, or the transverse ligament that anchors it in the bicipital groove. The elbow is flexed 90° with the forearm pronated. The patient now attempts to

Fig. 1.**30**   Yergason test to evaluate the long head of the biceps.

Fig. 1.**29**   Compression and rotation test. The patient is placed in the lateral position with the arm at the side and the elbow bent to 90°. The glenohumeral joint is compressed by applying downward pressure. The patient rotates the arm externally and internally. Pain and crepitation are signs of chondromalacia and/or degenerative joint diesease.

supinate the forearm and flex the elbow against resistance (Fig. 1.30). Lesions in any of these structures will cause pain in the bicipital groove.

Speed test. The speed test (palm-up test) is also used to demonstrate lesions of the long head of the biceps. The arm is in 90° forward flexion with the elbow extended and the forearm supinated. Attempt to press the extended arm down against the patient's active resistance (Fig. 1.**31**). If the test is positive, the patient will complain of pain in the anterior deltoid region.

Ludington test. Both arms are abducted and the palms placed on the head with the fingers interlocked. Voluntary contraction of the biceps will cause pain in the anterior deltoid region if the test is positive.

Heuter test. Under normal conditions, forceful flexion with the forearm pronated is achieved with the brachialis. The biceps contracts simultaneously, causing supination of the forearm. If this is not observed, then you should look for a lesion of the biceps or its tendons.

The long head of the biceps is directly palpated in the Lippman and De Anquin tests.

Additional tests. These tests may be useful in demonstrating specific pathology. In the **Lippman test**, the examiner palpates the bicipital groove approximately 3 cm distal to the shoulder with the patient's elbow flexed at a right angle. If the biceps tendon tends to sublux or dislocate, you can provoke dislocation or subluxation by palpation of the relaxed musculature. This is generally painful for the patient. In the **De Anquin test**, rotating the upper arm while palpating the biceps tendon in the bicipital groove will cause pain if the tendon is affected. In the **Gilcrest**

Fig. 1.**31**   Speed test to evaluate the long head of the biceps.

Fig. 1.**32** Stretching the long head of the biceps in the bicipital groove.

Fig. 1.**33** Compressing the long head of the biceps against the acromion.

test, reducing the subluxed or dislocated long biceps tendon while slowly adducting the arm will cause pain in the anterior deltoid region. The **Beru sign** demonstrates dislocation of the long head of the biceps tendon. If the long head dislocates, it can be palpated under the anterior deltoid when the biceps is voluntarily contracted. The **Duga sign** demonstrates an injury of the long head of the biceps tendon. In such an injury, the patient is unable to touch the contralateral shoulder with the hand of the affected arm.

Stretch test. Passive extension of the shoulder, extension of the elbow, and pronation of the forearm, or the patient's attempt to actively supinate the forearm, flex the elbow, or flex the shoulder forward from this position will cause pain in the anterior deltoid region (Fig. 1.**32**).

Compression test. Passive elevation of the arm to the end of the range of motion, and application of posterior pressure, causes pain in the tendon compressed between the acromion and humeral head (Fig. 1.**33**).

Clinical Tests for Glenoid Labral Lesions

O'Brien test. With the arm flexed 90° and adducted 10°, internally rotate the arm so that the thumb points down. The patient attempts to resist a downward force applied by the examiner. Pain in the acromioclavicular joint is a sign of acromioclavicular arthropathy. Pain projected to the superior part of the glenohumeral joint suggests a SLAP (Superior Labrum from anterior to posterior) lesion. Typically, the pain disappears when the arm is placed in external rotation with the palm up.

Compression and rotation test. With the arm abducted 90° and the elbow flexed 90°, apply com-

pression to the glenohumeral joint by pressing on the humerus while rotating the joint. As in the McMurray knee test, a snapping noise is a sign of damage to the labrum.

Anterior slide test. The patient is examined either standing or sitting, with the hands on the hips and thumbs pointing posteriorly. Place one hand across the patient's shoulder with the last segment of the index finger extending over the anterior aspect of the acromion at the glenohumeral joint. Place the other hand behind the patient's elbow and apply force in an anterosuperior direction. Instruct the patient to push back against this force. Sudden pain in the anterosuperior shoulder, corresponding to the pain typically experienced during exercise, or a palpable snap phenomenon is indicative of a SLAP lesion (Figs. 1.**34** and 1.**35**).

Clunk test. With the patient supine, place your hand on the posterior aspect of the shoulder directly under the humeral head. With the other hand, grasp the distal humerus and elbow condyles. The patient's affected arm is now brought from the extended position into forward flexion and external rotation. A snap phenomenon or clunk sound indicates damage to the labrum (Fig. 1.**36**).

Crank test. The crank test is used to demonstrate damage to the labrum and can be performed with the patient sitting or supine. With the patient's arm abducted 160° in the scapula plane, press along the longitudinal axis of the humerus while rotating the humerus with the other hand. The test is considered to be positive if:

Fig. 1.**34** Slide test. Position of the hands and arms for the anterior slide test.

Fig. 1.**35** Slide test. Application of force for the anterior slide test.

Fig. 1.**36** Clunk test for diagnosing anterior lateral tears.

— The patient experiences pain during rotation (typically during external rotation) with or without a click phenomenon.
— The test reproduces the typical symptoms experienced by the athlete.

It is often an advantage if the patient is supine as he/she will be significantly more relaxed in this position.

Specific Tests for Instability

Testing range of motion is especially crucial in a patient with suspected instability. Rotation should always be performed both in adduction and at 90° abduction. The first sign of anterior instability is often limited external rotation in both adduction and abduction. Flexion and abduction in the scapular plane are not usually limited. Occasionally, slight apprehension will be present during overhead motion. In addition to changes in the range of motion, parts of the infraspinatus and supraspinatus tendon are often sensitive to touch.

- **Differentiating between instability and laxity**
When evaluating shoulder instability, a clear distinction should be made between laxity and instability. Laxity refers to a hypermobile shoulder situation, such as can be demonstrated in the various translation tests, **without** any clinical symptoms. Laxity is often symmetric and is seen as part of generalized laxity. Instability refers to laxity **with** clinical impairment of the patient.

In North America, three acronyms are commonly used to classify shoulder instability. TUBS refers to **T**raumatic **U**nilateral **B**ankart lesion **S**urgery. AMBRII stands for **A**traumatic, **M**ultidirectional, **B**ilateral, **R**ehabilitation, **I**nferior capsular shift, **I**nterval repair. AIOS stands for **A**cquired, **I**nstability, **O**verstress, **S**urgery.

Anterior apprehension test. This test is positive in the presence of anteroinferior instability. The test is performed with the patient sitting or standing and the affected shoulder placed in 90° abduction and 90° external rotation. Continuing the external rotation while applying forward pressure to the humeral head with the thumb is met with muscular resistance as the patient feels that the shoulder is about to dislocate anteriorly (Fig. 1.**37**). The presence of pain alone should not be regarded as a positive test even though the muscular resistance can often appear simultaneously with the occurrence of pain. Patients will often indicate that "something bad is about to happen" or "it's starting to go out." This test can be performed in different degrees of abduction. Performing the test at 45° abduction evaluates the contribution of the medial glenohumeral ligament and the subscapularis tendon. In abduction of 90° and greater, the stabilizing effect of the subscapularis muscle is neutral-

Fig. 1.**37**   Anterior apprehension test.

Fig. 1.**38**   Posterior apprehension test.

ized and contribution of the inferior glenohumeral ligament is evaluated.

At 135° of abduction, the test primarily evaluates the anteroinferior joint capsule.

Occasionally, patients complain of pain in the posterior joint capsule. This is caused by the stretching of the joint capsule from the anterior translation of the humeral head.

A degenerative glenoid labrum with small tears can cause palpable and occasionally audible snapping during the apprehension test. Care should be taken with patients who have suffered multiple recurrent dislocations because dislocation can occur with the test. Performing the apprehension test with the patient supine is advantageous as the patient is in a more relaxed position.

Dead-arm sign. This refers to a situation in which the patient complains of a sudden stabbing pain with simultaneous or subsequent paralyzing weakness during the anterior apprehension test. This may be due to transitory pressure on the brachial plexus as the humeral head subluxes anteriorly.

Posterior apprehension test. This is helpful for diagnosing posterior instability. Place the patient's affected arm in 90° to 110° abduction at the shoulder and horizontally flex it approximately 20° to 30°.

Immobilize the scapula from above with your other hand. The fingers cover the scapular spine and the humeral head while the thumb reaches anteriorly to a point slightly lateral to the coracoid process. As horizontal flexion is slowly increased, the force along the longitudinal axis of the humerus will cause the glenohumeral joint to sublux posteriorly. Both the thumb lateral to the coracoid process and the fingers can palpate the translation of the humeral head. Occasionally, the humeral head will be visible inferior to the acromion as a slight prominence. An extension of 20° to 30° in the same horizontal plane will palpably reduce the humeral head (Fig. 1.**38**).

Evaluation of glenohumeral translation. Glenohumeral translation can be evaluated with the patient supine or sitting. This test provides a semiquantitative method of measuring the extent of laxity. The extent of translation is compared with the nonaffected shoulder.

Passive drawer test. When performing the test on a patient, place your contralateral hand on the patient's shoulder from posterior so that the index and middle finger lie anteriorly on the humeral head while the ring finger lies on the coracoid process. To test for a passive drawer, grasp the shaft of the humerus with the other hand and move it anteroposteriorly, noting the translation of the humeral head in relation to the coracoid process. With the same landmarks located, you can document an active drawer by having the patient perform active abduction and external rotation of the affected arm (see Fig. 1.**13**).

AP drawer test. This test can also be used to document AP laxity in the shoulder. The patient is positioned supine with the arm lying comfortably at the side. Attempt to stabilize the scapula while achieving AP translation of the humeral head without encountering muscular resistance form the patient.

In the classic anterior drawer test, stand facing the affected shoulder. To examine the right shoulder, grasp the upper third of the patient's arm with your right hand while immobilizing the patient's forearm and hand between your body and upper arm. In this position, flex the patient's upper arm approximately 20° and place it in slight external rotation. Immobilize the scapula with your other hand so that the fingers reach posteriorly to the scapular spine and the thumb anteriorly to the coracoid process. From this position, carefully translate the humeral head anteriorly. First perform the test at 50° abduction, repeating it at higher degrees of abduction up to 120°. This test can also produce a snapping phenomenon as a result of a torn or degenerative labrum.

Posterior drawer test. Hold the patient's shoulder in 20° to 30° flexion and 20° to 30° abduction with the elbow flexed 90°. When examining the right shoulder, stand superior to the patient, holding the patient's arm with your right hand and positioning your left hand so that the thumb is slightly lateral to the coracoid process and the long fingers stabilize the scapular spine posteriorly. Applying pressure with your thumb produces posterior translation.

Leffert test. This test is another way of obtaining quantitative information in the drawer test. Stand above the sitting patient and move the humeral head anteriorly. Anterior motion of your index finger in relation to the middle finger shows the translation of the humeral head (Figs. 1.**39a, b**).

Fukuda test. This test demonstrates a passive posterior drawer. With the patient sitting, place your thumbs on both scapular spines and your fingers anterior to the humeral head. Pressing posteriorly with the fingers creates a posterior drawer (Fig. 1.**40**).

Load-and-shift test. This test is performed similarly to the drawer test on the sitting patient. Immobilize the scapula with one hand, grasp the humeral head with the other, apply a medial force to the humerus, and translate the humerus anteroposteriorly.

Rowe test. In the Rowe test, the drawer test is performed with the patient standing and bending forward slightly. This allows the patient to fully relax the shoulder muscles as in the pendulum exercises (Fig. 1.**41**).

Sulcus sign. If multidirectional instability is present, a positive sulcus sign can be demonstrated. With the patient sitting or standing and the arm of the affected shoulder relaxed along the body, apply traction to the longitudinal axis of the humerus. This will widen the space between the acromion and the humeral head. A sulcus in the skin will appear in this region (Fig. 1.**42**).

Inferior apprehension test. For this test, place the patient's arm in 90° abduction. While supporting the arm with one hand, attempt to provoke inferior subluxation by applying pressure to the proximal upper arm with the other hand (Fig. 1.**43**).

Fulcrum test. The patient is positioned supine on the examining couch with the affected arm externally rotated 90° and abducted 90°. Continuing the external rotation while moving the humeral head anteri-

Figs. 1.**39a, b** Leffert test

Fig. 1.**40** Fukuda test

Fig. 1.**41** Rowe test. In the standing position, the patient bends slightly forward and the arm is relaxed. A gentle anterior–inferior translation is performed.

Fig. 1.**42** Sulcus sign

Fig. 1.**43** Inferior apprehension test.

orly will provoke muscular resistance by the patient, in combination with pain. Performing the same motion (external rotation) while moving the humeral head posteriorly is painless (Figs. 1.**44a, b**). This test is helpful in differentiating patients with a simple supraspinatus syndrome from those with tenosynovitis at the insertions of the rotator cuff as a result of hypermobility.

Thrower test. In this test, the patient performs a throwing motion against your resistance. This can reveal anterior subluxation during the throwing motion (Fig. 1.**45**).

Examination under anesthesia. Examining the shoulder under anesthesia permits both clinical and fluoroscopic documentation of joint laxity. The drawer tests described in the previous section may be used.

Occasionally, it is helpful to have an assistant stabilize the scapula. Snapping phenomena resulting from labrum pathology can be readily documented by compressing the humeral head into the glenoid fossa while simultaneously translating the bone (shift-and-load test). The extent of translation with the arm in external rotation should be documented with the arm in various degrees of abduction (60°, 90°, and 135°). Performing a bilateral examination is recommended to allow comparison of both sides. Posterior translation up to half the humeral head diameter can be normal. Anteriorly, the normal translation is significantly less and is usually one-third of the diameter of the humeral head.

Quantifying examination under anesthesia. AP translation is divided into four grades (Fig. 1.**46**).

- Grade 0: no palpable translation between the humeral head and the glenoid fossa.
- Grade I: the humerus can be moved up to the margin of the glenoid.
- Grade II: Subluxation of the humeral head past the margin of the glenoid with spontaneous reduction. This is the maximum considered normal during examination under anesthesia.
- Grade III: complete dislocation without reduction.

Figs. 1.**44a, b**   Fulcrum test. Moving the humerus anteriorly and rotating it exteriorly produces typical pain (**a**); external rotation with the head of the humerus centered can be achieved painlessly (**b**).

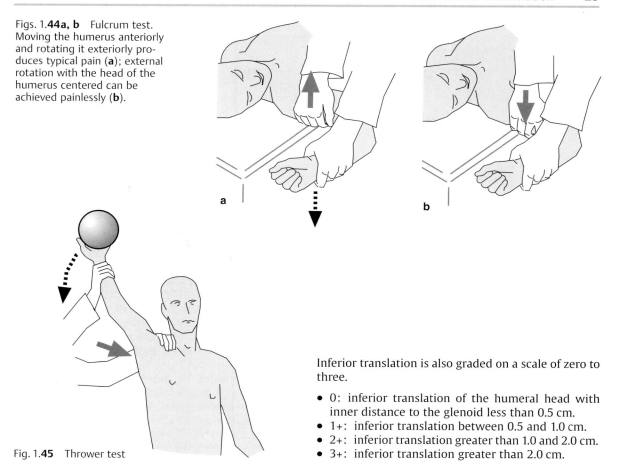

Fig. 1.**45**   Thrower test

Inferior translation is also graded on a scale of zero to three.

- 0: inferior translation of the humeral head with inner distance to the glenoid less than 0.5 cm.
- 1+: inferior translation between 0.5 and 1.0 cm.
- 2+: inferior translation greater than 1.0 and 2.0 cm.
- 3+: inferior translation greater than 2.0 cm.

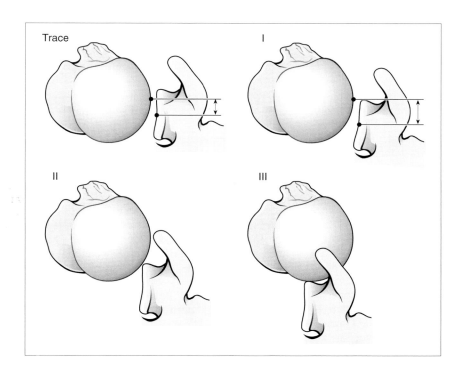

Fig. 1.**46**   Translation under anesthesia: humeral head translation is classified as types I–III.

Table 1.**8**   Muscle grading chart

Muscle gradation	Muscle reaction
0 = zero	No palpable contractility.
1 = trace	Evidence of slight contractility, but insufficient to move the extremity with gravity eliminated.
2 = poor	The muscle is able to move the extremity with gravity eliminated.
3 =fair	The muscle is able to move the extremity against gravity.
4 = good	The muscle moves the extremity against some resistance.
5 = normal	Normal muscle strength against resistance.

Neurologic Examination

The neurologic examination permits assessment of the individual muscle or muscle-group strength, testing reflexes and sensation. The examination can be performed with the patient standing or sitting.

Examining the Muscles

As in all other examinations, the strength of the muscle groups is compared with the opposite side. The chart shown in Table 1.**8** is recommended for objective evaluation and documentation.

Forward flexion. Testing evaluates the anterior part of the deltoid muscle (axillary nerve, C5) and the coracobrachialis muscle (musculocutaneous nerve, C5–C6), the secondary flexors, the clavicular head of the pectoralis major, and the biceps. Stand behind the patient and place one hand over the acromion and scapula and the other above the flexed elbow; the fingers are over the anterior segment of the arm and the biceps muscle. Here and in the following tests, instruct the patient to perform the respective motion (in this case flexion). Provide resistance that the patient can barely overcome.

Extension. Testing evaluates the latissimus dorsi (thoracodorsal nerve, C6), teres major (subscapular nerve, C5–C6), and the posterior portion of the deltoid (axillary nerve, C5–C6). The secondary extensors are the teres minor and the long head of the triceps. Extension is tested in a similar position to flexion except that the palm of the hand is now placed on the posterior aspect of the humerus. Instruct the patient to extend the arm posterior, and again provide resistance that the patient can barely overcome.

Abduction. The primary abductors are the middle portion of the deltoid (axillary nerve, C5–C6) and the supraspinatus (suprascapular nerve, C5–C6). The secondary abductors are the anterior and posterior portions of the deltoid and the serratus anterior. Stand behind or beside the patient, placing your hand over the acromion. Place the other hand beside the elbow and press against the lateral epicondyle of the humerus. Instruct the patient to abduct the arm, and determine the amount of resistance that the patient can barely overcome.

Adduction. The primary adductors are the pectoralis major (pectoral nerves, C5–T1) and the latissimus dorsi (thoracodorsal nerve, C6–C8); the secondary adductors are the teres major and the anterior portion of the deltoid. Test adduction in the same position as abduction. Grasp the arm with the resisting hand so that the fingers reach the medial side of the humerus.

External rotation. The primary external rotators are the infraspinatus (suprascapular nerve, C5–C6) and the teres minor (axillary nerve, C5). The posterior portion of the deltoid is the secondary external rotator. Stand beside the patient instructing him or her bend the elbow to 90° with the arm at the side in a neutral position. Place one hand on the elbow and provide resistance on the posterior distal forearm.

Internal rotation. The primary internal rotators are the subscapularis (subscapular nerve, C5–C6), pectoralis major (pectoral nerves, C5–T1), latissimus dorsi (thoracodorsal nerve, C6–C8), and the teres major (subscapular nerve, C5–C6). The anterior portion of the deltoid is the secondary internal rotator. Standing in the same position as for testing external rotation, place your resisting hand close to the radial styloid.

Scapular retraction. The primary retractors of the scapula are the rhomboid major (dorsal scapular nerve, C5) and the rhomboid minor (dorsal scapular nerve, C5). The secondary retractor is the trapezius muscle. Stand in front of the patient and place your hands on the patient's shoulders. Your palms should lie under the acromion with the fingers reaching around the patient's shoulders and touching the back. Have the patient retract the scapula while offering as much resistance as the patient can barely overcome.

Scapular protraction. The primary protractor of the scapula is the serratus anterior (long thoracic nerve, C5–C7). Stand behind the patient giving instructions to elevate the arm to 90° so that the humerus is parallel to the floor. Now instruct the patient to attempt to bend the elbow so that the hand touches the shoulder. Place one hand on the patient's spine; cup the patient's elbow with your resisting hand.

Scapular elevation. The primary elevators are the trapezius (spinal accessory nerve or cranial nerve XI) and the levator scapulae (C3–C4 and frequently the dorsal scapular nerve, C5). The secondary elevators are the rhomboid major and minor. Stand by the patient and place one hand on each acromion. Nor-

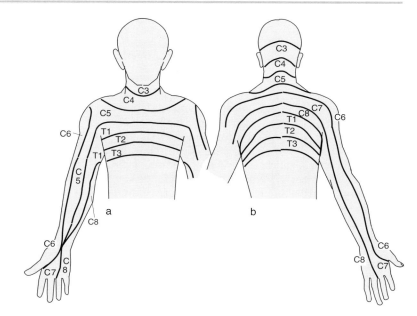

Figs. 1.**47a, b** Dermatomes in the upper extremity.

mally the elevators of the shoulder girdle are so strong you will hardly be able to overcome them.

Reflex Testing

Always test the deep tendon reflexes on both sides. Differences in response between the two sides suggest a neurologic process.

Biceps reflex. The patient's elbow should be flexed in a middle position and slightly pronated. Place your thumb on the distal portion of the biceps tendon and tap it. Normally the muscle will contract, causing flexion and supination of the forearm.

Triceps reflex. With the patient's elbow flexed approximately 90° and internally rotated, tap the triceps tendon proximal to the olecranon. Normally the muscle will contract, resulting in extension of the forearm.

Pectoralis major reflex. The patient abducts the arm by about 30°. Place your thumb on the pectoralis major tendon close to its insertion on the shaft of the humerus. Tapping the tendon will cause the muscle to contract, resulting in adduction and internal rotation of the arm.

Scapulohumeral reflex. The patient stands with the arm abducted 15° to 20°. Tap the inferior angle of the scapula with a slight lateral motion. Normally the arm will adduct and the scapula will move toward the spinal column.

Examining Sensation

Sensory nerve distribution is in band-shaped dermatomes. A few important landmarks are listed below:

— C5 (axillary nerve) is represented by an area of sensation the size of the palm of the hand.
— T1 is located on the medial upper arm.
— T2 is located in the axilla.
— T3 is located on the anterior wall, extending to the nipples.
— T4 is located inferior to the nipples.

Test sensation with a soft brush or a disposable pin. Differences between the sides in two-point discrimination also provide diagnostic information. Abnormal sensation (paresthesia) can take the form of increased sensation (hyperesthesia), decreased sensation (hypoesthesia), or total absence of sensation (anesthesia). Testing axillary nerve sensation after anterior shoulder dislocation is very important as this nerve can be injured, resulting in an area of decreased sensation. Shoulder injuries occasionally involve the brachial plexus. Paresthesia on the lateral forearm suggests involvement of the lateral cord of the brachial plexus. Impaired sensation in the medial forearm implicates the medial cord. If the small finger is affected in addition to the lateral forearm, expect involvement of the ulnar nerve.

Entrapment of the scapular nerve. In the presence of a clinically suspected scapular nerve entrapment syndrome, horizontal adduction with simultaneous maximum internal rotation can reproduce the clinical symptoms.

1.3 Radiology

Indications, Diagnostic Value, and Clinical Relevance

The shoulder comprises numerous structures that change their spacial relationships with different shoulder positions. It is not possible to visualize all of these structures in an AP radiograph in internal and external rotation. In no other part of the body is radiographic visualization in a single plane satisfactory. At the very least, AP *and* lateral radiographs are mandatory, and oblique projections are often required. However when it comes to the shoulder, some physicians are satisfied with only the AP radiograph in internal and external rotation. These two views are insufficient for imaging the shoulder joint; perhaps their only use is detecting calcific depositis in the rotator cuff.

The scapula is angled 30° to 45° off the axis of the chest. With this angular relationship, the glenohumeral joint is not well visualized in a standard AP protection. Optimum imaging of the glenohumeral joint demands that this angular relationship be taken into consideration.

Adequate radiographs in two planes may fail to image the shoulder satisfactorily. Projection of three-dimensional objects onto a two-dimensional image entails a loss of information. Special radiographic views have been developed in an effort to minimize this loss.

Standard Views

As in all other imaging of the musculoskeletal system, at least two films at right angles to each other are required. The AP and axial projections are the standard views.

a

b

c

Figs. 1.**48a–c**   Proper viewing of the glenohumeral joint (**a**) requires positioning the film cassette in relation to the plane of the scapula (**b**) and not in relation to the axis of the body (**c**).

Fig. 1.**49** Anteroinferior dislocation of the shoulder.

Fig. 1.**50** Infection of the right shoulder in a newborn, showing prominent soft-tissue shadows and lateral displacement of the humeral head.

Fig. 1.**52** Multiple loose bodies in enchondromatosis of the shoulder.

Fig. 1.**51** Avascular necrosis of the humeral head.

True AP view. The true AP radiograph may be taken with the patient standing or supine. The scapula is the reference plane for the glenohumeral joint and is at a 30° to 45° angle to the axis the body. The central ray in the AP radiograph must run parallel to the glenohumeral articular surface. Turn the patient's torso so that the plane of the shoulder blade lies parallel to the film cassette. The angle between the back and the film cassette will be about 30° to 45° (Figs. 1.**48a, b**).

The arm is in slight external rotation with the palm facing forward and the elbow extended. Rotation is best evaluated with the elbow flexed 90°. With the arm in external rotation, the greater tuberosity will appear on the lateral aspect of the humerus in profile. The central ray is aimed at the coracoid process and is angled 20° caudally. With the patient and cassette properly positioned, the glenohumeral joint is visualized parallel to the plane of projection, clearly demonstrating the joint space without any overlapping bony structures. For the projection, the humeral head and the glenoid fossa will only overlap if the shoulder is dislocated. The true AP view provides the basic study. These radiographs are suitable for identifying dislocations (Fig. 1.**49**), tumors, infections (Fig. 1.**50**), postinfectious conditions, avascular necrosis (Fig. 1.**51**), osteoarthritis of the shoulder, intra-articular loose bodies (Fig. 1.**52**), and fractures.

Axial view. The axial radiograph may be taken with the patient supine or sitting. It is most often taken as an inferosuperior projection with the patient supine. Towels or cushions are placed under the patient's head and affected shoulder to raise them approximately 10 cm. The affected arm should ideally be abducted 90° but pain will often prevent this. The film cassette is placed superior to the shoulder near the neck, with the central ray aimed perpendicularly through the axilla at the acromioclavicular joint (Figs. 1.**53a, b**).

Figs. 1.**53a, b**   Patient positioning for the axial view.

This view is difficult to obtain in patients with acute dislocations because it requires the patient to abduct the arm. In cases of acute trauma, the radiograph may be obtained from the opposite projection with the film placed in the axilla on a curved cassette or rolled film. The central ray is then aimed perpendicular to the acromioclavicular joint from above the shoulder.

The patient is positioned in a sitting position alongside the X-ray table. The upper arm is abducted with the elbow flexed at a right angle, and the forearm is placed on the top of the table. The patient leans over the table so that the shoulder overlies the cassette placed on the table. The radiograph is obtained in a craniocaudal projection with the central ray aimed at the glenohumeral joint.

The axial view is ideal to demonstrate the position of the humeral head in relation to the glenoid fossa. This view is useful in evaluation of a suspected posterior dislocation of the shoulder. In many cases, posterior dislocation cannot be reliably detected in the AP radiograph (see following section). Bony changes to the humeral head, such as a compression fracture or fractures of the greater and lesser tuberosities, can be demonstrated in this view, as can avulsion fractures of the glenoid (Fig. 1.**54**). The axial view can also identify fractures of the coracoid process and acromion, and can document an os acromiale (Fig. 1.**55**). The os acromiale is classified according to the ossification center as either preacromion, mesoacromion, metaacromion, or basiacromion (Fig. 1.**56**). The axial view can identify rotator cuff changes not seen on the true AP view.

If limited abduction precludes standard axial views, modified axial or transthoracic projections must be used to obtain images in the second radiographic plane.

Combinations of Standard Views for Specific Situations

Particularly in the shoulder, standard projections in two planes should not be deemed satisfactory.

The following views are recommended as a **standard series** for patients with **degenerative shoulder disorders.**

— AP view in internal rotation
— AP view in abduction
— Axillary view

A normal radiograph by no means exclude pathologic changes as most pathologic conditions of the shoulder involve soft-tissue injuries that are not visualized on radiographs. Radiographic changes appear only in advanced stages of disorders, for example in chronic tears of the rotator cuff. On the other hand, there is no clear correlation between the extent of bony changes, clinical symptoms, or response to therapy. Calcifications may be conspicuous, but they are not always responsible for symptoms.

Characteristic changes that occur after **shoulder instability** can be detected in suitable radiographs (**instability series**). If typical findings are visualized, anterior instability can be clearly distinguished from posterior instability. These projections include:

— AP view in internal rotation
— West Point axillary view
— Modified axillary view (such as the Stryker notch view)

A **trauma series** may be prepared for patients presenting with intense pain and **suspected fractures.** this series includes three projections at right angles to each other that can be obtained with minimal manipulation of the injured extremity.

Fig. 1.**54** Axial view showing a posterolateral Hill–Sachs lesion on the humeral head and bony Bankart lesion of the glenoid.

Fig. 1.**55** Axial view of an os acromiale.

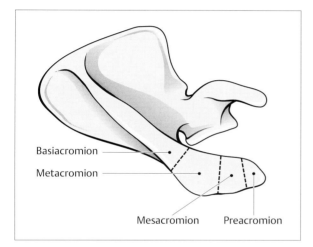

Basiacromion

Metacromion

Mesacromion   Preacromion

Fig. 1.**56** Os acromiale: different types.

– AP view in a neutral position
– True lateral view (scapular Y position)
– Axillary view

These radiographs can be used to determine the precise relationship of the fragments to each other and to the glenoid fossa, which is crucial for treatment and further prognosis of the injury.

Special Views for Degenerative Changes

Radiographic changes of subacromial pathology can manifest themselves in different ways. These include:

- Degenerative changes in the greater tuberosity with sclerosis, cysts, resorption grooves, flattening, and osteophytes.
- Subacromial spurs with osteophytes on the anterioinferior margin of the acromion. Calcification will occasionally be present in the coracoacromial ligament.
- Arthritis of the acromioclavicular joint with inferior osteophytes on both the acromion and clavicle.

Fig. 1.**57** Calcifications in the rotator cuff.

- Degenerative changes on the inferior aspect of the acromion with sclerosis as a result of inferior impingement of the humeral head. Articulation between the humeral head and the inferior aspect of the acromion is occasionally observed in massive chronic tears of the rotator cuff.
- Arthropathy from a defect in the rotator cuff, seen as secondary osteoarthritis of the shoulder in long-term chronic tears of the rotator cuff.
- Calcifications, often found in asymptomatic patients.

AP projection. Radiographs may be obtained in external rotation, internal rotation, or neutral position. The patient may be positioned sitting or supine but it is important for the plane of the shoulder blade

Fig. 1.**58** Superior migration of the humeral head in a chronic tear of the rotator cuff with severe degenerative joint disease.

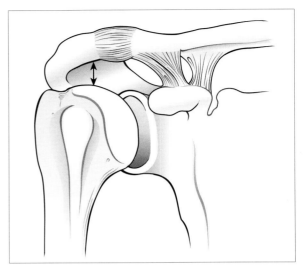

Fig. 1.**59** In the normal acromiohumeral internal (AHI) the distance between the superior surface of the humerus and the undersurface of the acromion ranges between 12 and 14 mm.

Fig. 1.**60** Patient positioning for the abduction view.

Fig. 1.**61** Superior migration of the humeral head during active abduction (Leclercq).

to be parallel to the film cassette. In applicable cases, AP views in varying rotation can help to localize calcifications in the specific portions of the rotator cuff (Fig. 1.**57**). Cystic or sclerotic changes in the greater tuberosity and acromion are identified. Superior migration of the humeral head indicates a tear of the rotator cuff (Fig. 1.**58**). Measuring the acromiohumeral interval (AHI) allows one to infer the condition of the rotator cuff. This interval is normally between 12 and 15 mm. In a complete tear of the rotator cuff, this distance is 6 to 7 mm. If the interval is less than 3 mm, one can diagnose a chronic massive tear where

the edges of the rotator cuff tendons have retracted (Fig. 1.**59**). Only rarely will the inferior glenoid lesions associated with instability be seen on the true AP radiograph.

True AP in external rotation. With the hand supinated and the arm slightly abducted, the plane of the epicondyles lies parallel to the film cassette. This projection demonstrates the glenohumeral joint in relation to the subacromial space, the greater tuberosity, and the humeral insertion of the supraspinatus tendon.

Fig. 1.**63**   Positioning for inferosuperior view of the bicipital groove.

Fig. 1.**62**   Positioning for superoinferior view of the bicipital groove.

Bicipital groove (superoinferior projection). The patient stands and bends over the X-ray table with the elbow flexed and the supinated forearm placed on the table. The film cassette is placed on the forearm and held in the patient's supinated hand, or supported by sandbags or towels in a horizontal position. The patient then bends so that the longitudinal axis of the humerus is 10° to 15° to the axis of projection. The bicipital groove is palpated and marked. The central ray enters the marked area vertically, producing an unobstructed projection of the bicipital groove (Fig. 1.**62**).

Bicipital groove (inferosuperior projection). A simpler, more practical method is the inferosuperior projection. The patient is positioned supine, the affected arm slightly abducted, and the upper arm supported in external rotation. The central ray parallels the axis of the humerus and is centered on the anterior margin of the humeral head. The film cassette is placed above the affected shoulder and is held by the patient (Fig. 1.**63**).
Both projections of the bicipital groove only provide reliable information if the central ray enters precisely tangential to the groove at its deepest point (Fig. 1.**64**). In actual clinical practise this is often not achieved, resulting in poorly projected images that are difficult to evaluate. If the radiographic visualization of the bicipital groove is vital, we recommend spot views via fluoroscopy. Ultrasound in the hands of an experienced examiner can provide the desired information.

Visualization of the subacromial space. The patient is positioned for the AP view in external rotation except that the central ray is angled 50° caudally. This view readily demonstrates calcifications of the coracoacromial ligament.

Coracoid process position. An inferosuperior projection shows the contour of the coracoid process. The patient is positioned supine with the arms at the sides, and the film cassette is placed under the patient's shoulder approximately 3–5 cm proximal to

True AP in neutral rotation. With the palms of the hands placed on the thighs, the plane of the epicondyles is now at a 45° angle to the cassette and the humeral head is in neutral. This demonstrates the greater tuberosity and the posterior insertion of the supraspinatus tendon.

True AP in internal rotation. With the elbow and the arm internally rotated, the axis of the epicondyles is perpendicular to the film cassette; the upper arm is abducted. This projection shows the subacromial space and may demonstrate a Hill–Sachs lesion.

Abduction view. This can document the contribution of glenohumeral motion to total abduction. It can also show an unobstructed view of the acromioclavicular joint. The patient stands at a right angle to the film cassette with the affected shoulder abducted 90° and the elbow flexed. In the AP projection, the central ray is aimed at the coracoid process (Fig. 1.**60**).

Leclercq view. Normally the humeral head will be centered in the glenoid fossa in an AP view. If there is a tear in the rotator cuff, the humeral head will be displaced superiorly when the patient actively abducts the arm against resistance (Fig. 1.**61**).

Fig. 1.**64**   Radiographic image of the bicipital groove.

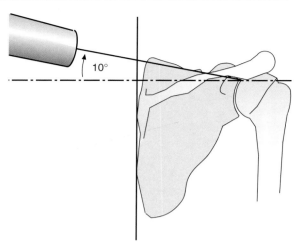

Fig. 1.**65**   Radiographic positioning for demonstrating the supraspinatus tunnel.

the coracoid process. The arm is slightly abducted with the hand supinated. The central ray is aimed at the coracoid process angled 15° to 30° cranially. In round-shouldered patients, this angle is greater than in flat-shouldered patients.

Supraspinatus outlet view. This demonstrates the shape of the acromion in the sagittal plane. The patient stands so that the body of the scapula is perpendicular to the film cassette. The scapular spine is positioned parallel to the floor, and the humerus is in neutral. The central ray is angled 15° caudally and aimed at the acromioclavicular joint (Fig. 1.**65**). This technique images the coracoacromial arch with the supraspinatus tendon beneath it and may be used to demonstrate changes in the anterior margin of the acromion. Bigliani has identified three acromial shapes (Figs. 1.**66 a–c**):

- Type I: flat acromion
- Type II: curved acromion
- Type III: anterior-to-inferior hook

However, the angle of inclination of the acromion appears to be more important in subacromial stenosis (Fig. 1.**67**).

Rockwood view. Routine AP views will not generally show calcifications of the coracoacromial ligament or inferior osteophytes on the acromion. Rockwood uses the 30° caudal projection. With the patient standing, an AP radiograph is taken with the central ray aimed 30° caudally (Fig. 1.**68**). This view detects changes in the subacromial area.

Special Views for Instability

Anterior dislocation of the shoulder can produce bony changes in the anteroinferior glenoid fossa (Bankart lesions or capsular calcifications) and on the posterolateral humeral head (Hill–Sachs lesion). Standard radiographs will often fail to detect both these lesions; special views are necessary to document them. However, standard radiographs can provide

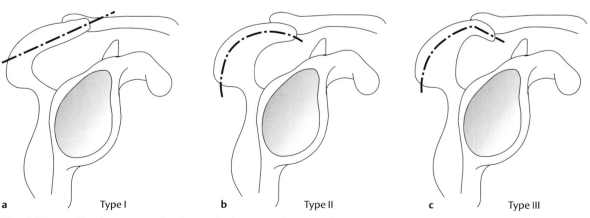

a   Type I   b   Type II   c   Type III

Figs. 1.**66a–c**   The three types of acromion in the supraspinatus outlet view.

Fig. 1.**67** The increase in acromial inclination decreases the supraspinatus outlet.

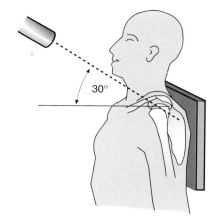

Fig. 1.**68** Visualization of the subacromial space in the Rockwood view.

important information in the presence of shoulder instability. True AP radiographs can provide information about the direction of dislocation and about accompanying injuries. An axial radiograph should always be obtained since this is the only way to positively exclude posterior dislocation (Figs. 1.**69a, b**). Even chronic dislocation with its typical associated injuries can be clearly documented in the axial projection (Fig. 1.**70**).

After reduction, or in the presence of, recurring instability, the AP view provides information about associated bony injuries (Hill-Sachs defects or Bankart lesions), possible muscular deficits (Figs. 1.**71a, b**), and secondary osteoarthritis of the shoulder.

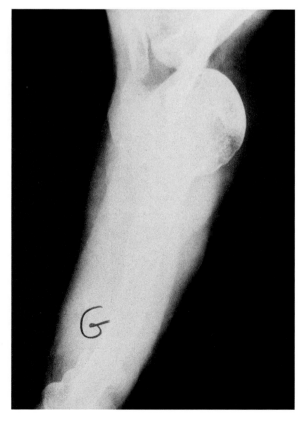

Figs. 1.**69a, b**   Chronic posterior dislocation in the AP (**a**) and axial (**b**) views.

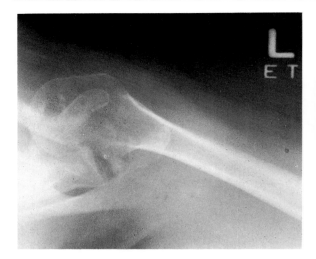

Fig. 1.**70** Chronic anterior dislocation in the axial projection.

a   b

Figs. 1.**71a, b** Inferior subluxation of the humeral head (**b**) compared to a normal shoulder (**a**).

Views of the Bony Margin of the Glenoid

West Point view. This technique demonstrates the anteroinferior bony margin of the glenoid in a PA projection. The patient is positioned prone with the arm abducted 90°; the elbow is flexed to allow the forearm to hang down over the side of the table. The affected shoulder is raised approximately 8 cm, and the head and neck are inclined toward the contralateral side. The film cassette is placed above the shoulder and the central ray is aimed directly at the axilla, angled 25° down from horizontal and 25° medially (Figs. 1.**72a, b**). Properly positioned, this will provide a tangential view of the anterior inferior glenoid fossa (Fig. 1.**73**). Over 90% of patients with recurrent anterior shoulder dislocation will show erosion, irregularities, or capsular calcifications in this region.

Apical oblique projection. This view is helpful in diagnosing shoulder instability. The patient is positioned sitting, with the injured shoulder in contact with the film cassette. This may be done using a sling to immobilize the shoulder. The patient's torso is rotated approximately 45° to align the plane of the shoulder blade parallel to the film cassette. The central ray is also angled 45° caudally and is aimed at the base of the coracoid process; it runs parallel to the body of the scapula which is held at this angle to the chest with the extremity at rest or adducted (Figs. 1.**74a, b**).

When evaluating radiographs obtained in this projection, it is helpful to use the base of the coracoid process as an anatomic landmark. This structure lies between the anterior and posterior margins of the glenoid. Structures demonstrated in this projection

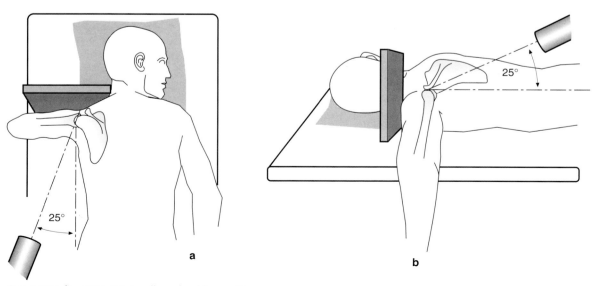

25°

25°

a   b

Figs. 1.**72a, b** West Point axillary shoulder position.

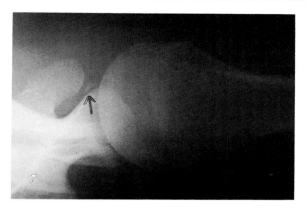

Fig. 1.**73** Bony Bankart defect in the West Point projection.

Fig. 1.**75** Positioning for the 60° internal rotation view for visualizing a Hill–Sachs lesion.

include the anterior and posterior margins of the bony glenoid as well as intra-articular fractures.

Views of Hill–Sachs Lesions

Standard views are not suitable for visualizing Hill–Sachs lesions and for this reason various special views are commonly used.

AP view at 60° internal rotation. Probably the simplest radiograph for demonstrating a Hill–Sachs is the AP projection in maximum internal rotation since the posterolateral compression fracture of the humeral head only appears in profile with the arm in internal rotation. This projection is not intended to visualize the glenohumeral joint parallel to the plane of projection, but rather demonstrates the posterolateral contour of the humeral head. The patient stands with his or her back to the film cassette. The central ray is aimed at the coracoid process, at a right angle to the coronal plane. With the elbow flexed 90°, the 60° internal rotation is easily verified (Fig. 1.**75**).

a   b

Figs. 1.**74a, b** Patient positioning for the apical oblique projection.

Fig. 1.**76**   Positioning for the Stryker notch view.

Fig. 1.**77**   Positioning for the Didiée shoulder view.

Fig. 1.**78**   Positioning for the Hermodsson view.

Stryker notch view. This technique is used to image the Hill–Sachs lesion longitudinally. With the patient supine, the upper arm is raised, the elbow flexed, and the hand placed on the head, with the heel of the hand resting at the top of the back of the head. The shaft of the humerus is parallel to the sagittal axis of the body. The upper arm is flexed over 90° and slightly internally rotated. The central ray is angled 10° cranially and aimed at the coracoid process, with the film cassette placed under the patient's shoulder (Fig. 1.**76**).

Didiée shoulder position. The Didiée view visualizes the anteroinferior margin of the glenoid and can demonstrate the presence of a Hill–Sachs lesion. The patient is prone, with the arm and back of the hand

placed on the posterior iliac crest. The elbow is flexed. The film cassette is under the injured shoulder, and the central ray is angled 45° lateromedially with respect to the floor and aimed at the humeral head (Fig. 1.**77**). In this view a Hill–Sachs lesion may appear distorted, making it difficult to determine its actual size.

Hermodsson view. This view can demonstrate a posterolateral compression fracture of the humeral head. The patient is supine or standing with the affected arm in internal rotation and the elbow flexed 90°. The hand is placed on the patient's back, or between the back and table, with the palm touching the table. The central ray is aimed at the humeral head at an angle of 30° to the longitudinal axis of the humerus (Fig. 1.**78**).

Saxer and Johner posterior tangential view. This technique can demonstrate the width and depth of Hill–Sachs lesions. The patient is supine and the elbow flexed 90°; the forearm is placed on the chest so that the fingertips touch the contralateral shoulder. The film cassette is placed superior to the affected shoulder. The central ray is aimed at the glenohumeral joint in a caudocranial projection, angled 20° laterally in the coronal plane and 20° posteriorly in the sagittal plane.

Views for Subluxation of the Glenohumeral Joint

Cephaloscapular projection. The cephaloscapular projection can be helpful in diagnosing subluxation of the glenohumeral joint. This projection will demonstrate the acromion, glenoid, humeral head, and coracoid process (overlapped and only slightly obscured by the clavicle). The patient is positioned standing or sitting and bending forward 45° so that the coracoid

Figs. 1.**79a, b**   Positioning for the cephaloscapular view.

process and acromion form a vertical plane. The film cassette is placed behind the patient parallel to this plane, with the central ray aimed at the glenohumeral joint and entering horizontally. If radiographs at rest are to be obtained, the elbows is flexed and the pronated forearm is placed on the table in a relaxed position (Figs. 1.**79a, b**). If posterior stress is desired to demonstrate posterior subluxation, this is achieved by using the patients body weight. Anterior stress is induced by allowing the forearm to hang down and by loading it with weights.

Signs of Posterior Dislocation on the AP Radiograph

Although the AP radiograph must be supplemented by an axial view whenever dislocation is suspected, it can provide evidence of posterior dislocation of the shoulder.

Cisternios compression line. The anteromedial compression fracture caused by posterior dislocation will appear as a sclerotic line lateral to the articular surface of the humeral head.

Pear sign. Since posterior dislocation will always force the joint into internal rotation, the greater tuberosity will be rotated anteriorly in such cases and no longer appear in focus. This gives the humeral head the shape of a pear in the AP radiograph.

Rim sign. In a posterior dislocation, the distance between the margin of the head and the margin of the glenoid fossa will exceed 6 mm.

Missing half-moon. If the glenohumeral joint is not visualized exactly parallel to the plane of projection, the contours of the humeral head and the glenoid fossa will overlap to form a shadow in the shape of a half-moon. This half-moon figure will not be present in a posterior dislocation.

Special Views for Trauma

In many dislocations and fractures, pain renders the positioning of the patient for a standard axial radiograph difficult or impossible. The following views can be used for the second imaging plane.

Transthoracic lateral view. With the patient sitting or standing, the lateral side of the affected shoulder is placed against the film cassette, and the contralateral arm is raised so that the supinated forearm is lying on top of the patient's head. The upper torso is rotated posteriorly. The central ray is perpendicular to the film cassette, aimed between the spine and sternum at a point slightly inferior to the coracoid process (Fig. 1.**80**). This radiographic projection is difficult to interpret due to overlapping structures, although the scapulohumeral arc (Moloney's line) is helpful in determining the position of the humeral head in relation to the glenoid fossa. In normal anatomy Moloney's line, formed by the

Fig. 1.**80**   Positioning for the transthoracic lateral view.

Fig. 1.**82**   Positioning for the scapular Y view.

shaft of the humerus and the axillary margin of the scapula, appears as a smooth continuous curve. In the posterior dislocation of the humeral head, it will be at an acute angle; in anterior dislocation, the angle will be very obtuse (Figs. 1.**81a–c**).

True lateral (scapular Y) shoulder position. Another technique for obtaining radiographs in the second imaging plane with a painful shoulder is to use the scapular Y position. The painful shoulder may be in

internal rotation in a sling. The patient stands with the affected shoulder against the film cassette, with the body and the affected shoulder forming an angle of approximately 60°. The cassette is against the anterolateral region of the affected shoulder. The central ray is directed tangentially along the posterolateral margin of the rib cage in line with the scapular spine and perpendicular to the cassette (Fig. 1.82). This positioning produces a true lateral image of the scapula and the glenohumeral joint, demonstrating the

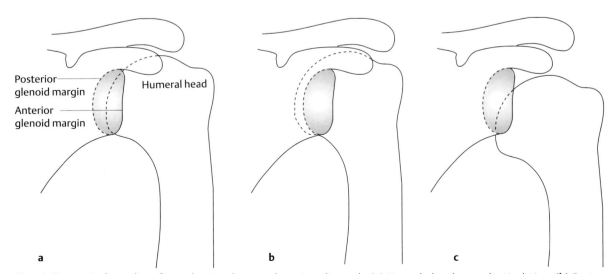

Figs. 1.**81a–c**   Moloney lines for evaluating the transthoracic radiograph. (**a**) Normal glenohumeral articulation. (**b**) Posterior dislocation showing an acute angle. (**c**) Anterior dislocation showing an obtuse angle.

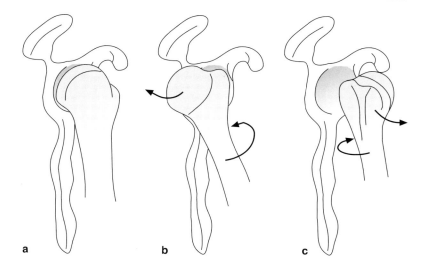

Figs. 1.**83a–c** Evaluation of the scapular Y radiograph. Normal articulation (**a**), posterior dislocation (**b**), anterior dislocation (**c**).

Fig. 1.**84** Positioning for the Velpeau view.

and the humeral head will normally appear centered within it. In an anterior dislocation, the humeral head will appear inferior to the coracoid process in front of the glenoid fossa; in a posterior dislocation it will be displaced posteriorly relative to the glenoid fossa (Fig. 1.**83a–c**). Fracture dislocations involving the greater tuberosity can be seen in this view, although fractures of the anterior or posterior glenoid margin will not be detected.

The combination of scapular Y, AP, and axillary views image the shoulder in perpendicular planes and provide maximum diagnostic information.

Velpeau view. This view is a further modification of the axillary projection. It can be used to obtain an axillary view in a patient with a shoulder immobilized in a sling, without abducting the arm. With the arm in a Velpeau bandage or sling, the patient stands with his or her back to the X-ray table and leans backward approximately 30° so that the affected shoulder lies above the film cassette placed on the table. The central ray is centered on the glenohumeral joint in a craniocaudal projection (Fig. 1.**84**). This technique clearly demonstrates the position of the humeral head relative to the glenoid fossa. Interpretation of the radiograph requires experience as it significantly distorts the size of the humeral head and glenoid fossa. This distortion does not diminish the value of this technique to demonstrate a dislocation.

Cuillo axillary view. This technique allows the supine positioning of a trauma patient without removing the arm from a sling. The patient is supine with the arm internally rotated and the elbow resting on radiolucent cushion material so that the shoulder is flexed approximately 20°. The central ray is aimed at the acromioclavicular joint, entering through the axilla (Fig. 1.**85**). This view demonstrates the anterolateral margin of the glenoid particularly well since it is unobstructed by interposed tissue.

position of the humeral head relative to the glenoid fossa. The scapula itself appears as a Y with the scapular body forming the vertical portion. The two upper limbs are formed anteriorly by the coracoid process and anteriorly by the scapular spine and acromion. The glenoid fossa lies at the center of these three lines

Fig. 1.**85** Positioning for the Cuillo view.

Fractures of the Proximal Humerus

Neer classification (Fig. 1.**86**) has become an established method for distinguishing fractures of the proximal humerus. This classification uses fragment identification and considers anatomic and biomechanical forces.

— Fracture of the anatomic neck of the humerus
— Fracture of the lesser tuberosity
— Fracture of the greater tuberosity
— Fracture of the surgical neck of the humerus

Injuries in which the fragments are either separated more than 2 cm or are at an angle exceeding 45° are referred to as displaced fractures; injuries involving lesser degrees of displacement are referred to as non-displaced or one-segment fractures. There are fracture dislocations when the head is displaced outside the joint space, not merely rotated.

Clavicular Fractures

Neer divides clavicular fractures into three groups:

— Fracture in the middle third (80% of all fractures)
— Fracture in the lateral third (15% of all fractures)
— Fracture in the medial third (85% of all fractures)

Group	Fragment 2	Fragment 3	Fragment 4
II True neck of humerus			
III Surgical neck of humerus			
IV Greater tuberosity			
V Lesser tuberosity			
VI Dislocation fracture anterior			
posterior			

Fig. 1.**86** Neer's four-segment classification Group I (minimal or no displacement not shown).

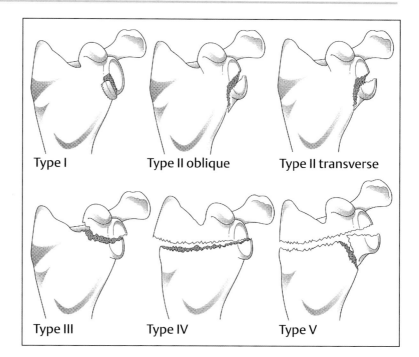

Fig. 1.87 Classification of fractures according to Ideberg.

Subdivisions according to neer are as fellows:

I: minimal displacement, interligamentous (cora-coclavicular-acromioclavicular [CC–AC])
II: fracture medial to CC ligaments
IIa: both ligaments attached to distal fragment
IIb: conoid ligament torn, trapezoid ligament attached to distal fragment
III: fracture involving the AC joint

These fractures are usually transverse and diagonal; rarely are they comminuted fractures or fractures involving loss of a segment.

Scapular Fractures

Zdravkovic and Damholt classify scapular fractures as follows:

— Fractures of the scapular body
— Fractures of the apophysis (including coracoid and acromion)
— Fracture of the superior lateral angle, including the neck and glenoid

Ideberg subdivides glenoid fractures themselves into five groups (Fig. 1.87).

Special Views of the Acromioclavicular Joint

To best image the acromioclavicular joint, remind the X-ray technologist to reduce peak kilovoltage by about 50%. This will significantly improve the image quality because the acromioclavicular joint is overexposed at standard X-ray unit settings.

Zanca view of the acromioclavicular joint. Often the acromioclavicular joint will be obscured by the scapular spine in the AP view. Possible solutions include an abduction or Zanca view. Aim the central ray at the acromioclavicular joint and angle it 10° cranially (Fig. 1.88). This technique is often the only way to demonstrate changes in the lateral clavicle, acromion, or coracoclavicular ligaments.

Acromioclavicular stress view. This is used to confirm separation of the acromioclavicular joint that presents with superior displacement of the lateral end of the clavicle. The patient sits with the back against an upright film cassette. The cassette should be wide enough to image both acromioclavicular joints simultaneously. Both arms are weighted with about 10 kg. The weights are suspended by wrist straps, not held by the patient. This eliminates any stabilizing effect of the shoulder muscles on the acromioclavicular joints. If the acromioclavicular joint is separated, the clavicle on the affected side will be superiorly displaced relative to the acromion and coracoid process (Figs. 1.89a, b). This study is very painful in the case of an acutely injured acromioclavicular joint.

Alexander lateral projection of the scapula. Patient positioning, image size, and film cassette are the same as for the lateral scapula Y projection. The patient attempts to thrust both shoulders as far forward as possible. Films are taken of the acromioclavicular joint in a relaxed and forward thrust position. In a separated acromioclavicular joint, the acromion will be visible anteriorly and inferiorly under the distal

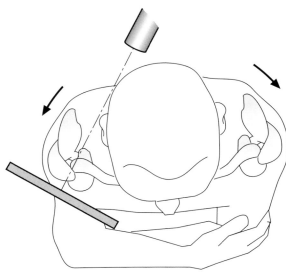

Fig. 1.**90**   Lateral Alexander view of the acromioclavicular joint.

Fig. 1.**88**   Positioning for the Zanca view.

end of the clavicle when compared with the relaxed position view (Fig. 1.**90**). The uninjured side can be used as a comparison view.

The Rockwood classification of dislocations in the acromioclavicular joint is as follows (Fig. 1.**91**).

- Type 1: strain of the acromioclavicular and coracoclavicular ligaments with pain and localized swelling. The ligaments are intact; the acromioclavicular joint is stable.
- Type II: tear of the acromioclavicular ligament and strain of the coracoclavicular ligaments. Instability in the AP plane. Minimal upward displacement of the distal clavicle.
- Type III: tear of the acromioclavicular and coracoclavicular ligaments with significant superior displacement of the lateral end of the clavicle.
- Type IV: same as type III but with posterior displacement of the lateral end of the clavicle.
- Type V: exceeds type III with massive dislocation.
- Type VI: rare form with dislocation of the clavicle under the acromion accompanied by intense swelling.

Figs. 1.**89a, b**   (**a**) Positioning for the acromioclavicular projection with weights. (**b**) Radiograph showing separation of the acromioclavicular joint. Note the position of the weights suspended from the wrists.

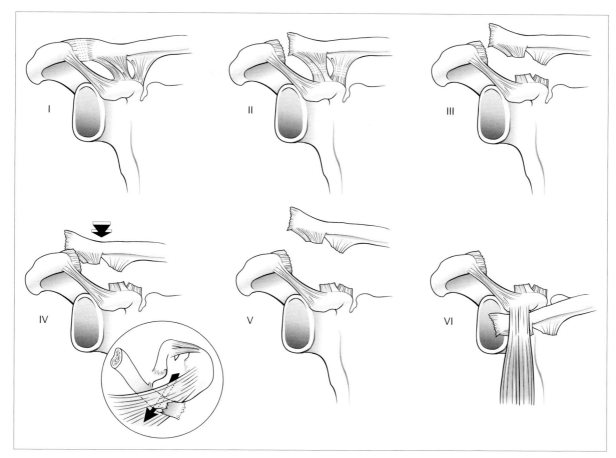

Fig. 1.**91**   Rockwood classification of AC joint injury
Type I: sprain of AC ligament, AC joint intact, CC ligament intact, deltoid and trapezius muscles intact.
Type II: AC joint disrupted, AC joint wider; may be a slight vertical separation when compared with the normal shoulder; sprain of CC ligaments; coracoclavicular interspace might be slightly increased; deltoid and trapezius muscles intact.
Type III: AC ligaments disrupted; AC joint dislocated and the shoulder complex displaced inferiorly; CC ligaments disrupted; coracoclavicular interspace greater than the normal shoulder (i.e., 25% to 100% greater than the normal shoulder); deltoid and trapezius muscles usually detached from the distal end of the clavicle.
Type IV: AC ligaments disrupted; AC joint dislocated and clavicle anatomically displaced posteriorly into or through the trapezius muscle; CC ligaments completely disrupted; coracoclavicular interspace may be displaced, but may appear to be the same as the normal shoulder; deltoid and trapezius muscles detached from the distal end of the clavicle.
Type V: AC ligaments disrupted; AC joint dislocated and the shoulder complex displaced inferiorly, CC ligaments disrupted; coracoclavicular interspace greater than the normal shoulder (i.e., 100% to 300% greater than the normal shoulder); deltoid and trapezius muscles detached from the distal end of the clavicle.
Type VI: AC ligaments disrupted; CC ligaments disrupted; AC joint dislocated and the clavicle displaced inferior to the acromion or the coracoid process; coracoclavicular interspace reversed with the clavicle being inferior to the acromion or the coracoid; deltoid and trapezius muscles are detached from the distal end of the clavicle.

Special Views of the Sternoclavicular Joint

Rockwood sternoclavicular view: This is also called the serendipity view, as Dr. Rockwood incidentally noted the value of this projection. The patient is supine on the X-ray table, with the arms at the sides and palms facing the table. A 28×35 cm film cassette is placed beneath the patient's neck and shoulders. The X-ray is angled 40° cranially from vertical, with the central ray entering at the sternal angle. Attempt to project at least the medial halves of both clavicles onto the middle of the film. The distance between the X-ray tube and film cassette should be 100 cm in children and 140 cm in adults (Figs. 1.**92a–d**). Normally, both clavicles will be located in the same horizontal plane. Anterior deviation of a clavicular axis is a sign of an anterior dislocation of the joint, posterior deviation of posterior dislocation. Degenerative or other processes can also be imaged in this projection, although tomography will provide more information in many situations (Fig. 1.**93**).

Fig. 1.**93**   Tomogram of the sternoclavicular joint.

Figs. 1.**92a–d**   (**a**) Rockwood sternoclavicular projection. (**b**) Normal sternoclavicular articulation. (**c**) Anterior dislocation. (**d**) Posterior dislocation.

Hobbs sternoclavicular view. In this technique, the patient stands at the end of the X-ray table, bending forward so that the cervical spine is almost parallel to the table. The central ray is aimed at the sternoclavicular joint from posterior (Fig. 1.**94**).

Dislocation most frequently occurs anteriorly; posterior dislocation is rare. The injuries are roughly classified as follows:

— Mild sprain
— Moderate sprain (subluxation)
— Severe sprain (dislocation)

1.4 Ultrasound

Indications, Diagnostic Value, and Clinical Relevance

Ultrasound extends the range of shoulder imaging modalities and has demonstrated its value in diagnosing rotator-cuff lesions and shoulder instability. Ultrasound and plain radiography are primary imaging modalities that complement each other and they can often confirm tentative clinical diagnoses. Ultrasound studies alone are often able to confirm a complete tear of the rotator cuff. They can be used to verify and quantify fragment dislocation in avulsion fractures of the tuberosities.

Normal Findings

Certain transducer positions have been defined in the interest of standardizing the examination technique. These positions are named according to the anatomic orientation relative to the musculoskeletal system. A complete examination of the shoulder should be performed using the following standard projections:

— Anterior transverse plane
— Coracoacromial window
— Lateral coronal plane
— Posterior transverse plane

Fig. 1.**94**   Positioning for the Hobb's sternoclavicular projection.

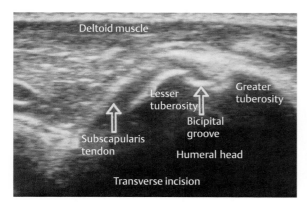

Fig. 1.**95**   Anterior transverse imaging plane.

Fig. 1.**96**   Coracoacromial window.

If pathologic findings are detected in standard projections, they should be documented in a second imaging plane perpendicular to the initial projection.

Anterior transverse plane. The anterior transverse plane is located anterior to the shoulder as a transverse section taken through the bicipital groove. This projection demonstrates the medial portions of the subscapularis tendon as far as its insertion at the lesser tuberosity and, laterally, the long biceps tendon. The long biceps tendon is evaluated in the bicipital groove that is bounded medially by the lesser tuberosity and laterally by the greater tuberosity (Fig. 1.**95**). The long biceps tendon appears as an echogenic structure; usually the transducer must be inclined slightly to obtain hyperechoic image. Within the bicipital groove, the tendon courses not quite parallel to the surface of the skin. These portions of the tendon can only be imaged perpendicular to the direction of sound propagation by tilting the transducer laterally to vary the angle of incidence until the tendon is visualized as an echogenic structure. The dynamic action of the subscapularis tendon should be evaluated in external and internal rotation.

The coracoacromial window. The coracoacromial window is located by placing the transducer on the contour of the shoulder lateral and parallel to the axis of the coracoacromial ligament. In this imaging plane the rotator cuff can be evaluated initially with the arm in a neutral position, then in internal rotation with extension, and finally with the arm in external rotation. The coracoid process and the convex arc of the humeral head with its typical posterior acoustic shadow appear as echogenic structures along the boundaries of the coracoacromial window; these structures serve as bony landmarks. Above the echogenic contour of the humeral head lies echogenic articular cartilage; above this is the rotator cuff, appearing as a moderately hyperechoic region. The upper boundary layer of the cuff cannot be distinguished from the lower lamina of the subdeltoid bursa; these two structures appear as a single echo-

genic arc of reflection. A narrow hypoechoic halo is discernible above this combined boundary layer, corresponding to the actual subdeltoid bursa. The upper lamina of the bursa combines with the lower fascia of the deltoid muscle to form a sharp, echogenic arc of reflection. This typical sequence of layers is referred to as a wheel pattern, with the contour of the humeral head forming the rim, the rotator cuff the tire, and the line of the bursa representing the tread (Fig. 1.**96**).

Different portions of the rotator cuff can be examined through the coracoacromial window by changing the rotation of the arm. The long tendon of the biceps is defined as the border structure between the supraspinatus and subscapularis tendon. The subscapularis tendon lies medial to the biceps tendon, and the supraspinatus tendon lateral to it. The examination in internal rotation with extension brings the insertion of the tendon into the imaging plane in front of the bony margin of the acromion. In normal ultrasound anatomy, the supraspinatus tendon will appear as a band-shaped, moderately echogenic structure above the narrow, hypoechoic layer of articular tissue and the hyperechoic contour of the humeral head.

Lateral coronal plane. In the lateral coronal plane, the transducer lies medially on the acromion and laterally on the deltoid. Particularly in abduction movements, this position permits evaluation of the gliding action of the supraspinatus tendon as well as imaging of the lateral portion of the subdeltoid bursa. It is also used for documenting craniocaudal hypermobility. The typical hypoechoic boundary layers of the bony margins of the acromion and humeral head with its posterior acoustic shadow serve as anatomic landmarks. The moving supraspinatus tendon lies laterally on the humeral head, extending to its insertion on the greater tuberosity. The halo of articular cartilage is visible as a hypoechoic region beneath the tendon. The echo structure formed by the subdeltoid bursa and the lower deltoid fascia is clearly discernible above it (Fig. 1.**97**).

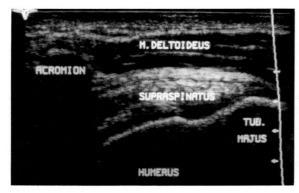

Fig. 1.**97**   Coronal lateral imaging plane.

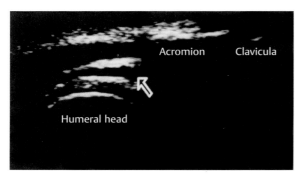

Fig. 1.**99**   Double contour of the bursa with an effusion in the subacromial bursa.

Posterior transverse plane. In the posterior transverse plane, palpate the scapular spine and place the transducer immediately inferior to it, aiming the transducer horizontally. The hyperechoic bony boundary layer of the posterior glenoid and the contour of the humerus should be sharply distinguished in the image. The triangular hyperechoic glenoid labrum rests on the margin of the glenoid. As in the wheel pattern in the anterior imaging planes, the musculotendinous portion of the infraspinatus muscle lies on the contour of the humerus in the posterior transverse plane. Moving the arm into external rotation permits static and dynamic imaging of this tendon as far as its insertion on the greater tuberosity (Fig. 1.**98**).

Pathologic Findings in the Presence of Degenerative Changes

Changes in the Subacromial Bursa

Irritation of the subdeltoid bursa and subacromial bursa accompanies many changes in the subacromial space. This irritation will appear in the sonogram as a hypoechoic region correlating with an effusion. Extensive accumulations of fluid cause what is known as relative enhancement behind the affected area due to the reduced attenuation in the fluid. Acute bursitis

Fig. 1.**98**   Posterior horizontal imaging plane.

usually leads to massive effusion with clearly discernible separation of the bursa laminae (Fig. 1.**99**).

Tear of the Rotator Cuff

Tears in the rotator cuff are divided into two categories. **Safe geometric tear signs** are differentiated from **unsafe structural tear signs** that specifically include changes in the echogenicity of the tendons (Table 1.**9**).

- **Safe geometric tear sign**
- **Missing rotator cuff.** It has become common to refer to a "bald head" in describing a complete tear of the rotator cuff. In the coracoacromial window sonogram, the typical wheel pattern of the cuff will be missing above the contour of the humeral head; the deltoid is in direct contact with the contour of the humeral head (Fig. 1.**100**). These findings are particularly striking when the opposite shoulder is imaged. This is a sign of a complete rotator-cuff tear. In the anterior transverse plane, positive diagnosis of a complete tear of the subscapularis tendon is also possible. The supraspinatus tendon tear is characterized in the lateral imaging plane by direct contact between the deltoid muscle and the contour of the humeral head; the contour of the cuff will be missing completely.

Table 1.**9**   Safe and unsafe signs of rotator cuff pathology in ultrasound

Safe geometric tear signs
- missing rotator cuff ("bald head")
- segmental narrowing with reversed contour
- abrupt change in diameter
- step sign

Unsafe structural tear signs
- hyperechoic zone
- hypoechoic zone
- combined hypoechoic and hyperechoic zone

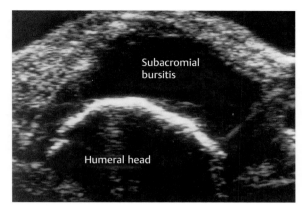

Fig. 1.**100** "Bald" humeral head with massive effusion beneath the deltoid. The contour of the rotator cuff is missing completely.

Fig. 1.**101** Flattened wheel pattern with reversed contour of the rotator cuff (left) compared with the normal contralateral side (right).

Fig. 1.**102** Echogenic zone within the rotator cuff.

— **Segmental narrowing with reversed contour.** Segmental narrowing and flattening of the rotator cuff by over 50% compared with the contralateral side, combined with a dip in the normally convex contour, is also to be regarded as a sign of a tear. However, this sign is not as clear as the presence of a completely "bald head." Segmental narrowing of the cuff is referred to when the tendinous plate medial and lateral to the affected area is of normal width. The decisive criterion is the reversed contour of the cuff boundary, i.e., the region with a concave depression in the tendon structure (Fig. 1.**101**).

— **Abrupt change in diameter.** Narrowing may take the form of an abrupt change in the diameter of the supraspinatus tendon, extending laterally to the point of insertion.

— **Step sign.** Less frequently, a step sign is encountered in which the hyperechoic boundary of the bursa is interrupted. This is a sign of a tear in the rotator cuff. Such a sign is seen in either a partial or complete tear of the rotator cuff and is primarily observed with traumatic tendon defects.

- **Inconclusive structural signs of a tear and changes in echogenicity**

Changes in the echogenicity of the tendon structure that are not accompanied by changes in geometry are inconclusive signs that may indicate a tear in the rotator cuff. Positive diagnosis of a tear in the rotator tendons requires a change in tendon geometry; a change in echogenicity alone is not sufficient.

Hyperechoic zones in the supraspinatus tendon are best detected in the coracoacromial window in internal rotation with extension (Fig. 1.**102**). It is essential to distinguish such a hyperechoic zone from a central echo that frequently occurs in the normal tendon as it is imaged horizontally, and from the long head of the biceps tendon coursing beneath it. Dynamic examination is helpful here. The hyperechoic zone should always be demonstrated in a second imaging plane. For example, after the initial examination of the coracoacromial window, imaging findings should be confirmed in the longitudinal section of the supraspinatus. A hyperechoic zone may be a sign of degenerative changes in the rotator cuff. Other possible causes can include inflammatory processes such as calcific tendonitis, tendon fibrosis, or scarring from a tear in the rotator cuff accompanied by formation of granulation tissue.

When evaluating changes in echogenicity be aware that ultrasonography does not permit histologic differentiation. Ensure that the description of image data is strictly separated from the final evaluation of these findings.

A combination of a hyperechoic and hyperechoic zone is encountered far more frequently than an isolated hyperechoic area. This phenomenon can occasionally occur in calcific tendinitis with accompanying inflammation of portions of the rotator cuff. Hypoechoic zones in the rotator cuff can occur on the bursa side, joint side, or within the tendons (Fig. 1.**103**). They are frequently encountered together with geometric changes.

Fig. 1.**103**   Echogenic zone within the rotator cuff.

Fig. 1.**105**   Posterior dislocation of the shoulder in the posterior horizontal imaging plane (right) compared with the normal contralateral side (left).

● **Typical problems in evaluating the rotator cuff**

In light of the numerous sources of error, ultrasound image phenomena must fulfill special requirements before they are regarded as genuine findings. These always include:

— Detection of the phenomenon in a second imaging plane
— Verification of the image phenomenon in a dynamic examination.
— Presence of morphologic changes in the sonogram; differences in echogenicity alone are not sufficient.

Only when all of these conditions have been met should one refer to normal or pathologic ultrasound findings.

Changes in the Long Head of the Biceps Tendon

Tear in the biceps tendon. A tear in the long head of the biceps tendon can be diagnosed from the lack of a normal, hyperechoic tendinous structure in the bicipital groove in the anterior transverse plane. Naturally, this finding must be reproducible in the anterior longitudinal plane.

Fig. 1.**104**   Biceps halo (left) compared with the normal contralateral side.

Tendinitis of the biceps tendon. Tendinitis of the biceps tendon usually results in increased accumulations of fluid in the tendon sheath. The resulting widening of the tendon sheath is detectable in the anterior transverse sonogram as a hypoechoic halo around the hyperechoic sheath. This phenomenon is referred to as a biceps halo (Fig. 1.**104**). A biceps halo can also occur without any irritation of the tendon when effusion into the shoulder joint continues into the tendon sheath. In this case the condition is attributable to pathology of the glenohumeral joint itself.

Pathologic Findings in the Presence of Instability

Ultrasound studies of bony surfaces for diagnosing instability require different settings than for soft tissue, where gray-scale values are important. Bony margins produce maximum reflection, resulting in a hyperechoic image. Sonograms for diagnosing the stability of the glenohumeral joint are obtained in two imaging planes. Anterior and posterior can be examined in the posterior transverse plane. Inferior instability can be verified by a stress test in the lateral coronal plane. Systematic examination of active and passive joint motion can provide information on the direction of instability.

Dislocation

The extent and direction of instability can be determined by changing the normal relation between the humeral head and the glenoid. In acute or chronic dislocation, the position of the humeral head can be imaged in relation to the glenoid fossa. Since no special positioning is required, the patient is not only spared radiation exposure but also the painful positioning needed to obtain radiographs. Pregnant patients can be examined perfectly safely. In posterior dislocations, the humeral head will lie significantly posterior to the posterior margin of the glenoid fossa (Fig. 1.**105**). Imaging the contralateral shoulder will confirm the diagnosis, even for an inexperienced examiner. In an anterior dislocation, the posterior margin of the humeral head will lie anterior to the

Fig. 1.**106** Anterior dislocation of the shoulder in the posterior horizontal imaging plane (right) compared with the normal contralateral side (left).

Fig. 1.**108** Bilateral Hill–Sachs lesion in the posterior horizontal imaging plane.

Fig. 1.**107** Inferior drawer (sulcus sign) in the lateral coronal imaging plane (right) compared with the normal position (left).

posterior margin of the glenoid. Voluntary dislocations can be documented under ultrasonographic control (Fig. 1.**106**).

Ultrasound is particularly advantageous in diagnosing dislocations in newborns. Traumatic dislocations of the glenohumeral joint can even occur during birth. Since the shoulder of the newborn consists almost entirely of cartilaginous structures, radiography is extremely difficult. As with the hip, diagnostic ultrasound can be used in newborns to determine the relative position of the two articular surfaces.

Inferior instability. Inferior instability is evaluated in the lateral coronal plane; a groove test is performed under ultrasonographic control. The hyperechoic contour of the acromion and the contour of the humeral head, which disappears medially in the acoustic shadow of the acromion, serve as bony anatomic landmarks. The distance from the superior margin of the acromion to the contour of the humerus is initially measured with the arm in a neutral position. A distal stress is then applied to the relaxed arm as in clinical testing for the sulcus sign and the results are documented in a second sonogram (Fig.1.**107**). Occasionally, the humeral head can be moved more than 2 cm out of the glenoid fossa. The sulcus test under ultrasonographic control is more sensitive and objective than the clinical test which, when positive, is itself characteristic proof of multidirectional joint instability. In demonstrating inferior instability and permitting quantitative documentation of findings, the ultrasound test is important in the differential diagnosis of instability because it can distinguish

multidirectional instability from unidirectional forms.

Hill–Sachs Lesions

Ultrasound can detect the compression fracture in Hill–Sachs Lesions. The shoulder is first examined in the posterior transverse plane with the arm in a neutral position, and the convexity of the humerus is examined for irregularities and interruptions in its contour. Here, pay particular attention to the layer of cartilage. Continue the ultrasound examination by instructing the patient to slowly lift the arm to 90° flexion while you guide it. This allows examination of an entire posterosuperior humeral convexity. Typically, a Hill–Sachs lesion can be recognized as an approximately triangular depression in the contour of the humerus with an echo at its base (Fig. 1.**108**). Compression in the bone should not be confused with the physiologic transition between the greater tuberosity and the humeral head. Ultrasonography permits exact measurement of the Hill–Sachs lesion.

Other Pathologic Findings
Fractures of the Humeral Head

Ultrasound can be used as a supplementary modality in support of radiographic studies in fractures of the humeral head. These studies concentrate primarily on the rotator cuff when secondary injuries to the cuff are suspected. However, ultrasound can also be used in evaluating the fracture itself, particularly in the case of isolated avulsion fractures of the greater tuberosity. Traction of the infraspinatus and supraspinatus causes the greater tuberosity to migrate superoposteriorly. Because imaging can be freely directed in ultrasound studies, the course of the fracture cleavage can be followed during the imaging processes. This makes it possible to precisely evaluate the relationship between the fracture fragments. Step-offs in

Fig. 1.**109**   Intra-articular effusion in the posterior horizontal imaging plane.

Fig. 1.**110**   Suppurative arthritis in the coracoacromial window.

the surface contour of the humerus are more readily discernible on the sonogram than on the radiograph. Frequently the fragment of the greater tuberosity will be seen to have migrated superiorly; comparison with the opposite shoulder will reveal significant superior displacement and a step-off in the contour of the humeral head. The narrow band of soft tissue contracted toward the acromion will be discernible even with the arm in a neutral position. In abduction, the fragment of the greater tuberosity presses the supraspinatus tendon against the inferior aspect of the acromion. Here, ultrasound studies are a valuable supplement to standard radiographs.

Diagnosis of Effusion and Proliferative Changes

Intra-articular and extra-articular effusion. Intra-articular effusion of the glenohumeral joint is characterized by a hypoechoic expansion of the capsular space, primarily in the posterior transverse plane (Fig. 1.**109**). The fluid is often conducted to the sheath of the biceps tendon, causing the familiar biceps halo. In the presence of shoulder irritation of uncertain cause, ultrasound studies can differentiate between intra-articular and extra-articular fluid accumulations.

Intra-articular effusion with hypoechoic expansion of the intra-articular space can result in the rotator cuff being lifted off the contour of the humeral head. This superior migration can be identified in the lateral coronal plane. Extra-articular fluid accumulations lie above the rotator cuff near the transducer and can be distinguished from the intra-articular space (Fig. 1.**110**).

1.5 Arthrography

Indications, Diagnostic Value, and Clinical Relevance

For a long time, arthrography was the only diagnostic modality available for imaging the intra-articular space and the surrounding soft-tissue structures of the shoulder. The method was first described in 1933 and most examiners injected air as a contrast medium. During the 1950s a single-contrast process using a water-soluble contrast medium became popular. The first double-contrast arthrographic studies of the shoulder were described in 1942. However, this technique was slow in becoming established. While the double-contrast method makes it possible to visualize more structures than in single-contrast arthrography, the numerous overlapping structures often make evaluation quite difficult. Occasionally, the double-contrast technique can be used to obtain more detailed information on such phenomena as intra-articular loose bodies and to evaluate articular surfaces or the underside of the rotator cuff. Bursography of the subacromial bursa is also performed. Arthrography may be indicated for both traumatic and degenerative changes (Table 1.**10**). Invasive arthrography should come at the end of the diagnostic imaging sequence.

Serious complications are rare in arthrography. A known history of allergy to contrast media can be a contraindication to arthrography, as can the presence of an acute infection in the shoulder or surrounding soft tissues. Genuine contrast-medium allergies are extremely rare in shoulder arthrography. One author found only 318 incidents in a retrospective evaluation of 126 000 arthrographic studies. No deaths were observed. Serious complications included one air embolism, four cases of severe hypotention, one case of laryngeal edema, and three instances of infection. The most frequent complications included chemical

Table 1.**10**   Indications for arthrography

Traumatic changes
— Complete tear of the rotator cuff
— Partial tear of the rotator cuff
— Defects in the capsular ligaments after dislocation
— Tears of the long head of the biceps tendon
— Dislocation of the long head of the biceps tendon
— Intra-articular loose bodies

Degenerative changes
— Complete tear of the rotator cuff
— Partial tear of the rotator cuff
— Adhesive capsulitis
— Tendinitis of the long head of the biceps tendon
— Synovitis of the glenohumeral joint
— Osteoarthritis of the shoulder
— Atraumatic shoulder instability

Fig. 1.**111**   Normal arthrogram.

synovitis (0.15%), vasovagal reactions (<0.1%), and urticaria (<0.01%).

Although the clinical importance of arthrography has diminished in recent years with the increase in the use of ultrasound and the development of MRI, it remains a reliable method for imaging rotator-cuff pathology in complete tears and partial tears on the joint side. It clearly demonstrates the extent of capsular shrinkage in adhesive capsulitis. Due to its high degree of diagnostic certainty, it remains the "gold standard" diagnostic test.

Technique and Examination Procedure

Contrast medium. Water-soluble ionic and nonionic contrast media containing iodine are used as positive contrast medium, and room air is used as a negative contrast medium. Adding epinephrine delays absorption and is done when maximum contrast duration is required, as is the case for conventional tomography or computed tomography.

Image documentation. Examination under fluoroscopic control is a key element of shoulder arthrography. This is initially done before injecting the contrast medium. Calcification can be identified or excluded with the arm in various rotational positions.

The stability of the glenohumeral joint can be tested in the axial view. The next important step is to evaluate the shoulder joint after contrast-medium injection. Pain occurring immediately after injection and significant joint resistance that can be felt even after the first few millimeters are signs of adhesive capsulitis. After injection of the contrast medium, it is important to move the shoulder passively in every direction. This ensures that even minor tears of the rotator cuff are impregnated with contrast medium. Final functional testing under fluoroscopic control will permit conclusions to be drawn about the location of a possible tear or about instability of the long biceps tendon with the arm in internal and external rotation.

Radiographs are then prepared in five planes:

— AP projection in internal rotation
— AP projection in external rotation
— AP projection in abduction
— Axial view
— Bicipital groove view.

When examining pathology of the rotator cuff, radiographs should be prepared using soft-tissue technique. This permits superior evaluation of lateral structures, particularly the region of the tendinous insertions of the rotator cuff on the greater tuberosity. The radiographs should be obtained within 20 minutes because the small volumes of contrast medium are quickly absorbed for example in the presence of adhesive capsulitis, and image quality rapidly deteriorates.

Normal Findings

In the AP projection with the arm in external rotation, the contrast medium surrounds the articular surface of the humeral head, extending as far as the insertion of the capsule at the anatomic neck. Since the subscapularis tendon is taut in external rotation, the subscapular bursa will only partially fill. The sheath of the long head of the biceps tendon is located on the lateral portion of the humeral head and is also filled with contrast medium. The biceps tendon itself causes a filling defect in the tendon sheath. The image in internal rotation shows the humeral head surrounded by contrast medium, and its hemispheric shape is clearly visible. The inferior capsular pocket is filled with contrast medium. The biceps tendon and the filled tendon sheath now lie further medially, and their course can be followed distally (Fig. 1.**111**). In abduction, the contrast medium is again pressed out of the subscapular bursa and in particular the inferior

Fig. 1.**112**   Contrast medium escapes from the glenohumeral joint into the subacromial bursa in a complete rotator cuff tear.

Fig. 1.**113**   Contrast medium escapes into the subacromial bursa, spreading as far as the acromioclavicular joint (geyser sign).

recess that is now under tension. Both structures are less discernible. The axial view clearly shows the filled subscapular recess at the base of the coracoid process. The filled sheath of the biceps is visualized, as is the posterior recess of the joint that is visible in this position because the joint capsule is flaccid. The contrast medium flows around the articular surfaces of the glenoid fossa and the humeral head. The inferior recess is compressed and is not visible because the joint capsule is under tension. The anterior and posterior portions of the glenoid labrum appear as filling defects.

The bicipital groove now shows the tendon sheath filled with contrast medium and the long head of the biceps tendon as a filling defect between the greater and lesser tuberosities. There are two particularly weak points in the joint capsule. One is the subscapular bursa and the other is the sheath of the long head of the biceps tendon. Overfilling the joint with contrast medium or performing vigorous motions to disperse the contrast medium can cause it to leak out at these locations. In addition to diminishing the quality of the arthrogram, this also causes pain.

Pathologic Findings in the Presence of Degenerative Changes

Complete Tear of the Rotator Cuff

Leakage of contrast medium from the glenohumeral joint into the subacromial bursa is a clear sign of a complete tear of the rotator cuff. Arthrography has 95–100% accuracy in diagnosing complete tears of the rotator cuff. In addition to visualizing the joint cavity, it also visualizes the subacromial bursa. Soft-tissue technique is particularly suitable for imaging contrast-medium leakage (Fig. 1.**112**). However, neither the rotator cuff itself nor the tear can be clearly imaged. Double-contrast techniques may be helpful here.

If the bursa fills only as the shoulder is moved, it may be presumed that the tear is small. Occasionally,

there will be a space between the bursa and the joint space that is free of contrast medium. This shows that rotator-cuff tissue is still interposed between the head and the acromion, meaning that the tear is not yet severe ("bald" humeral head). More extensive chronic rotator-cuff tears can lead to degenerative processes in the subacromial space. This will be seen on the plain radiographs as superior displacement of the humeral head. Occasionally, the joint space of the acromioclavicular joint will communicate with the subacromial bursa. This will lead to what is known as the "geyser sign" in arthrography (Fig. 1.**113**).

The diagnostic value of arthrography in evaluating complete tears of the rotator cuff depends on various factors. These include the time that the image documentation was obtained, radiographic parameters such as screen-film system, image definition, clarity of detail, contrast density, and radiographic projections. After the successful repair of a rotator-cuff tear, contrast-medium leakage can be demonstrated. For this reason, an arthrogram after rotator cuff surgery with persisting symptoms will not be conclusive.

Partial Tear of the Rotator Cuff

Partial tears of the rotator cuff that are limited to the bursal side or an intratendinous tear cannot be demonstrated with arthrography. Since the defect does not go through the entire thickness of the tendon, there is no communication with the subacromial bursa and no leakage of contrast medium into the bursa. However, most partial tears lie on the undersurface of the tendon and can be detected in an arthrogram. Irregularities of the underside will appear. If severe degeneration is present, contrast medium will also leak into the substance of the rotator cuff, and small depots of contrast medium will appear in the tendon itself. In such cases, it is important to move the shoulder through a range of motion after injecting contrast medium to press the contrast medium into the defects in the tendon (Fig. 1.**114**).

Fig. 1.**114** Partial inferior tear of the rotator cuff showing contrast medium escape into the tendinous tissue.

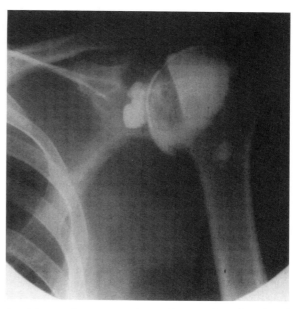

Fig. 1.**115** Adhesive capsulitis with a significantly reduced capsule volume.

These ulcerated or crater-shaped contrast-medium depots in the tendon generally appear laterally at the greater tuberosity and are referred to as a "rooster's comb" phenomenon.

If the tears or degenerative changes are only present on the outer or bursal surface of the rotator cuff, they will not be demonstrated at arthrography. **Bursography,** in which the subacromial bursa is selectively filled with contrast medium, can be useful in these cases. This method is used to evaluate the condition of the bursa. The examiner should note the filling volume and the visualization of the synovial surfaces. A normal subacromial bursa will accommodate between 5 mL and 10 mL of contrast medium. In patients with subacromial bursal pathology, the filling volume is reduced to 1–2 mL.

Changes in the Biceps Tendon Sheath

The long head of the biceps tendon lies between the greater and lesser tuberosities and is best imaged in tangential views. Generally, arthrography will reveal communication between the glenohumeral joint and the sheath of the long biceps tendon, with contrast medium in the tendon sheath.

Simple tears of the long head of the biceps tendon can be detected on an arthrogram. In such a case, the contrast-medium defect in the tendon sheath will be missing. Leakage of contrast medium from the tendon sheath is frequently observed but cannot be regarded as a specific sign of a tear. Contrast-medium leakage can result from excessive injection pressure.

The displacement of the tendon can also be demonstrated in tendon dislocations. In such a case, the bicipital groove projection will show an empty groove and displacement of the tendon and its sheath; the projection in external rotation will frequently show the tendon and sheath medial to the bicipital groove. Irritation or inflammation of the tendon and its sheath will appear as irregular contrast-medium fill-

ing. Other causes for the tendon not filling include adhesive capsulitis or failure to move the joint sufficiently after injection. However, the sheath of the long head of the biceps tendon will not always be visualized on the arthrogram, so no diagnostic conclusions can be drawn if filling of the sheath is not detected.

Adhesive Capsulitis and Therapeutic Arthrography

Intra-articular placement of the needle is difficult in adhesive capsulitis. The normal capacity of the joint space is reduced to 5–6 mL. Attempting to expand the fibrotic joint capsule any further will often cause pain. In its early stages, the disorder is visualized as a furrowed capsular margin with near normal filling volume. In the later stages, the joint space becomes progressively smaller, and the subscapular recess and axillary recess merge. The AP radiographs show tight capsular ligaments. In external rotation, the inferior recess will appear very small and will occasionally be missing entirely (Fig. 1.**115**). In internal rotation, the subscapular bursa and the extremely tight sheath of the long head of the biceps tendon will fill slightly with contrast medium. The biceps tendon will appear lateral and slightly superior to the humeral head and is easily confused with a rotator cuff tear.

Therapeutic arthrography. In adhesive capsulitis, one may attempt therapeutic arthrography. The goal of this procedure is to improve the range of motion of the shoulder by distension arthrography with precisely targeted injection of local anesthesia (possibly in combination with steroids), and to improve this range of motion with a subsequent program of specific mobilization. However, this technique has not proven very valuable since capsular rupture almost always occurs at the subscapular bursa. While this region represents the weak point of the capsule, it is not the reason for limited motion in adhesive capsulitis.

Pathologic Findings with Instability

Patients with recurrent shoulder dislocations frequently evidence an enlarged anteroinferior recess. This is particularly evident in internal rotation and on the axial radiograph. For example, when a capsular tear is present following a traumatic anteroinferior dislocation, the extravasation will frequently develop in this area. Occasionally a displaced glenoid labrum can be directly visualized on the glenoid or the scapula. Labral pathology is only reliably demonstrated with tomograms of the joint. In addition to conventional contrast medium, air can be used to produce a pneumotomogram of the joint. The following changes can be visualized in an acute dislocation or chronic shoulder instability:

— Leakage of contrast medium in capsule and ligament tears. This phenomenon can only be demonstrated within the first 2 days after trauma (6–48 hours) since these defects close relatively rapidly.
— Anteriorly and medially widened joint capsule.
— Absence of the glenoid labrum or penetration of contrast medium into the substance of the labrum.
— Intra-articular loose bodies.
— Rotator cuff tear.

Today, arthrography and joint tomography have been largely replaced by CT arthrography in diagnosing instability. The role of MRI in shoulder imaging has largely displaced arthrography.

Other Pathologic Findings

Intra-articular Loose Bodies

Occasionally, intra-articular loose bodies are detected with arthrography. Usually they are better visualized using a double-contrast technique. They can occur in every joint compartment, and are even encountered in the sheath of the long head of the biceps tendon.

Synovitis

In synovial inflammation, irregular filling of the entire joint will occur with bubble-like contrast-medium filling defects. Irregularities on the underside of the rotator cuff are seen as in an incomplete tear.

Problems, Sources of Error, and Difficulties

Despite the high accuracy of this method in diagnosing tears of the rotator cuff, discrepancies are often encountered between arthrographic and intraoperative findings, most of which are false positives. **False positive findings** can be caused by intratendinous calcifications that may be confused with contrast-medium leakage. Such errors can be avoided if the plain radiographs in various rotational positions are correctly interpreted. In rare cases, contrast medium can leak out of the joint through a physiologic gap in the rotator cuff between the supraspinatus and subscapularis tendons. This is a rarely encountered anatomic anomaly seen especially in hypermobile joints. Other misinterpretations can arise when contrast medium is mistakenly injected into the subacromial bursa. Contrast-medium deposition in the subacromial bursa can result when the needle is withdrawn from the joint and pressure is applied to the plunger. In the external rotation image, it is also possible for a filled biceps tendon sheath to simulate contrast-medium leakage. This error is easily corrected by evaluating the image in internal rotation. Often there will be a small superomedial recess superior to the insertion of the biceps tendon at the glenoid labrum, which also can simulate contrast-medium leakage.

False negative findings are attributable to post-infectious or posttraumatic adhesions and to substance defects filled with granulation tissue. This can also prevent the subacromial bursa from filling. Insufficient quantities of contrast medium or failure to move the shoulder sufficiently after contrast medium can also lead to false negative findings.

1.6 Nuclear Medicine Studies

Principles, Indications, Diagnostic Value, and Clinical Relevance

Those disorders that can be visualized in nuclear medicine studies have a relatively uniform appearance regardless of their location. With few exceptions, the underlying metabolic disorders progress similarly. This section is organized by disease entities in which nuclear medicine studies are used.

There are many pathophysiologic situations where nuclear medicine studies can provide information that morphologic imaging modalities cannot. The metabolic information often complements the structural information provided by other imaging techniques. Often a diagnosis can be confirmed by combining methods.

Plain-film radiography, CT, and MRI usually focus on a single area. Nuclear medicine imaging offers significant advantages because it can visualize the entire body simply, quickly, and cost-effectively with comparatively little radiation exposure. However, despite significant improvements in nuclear medicine imaging, it cannot approach the detailed anatomical visualization provided by CT or MRI. The skeleton and joints are not rigid or static systems, rather they are in dynamic equilibrium where metabolic changes can frequently be visualized before the onset of structural changes.

The following section discusses indications for nuclear medicine studies relevant to orthopedics.

Technique, Instrumentation, and Examination Procedure

The basic study in nuclear medicine imaging is a bone scan with technetium-99m-labeled phosphonates. The osteotropic radiopharmaceutical uptake is a function of perfusion and vascular permeability. The majority of disorders involve metabolic dysfunction. Changes in metabolic function can be imaged early with high sensitivity, generally before structural changes can be detected.

Following intravenous injection of a technetium-99m-labeled phosphonate complex, late images are obtained after approximately 3 hours. In children, dosages are reduced according to age and weight (Müller-Schauenburg and Feine, 1988).

Whole-body images provide an overview of the entire skeletal system. The metabolic activity of individual joints can be compared, and this in turn can be compared with the axial skeleton, that is normally in a state of equilibrium. If only coned-down views are obtained and an incorrect selection of acquisition parameters occurs, misdiagnosis of the metabolic state of a joint can occur. On the other hand, local views provide important details and should be obtained after the whole-body images.

Modern double-headed gamma camera systems are available for whole-body imaging. They provide high-quality anterior and posterior images of the entire skeleton within 15 minutes, visualizing most joints. Local views can be obtained in any imaging plane using high-resolution collimators or pinhole collimators.

A detailed history should be taken. In addition to the tentative clinical diagnosis, this should include questions about previous surgery, trauma, exposure to radiation, and medications, especially after chemotherapy and previous bone scans. This information is required to interpret the images properly. The patient does not have to refrain from eating or training prior to the examination, and allergic side effects are not expected. The waiting period between intravenous injection of the radiopharmaceutical and acquisition must be sufficiently long to achieve good contrast between bone and soft tissue and sufficient concentration in the organ being imaged. The optimum ratio between bone and soft-tissue activity for a bone scan is achieved approximately 3 hours after injection.

In the second half of the waiting period, the patient should be given sufficient water. The bladder should be emptied before acquisition and again before individual images or SPECT (single photon emission CT imaging) of the pelvis. Any metallic clothing should be removed.

Three-phase bone scans are recommended for joint disorders. The three phases measure perfusion (vascular phase), blood-pool activity (blood-pool phase), and bone metabolism (bone phase). Vascular images of the affected area are obtained over a period of 60 seconds following bolus injection of the radiopharmaceutical. Blood-pool images are obtained 2–5 minutes after injection, and bone metabolism is visualized approximately 3 hours after injection. Acquisition should include qualitative and quantitative studies, i.e., analog and digital studies. This permits quantification of perfusion, soft-tissue activity, and bone metabolism where necessary.

The site of the disorder should be known when performing a three-phase bone scan. Where clinical findings are inconclusive, it is best to select one region to be visualized because the field of view will be limited, at least in the vascular phase. Global visualization of soft-tissue activity throughout the entire joint system is possible in the blood-pool phase by obtaining a rapid series of individual images or by whole-body acquisition.

Acquisition usually involves obtaining planar images. Planar acquisition may fail to visualize certain changes because of the summation imaging effect. Therefore, SPECT (single-photon emission computed tomography) should be used for the torso and large joints. Modern SPECT systems with multiple detector heads achieve spatial resolution of approximately 6 mm with acceptable acquisition times.

Pinhole imaging is a valuable technique but is underutilized. Pinhole magnification images can visualize details that conventional images fail to detect. This is useful in joint disorders, which require detailed images, and particularly helpful in children and when imaging small joints (Bahk, 1994).

The bone scans described above are adequate in most orthopedic settings. The method is highly sensitive, but with low specificity because bone metabolism reacts early yet relatively uniformly to various stimuli.

With inflammatory disorders, different radiopharmaceuticals can be used to provide a wide range of information about joint function. A broad range of radiopharmaceuticals with widely varying uptake is available for imaging inflammatory and infectious processes. Examples from the group of tracers with unspecific uptake (for visualizing exudates or phagocytosis) include gallium-67 citrate, technetium-99m Nanocoll, or technetium-99m-labeled immunoglobulins. When infection is suspected, more specific metabolic visualization is possible using leukocyte scans, for example with autologous separated granulocytes, labeled with indium-111 or technetium-99m-Hexa-

Fig. 1.**116**   Chronic osteomyelitis of the left tibial head. Two different radiopharmaceuticals are used. The weak, unspecific uptake pattern in the technetium-99m Nanocoll image (left) tends to exaggerate the extent of the infection. The intensive uptake in the image obtained with technetium-99m-labeled monoclonal antigranulocyte antibodies (right) clearly demarcates the focus of the infection.

Other radiopharmaceuticals are beyond the scope of this discussion. Detailed consultation with the nuclear medicine department is always appropriate.

In the examination methods discussed, the structures are imaged indirectly; the radiopharmaceutical is transported via the vascular system. Scintigraphy involving injection of a radiopharmaceutical directly into the joint is not common, although in settings such as periprosthetic infection it has some utility.

A detailed history covering complaints, previous surgery, radiation therapy, trauma, medication, immobilization, etc. should always be obtained and a brief clinical examination performed prior to the scan. Clinical and laboratory findings and the results of other diagnostic imaging studies should be considered. Without this information, evaluation of the scan remains purely descriptive and provides significantly less information.

Osteoarthritis

Degenerative joint changes or osteoarthritis are a frequent clinical indication for radiologic examination. Degenerative changes can be observed in varying severity in almost every older patient and are usually an incidental finding during nuclear medicine studies. Degenerative processes lead to osteoblastic activation and reactive bone formation, which can be detected early in nuclear medicine studies (Fig. 1.**117**).

Although these changes are usually incidental findings, they must be distinguished from other causes of bone metabolism such as metastases, fractures, or inflammatory changes. Parameters such as the phase of uptake, the intensity of uptake, the topographic location of increased metabolism in detailed images (pinhole or SPECT), and correlation with radiographic findings help clarify the etiology of these changes.

Occasionally, nuclear medicine studies are performed to document the metabolic activity of lesions identified on radiographs where degenerative causes must be distinguished from other causes of arthropathy.

Fig. 1.**117**   Typical appearance of Heberden's nodes and severe interphalangeal osteoarthritis.

methyl propyleneamine oxime (HMPAO). In place of this relatively complicated multi-step procedure, a comparatively simple method can now be used. This involves the use of a technetium-99m-labeled monoclonal murine antibody against the granulocyte surface antigen NCA 95 (Fig. 1.**116**). This method requires only intravenous injection of the labeled antibody. It also permits specific identification of granulocyte infection foci. In osteomyelitis, the sensitivity and specificity are equivalent to the multi-step procedure.

The most intense increase in bone metabolism often occurs in the region of subchondral cysts where pressure is high, in areas of bone remodeling, and less so in matured osteophytes. Therefore, it is not surprising that the intensity of increased uptake does not always correlate with the most prominent site of degenerative changes in the radiograph. However, the intensity of metabolic activity in bone scans may correlate with the clinical pattern of symptoms (Merrick, 1992).

Metabolic changes can be visualized long before there is any radiographic evidence of destruction. In the setting of medial compartment arthritis of the knee where a high tibial osteotomy is contemplated, this is crucial information. Only about 30% of areas of increased metabolism in nuclear medicine studies of the knee correlate with findings in conventional radiographs. If, in varus gonarthrosis, increased uptake is observed in the lateral compartment and radiographic findings are normal, the prognosis for successful osteotomy will be poorer than if the lateral compartment is both radiographically and scintigraphically normal.

Nuclear medicine can provide important information in the evaluation of osteoarthritis in the temporomandibular joint (Fig. 1.**118**) and the small vertebral joints, for example in the evaluation of facet syndrome and back pain of uncertain cause (see also chapter 8, p. 380, Spine) (Holder, 1990; Holder et al, 1995.)

Inflammatory Joint Disorders and Joint Infection

Diagnostic imaging studies play a special role in the evaluation of rheumatic joint disorders. Individual imaging modalities are important in answering the following questions:

1. Is an inflammatory joint disorder present?
2. Which joint disorder is present?
3. How big is the affected area and what is the pattern of involvement?
4. How intense is the inflammatory activity?
5. Are complications present?
6. How is the disorder progressing, particularly under medication?
7. Is surgical intervention indicated?
8. Are postoperative complications present?

Nuclear medicine studies can provide important diagnostic information with regard to several of these questions (Kaye, 1990).

Where clinical and laboratory findings are inconclusive, nuclear medicine studies can detect an inflammatory joint disorder in its early stages before any changes appear in radiographs. Bone scans should always be performed as three-phase studies in this setting since the early phase in articular images shows inflammatory infiltration and synovial activity (Fig. 1.**119**). Positive findings in such studies are an important sign of the inflammatory nature of the disorder.

Fig. 1.**118** Severe arthritis in the temporomandibular joint.

The examination should be designed to provide an overview of the state of inflammatory activity in as many joints as possible in the early phase. Inaccurate information could be obtained if clinicians rely only on the bone phase of a study. The bone phase visualizes the reactive bone metabolism, which however will respond to synovial inflammation at an early stage. This is important e.g. in the early diagnosis of sacroileitis (see chaps 8 and 9, Spine and Pelvis).

The early phases can provide important information in the presence of arthropathy of uncertain cause by differentiating between inflammatory and noninflammatory disorders. However, this distinction is not completely accurate as active chronic osteoarthritis can simulate acute arthritis. Since the field of view is limited in the first two phases (or at least in the first phase), the clinically more significant joint is imaged. If no one joint is primarily affected, the hands are imaged for documentation purposes since they are a frequent site of the disorder.

Aside from the high sensitivity of nuclear medicine studies, visualization of the entire skeletal system offers a major advantage. Radiologic studies focus on one area or joint; nuclear medicine studies can document all areas or joints with relatively short examination times. Often significantly more areas or joints are affected than clinical findings would indicate.

Identification of specific disease entities is not possible. Only the pattern of involvement may provide information on the underlying arthritic condi-

Fig. 1.**120** Rheumatoid arthritis in the knee. The unspecific uptake in the bone scan in the upper series of images exaggerates the inflammatory process. In the labeld leukocyte study in the lower series of images, uptake is primarily seen where inflammation has infiltrated the synovia.

Fig. 1.**119** Florid rheumatoid arthritis. The vascular phase (5 minutes after injection) visualizes the inflammatory activity in the individual joints. In the bone phase (3 hours after injection), changes in bone metabolism are visualized as well.

tion. Usually the cause of the increased uptake can be identified with greater certainty by other means.

Early detection, estimation of inflammatory activity, and visualization of the pattern of involvement are three major areas in which bone scans can provide useful information. These studies are also an important instrument for excluding an inflammatory joint disorder. A completely normal bone scan is usually reliable evidence in this case. In general, the false negative rate of nuclear medicine studies is quite low.

Detection and quantification of the activity of the disorder are crucial to therapeutic management. For this reason, substances have been sought that permit specific quantitative information in addition to the unspecific visualization of synovial inflammation. Blood-pool markers such as technetium-99m albumin, technetium-99m-DPTA, or technetium-99m pertechnetate have failed to provide significant advantages. Labeled and separated autologous leukocytes provide more specific information that indicates the degree of cellular infiltration in the pannus (Fig. 1.**120**). Although the uptake mechanism is not known (presumably unspecific bonding to Fc receptors on polymorphic leukocytes, lymphocytes, and macrophages and via increased vascular permeability), the

uptake intensity of technetium-99m-labeled polyclonal human immunoglobins correlates well with the degree of inflammation found in histopathologic studies. This method has utility in the detection, evaluation, and monitoring therapy of chronic inflammatory joint disorders (DeBois et al, 1995).

Antibodies such as technetium-99m-CD3 anti-T-lymphocytes or technetium-99m-CD4 anti-T-helper lymphocytes detect very specific cellular immune reactions. These substances are currently in the process of further clinical testing.

Rheumatoid joint disorders must be distinguished from septic arthritis and osteomyelitis close to the joint. Nuclear medicine studies can visualize both situations with high sensitivity. However, unspecific activated bone metabolism is seen in both infectious and inflammatory settings. Reactive bone metabolism can also remain once infections have healed. Excluding other causes of increased bone metabolism can also be difficult. For these reasons, specific leukocyte studies are often indicated (Fig. 1.**121**). This method can achieve accuracy of about 90% outside the axial skeleton. Usually these studies identify and specifically visualize the infected area. Nuclear medicine studies are usually combined with MRI where more precise anatomical correlation of the extent of infection is required, for example in determining joint involvement in epiphyseal and metaphyseal osteomyelitis.

In some settings it may not be possible for nuclear medicine studies to distinguish non-bacterial and rheumatoid inflammation from bacterial infection.

Fig. 1.**121** Osteomyelitis of the patella. The bone scan in the right image shows uptake in all bony structures, whereas the labeled leukocyte study in the left image correctly limits the area of increased focal uptake to the infected patella. This excludes arthritis.

Fractures

Conventional radiographs and CT are the primary imaging modalities for evaluating injuries. In specific settings, nuclear medicine studies can be indicated. Often the significance of these studies in evaluating trauma is underestimated. Applications include normal radiographic findings in the presence of trauma sufficient to produce injury and suspicious clinical findings, detection or exclusion of stress fractures, detection or exclusion of child abuse, determination of the relative age of a fracture, and posttraumatic and post-treatment follow-up (Spitz et al, 1989).

Extensive studies have demonstrated the high sensitivity of bone scans in the diagnosis and evaluation of fractures: this method diagnosed 95% of all fractures in patients less than 65 years old within 24 hours of injury. Seventy-two hours after injury it was able to demonstrate 100% of all fractures in patients less than 65 years old and 95% of all fractures in patients over 65 years old (Matin, 1988). More recent data show that these results vary according to location; the speed and probability of diagnosis decrease from the periphery to the axial skeleton. A well-known indication is early confirmation of the diagnosis of a scaphoid fracture in the presence of normal radiographic findings (Fig. 1.**122**). Fractures of the spine, cranial vault, and hips are difficult to evaluate in older patients with significant osteoporosis.

Bone scans are important both for diagnostic and forensic purposes in excluding or confirming fractures in cases of child abuse. Similarly, the method can be easily used in adults with multiple trauma to detect occult fractures in the presence of clinical findings with negative radiographic findings.

It can be important to determine the age of a fracture, even in a non-forensic setting. Vascular images will return to normal within 3–4 weeks of an

Fig. 1.**122** The images shows an acute navicular fracture that did not show up in the radiographs. The soft-tissue phase (upper image) and bone phase (lower image) reveal abnormal findings.

acute fracture; soft-tissue activity will be normal after about 8–12 weeks. Bone metabolism changes its configuration and intensity over time. Follow-up examinations at short intervals within 10 days can be used to document quantifiable changes in intensity in acute fractures that will be absent in chronic fracli. lat.

Fig. 1.**123** Stress fracture of the tibia.

Avascular Necrosis

With the advent of MRI, nuclear medicine studies are no longer as important a method for detecting avascular necrosis as they once were.

There are many causes of avascular necrosis and many circumstances under which it can occur. These are not always obvious and can include trauma, steroids, radiation therapy, alcoholism, chemotherapy, kidney transplants, and many other causes. Common sites include the femoral head (known as Legg-Calve-Perthes disease in children), femoral condyles, humeral head, talus, lunate, scaphoid, and the first and second metatarsals.

The pathophysiologic process begins as the result of disturbed circulation, which leads to necrosis of the bone marrow and matrix cells. Repair processes result in revascularization via collateral circulation and reactive bone remodeling or apposition. Disintegration of the articular surfaces due to cartilage destruction may precipitate secondary degenerative changes (Tumeh, 1996). As a result, findings in nuclear medicine studies will vary depending on the stage of the disorder. The early stage is characterized by photopenia. This is often observed in traumatic avascular necrosis of the femoral head. In the revascularization stage, hyperemia can mask the defect and produce false negative findings. However, there will typically be a zone of increased perfusion, soft-tissue activity, and mineralization activity at the boundaries of the necrotic defect that appears as a cup-shaped sign. The repair stage is usually characterized by a circumscribed increase in bone metabolism. Since these changes can be very discreet, studies should be obtained using a multi-phase acquisition technique. Perfectly symmetric patient positioning is needed to permit comparison with the activity of the contralateral joint. Carefully prepared detailed images are important. These are best obtained as pinhole magnification images and, in large joints, as SPECT images (Fig. 1.**124**).

tures. After 2 years, 90% of all fractures will have returned to normal; moderately increased metabolism will persist throughout the patient's lifetime in the remaining fractures. Nuclear medicine studies play an important diagnostic role in evaluating occult fractures, periostitis, stress fractures, and in enthesopathy (Fig. 1.**123**). These studies may also be indicated to evaluate posttraumatic complications such as delayed fracture healing or malunion, pseudarthrosis, reflex sympathetic dystrophy, avascular necrosis, or infection.

Fig. 1.**124** SPECT image showing avascular necrosis in the left femoral head. There is a defect in the femoral head and reactive bone metabolism in the growth plate.

Fig. 1.**125**   Aseptic implant loosening in the left hip. Intensely increased metabolic activity is seen in the entire implant bed (right image), whereas the labeled leukocyte study (left image) reveals no abnormal findings.

Bone scans are a sensitive method that can demonstrate vascular lesions and osteonecrosis very early. In this regard they are significantly superior to plain-film radiography. Another advantage is whole-body imaging, which permits detection of lesions that are not yet symptomatic. Comparative studies have demonstrated that MRI is more accurate, particularly with respect to the early phases of avascular necrosis (Mitchell et al, 1986). However, these studies compared MRI and CT with planar nuclear medicine imaging without the pinhole technique.

Nuclear medicine imaging remains a useful modality when MRI findings are inconclusive and when lesions to bony structures are to be excluded. Pain of uncertain origin that may stem from a variety of causes represents a further indication. These include differentiating avascular necrosis of the femoral head from inflammation of the hip or transitory osteoporosis. Aspects such as availability, cost, or whole-body imaging also influence the choice of imaging modality.

Postoperative Follow-up after Joint Replacement

Implant loosening and infection are serious postoperative complications that lead to revision arthroplasty. Infection of the periprosthetic bone usually requires removal of the implant and the infected periprosthetic tissue, local antibiotic treatment, and placement of an implant in a second procedure. Therefore, precise preoperative diagnosis and differentiation between septic and aseptic implant loosening is crucial. Conventional radiography does not usually allow this degree of differentiation. Metallic artifacts make it difficult to obtain CT imaging. Nuclear medicine imaging can be helpful in visualizing the periprosthetic tissue in this setting. The sensitivity of bone scans in detecting osteoblastic activity due to loosening or infection is so high that a normal bone scan

nearly excludes these two possibilities (Al Sheikh et al, 1985). False negative findings occur only where the infection is located in the periprosthetic soft tissue and does not involve the bone matrix. However, increased osteoblastic activity is an unspecific reaction of bone to a wide variety of influences. The specificity of static nuclear medicine imaging is low in differentiating septic from aseptic implant loosening (Williamson et al, 1979). Increased metabolism in the periprosthetic bone can also persist for months or years postoperatively as a physiologic result of healing processes. This is often observed in uncemented implants.

Leukocyte studies are a more specific method with significantly higher accuracy in detecting septic implant loosening (Fig. 1.**125**). This method primarily utilizes autologous granulocytes, which are labeled with indium-111 oxinate or Tc-99m-HMPAO after separation (Palestro et al, 1990). Comparative studies with gallium-67 citrate, which can also detect infection, have shown leukocyte imaging to be the superior method (Schauwecker et al, 1984).

Instead of these quite complicated methods, one can achieve comparable results (i. e., about 85% accuracy) using technetium-99m-labeled monoclonal antibodies. This method is always available, does not require cell separation, and can be performed with a single intravenous injection. Where the bone scan is evaluated simultaneously, this method achieves a sensitivity of about 89% and a specificity of about 84% (Sciuk et al, 1992). Findings should be compared to the bone or marrow scintigram to reduce the rate of false positive findings.

Where aseptic granulocyte accumulation is present in the periprosthetic tissue, one should consider a body rejection reaction, granuloma, hematoma, unspecific reaction to abraded particles from the implant surface, or reaction to metal. Comparison with the bone scan is of little help in these cases because increased bone metabolism may also be expected. Another diagnostic pitfall that can produce false positive findings is periprosthetic islands of bone marrow. Due to their physiologic uptake mechanism, the antibodies will mark these islands of marrow as they bond to the precursor cells of granulopoiesis. This may be misinterpreted as increased uptake due to infection. Comparing the leukocyte scan with a technetium-99m-sulfur colloid image has been suggested to avoid this type of misinterpretation. However, incongruent visualization may be expected in the presence of infection and congruent visualization in the presence of a marrow island because this colloid will mark bone marrow but not the site of an infection (Palestro et al, 1990). Comparison with the bone scan is also helpful in distinguishing a marrow island from an infection. The marrow island will show normal perfusion, normal soft-tissue activity, and a degree of mineralization identical to that of the rest of the skeleton, whereas bone metabolism will be increased in infected parts of the skeleton. Sites of infection along the femoral components of a total hip implant appear as areas of increased uptake in the leukocyte scan. Infections, and particularly chronic infections in the acetabular component lead to decreased uptake (cold lesions). The cold areas are an unspecific sign of bone marrow depression. They can be regarded as both a sequela of infection and as postoperative destruction of the bone marrow in the acetabulum.

In summary, nuclear medicine studies are seen to play an important role in the evaluation of postoperative complications of total joint arthroplasty such as implant loosening and infection.

References

Al Sheikh W, Sfakianakis GN, Mnaymneh W, et al. Subacute and chronic bone infections: diagnosis using In-111, Ga-67 and Tc-99m MDP bone scintigraphy and radiography. *Radiology.* 1985; 155: 501–506.

Bahk YW. *Combined scintigraphic and radiographic diagnosis of bone and joint diseases.* Berlin–Heidelberg: Springer 1994.

DeBois MHW, Pauwels EKJ, Breedveld FC. New agents for scintigraphy in rheumatoid arthritis. *Eur J Nucl Med.* 1995; 22: 1339–1346.

Holder LE. Clinical radionuclide bone imaging. *Radiology.* 1990; 176: 607–614.

Holder LE, Machin JL, Asdourian PL, Links JM, Sexton CC. Planar and high-resolution SPECT bone imaging in the diagnosis of facet syndrome. *J Nucl Med.* 1995; 36: 36–44.

Kaye JJ. Arthritis: roles of radiography and other imaging techniques in evaluation. *Radiology.* 1990; 177; 601–608.

Matin P. Basic principles of nuclear medicine techniques for detection and evaluation of trauma and sports medicine injuries. *Semin Nucl Med.* 1988; 18 (2): 90–112.

Merrick MV. Investigation of joint disease. *Eur J Nucl Med.* 1992; 19: 894–901.

Mitchell MD, Kundel HL, Steinberg MEL, Kressel HY, Alavi A, Axel L. Avascular necrosis of the hip: Comparison of MR, CT and scintigraphy. *AJR.* 1986; 147: 67–71.

Müller-Schauenburg W, Feine U. Qualitätskontrolle in vivo: Skelett. In: Schober O, Hundeshagen H: Qualitätskontrolle in vivo. *Nucl Med.* 1988; 27: 163–164.

Palestro CJ, Kim CK, Swyer AJ, Capozzi JD, Solomon RW, Goldsmith SJ. Total-hip arthroplasty: periprosthetic indium-111-labeled leukocyte activity and complementary technetium-99m-sulfur colloid imaging in suspected infection. *J Nucl Med.* 1990; 31: 1950–1955.

Schauwecker DS, Park HM, Mock BH, et al. Evaluation of complicating osteomyelitis with Tc-99m MDP, In-111 granulocytes, and Ga-67 citrate. *J Nucl Med.* 1984; 25: 849–853.

Sciuk J, Puskás C, Greitemann B, Schober O. White blood cell scintigraphy with monoclonal antibodies in the study of the infected endoprosthesis. *Eur J Nucl Med.* 1992; 19: 497–502.

Spitz J, Tittel K, Weigand H. Szintimetrische Untersuchungen zum Nachweis und zur Verlaufskontrolle von Frakturen. In: Feine U, Müller-Schauenburg W, *Skelettszintigraphie.* Nürnberg; Wachholz: 1989: 181–190.

Tumeh SS. Scintigraphy in the evaluation of arthrography. *Radiol Clin North Am.* 1996; 34(2): 215–231.

Williamson BRJ, McLaughlin RE, Wang GJ, Miller CW, Teates D, Bray ST. Radionuclide bone imaging as a means of differentiating loosening and infection in patients with a painful total hip prosthesis. *Radiology.* 1979; 133: 723–725.

1.7 Computed Tomography

Indications, Diagnostic Value, and Clinical Relevance

Indications for plain CT are bony lesions that are difficult to evaluate on plain radiographs (Table 1.**11**). Due to the overlapping structures in the shoulder, determining the exact location and orientation of fragments and possible articular surface involvement is not always possible with radiographs. Plain CT can provide information for planning therapy by precisely visualizing fractures of the proximal humerus and glenoid and by visualizing bony defects after dislocations.

If soft-tissue injuries are suspected, CT arthrography is indicated. The primary indication is a defect in the glenoid labrum. CT arthrography can be used to evaluate the joint capsule. Together with MRI, CT arthrography is the method of choice for visualizing labral lesions. In deciding between imaging modalities, the availability of CT scanning systems compared with MRI scanning systems should be weighed against the disadvantage of CT arthrography as an invasive procedure.

Visualization of rotator cuff pathology is another possible indication. However, modalities such as ultrasound and arthrography are superior due to their lower cost.

Technique, Instrumentation, and Examination Procedure

Plain CT. The patient is positioned supine. To image the joint in a neutral position, instruct the patient to hold the hand flat on the hip. The patient must not place his or her arm on the abdomen because respiratory excursion will produce motion artifacts. For images in internal rotation, the patient places the

Table 1.**11** Indications for CT

Plain CT	CT arthrography
Fracture of the proximal humerus	Labral lesion
Scapular fracture	Imaging the joint capsule
Glenoid fracture	Rotator cuff pathology
Bony Bankart lesion	Biceps tendon pathology
Hill–Sachs lesion	
Arthritis of the glenohumeral joint	
Arthritis of the acromioclavicular joint	
Calcific tendinitis	

hand and forearm beneath the buttocks. After obtaining a topographic image, tomograms are obtained from the acromioclavicular joint to the inferior recess. The images are evaluated with both the soft-tissue windows and bone windows.

CT arthrography. As in conventional shoulder arthrography, contrast medium is injected into the joint under sterile conditions and fluoroscopic control. Adding epinephrine to the contrast medium is recommended to delay absorption. The joint is aspirated from the side opposite the direction of instability to prevent artifacts from escaping air and/or contrast medium and iatrogenic damage to the joint capsule. After contrast medium is injected, air is injected. Afterwards, carefully move the shoulder through its range of motion to achieve uniform contrast-medium dispersion. Next, imaging studies are obtained as in a plain CT scan.

Normal Findings

Normal findings in a plain CT scan show the humeral head in its relation to the glenoid fossa in the transverse plane. The bony contour of the humerus, scapula, clavicle, and acromion can also be evaluated. In addition, plain CT scans can be used for measuring angles that may be relevant in assessing a dislocation tendency.

Normal findings in CT arthrography include simultaneous visualization of all parts of the image; the intra-articular air with low signal intensity, the glenoid labrum showing the density of soft tissue, the dense contrast medium, and the contours of the bones. This generally requires a specific selection of windows to achieve a compromise between a pure soft-tissue window and a bone window.

Pathologic Findings in the Presence of Degenerative Changes

Arthritis

Arthritic changes in the humeral head after trauma or avascular necrosis of the head can be clearly demonstrated with CT.

Fig. 1.**126** Contrast medium escaping into the subacromial bursa in a CT arthrogram.

Calcific Tendinitis

CT permits more exact localization of calcifications than is possible with plain radiographs. The boundary of the surrounding tissue is also precisely imaged. Some authors believe the sharpness of this boundary is indicative of the extent of the resorptive processes. However, the importance of CT in this setting is minimal as it does not contribute significant information in addition to radiographic and ultrasound studies.

Disorders of the Rotator Cuff

Plain CT or CT arthrography is rarely indicated for degenerative changes in the subacromial space. Calcific tendinitis, rotator-cuff tears, and muscle atrophy are mentioned as indications. The high resolution of radiodense structures with CT allows imaging and localization of calcifications. This may permit differentiation between degenerative and reactive calcifications and formation and resorption phases. It will sharply delineate a deposit and determine its size, location, and density. This information is important for aspiration, but the same information can be obtained from plain radiographs, with the joint in different rotational positions, and from ultrasound studies. CT diagnosis of rotator cuff lesions requires injection of contrast medium (Fig. 1.**126**). Studies describe discontinuity, asymmetry, and triangular or drawstring configurations as signs of severe damage to the rotator cuff. In this system, exact classification of the cause of pathology is contingent on demonstrated atrophy of the supraspinatus.

Despite the capabilities discussed here, CT is not very helpful in routine diagnostic imaging of rotator cuff disorders. Although leakage of contrast medium into the subacromial bursa can demonstrate a tear in the rotator cuff and provide some preoperative infor-

Fig. 1.**127**   V-shaped posterolateral Hill–Sachs lesion.

Fig. 1.**128**   Bony Bankart lesion in a typical anteroinferior location.

Fig. 1.**129**   CT arthrogram showing separation of the anterior capsule labrum complex (Bankart lesion).

mation about the extent of the tear, equivalent diagnostic information can be obtained with less costly examination methods that are more suitable for routine use.

Disorders of the Biceps Tendon

In CT arthrography, a tear of the biceps tendon is demonstrated by an empty bicipital groove. Dislocation of the tendon is associated with a rupture of the transverse ligament and a tear in the subscapularis tendon near its insertion. In such cases, leakage of contrast medium clearly demonstrates the pathologic condition.

Pathologic Findings in the Presence of Instability

Hill–Sachs Lesions

Hill–Sachs lesions are reliably demonstrated in CT scans (Fig. 1.**127**). Even minor Hill–Sachs lesions are discernible. Plain radiographs will not detect changes in the cartilaginous region of the humeral head, whereas CT clearly demonstrates even minor defects. This modality can also be used to determine preoperatively the extent of the compression fracture in three planes so that the surgeon can plan the reconstruction in applicable cases. However, since CT is complicated, costly, and may require invasive testing, it is not commonly used to document Hill–Sachs lesions.

Bankart Lesion

Bony Bankart lesions and capsular calcifications can also be more clearly visualized than in plain radiographs (Fig. 1.**128**). However, it must be ensured that both shoulders are imaged in the same position. Otherwise it will not be possible to compare the injured shoulder with the normal shoulder. Soft-tissue changes in the anterior capsular ligaments such as a patulous capsule can be demonstrated with contrast medium in CT arthrography. The crucial question of whether the labrum is damaged can only be answered by a CT arthrogram (Fig. 1.**129**). Bankart lesions can be visualized in this manner, as can subperiosteal separation of the capsule along the anterior glenoid. The wide range of normal anatomical variants of the glenoid labrum make conclusive evaluation difficult. Failure to visualize the labrum and tears in the labrum at typical locations (anteroinferior glenoid) are relatively conclusive signs. Changes in the superior portions of the labrum are frequently the cause of false diagnoses.

Fig. 1.**130**   Chronic posterior dislocation.

Fig. 1.**131**   Fracture of the greater tuberosity with posterior dislocation of the fragment.

Bony Abnormalities Contributing to Dislocation (Angle of the Glenoid Fossa, Angle of the Shaft of the Humerus)

These are standard parameters that predispose some patients to instability. They include:

● **The transverse glenohumeral index (TGHI).** This is calculated from the ratio of the maximum diameter of the glenoid fossa to the maximum diameter of the humeral head. This index is regarded as a measure of the stability of the joint.

● **The angle of the opening of the glenoid fossa.** This is used to assess the extent of dysplasia of the glenoid fossa, thought to be a factor predisposing to increased dislocation. The angle refers to pathologic flattening of the fossa. A distinction must be made between the bony and cartilaginous angle of the opening of the glenoid fossa.

● **The angle of inclination of the glenoid fossa.** A distinction is made between the angle of the scapula to the glenoid fossa (inclination of the fossa relative to the scapula) and the horizontal angle of glenoid fossa inclination (inclination of the fossa in the horizontal plane of the body). Retroversion is posterior inclination of the glenoid fossa; anteversion is anterior inclination.

● **The version of the humeral head.** This is the angle between the axis of the head and neck and the axis of the epicondyles. Normally, the head is inclined slightly posteriorly, i.e., it exhibits physiologic retroversion. Reduced retroversion is observed in recurrent shoulder dislocations.

● **The pectoralis–glenoid fossa angle.** The angle between the pectoralis and the glenoid is another predisposing factor cited in shoulder instability. This angle describes the inclination of the glenoid fossa relative to the direction of pull of the pectoralis muscle.

Chronic Dislocation

In a chronic dislocation, the CT will clearly demonstrate the position of the humeral head. The head usually appears locked on the glenoid with an obvious Hill–Sachs lesion. Aside from documenting the dislocation, CT can visualize associated injuries to the articular surfaces (Fig. 1.**130**).

Other Pathologic Findings

Fractures of the Proximal Humerus

In fractures of the proximal humerus, CT clearly demonstrates the fractures. In this type of injury, the number of fragments is less important in the prognosis than the degree of displacement and rotation. Fragments that are displaced less than 1 cm and rotated less than 45° minimally influence the prognosis. Fragments widely separated from their surrounding structures increase the risk of avascular necrosis of the humeral head. The number and position of the bone fragments with respect to each other and their position relative to the glenoid can be demonstrated in CT scans (Figs. 1.**131** and 1.**132**). These can provide additional information for prognosis, the clinical course of the disorder, and the treatment.

Fractures of the Glenoid Fossa

Here, CT is superior to conventional radiographs (Fig. 1.**133**). In addition to showing the number of fragments, it is possible to image the intra-articular course of the fracture line. This information can determine further treatment, the clinical course of the injury, and the prognosis.

When evaluating fractures and the displacement of fracture fragments, it is always useful to obtain scans of the uninvolved side. Three-dimensional reconstruction is possible to image avulsed fragments of the glenoid (Fig. 1.**134**). However, since these images do not offer any additional advantages for

Fig. 1.**132**   Humeral-head fracture with multiple fragments.

Fig. 1.**133**   Fracture of the glenoid fossa.

Fig. 1.**134**   Three-dimensional CT reconstruction of a glenoid fracture.

determining treatment, three-dimensional reconstruction has not gained general acceptance.

1.8 Magnetic Resonance Imaging

Indications

The most frequent indications of an MR examination of the shoulder are, as for all other joints, the visualization and documentation of traumatic lesions and degenerative changes (Table 1.**12**). For tumorous conditions, MRI primarily serves to determine the extent of the tumors and to visualize the affected tissue. Determining the type of tumor is rather limited, as is true for all other imaging methods. Except for the usual contraindications, there are no further contraindications.

MRI is equivalent to CT arthrography in evaluating the rotator cuff but is superior for assessing extracapsular changes. Osseous changes are equally well diagnosed with either modality. Position and size of osseous fragments, however, are better determined by CT, while so-called occult osseous lesions are better detected by MRI.

Technique, Instrumentation, and Examination Protocol

Care should be taken that the patient is positioned comfortably. Normally, the patient lies supine with the arm slightly internally rotated and adducted. Vacuum cushions or foam wedges can be used for stabilization. The resonance signal is generally acquired with surface coils adapted to the shoulder.

The planes are selected to suit the structures to be examined. The shoulder is generally examined in three planes with the glenoid fossa used as the structure of reference. The oblique sagittal sections are parallel to the glenoid fossa and should include the supraspinous fossa for evaluation of the supraspinatus muscle. The transverse and coronal sections are

Table 1.**12**   Possible indications for MRI

Rotator cuff	Instability	Other
Bursitis	Labral lesions	Tumors
Intratendinous degeneration	Capsule lesions	Fractures
Partial tears of the rotator cuff	Bony Bankart defects	Avascular necrosis
Complete tears of the rotator cuff	Hill–Sachs defects	Inflammation
Muscle fibrosis and atrophy	Rotator cuff lesions	
Arthritis of the acromioclavicular joint		

placed perpendicular to this plane. The transverse sections should encompass the acromioclavicular joint. To improve the delineation of the tendon of the supraspintus muscle, the coronal sections must be aligned to the orientation of the tendon, which is determined by the rotation of the humerus and noted on the transverse image. Analogous to the visualization of the other joints, proton density weighted sequences are used for general orientation. The evaluation of pathologic changes requires T2 and T2*-weighted sequences as well as fat suppression. Enhancement after intravenous injection of a gadolinium-based contrast medium is best appreciated on fast GRE sequences or on fat-suppressed T1-weighted sequences. Intra-articular instillation of contrast medium generally is not necessary, though it is favored by some investigators.

Normal Findings

In craniocaudad direction, the transverse sections delineate the trapezius muscle and its insertion at the acromion and the clavicle. The acromioclavicular joint, together with its capsule and cartilage, is well visualized on slightly T1-weighted GRE sequences. Using high-resolution techniques, the small intra-articular disk can be identified. The stabilizing ligaments, comprising coracoclavicular, acromioclavicular, and coracoacromial ligaments, are difficult to identify in this plane and lesions can be assigned to the ligaments on the basis of their topography only. Further caudally, the transverse sections delineate the glenohumeral articulation (Fig. 1.**135**). While the humeral head and the glenoid fossa are covered with hyaline cartilage, the ring-like enforcement of the glenoid fossa — the glenoid labrum — consists of fibrocartilage, which usually blends with the joint capsule. The labrum is of variable thickness. In the middle anterior portion, it appears to sit like at a triangle on the glenoid labrum, separated from it by a layer of hyaline cartilage. Owing to its fibrous structure, it has a lower signal intensity than the hyaline cartilage. In about 20% of cases the capsule inserts medially to the labrum, and in about 10% of cases even more medially at the scapular neck. Between the anterior labrum and the capsule, the capsule is reinforced by the glenohumeral ligament, with its middle portion generally recognized on the transverse sections. The long biceps tendon is seen on cross-section as a thick, almost signal-void structure in the intertubercular sulcus. Likewise, the nearly signal-void structures of the tendinous extension of the infraspinatus and subscapular muscles can be followed to their insertion at the major and minor tuberosities. T1-weighted sequences display the fat beneath the deltoid muscle as a fine, high-signal band. T2-weighted images visualize the subdeltoid bursa as a homogenously bright band, especially if a joint effusion is present.

The sections perpendicular to the plane (Fig. 1.**136**) of the glenoid fossa show in posteroanterior

Fig. 1.**135** Transverse image (SE 500/20) showing normal glenohumeral joint.

order the infraspinatus muscle and teres minor with their tendon extending to the major tuberosity. Since the glenoid fossa is not always strictly perpendicular to the scapula, the oblique coronal sections must follow the course of the muscle and tendon as seen on the transverse sections for the evaluation of the supraspinatus muscle. The tendon of the supraspinatus muscle can display a medium signal intensity on the T1-weighted images. This increase in signal intensity is imparted by interference of the tendinous structure with the main magnetic field, whenever tendon and field are at a certain angle to each other ("magic angle"). The subacromial fat is seen as a bright band above the tendon. On heavily T2-weighted sequences, the subacromial and subdeltoid bursae are delineated, especially in the presence of an effusion. This plane also visualizes the long biceps tendon, but usually only its distal intra-articular segment. To visualize the tendon in its entirety, the sections must accommodate the intra-articular course, as seen on the transverse sections. To avoid partial volume effects, the section thickness should not exceed 3 mm. The superior and inferior labrum appear rounded in comparison with the anterior labrum. The inferior portion of the capsule is folded when the humerus is in typical adduction.

The third, sagittal, plane, which is parallel to the glenoid fossa, shows, in mediolateral order, the characteristic-shape of the scapula with the supraspinatus fossa, and the subscapular muscle along the anterior surface of the y-shaped scapula (Fig. 1.**137**). The trapezius is dissected superior to the supraspinatus muscle and separated from it by a thick layer of fat. Inferior and lateral to the infraspinatus muscle, the teres minor extends from the infraspinous fossa and lateral margin of the scapula to the major tuberosity. The teres major originates inferiorly along the lateral scapular margin and attaches to the minor tuberosity. Anteriorly, the tendon of the pectoralis minor is seen converging to the coracoid process, and the pectoralis major converging to the minor humeral tuberosity. Diagnostically important is the section

Fig. 1.**136**   Coronal oblique image (SE 500/20) showing normal glenohumeral and acromioclavicular joints.

Coracoclavicular ligament

Fig. 1.**137**   Sagittal oblique image (SE 500/20) showing normal glenohumeral and acromioclavicular joints. Note the coracoclavicular ligament.

Coracoacromial ligament

Origin of the long biceps tendon

Fig. 1.**138**   Sagittal oblique image (SE 500/20) showing normal glenohumeral and acromioclavicular joints. The coracoacromial ligament is partially visible. Note the origin of the long biceps tendon.

Tendon of supraspinatus

Tendon of subscapularis

Tendon of infraspinatus

Fig. 1.**139**   Sagittal oblique image (SE 500/20) showing the rotator cuff, consisting of tendons of the subscapularis, supraspinatus and infraspinatus muscles.

that traverses the acromioclavicular joint, showing the cross section of the subacromial supraspinatus muscle and its tendon. Between the anteriorly located coracoid process and the acromion stretches the coracoacromial ligament. The origin of the long biceps tendon is identified at the anterosuperior circumference of the glenoid (Fig. 1.**138**). The transition where the tendons of the subscapular, supraspinatus, and infraspinatus muscles form the rotator cuff is further lateral. It retains the humeral head (Fig. 1.**139**).

Pathologic Findings of Degenerative Changes

Degenerative Changes of the Rotator Cuff

Impingement is the major cause of degenerative changes involving the rotator cuff. Impingement is associated with morphologic variations of the acromion, especially an inferiorly curved process, by oste-

ophytes that arise anteroinferiorly from the acromion, and by hypertrophy of the acromioclavicular joint. Three stages are distinguished. Stage 1: mild intratendinous edema and possible hemorrhage. Stage 2: tendinitis of the rotator cuff, fibrosis, and thickening of the tendon. An effusion is seen in the acromial and subdeltoid bursa. Stage 3: partial and complete tears of the rotator cuff. These stages correspond to the three grades that categorize the MR findings of the rotator cuff. Grade I: diffuse increase in the signal intensity on the T1-weighted and proton-density image. An increased signal intensity is often better appreciated on the T1-weighted fast SE sequence or on a T2*-weighted GRE sequence. Grade II: increased signal intensity in all sequences, best seen on the T2*-weighted and fast SE images. The supraspinatus tendon is thinned and irregular in outline (Fig. 1.**140**). Grade III: partial or complete defect in the tendon, with increased signal intensity in all sequences. The tears are also well detected on the T2-weighted images due to intrusion of synovia into the created clefts. Inflammatory tissue is characterized by locally expanded extracellular space. After intravenous injection of gadolinium-based contrast medium, the damaged soft-tissue structures enhance

Degeneration

Fig. 1.**140** Coronal oblique image (GRE 500/11 out of phase) showing grade II degeneration of the supraspinatus tendon.

Degeneration

Subchondral avascular necrosis

Fig. 1.**141** Coronal oblique image (GRE 500/11 out of phase after application of intravenous gadolinium contrast medium) showing degeneration of the supraspinatus tendon and subchondral avascular necrosis in the humeral head.

Tear of the supraspinatus tendon

Fig. 1.**142** Coronal oblique image (GRE 500/11 out of phase after application of intravenous gadolinium contrast medium) showing a complete tear of the supraspinatus tendon with retraction of the muscle.

Necrosis

Fig. 1.**143** Transverse image (STIR 3800/160) showing stress necrosis at the insertion of the rotator cuff.

on the T1-weighted images, even more so on T1-weighted fast GRE sequences. Moreover, the irritated synovial membrane enhances due to hyperemia and intensified secretory activity (Fig. 1.**141**).

Grade I is frequently associated with a decrease in the subacromial fat plane, best seen on the T1-weighted images. On the T2-weighted or STIR image, a small amount of fluid is occasionally observed in the subacromial-subdeltoid bursa. Grade II shows more often a bursal fluid accumulation and an obliterated fat plane. Grade III is, in the case of a completely torn rotator cuff (Fig. 1.**142**), always accompanied by an effusion in the glenohumeral joint and bursa through the concomitant communication between joint capsule and bursa. With progression of the disease, the supraspinatus muscle retracts, and atrophy and fatty degeneration develop, best diagnosed on the T1-weighted image. Massive tears can lead to inactivity atrophy of the remaining shoulder muscles with resultant instability and upward migration of the humeral head. Vascular changes of the humeral head, contributed by the loss of joint fluid, induce subchondral osseous necrosis (Fig. 1.**143**), cartilage degeneration, and loss of cartilage.

Cartilaginous changes are best recognized on T2*-weighted sequences or on T1-weighted fast SE sequences.

Enthesopathy of the Rotator Cuff

In athletes whose activities include overhead motions, changes at the osseous insertion of the rotator cuff can be occasionally observed. The tendon shows a few areas of increased signal intensities or even tears as found in the more proximally located degenerative tendon changes. This is accompanied by small cortical to subcortical lesions that are of increased signal intensity on the T2-weighted images, and centrally increased signal intensity surrounded by a rim of decreased signal intensity on the T1-weighted sequences. The T1-weighted image delineates these lesions as areas of decreased signal intensity (Fig. 1.**144**). After intravenous injection of gadolinium-based contrast medium, a distinct central enhancement is usually observed (Fig. 1.**145**). In addition, the distal segment of the tendon frequently enhances. These changes are summarized under the term "overuse enthesopathy."

Partial tear of
the supraspinatus
tendon

Fig. 1.144 Coronal oblique image (GRE 500/11 out of phase) showing stress necrosis at the insertion of the rotator cuff and partial tear of the supraspinatus tendon.

Stess necrosis with
contrast medium
enhancement

Fig. 1.145 Coronal oblique image (GRE 500/11 out of phase after application of intravenous gadolinium contrast medium) showing stress necrosis at the insertion of the rotator cuff. The contrast medium enhancement through the compromised blood-tissue barrier is a sign of vital tissue.

Empty bicipital
groove

Biceps tendon

Infraspinatus-
tendon

Fig. 1.146 Transverse image (GRE 500/11 out of phase after application of intravenous gadolinium contrast medium) showing a tear of the long biceps tendon. The infraspinatus tendon is displaced, and the bicipital groove is empty.

Calcification

Subdeltoid bursitis

Fig. 1.147 Transverse image (STIR 3800/160) showing calcification at the insertion of the rotator cuff and subdeltoid bursitis.

Changes of the Long Head of the Biceps Tendon

Repetitive impingement, steady overuse, recurrent subluxations, and chronic arthritis lead to degenerative changes of the long head of the biceps tendon. These changes are displayed on MRI as thinning of the tendon with increasing signal intensities — initially on the intermediate protein density images and on the T1-weighted images, later also on heavy T2-weighted images. With progression of the degenerative changes, synovia accumulates in the tendon sheaths, best seen on T2-weighted or fat suppression (STIR) images.

In severe degenerative changes of the rotator cuff, minor trauma can cause tears of the long biceps tendon (Fig. 1.**146**). The tear commonly occurs where the tendon leaves the sheath. In most labral lesions with superior anterior to posterior extension (SLAP lesions), the long biceps tendon is detached from the glenoid. The intracapsular segment of the torn tendon can displace the subscapular muscle. The tendon sheath is filled with fluid and no tendon components are found in the intertubercular sulcus. The tear itself generally is often difficult to visualize owing to the curved course of the tendon. An empty sulcus is also observed with medial dislocations of the long biceps tendon.

Calcifying Tendinitis

The calcifications of chronic inflammatory arthritis cannot be directly visualized. Areas with a signal void in all weightings and with artifacts on GRE images, together with increased signal intensities on T2 or STIR sequences as seen in inflammatory tissues, allow the diagnosis of calcifying tendinitis (Figs. 1.**147** and 1.**148**). Postoperative artifacts caused by metallic particles compromise the evaluation considerably.

Synovial membrane with contrast-medium enhancement

Calcification

Fig. 1.**148** Coronal oblique image (GRE 500/11 out of phase after application of intravenous gadolinium contrast medium) showing calcification at the insertion of the rotator cuff. Contrast-medium enhancement is seen in the synovial membrane with subdeltoid bursitis.

Thickening of the capsule with contrast-medium enhancement

Erosion of the acromion

Rotator cuff tear

Fig. 1.**149** Sagittal oblique image (GRE 500/10 out of phase after application of intravenous gadolinium contrast medium) showing arthritis of the acromioclavicular joint with inflammation and thickening of the capsule in osteoarthritis of the shoulder with a rotator cuff tear.

Thickening of the capsule

Erosion of the acromion and the clavicula

Fig. 1.**150** Coronal oblique image (GRE 500/11, out of phase, after administration of intravenous Gd contrast medium), showing irregularity of the joint surface and thickening of the capsule.

Fig. 1.**151** Transverse image (STIR 1900/125) showing separation of the glenoid labrum without dislocation (type II Bankart lesion).

Changes of the Acromioclavicular Joint

Severe degenerative changes of the glenohumeral joint are often associated with degenerative changes of the acromioclavicular joint. These changes consist of a thickened capsule with high signal intensity on T2-weighted images, and marked enhancement (Fig. 1.**149**). Furthermore, an irregularly outlined joint surface and, in long-standing arthropathy, subchondral sclerosis are found in the clavicle and acromion, visualized especially well on GRE sequences. The enhancement observed in these subchondral lesions indicates increased bone turnover (Fig. 1.**150**).

Pathologic Findings in Instabilities

Changes of the Labrum (Bankart Lesion)

In shoulder instabilities, lesions of the labrum are invariably detectable. They are classified as follows:

— Type I, constituting degenerative changes with increased signal intensity centrally on the proton-density and T1-weighted phase-contrast images.
— Type II (Fig. 1.**151**), consisting of tears, primarily at the base, again recognized by the increased signal intensity, but also on the T2-weighted image.
— Type III (Fig. 1.**152**), consisting of tears with dislocation of the labral fragment.
— Type IV (Fig. 1.**153**), consisting of tears with subperiosteal elevation of the capsule and possible fissure even in the glenoid. Fissures are clearly delineated in fat-suppressed sequences (e. g., STIR).

In athletic activities with overhead motions, the labral lesion occurs commonly in the anterosuperior region and extends posteriorly (SLAP lesion).

Intravenous administration of gadolinium-based contrast medium does not improve sensitivity and specificity of the MR examination for the detection of labral lesions. Enhancement at the base where the

Fig. 1.**152** Transverse image (STIR 1900/125) showing separation of the glenoid labrum with dislocation (type III Bankart lesion).

Fig. 1.**153** Transverse image (GRE 500/10 out of phase after application of intravenous gadolinium contrast medium) showing separation of the glenoid labrum with a fracture of the anterior glenoid (type IV Bankart lesion).

Fig. 1.**155** Transverse image (STIR 3800/160) showing a Hill–Sachs lesion.

Fig. 1.**154** Transverse image (STIR 3800/160) showing a tear of the anterior capsule with leakage of synovial fluid.

labrum rests on the glenoid and in the region of the detached capsule indicates an acute injury.

Changes of the Joint Capsule

Tears in the joint capsule are indirectly detected through the leak of synovia, primarily on the T2-weighted image. The irritated synovial membrane, either by trauma or by primary inflammatory processes, always enhances after intravenous administration of gadolinium-based contrast medium (Fig. 1.**154**).

Hill–Sachs Lesion

This is defined as a compression fracture of the dorsolateral humeral head, generally following an anterior dislocation. The transverse sections show the corresponding impression of the humeral head, with perifocally decreased signal intensity on the T1-weighted and increased signal intensity on the T2-weighted images. These signal changes are due to bone marrow edema and can even be found at this site without impression, presumably representing trabecular fractures caused by the same pathomechanism (Fig. 1.**155** and 1.**156**).

Fig. 1.**156** Transverse image (GRE 500/11 out of phase) showing a Hill–Sachs lesion and a Bankart lesion.

Fig. 1.**157** Sagittal image (SE 600/20 after application of intravenous gadolinium contrast medium) showing an impacted fracture.

Fig. 1.**158** Transverse image (GRE 500/11 out of phase after application of intravenous gadolinium contrast medium) showing a fracture of the greater tubercle of the humerus.

Fig. 1.**159** Transverse image (STIR 3800/150) showing bone avascular necrosis following a fracture.

Fig. 1.**160** Transverse image (GRE 500/11 out of phase after application of intravenous gadolinium contrast medium) showing avascular necrosis with central contrast-medium enhancement following a fracture.

Fig. 1.**161** Transverse image (STIR 1900/125) showing a Ewing's sarcoma of the humeral head.

Other Pathologic Findings

Fractures of the Proximal Humerus

Fractures of the humeral head are almost always diagnosed on conventional radiographic examination. So-called occult fractures are disclosed on MRI as linear-to-patchy areas of increased signal intensity, best seen on fat-suppression sequences. After intra-venous contrast medium, enhancement is seen along the fracture line or as patchy areas in fractures confined to the trabecular bone. In addition, the accompanying soft-tissue injuries can be visualized by MRI (Figs. 1.**157** and 1.**158**).

Avascular Necrosis

Avascular necrosis is the most frequent complication after fractures of the humeral head (Figs. 1.**159** and 1.**160**). Corticosteroid medication, alcoholism, sickle cell anemia, and caisson disease are nontraumatic causes. Analogous to other joints, the area of necrosis is marked by a well-demarcated decreased signal on the T1-weighted image that extends to the articular surface. The T2-weighted image shows increased signal intensity centrally. Enhancement depends on the age of the necrosis and is peripheral for old and central for acute necrotic lesions.

Tumors

Tumors in the region of the shoulder are well delineated and localized on MRI (Figs. 1.**161** and 1.**162**).

Ewing's sarcoma of
the humeral head

Fig. 1.**162**   Coronal image (SE 500/20) showing a Ewing's sarcoma of the proximal humerus.

A specific diagnosis can only be made with considerable reservation. For instance, a small enchondroma cannot by distinguished with certainty from a fibrosarcoma, unless the cortex is destroyed. Even with cortical involvement, the differential diagnosis can be difficult if it represents a secondary fracture. Furthermore, the enhancement pattern does not permit a definitive differentiation between malignant and benign tumorous osseous lesions.

References

Axel L. Chemical Shift Imaging. In: Stark DD, Bradley WG. *Magnetic Resonance Imaging.* St. Louis: CV Mosby; 1988: 201–28

Bankart ASB. Recurrent or habitual dislocation of the shoulder. *Br Med J.* 1923; 2: 1132

Bankart ASB. The pathology and treatment of recurrent dislocation of the shoulder joint. *Br J Surg.* 1938; 26: 23

Barry LE, Wolf GL. Contrast Agents. In: Stark DD, Bradley WG. *Magnetic Resonance Imaging.* St. Louis: CV Mosby; 1988: 161–181

Bigliani LU, Morrison DS, April EW. The morphology of the acromion and its relationship to the rotator cuff tears. *Orthop Trans.* 1982; 10: 228

Bradley WG. Flow Phenomena. In: Stark DD, Bradley WG. *Magnetic Resonance Imaging.* St. Louis: CV Mosby; 1988: 108–137

Bydder GM, Young IR. Clinical Use of the Partial Saturation and Saturation Recovery Sequences in MR Imaging. *J Comput Assist Tomogr.* 1985; 9: 1020–1032

Bydder GM, Young IR. MR Imaging: Clinical Use of the Inversion Recovery Sequence. *J Comput Assist Tomogr.* 1985; 9: 659–675

DePalma AF. *Surgery of the Shoulder.* Philadelphia: Lippincott; 1983

Fullerton GD. Physiologic Basis of Magnetic Relaxation. In: Stark DD, Bradley WG. *Magnetic Resonance Imaging.* St. Louis: CV Mosby; 1988; 36–55

Graf R, Schuler P. *Sonographie am Stütz- und Bewegungsapparat bei Erwachsenen und Kindern.* Weinheim: Chapman; 1994

Habermeyer P, Krueger P, Schweiberer L, ed. *Schulterchirurgie.* Munich–Vienna–Baltimore: Urban & Schwarzenberg; 1990

Harland U, Sattler H. *Ultraschallfibel Orthopädie, Traumatologie, Rheumatologie.* Berlin–Heidelberg–New York: Springer; 1991

Hedtmann A, Fett H. *Atlas und Lehrbuch der Schultersonographie.* Stuttgart: Enke; 1991

Hendrick RE. Image Contrast and Noise. In: Stark DD, Bradley WG. *Magnetic Resonance Imaging.* St. Louis: CV Mosby; 1988: 66–83

Hill HA, Sachs MD. The grooved defect of the humeral head. A frequently unrecognized complication of dislocations of the shoulder joint. *Radiology.* 1940; 35: 690

Jerosch J. *Bildgebende Verfahren in der Diagnostik des Schultergelenkes.* Zülpich: Biermann; 1991

Jerosch J, Marquardt M. *Sonographie des Bewegungsapparates. Ein Handbuch für die Praxis.* Zülpich: Biermann; 1993

Katthagen B-D. *Schultersonographie.* Stuttgart: Thieme; 1988

Köhler/Zimmer; Schmidt H, Freyschmidt J, eds. *Grenzen des Normalen und Anfänge des Pathologischen im Röntgenbild des Skeletts.* Stuttgart–New York: Thieme; 1989

Neer CS. Displaced proximal humeral fractures. *J Bone Joint Surg.* 1970; 52-A: 1077

Neer CS. Anterior acromioplasty for the chronic impingement syndrome in the shoulder. *J Bone Joint Surg.* 1972; 54-A: 41

Neer CS. *Shoulder Reconstruction.* Philadelphia: Saunders, 1990

Post M. *The Shoulder — Surgical and Nonsurgical Management.* Philadelphia: Lea & Febinger; 1988

Rockwood C, Matsen F. *The Shoulder.* Philadelphia: Saunders; 1990

Smith HJ, Ranallo FN. *A Non-Mathematical Approach to Basic MRI.* Madison (Wisconsin): Medical Publishing Corporation; 1989

Wehrli FW. Principles of Magnetic Resonance. In: Stark DD, Bradley WG. *Magnetic Resonance Imaging.* St. Louis: CV Mosby; 1988: 3–23

2 | Elbow

2.1 Introduction

The elbow joint is a complex structure consisting of three separate articulations: the humerus and ulna, humerus and radius, and ulna and radius. Although it is often considered a hinge joint, the elbow allows rotation of the forearm at the radioulnar joint. Elbow stability and function are maintained by ligamentous structures.

The elbow is important to the function of the upper extremity as is used to establish contact between the hand and the body from head to toe. Even with a limited range of motion in the shoulder, most activities in daily life can be performed with a mobile elbow.

Capable of both hinged and rotary motion, the elbow is susceptible to degenerative changes and acute injuries. One need only think of the motions in sports such as tennis, gymnastics, squash, or javelin throwing. That create asymmetric stresses that could lead to damage both in the joint and in the surrounding soft-tissue cuff. Examples common are tennis elbow or golfer's elbow. Activities such as skiing, motorcyle riding, handball, or pitching, are particularly likely to result in elbow injuries. In sports where the participant can fall on the outstretched upper extremity, the elbow often bears the weight of the entire body. Fractures, dislocations, and ligament tears can occur.

2.2 Clinical Examination

Standard Examination

After taking a detailed history, the axis and position of the joint and the joint contours are inspected. Stand beside the patient and hold the anterior lateral upper arm when palpating the elbow. Palpate the medial epicondyle, the medial supracondylar line of the humerus, the olecranon, the posterior ulnar border, the olecranon fossa, the lateral epicondyle of the humerus, the lateral margin of the humerus, the radial head, and the various soft-tissue regions of the elbow. Motion in flexion and extension as well as pronation and supination is tested and recorded. Strength and sensation are evaluated after functional tests have been performed.

Patient History

Clinical examination of the elbow begins with taking the patient's history. Various disorders can be caused by acute injuries, chronic stressors, degenerative changes, and systemic disorders. Finding the problem is easiest in patients with recent trauma who can precisely describe how the accident occurred. With degenerative disorders or the sequelae of chronic stressors, obtaining a precise description of events long past is of great importance. Systemic disorders that can involve the joints should not be overlooked. A knowledge of injuries to the elbow sustained in the past and of how they were treated is also important. The patient's age has a bearing on clinical considerations. An elbow injury in a 40-year-old weekend athlete may be treated differently to one in a 25-year-old professional athlete.

Aside from age, the patient's occupation and athletic activities are crucial aspects of the history. This information is generally helpful in evaluating chronic symptoms. Knowledge of the precise motions involved in the various activities is important; by asking specific questions the problem can be rapidly ascertained. Tennis elbow is one example of how repetitive motion can contribute to the onset of a clearly defined clinical syndrome, whether the patient is an electrician, carpenter, or tennis player.

With chronic symptoms, it is important to inquire specifically how the pain radiates, where it is localized, at what time it usually occurs (nighttime pain or motion-dependent pain), as well as about the quality of pain.

In acute trauma, a precise reconstruction of the mechanism of injury should be attempted. This is very helpful in determining whether the trauma is direct or indirect. For example, it should be determined whether the patient fell on the hand with the elbow extended or fell with his or her full body weight on the flexed joint.

Observation

Inspection and the remainder of the clinical examination should be performed with the patient undressed. Both arms should be visible from midclavicle to fingertips. This is the most reliable way to evaluate possible asymmetry or pathologic position. Often patients will exhibit pathologic patterns of motion while undressing.

Fig. 2.**1**   Olecranon bursitis

In full extension, the longitudinal axes of the upper arm and forearm form a lateral valgus angle (carrying angle). The physiologic range for this angle is between 10° and 15° in women, and 5° in men. The valgus angle allows the elbow to fit closely into the waist, usually slightly superior to the iliac crest.

A valgus angle exceeding the normal range of 5° to 15° is referred to as cubitus valgus. A frequent cause of this is epiphyseal damage secondary to a fracture of the lateral epicondyle. In cubitus varus, the angle is less than 5°. This is often a result of childhood trauma, such as a supracondylar fracture where the distal humerus heals with malunion or with early physeal closure.

In addition to limitations in motion, observation should also focus on contour changes in the elbow joint. Swelling may be local or diffuse. It can be so extensive that the elbow is held at 45° flexion, the position in which the volume of the joint capsule is greatest. Frequent causes for this are crush injuries or fractures. The possibility of joint inflammation, particularly in the presence of additional erythema, should also be considered, Localized swelling above the olecranon also occurs when the olecranon bursa is swollen (Fig. 2.**1**).

Scars should be noted. Often they may be the cause of restricted motion or even contractures.

Palpation

To palpate the elbow, stand beside the patient, holding the anterior lateral aspect of the upper arm. Place the elbow in approximately 90° flexion by extending and abducting the upper arm (Fig. 2.**2**). Crepitus that occurs during this motion may be caused by a fracture, arthritis, thickened synovia, or a bursa. Be sure to note any pain or swelling.

• Medial epicondyle
First palpate the medial epicondyle on the medial side of the humerus. It defines the contour of the medial elbow and is susceptible to fracture, particularly in children.

• Medial supracondylar line of the humerus
The medial supracondylar line can be palpated superior to the medial epicondyle. It is the structure onto which the wrist flexors insert. Occasionally a small

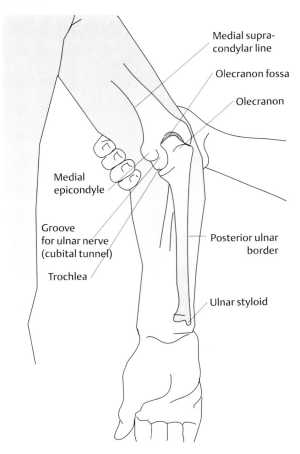

Fig. 2.**2**   Palpable structures in the elbow region

bony prominence will be palpable in this region, which can produce compression of the median nerve.

• Olecranon
The olecranon is easily palpated in flexion as the proximal end of the ulna within the olecranon fossa. Neither the bursa nor the triceps tendon interfere with palpation. The skin over the olecranon is extremely loose and permits flexion of the elbow.

• Posterior ulnar border
Palpate the posterior ulnar border from the olecranon to the ulnar styloid at the wrist.

• Olecranon fossa
The olecranon fossa is located at the distal end of the posterior humerus. When the arm is extended, the olecranon disappears into a groove filled with fat and a portion of the aponeurosis of the triceps muscle. Palpation is difficult.

• Lateral epicondyle of the humerus
The lateral humeral epicondyle lies lateral to the olecranon. It is smaller than the medial epicondyle and thus more difficult to define.

- **Lateral supracondylar line**

This bony margin may be palpated on the lateral humerus almost as far as the deltoid tuberosity.

Placing the thumb on the medial epicondyle, the index finger on the olecranon, and the middle finger on the lateral epicondyle, you will note that the lines connecting your fingers form an isosceles triangle when the elbow is flexed 90°. When the elbow is extended, the fingers will form a straight line. Any deviation from this geometric alignment requires further examination.

- **Radial head**

Examine this structure with the elbow flexed 90°. The radial head will be palpable approximately 2.5 cm distal to the lateral epicondyle of the humerus through the muscle mass of the wrist extensors. If the radioulnar joint can move through its full physiologic range of motion, almost three-quarters of the radial head will be palpable. The radial head is more easily palpable if dislocated.

To examine the soft tissue, the elbow should be divided into four regions.

- **Medial aspect**

The arm should be slightly abducted and the elbow flexed 90° for this examination.

Ulnar nerve. This is located in the groove between the medial epicondyle of the humerus and the olecranon. It can be palpated as it is gently rolled under the index and middle fingers. Thickening in this region due to scar tissue sometimes causes a tingling sensation in the patient's ring and little fingers because of nerve compression. Injury to the ulnar nerve often occurs in supracondylar or epicondylar fractures, or as a result of direct trauma.

Wrist flexors and pronators. The pronator teres, flexor carpi radialis, palmaris longus, and flexor carpi ulnaris originate from the medial epicondyle as a common structure. These muscles should first be palpated as a group and then individually from radial to ulnar. Proceeding systematically from the medial epicondyle of the humerus to the wrist on the flexor side, tender areas can often be located above the insertion of the muscle or along its course (Fig. 2.3). Tennis, golf, or regular use of a screwdriver can often provoke painful changes in this area.

Medial collateral ligament. This is a primary stabilizer of the humeroulnar joint. It arises from the medial epicondyle of the humerus and extends in a fan-shaped pattern to the medial margin of the trochlear notch of the ulna. This structure cannot be palpated, but pathologic changes such as valgus stress can produce tenderness.

- **Posterior aspect**

The olecranon defines the contour of this region.

Fig. 2.3   Palpating the wrist flexors and pronators

Olecranon bursa. This structure is only palpable in the presence of acute inflammation when it will be thickened and mobile.

Triceps muscle. Spanning two joints, the triceps with its three heads is essential for extending the elbow. The long head from its origin to the common muscle mass will be palpable along with the lateral head in the posteromedial upper arm when the muscle is slightly contracted. The lateral head of the triceps is also easily palpated in the posterolateral upper arm. All three heads of the triceps are joined in an aponeurosis proximal to the olecranon and are readily palpable as a wide thin structure. This region should be examined carefully in patients who have fallen on the elbow.

- **Lateral aspect**

Wrist extensors. The brachioradialis, extensor carpi radialis longus, and extensor carpi radialis brevis commonly originate from the lateral epicondyle of the humerus and the lateral supracondylar line. At the elbow they appear as a single unit that splits into two distinct palpable structures, the brachioradialis and the wrist extensors, on the extensor side of the forearm. The brachioradialis can be examined for tenderness and lesions up to its insertion on the ulnar styloid. As wrist extensors, these three muscles are thought to be crucial to the development of tennis elbow. Patients with this disorder will show evidence of tenderness at the common origin of these muscles (Fig. 2.4).

Lateral collateral ligament. This extends from the

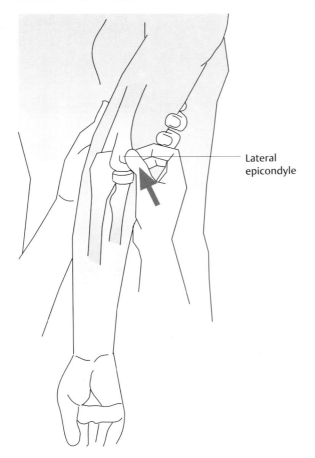

Fig. 2.**4** Palpating the lateral epicondyle and the wrist extensors

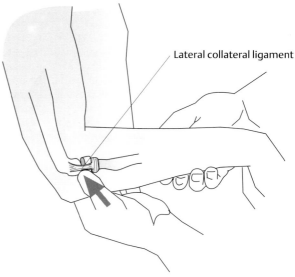

Lateral collateral ligament

Fig. 2.**5** Palpating the annular ligament

lateral epicondyle to the annular ligament. Varus stress will make it tender to palpation.

Annular ligament. This ligament surrounds the capitellum and radial neck. It will only be palpable in the presence of pathologic changes in the ligaments themselves or in the radial head (Fig. 2.**5**).

- **Anterior aspect**

Cubital fossa. The cubital fossa is the triangular region bordered laterally by the brachioradialis and medially by the pronator teres. The biceps tendon, brachial artery, and the median and musculocutaneous nerves pass through this region from lateral to medial.

Biceps tendon. The biceps tendon is palpable from the muscle mass to its insertion on the radius in flexion and supination. In a distal tear the muscle and tendon retract into the upper arm, where they are visible as significant swelling.

Brachial artery. The pulse of the brachial artery is palpable in the cubital fossa medial to the biceps tendon.

Assessing Range of Motion

The range of motion in the elbow consists of four movements: flexion, extension, supination, and pronation. Flexion and extension are effected primarily by the humeroradial and humeroulnar joints, while supination and pronation are effected in the proximal and distal radioulnar joints.

Active range of motion. The patient may stand or sit for this examination. Testing the active range of motion supplies information on the patient's ability to move the elbow without assistance.

Flexion (135°) and extension (0° or –5°). Instruct the patient to touch the shoulder with the anterior aspect of the forearm. The musculature of the upper arm usually limits flexion. Extension is limited by the olecranon, which strikes the olecranon fossa. Normal extension in men is 0°; in women up to 5° of hyperextension is normal.

Supination (90°) and pronation (90°). The supination test should be performed with the elbow in 90° flexion and the upper arm in adduction to prevent shoulder movement. From the neutral position, the patient turns the palms upward in supination and downward for pronation. The radius should rotate 180° around the ulna.

Passive range of motion. Instruct the patient to place the elbow on his or her hip while you cup the olecranon with one hand and move the forearm with the other.

Flexion and extension. Flex and extend the elbow from the neutral position as described above. Note

Fig. 2.**6**   Evaluating the collateral ligaments

the range of motion and the quality of the endpoint of motion.

Supination and pronation. Now move your hand from around the patient's forearm to grasp the patient's hand. Slowly move the joint into supination and pronation. Here too, note the range of motion and the quality of the endpoint of motion.

Specific Tests

Ligament instability. To evaluate the lateral and medial collateral ligaments, grasp the posterior aspect of the elbow with one hand and the wrist with the other (Fig. 2.**6**). While immobilizing the elbow, apply a varus or valgus stress with the hand around the patient's wrist. With one finger of the hand mobilizing the elbow, evaluate the size of the joint cavity laterally and medially and check for tenderness.

Tinel sign. Tapping the ulnar nerve in its groove between the medial condyles and olecranon can produce a tingling sensation in the area supplied by this nerve if it is compromised.

Tennis elbow. Immobilize the patient's elbow with one hand while palpating the origins of the wrist extensors over the lateral humeral epicondyle with the thumb. Instruct the patient to extend the wrist against resistance. In tennis elbow (lateral epicondylitis) the patient will experience pain at the site of the origins of the wrist extensors.

Posterolateral instability. With the upper arm immobilized and adducted, move the forearm into supination and valgus position at 20° to 30° flexion. Applying axial compression in this matter will provoke visible and palpable subluxation in the elbow in the presence of posterolateral instability. The same procedure is also possible with the shoulder in maximum extension.

Neurologic Examination

The neurologic examination consists of motor strength, reflex testing, and sensation testing.

Examining the Muscle

As in the range of motion tests, the examination covers flexion, extension, supination, and pronation. Muscle strength is classified according to the system described in the shoulder chapter (Table 1.**8**, p. 24). The patient can either stand or sit during this examination.

Flexion. The brachialis (musculocutaneous nerve, C5, C6) and, with the forearm in supination, the biceps (musculocutaneous nerve, C5, C6) are tested as primary flexors, and the brachioradialis and supinator as secondary flexors. Stand in front of the patient, stabilizing the elbow with one hand while grasping the patient's distal forearm with the other. Now instruct the patient to flex the forearm against resistance.

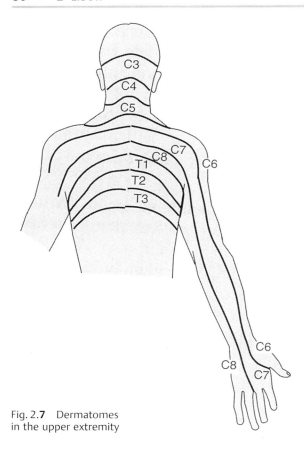

Fig. 2.**7** Dermatomes
in the upper extremity

supply to the elbow are the biceps reflex, brachioradialis reflex, and triceps reflex.

Biceps reflex (C5). The patient's elbow is flexed in a middle position and slightly pronated. Place your thumb on the distal portion of the biceps tendon and tap the tendon. The normal response will be for the muscle to contract, causing flexion and supination of the forearm.

Brachioradialis reflex (C6). The arm is positioned as when testing the biceps reflex. Tap the brachioradialis tendon at the distal end of the radius with the flat side of the reflex hammer.

Triceps reflex (C7). The patient holds the elbow approximately 90° flexed and internally rotated. Tap the triceps tendon proximal to the olecranon. The normal response will be for the muscle to contract, extending the forearm.

Examining Sensation

There are four dermatomes that provide elbow sensation (Fig. 2.**7** see also Fig. 1.**47 a, b**, p. 25).

— C5: anterior forearm, sensory branches of the axillary nerve.
— C6: lateral forearm, sensory branches the musculocutaneous nerve.
— C8: medial forearm, antibrachial cutaneous nerve.
— T1: medial arm, brachial cutaneous nerve.

2.3 Radiology

Indications, Diagnostic Value, and Clinical Relevance

Often the diagnosis of an elbow fracture can be reached on the basis of the patient's history and clinical examination. Only radiographs will allow one to precisely evaluate the type of fracture or dislocation, the direction of the fracture line, the position of the fragments, or accompanying soft-tissue injuries.

When an injury to the elbow is suspected, radiographs are normally prepared in AP and lateral projection. These may be supplemented by oblique projections in internal and external rotation.

Standard and Special Views

AP radiograph. To obtain the routine AP radiograph, the arm is supinated and the elbow completely extended. The central ray is aimed perpendicular to the cassette through the midpoint of the elbow (Fig. 2.**8**). This projection is usually sufficient to demonstrate injuries to the medial and lateral humeral epicondyles, the olecranon fossa, the capitellum, the humeral trochlea, and the radial head (Fig. 2.**9**). This

Extension. The triceps (radial nerve, C7) is tested as the primary extensor, and the anconeus as the secondary extensor. The arm is positioned the same way as in the flexion test. Instruct the patient to extend the arm from a flexed position against resistance.

Supination. The biceps and supinator (musculocutaneous nerve, C5, C6, and radial nerve, C6) are the primary supinators of the forearm; the brachioradialis is the secondary supinator. For clinical evaluation of muscle strength, immobilize the patient's adducted arm at the body with one hand and grasp the flexed forearm from the outside. Instruct the patient to supinate from a zero position against resistance.

Pronation. The pronator teres (median nerve, C6) and the pronator quadratus (anterior interosseous branch of the median nerve, C8, T1) are tested as the primary pronators, and the flexor carpi radialis as the secondary pronator. The initial position is the same as in the supination test. Grasp the forearm from the inside.

Reflex Testing

The two sides are compared during testing. The three reflexes that provide information about the nerve

Fig. 2.**8**   Patient positioning for the AP view

Fig. 2.**9**   Standard AP radiograph

Fig. 2.**10**   Patient positioning for the lateral view

Fig. 2.**11**   Lateral radiograph showing the olecranon, the anterior aspect of the radial head, and the humeroradial joint

view is also well suited for demonstrating the carrying angle of the elbow, the angle between the axes of the upper arm and forearm. A valgus angle of 10° to 15° is regarded as anatomically normal. In children, the four ossification centers of the distal humerus are also discernible in the AP radiograph: the capitellum, medial condyle, lateral epicondyle, and humeral trochlea. Knowing at what age these ossification centers close can provide important information for evaluating elbow injury. In evaluating pediatric elbow trauma, a view of the uninjured side for comparison is extremely helpful.

Lateral view. The elbow is flexed 90° with the ulna on the film cassette, and the hand is placed with the thumb up and the fingers flexed. The central ray is aimed perpendicular to the cassette at the radial head (Fig. 2.**10**). This projection is well suited for evaluating the olecranon, the anterior aspect of the radial head,

and the humeroradial joint. However, visualization of the posterior half of the radial head and the coronoid process of the ulna is less than optimal because the two are superimposed (Fig. 2.**11**). This projection provides important information about the shape and relative position of bony structures. In children the distal humerus is shaped like a hockey stick, with an angle of 140°. Interruption of this shape is a sign of a supracondylar humeral fracture. The position of the capitellum in relation to the distal humerus and proximal radius is also significant. The lateral view reveals a longitudinal axis running through the proximal radius and the center of the capitellum. A line is present along the anterior cortex of the distal humerus. If this line is extended through the joint, it intersects

Fig. 2.**12** Patient positioning for the radial head--capitellum view (oblique projection)

Fig. 2.**13**   Radial head–capitellum view for demonstrating the radial head unobscured by overlapping shadows

Fig. 2.**14**   Fracture of the distal humerus

the middle third of the capitellum. An elbow injury can cause significant displacement of the cushion of fatty tissue, the "anterior sail" sign. The cushion of fatty tissue deep in the olecranon fossa is not normally visualized in the lateral view; if it is visible, this is a sign often associated with a fracture and is referred to as the "posterior sail" sign.

Radial head–capitellum view. This variation of the lateral view is used to obtain an unobscured image of the radial head. As in the lateral view, the patient is positioned with the ulna on the cassette, the elbow flexed 90°, the thumb up, and the fingers flexed. The central ray is aimed at the radial head at an angle of 45° to the forearm (Fig. 2.**12**). In addition to projection of the radial head, this view clearly demonstrates the capitellum, humeroradial joint, and humeroulnar joint (Fig. 2.**13**).

Trauma view. In case of suspected fracture, views in two perpendicular projections are sufficient.

Pathologic Findings

Fractures

Distal humeral fractures. Fractures of the distal humerus are classified as supracondylar, transcondylar, intercondylar, condylar, or epicondylar. In adults the AP and lateral radiographs are generally sufficient to evaluate fractures of the distal humerus (Fig. 2.**14**). Occasionally, tomography is used for more precise localization of fragments in comminuted fractures. The AO/ASIF classification has type A, type B, and type C fractures (Fig. 2.**15**).

Diagnostic studies are more difficult in children. The two standard views are usually sufficient to visualize the variations in the position of the ossification centers, although it is often difficult to identify the exact fracture line. Supracondylar fractures resulting from a fall on the extended hand account for approximately 95% of all cases. The lateral view demonstrates the loss of the typical hockey-stick shape and displacement of the anterior humeral line. A positive "sail" sign is often seen. Obtaining a radiograph of the contralateral elbow is common practise.

Radial head fracture. This is the fracture most frequently encountered in the elbow region (Fig. 2.**16**).

Fig. 2.**15** A = extra-articular fracture, B = partial articular fracture, C = complex articular fracture

AP and lateral radiographs are mandatory. A radial head–capitellum view should be obtained for demonstrating fractures in which the fragments are not displaced. Determining the extent of the fracture line is crucial for therapy. The injury is treated closed or open, depending on displacement of the fragments.

Fig. 2.**16**   Fracture dislocation of the radial head

Fig. 2.**17**   Osteochondritis dissecans of the capitellum

head–capitellum view. As the disease progresses, the tissue separates from its bed in the capitellum. In this phase one refers to an "in situ" lesion. If the tissue separates, it may be seen as an intra-articular loose body (Fig. 2.**17**).

CT arthrography is particularly well suited for diagnosing osteochondritis dissecans. This modality can demonstrate the cartilage defect in the capitellum and distinguish between an in situ lesion and an intra-articular loose body.

Elbow Dislocations

There are three major types of elbow dislocation:

— The radius and ulna dislocate anteriorly, posteriorly, medially, or laterally (or combinations thereof).
— The ulna dislocates anteriorly or posteriorly.
— The radius dislocates anteriorly, posteriorly, or radially.

Posterior or posterolateral dislocations are encountered most frequently. Standard radiographs are generally obtained to demonstrate dislocation of the elbow. However, we recommend obtaining radiographs of the forearm in two planes to exclude the risk of overlooking a simultaneous fracture of the ulna (Figs. 2.**18a, b**).

2.4 Ultrasound

Indications, Diagnostic Value, and Clinical Relevance

Although the clinical examination and radiographic studies generally permit a diagnosis, ultrasound is an additional, low-cost, noninvasive diagnostic modality.

Fracture of the coronoid process. This injury is frequently encountered in conjunction with posterior dislocation of the elbow. The required studies usually include a radial head–capitellum view and an oblique view in addition to the standard radiographs in two planes.

Monteggia Fracture

The classic description of a Monteggia fracture is a fracture at the junction of the proximal and middle ulna in combination with anterior dislocation of the radial head (type I). Generally, the forearm will be shortened and the fractured ulna angled anteriorly.

Additional types of Monteggia fractures include:

— Type II: proximal ulnar fracture with posterior angling of the proximal fragment, posterior or posterolateral dislocation of the radial head.
— Type III. proximal ulnar fracture with lateral or anterolateral dislocation of the radial head.
— Type IV: fracture of the proximal end of the radius and ulna with anterior dislocation of the radial head (rare).

The AP and lateral radiographs are sufficient for diagnosis.

Osteochondritis Dissecans of the Capitellum (Panner Disease)

In its initial stages Panner disease does not display any unique radiographic findings. The only sign may be a slight flattening of the capitellum in the radial

Fig. 2.**19**   Normal findings in the humeroradial longitudinal plane

Figs. 2.**18a, b**   Dislocation of the radial head

Fig. 2.**20**   A ganglion appears as a hypoechoic structure with a hyperechoic internal reflection pattern

Indications generally include distinguishing between solid and cystic masses (cysts, tumors, and ganglia). Less common uses include evaluation of effusions, intra-articular loose bodies, bursitis, tenosynovitis at the muscular insertions, instability, fractures, and dislocations of the radial head.

Ultrasonography may be helpful in the diagnosis and treatment of "nursemaid's elbow" injuries in children since the joint structures are still largely cartilaginous.

Normal Findings

Various transducer positions are required for examining anterior and posterior aspects of the joint.

In the **humeroradial longitudinal plane,** the proximal humeral shaft and the capitellum are identified as bony landmarks. At the capitellum, the cartilage covering is readily discernible as a hypoechoic strip over the hyperechoic boundary reflection of the bone. Further distal, the radial head is another bony landmark whose behavior should be observed, especially during the pronation and supination move-

ments in the dynamic examination. The joint space appears as a hypoechoic area between these two landmarks. The joint capsule is discernible as a narrow hyperechoic band above the interior of the joint. Above this is a muscular layer consisting of the forearm flexors, biceps, brachialis, and brachioradialis (Fig. 2.**19**).

Pathologic Findings

Effusion

With an effusion, the image in the anterior humeroradial plane will reveal a hypoechoic zone above the hyperechoic bony landmarks. The narrow hyperechoic joint capsule will be visible above this, indicating distension of the capsule.

Ganglia and Cysts

A ganglion appears as a hypoechoic structure, with an internal reflection pattern that is occasionally hyperechoic (Fig. 2.**20**).

Cysts are also recognizable as hypoechoic masses. Often the tail of the cyst will be seen to communicate with the joint.

Tumors

Tumors can appear as hyperechoic or hypoechoic masses in any location. Preoperative ultrasound examination can demonstrate the position of the tumor and its proximity to important vascular structures. However, ultrasonography does not permit histologic differentiation.

Instability

Ligament structures cannot be directly visualized here either. The ultrasound examination can only demonstrate that the joint can be opened further than the contralateral side under varus or valgus stress.

Fig. 2.**21**   Normal findings at arthrography

Dislocation of the Radial Head

In radial head dislocations in both children and adults, ultrasound can clearly demonstrate the position of the dislocated radial head. Even after reduction, a hypoechoic halo around the radial head will be discernible. This is a sign of a hematoma, which is generally present.

Fracture of the Radial Head

A hypoechoic halo will appear in a fracture of the radial head. This is indicative of effusion.

2.5 Arthrography

Indications, Diagnostic Value, and Clinical Relevance

Arthrography of the elbow provides information about the size of the capsule and the condition of the articular surfaces. The most frequent indication is to confirm the presence of intra-articular loose bodies or a capsule tear. Intra-articular loose bodies may be attributable to either osteochondritis dissecans or an acute injury. Arthrography is occasionally indicated for chronic instability with a patulous joint capsule or tears of the ligaments and/or capsule.

Technique

Air, a positive contrast medium, or a combination of the two may be used. Double-constrast arthrography is recommended for most cases. Use of a contrast medium is recommended for a suspected capsule tear or synovial cyst. The contrast is injected into the sitting patient through a lateral portal under fluoroscopic control.

Normal Findings

The normal arthrogram will image the anterior, posterior, and periradial joint recesses in addition to the humeroradial, humeroulnar, and radioulnar joints. The articular surfaces and synovia will appear even more clearly if the double-contrast technique is used (Fig. 2.**21**).

Pathologic Findings

Intra-articular Loose Bodies

Double-contrast arthrography is particularly suitable for demonstrating intra-articular loose bodies. These bodies either move freely in the joint or are suspended in the synovia. Often the site that the loose bodies arose from is visible. Contrast medium may collect in the depression.

Capsule Tear

Single-contrast arthrography is usually sufficient for this examination. Leakage of the contrast medium from the joint capsule is a sign of a tear or partial tear of the capsule. In arthrography, care should be taken not to insert the needle near the expected site of the tear.

2.6 Nuclear Medicine Studies

See chapter 1 (Shoulder, p. 54) for a general discussion on the utility of nuclear medicine studies.

2.7 Computed Tomography

Indications, Diagnostic Value, and Clinical Relevance

CT of the elbow may be performed as an additional study for diagnosing persistent symptoms and clarifying inconclusive radiologic findings. CT has an advantage over other imaging modalities in that it can permit simultaneous evaluation of bone and soft tissue.

In evaluating a limited range of motion or locked joint, CT is particularly suitable to localize intra-articular loose bodies and osteochondral defects in the articular surfaces. CT arthrography can also be used for this purpose. Even small intra-articular bodies appear in sharp distinction to the dark intra-articular air. This simplifies the selection of the surgical approach.

Pathologic Findings

Fractures and dislocations

Studies can be used to evaluate the relative positions of fragments and to determine soft-tissue interposition. This can simplify preoperative planning. CT can also image associated soft-tissue injuries in fractures and dislocations. Where conventional studies are inconclusive, CT can confirm fractures in which small mobile fragments result in locking. CT studies after

Fig. 2.**22** CT image of a fracture of the distal humerus

fracture healing can demonstrate sclerotic edges consistent with pseudarthrosis (Fig. 2.**22**).

Osteochondritis dissecans and intra-articular loose bodies

By definition, intra-articular loose bodies are mobile parts of the synovial tissue, cartilage, or bone fragments. Generally, plain views in two planes and spot views are sufficient to diagnose intra-articular loose bodies. If there are doubts as to the position of these bodies within the joint, CT arthrography may be used. Intra-articular loose bodies can be precisely located, and it is often possible to visualize the site of their origin.

Cubital tunnel syndrome

CT can identify compressing lesions. It can determine whether bony structures or soft tissue are responsible and can distinguish causes such as bony ridges or scarring. CT aids preoperative planning, particularly when the symptoms are due to compression by bone structures. CT studies also provide information on the severity of the damage.

Degenerative changes

In addition to changes seen in conventional radiographs, CT aids the identification of effusions, calcifications, and capsular changes.

2.8 Magnetic Resonance Imaging

Indications, Diagnostic Value, and Clinical Relevance

As with other joints, the indications rest on the superb soft-tissue differentiation and the high sensitivity for lesions of any type using fat suppression and intravenous administration of gadolinium-based contrast medium. The major indications to be mentioned are osteochondrosis dissecans, epicondylitis, arthritis, bursitis, tendon tears, fractures, osteomyelitis, and tumors.

Technique and Examination Procedure

The patient is supine with the upper and lower arm comfortably positioned and a surface coil applied to the elbow. To avoid any motion artifacts, the lower arm should not been placed on the body. The sections are sagittal and coronal to the upper and lower arm since the joint generally cannot be kept extended. Depending on the joint position, additional transverse sections are obtained. The sequences are the same as used for the other joints.

Pathologic Findings
Osteochondritis dissecans (Figs. 2.**23**, 2.**24**)

This condition primarily affects the humeral capitellum. As in the other joints, it is seen as a subchondral zone of decreased signal intensity on T1-weighted images and of high signal intensity on T2-weighted

Effusion

Desiccated tissue

Fig. 2.**23** Sagittal image (STIR 1800/125) showing osteochondritis dissecans of the humerus with effusion.

Cartilage defect

Hyperemic halo

Fig. 2.**24** Sagittal image (GRE 500/11 out of phase after application of intravenous gadolinium contrast medium) showing osteochondritis dissecans. The image demonstrates a cartilage defect, hyperemic halo along the bone lesion, and synovitis.

Fig. 2.**25**   Coronal image (GRE 500/10 out of phase after application of intravenous gadolinium contrast medium) showing epicondylitis with peritendinitis of the extensor tendon.

Fig. 2.**26**   Sagittal image (STIR 1900/125) showing osteoarthritis with joint effusion, a subchondral cyst in the humeral condyle, and narrowing of the joint cavity.

Fig. 2.**27**   Coronal image (GRE 500/10 out of phase after application of intravenous gadolinium contrast medium) showing rheumatoid synovitis.

images, often concurring with cartilaginous defects and fissures. The affected osseous fragment is usually sharply marginated. After the osseous-cartilaginous fragment has become detached, a usually well-demarcated halo of high signal intensity appears on the T2-weighted images, representing synovial extension. Intravenous application of gadolinium-based contrast medium reveals perifocal hyperemia and edema. When the fragment has become completely separated from its bed, it is frequently found as a loose body in the olecranon fossa or coronoid fossa. The coexisting joint effusion reveals the loose intra-articular body as dark defects in the bright fluid on T2-weighted images.

Epicondylitis (Fig. 2.**25**)

Stress causes irritation at the origin of the extensor tendons (in tennis players) or flexors (in golfers). The resultant edema is seen in the coronal plane as linear increase in signal intensity on the T2-weighted sequences. The tendons are thickened. The epicondyle can be involved in terms of osseous avulsions,

bone marrow edema or hyperemia, or, depending on the duration, accentuated sclerosis.

Osteoarthritis (Fig. 2.**26**)

This involves the humeroradial articulation to a greater extent than the humeroulnar articulation, and is the result of accidental or repetitive trauma. It is characterized by osteophytes and sclerosis on T1-weighted images and by joint space narrowing and subchondral cysts on T2-weighted images. In general, a more or less severe synovitis develops and is clearly seen on the T1-weighted phase contrast image after intravenous administration of gadolinium-based contrast medium.

Rheumatoid arthritis (Fig. 2.**27**)

This is characterized by inflammatory hypertrophy of the synovial membrane associated with joint effusion. Consequently, the images of choice are obtained with T2-weighted or STIR sequences, together with T1-weighted phase-contrast images after intravenous administration of gadolinium-based-contrast medium. This technique will also visualize osseous erosions.

Osteomyelitis (Fig. 2.**28**)

The affected osseous area is seen as high signal intensity on T2-weighted images. The outline is indistinct and the signal intensity decreases from the original nidus at the center to the periphery. Cortical defects are characteristic, with the defects exhibiting zones of increased signal intensity that extend deep into the periosteal soft tissues. A definite fluid accumulation is present. The T1-weighted images show the osseous lesions with decreased signal intensity. After intravenous administration of gadolinium-based contrast medium, scalloped enhancement demarcates the primary focus in the intraosseous space and outlines the surrounding abscess. Contrast enhancement in the

Fig. 2.**28** Sagittal image (GRE 500/10 out of phase after application of intravenous gadolinium contrast medium) showing osteomyelitis with sequestrum.

Fig. 2.**29** Sagittal image (GRE 500/10 out of phase after application of intravenous gadolinium contrast medium) showing nearly complete tear of the biceps tendon.

Fig. 2.**30** Image (GRE 500/10 out of phase after application of intravenous gadolinium contrast medium) showing fracture line in the radial head.

Fig. 2.**31** Sagittal image (STIR 1900/125) showing lymphangioma without involvement of the joint.

soft tissues reveals the inflammation-induced impairment of the blood-tissue barrier.

Tendon tear (Fig. 2.**29**)

The biceps tendon is most frequently involved, infrequently the triceps tendon. The dehiscence is well delineated on sagittal T1-weighted and T2*-weighted images. The retracted proximal tendon appears thickened on the transverse sections. At the radial insertion of the tendon, which is the most frequent site of the rupture, the lesion is seen as edema (high signal on T2-weighted or STIR images) and as hemorrhage (high signal intensity on T2-weighted images).

Fractures (Fig. 2.**30**)

Fractures of the radial head can be divided into fractures with or without dislocation and can be associated with fractures of the capitellum. The fracture is seen as a line that has decreased signal intensity on T1-weighted images and increased signal intensity on T2-weighted images.

Tumors (Fig. 2.**31**)

MRI primarily serves to determine the site and extent of the tumorous process and to identify the displaced or infiltrated tissue. A tissue diagnosis is only rarely attainable. As with tumors in the vicinity of other joints, the question of intra-articular extension must be addressed. In view of the complexity of these questions, the tumor must be visualized in all planes and generally in several differently weighted sequences. To delineate the tumor borders, the examination should be completed with images obtained after intravenous administration of gadolinium-based contrast medium.

References

Andrews JR. Bony injuries about the elbow in the throwing athlete. *Instr Course Lect.* 1985; 34: 323
Ballinger PW. *Merrill's atlas of radiographic positions and radiologic procedures.* St. Louis: Mosby; 1982
Bernau A, Berquist TH. *Postioning Techniques in Orthopedic Radiology. Orthopedic Postioning in Diagnostic Radiology.* Munich–Vienna–Baltimore: Urban & Schwarzenberg; 1983

Berquist TH. Magnetic resonance imaging: Preliminary experience in orthopedic surgery. *Magn Reson Imaging.* 1984; 2: 42

Godefray G et al. Arthrography of the elbow: Anatomical and radiological considerations and technical considerations. *Radiology.* 1981; 62: 441

Greenspan A, Norman A. The radial head, capitellar view. Useful technique in elbow trauma. *AJR.* 1982; 138: 1186

Greenspan A, Norman A, Rosen H. Radial-head capitellum view in elbow trauma: Clinical application and radiographic-anatomic correlation. *AJR.* 1984; 143: 355

Hempfling H. Die endoskopische Untersuchung des Ellbogengelenkes vom dorso-radialen Zugang. *Z Orthop.* 1983; 121: 331

Holland P, Davies AM. Real-time digital enhancement and magnification in the assessment of acute elbow injuries. *Br J Radiol.* 1991; 64: 591

Hoppenfeld S. *Klinische Untersuchung der Wirbelsäule und der Extremitäten.* Stuttgart–New York: G Fischer, 1982: 33

Jobe FW, Nuber G. Throwing injuries of the elbow. *Clin Sports Med.* 1986; 5: 621

Lorenz R. Frakturen im Bereich des Ellbogengelenkes. *Radiologie.* 1990; 30: 102

Manns RA, Lee JR. Critical evaluation of the radial head-capitellum view in acute elbow with an effusion. *Clin Radiol.* 1990; 42: 433

Morrey BF. *The Elbow and its Disorders.* Philadelphia: Saunders; 1985

Muhr G, Wernet E. Bandverletzungen und Luxation des Ellenbogengelenkes. *Orthopäde.* 1989; 18: 268

O'Driscoll SW, Bell DF, Morrey BF. Posterolateral rotary instablity of the elbow. *J Bone Joint Surg.* 1991; 73-A: 440

Wirth CJ, Kessler M. Sinnvoller Einsatz der radiologischen Diagnostik bei Sportschaden. *Radiologe.* 1983; 23: 389

Yocum LA. The diagnosis and nonoperative treatment of elbow problems in the athlete. *Clin Sports Med.* 1989; 8: 439

3 | Hand

3.1 Introduction

Injuries to the hand play a major role both in sports and in occupations. The hand is among the most frequently injured parts of the body. Although the injuries themselves are rarely life threatening, the loss of sensory and motor capabilities severely compromises a patient's well-being. Diagnosis of hand injuries can be difficult due to the close proximity of many anatomical structures, and particularly since symptoms can be subtle. This is especially true of the wrist. Differences in the motion of the carpal bones make the wrist subject to a wide range of injuries from acute and chronic stresses. Thorough familiarity with the functional anatomy and detailed knowledge of the patterns of motion in specific sports are required to make a precise diagnosis.

The primary functions of the hand are sensation and grasping. Sensation is especially crucial on the radial aspect of the index finger and on the ulnar aspect of the thumb, the surfaces primarily involved in grasping, feeling, and holding. Mobility of the hand and the entire upper extremity is important for grasping. The hand must be able to reach the mouth. The arm provides a balanced motor system that permits both forceful and fine coordinated motions.

Evolutionary specialization of the thumb as an opposable digit provides humans with exceptional motor abilities in the upper extremities. This specialization makes the thumb the most important digit of the hand; preservation of its function is one of the highest-priority goals in therapy.

3.2 Clinical Examination

Patient History

Clinical examination begins with systematically taking a history of all personal and medical data. The patient's age, occupation, and leisure and athletic activities often influence the indications for hand surgery, as do comorbidities, social background, and emotional disorders. The patient's general condition as well as cardiovascular problems, diabetes, coagulopathy and convulsive disorders can significantly influence decisions pertaining to surgical intervention. Chronic symptoms require a thorough history. The patient should discribe any previous illnesses or earlier injuries, and indicate the duration of present symptoms. Inquire when symptoms occur and whether they fluctuate over time. Have the patient describe patterns of pain and behavior of the hand in motion and under stress. A thorough history will provide sufficient information for a tentative diagnosis. For example, altered sensation and weakness in the index and middle fingers accompanied by nighttime paresthesia is often characteristic of carpal tunnel syndrome. Sudden, occasionally painful, snapping over the metacarpal heads when flexing and extending a finger is a typical sign of trigger finger. When evaluating chronic symptoms, inquire about previous periods of occupational disability. It is also important to determine which previous interventions were successful in alleviating symptoms.

In acute trauma, always document the time, site, and description of the accident. Record the type of injury. Differentiate between cuts, crush injuries, saw accidents, injuries from chemical action or burns, bite wounds, and closed trauma. This information can be important for determining subsequent diagnostic strategy. Do not underestimate the significance of seemingly minor injuries. It is important to determine the precise time of the accident since this has therapeutic consequences. This applies particularly to replantation and treatment of open wounds, but also to primary repair of a torn tendon, which will usually only be effective if performed within the first 10–14 days. The object that caused the injury should be known; this is important in evaluating the danger of infection in open wounds.

Often, the clinical suspicion developed while obtaining the history only requires confirmation in further diagnostic studies. If the patient has already consulted another physician, it is important to obtain precise information about prior treatment and the course of therapy to date.

Observation
General Observation

It is best to follow a routine when examing the patient, especially when preparing a medical opinion. Inspection begins as the patient enters the examining room. Valuable information about pain and compensatory posture can be obtained by observing the patient's spontaneous behavior. Compare both sides

Fig. 3.**1**   Ganglion on the extensor side of the wrist.

Fig. 3.**2**   Rheumatic hand with swan-neck deformity of the index finger, boutonnière deformity of the middle finger, and ulnar deviation of the long fingers.

when inspecting the patient, and include the entire upper extremity. Document the shape and posture of the hand first. The shape can be altered by generalized or localized swelling, congenital or acquired deformities involving position, contractures, and muscle atrophy. Localized swelling may be found with inflammation, tumors, after injury of the capsular ligaments, and in fractures. Ganglia originating either at the tendons, synovial lining, or the joints (Fig. 3.**1**) can cause swelling. Muscle atrophy occurs after prolonged periods of inactivity or as a sequelae of compressive neuropathy (thenar atrophy after prolonged compression of the median nerve in the carpal tunnel). Axial deformities suggest a fracture or dislocation; limp flexion of the distal phalanx of a finger suggests injury to an extensor tendon. Next, the skin is inspected. The color of the skin provides information on the current state of vascular supply to the hand. Color changes may occur as a result of bacterial infection (with localized hyperemia and erythema). They may also occur with systemic or metabolic disorders (shiny atrophic skin in progressive scleroderma; hyperpgimentation of the palmar furrows in Addison disease; palmar erythema in chronic disorders involving hyperglobulinemia, such as cirrhosis of the liver). Skin color may also change with inflammatory joint disorders (spotted erythema and cyanosis in rheumatoid arthritis).

The calluses on the palmar surface provide clues about occupation and physical exertion. Dominance of the hand (right or left-handed patient) should be taken into consideration. Inability to perspire is a sign of impaired nerve function in the hand or finger, particularly when clearly demarcated from the normal adjacent skin. Dry and scaly areas of skin are a sign of loss of nerve function in the hand or finger. The appearance of the fingernails (i.e., deformation, change in color, or change in consistency) can provide information about systemic disorders or metal intoxication. Hollow nails suggest iron-deficiency anemia; "half and half" nails suggest renal insufficiency and cirrhosis of the liver. Hourglass nails, often together with clubbed fingers, are seen in bronchial carcinoma and other lung disorders, cirrhosis of the liver, regional enteritis, and cyanotic heart defects. Mees

stripes are seen with thallium and arsenic poisoning. In postmenopausal women, posterolateral swelling is often observed in the distal interphalangeal joint. This is known as Heberden's nodes and can present as a painful flexion contracture of the distal joint. Arthritis of the proximal interphalangeal joint, referred to as Bouchard's nodes, is rare in comparison.

In addition to swelling of individual fingers and finger joints, symmetric swelling at the metacarpophalangeal and proximal interphalangeal joints can be observed in rheumatoid arthritis. Often, these joints (especially the metacarpophalangeal joints of the index and long fingers) are the first location in which the chronic inflammatory disorder will manifest itself. This can be accompanied by transient joint effusions and tenosynovitis. Women are most frequently affected (women:men = 3:1). Patients complain of typical morning stiffness in the affected joints, and pain during motion or palpation. Increasing destruction of the capsular ligaments, tendons, and articular surfaces in the further course of the disease can produce characteristic finger deformities. These include:

– Swan-neck flexion deformity of the metacarpophalangeal and distal interphalangeal joints with an overextended proximal interphalangeal joint (Fig. 3.**2**).
– Boutonnière deformity with flexion in the proximal interphalangeal joints and extension in the distal interphalangeal joint (Fig. 3.**2**).
– Deformity of the thumb with 90° flexion in the metacarpophalangeal joint and 90° hyperextension in the distal joint.
– Ulnar deviation of the fingers (Fig. 3.**2**).

Examination of a severely injured hand is difficult yet imperative. Often inspection of visible injuries permits an estimation of the degree of injury and subsequent diagnostic procedure. The location of the injury provides some information about the damaged structures. Palmar lesions primarily involve flexor tendons and neurovascular structures; dorsal lesions usually

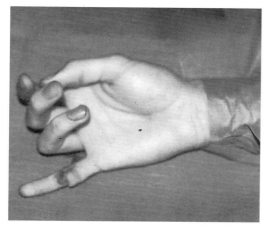

Fig. 3.**3**   Flexor tendon injury.

Fig. 3.**4**   Circular-saw injury.

Fig. 3.**5**   Syndactyly of the middle and ring fingers.

involve extensor tendons, bones, and joints. The position of injured fingers can be a sign of tendon injuries. Axial and rotational defects provide information about fractures and joint injuries, such as dislocations and tendon tears. In complex injuries, neurovascular bundles and tendon stumps can be inspected. It is also important to evaluate the degree of contamination of the hand (Figs. 3.**3** and 3.**4**).

Deformities

Congenital anomalies of the upper extremity are rare and are only found in one of 600 newborns. Approximately 10% of this number are estimated to be severe functional deformities. Polydactyly is the most frequent deformity of the hand, followed by syndactyly. Deformities can be caused by hereditary diseases such as trisomy 21 (Down syndrome) and exogenous factors such as thalidomide (Figs. 3.**5** and 3.**6**).

Fig. 3.**6**   Bilateral cleft hands.

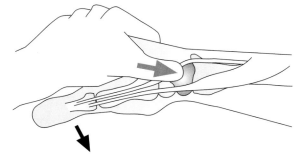

Fig. 3.**7** Palpation of the scaphoid.

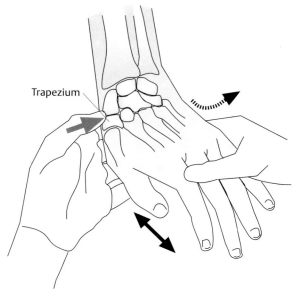

Fig. 3.**8** Palpation of the trapezium and the first metacarpal.

Palpation

Palpation complements the impression gained by inspection. Systematic palpation of the hand includes evaluation of soft tissue, bone, and joints. Turgor and perspiration of the hand are also assessed. The skin of the palm of the hand is significantly thicker than that of the dorsal hand. Numerous fibers radiate from the palmar aponeurosis as retinacula into the skin of the hollow of the hand, firmly connecting it to the aponeurosis. This makes it possible to firmly grip objects without the skin separating from the subcutaneous tissue. Evaluate the skin's surface texture (smooth or rough; dry or moist), mobility, and temperature. Swelling may be due to effusion or changes in the soft tissue or bone; evaluate swelling for consistency (soft, hardened, or fluctuant). Knotty changes or changes over a wide area detected in the connective tissue on the hollow of the hand can suggest a Dupuytren's contracture. Tender areas should be precisely localized; check for radiating pain. Nodular thickening in the annular ligaments that causes a snapping sound and transient locking during flexion or extension suggest a trigger finger. Abrasion injuries are examined by evaluating restoration of capillary flow.

Palpation should not be limited to the hand. The examination should include the elbow, shoulder, and cervical spine, particularly when pain radiates into the forearm. Be particularly alert to localized tenderness resulting from overuse (medial and lateral humeral epicondylitis) and peripheral nerve compression syndromes, including supinator syndrome, pronator teres syndrome, and cubital tunnel syndrome. Compare results with the contralateral side to confirm findings.

The major landmarks for palpation of the hand include:

Radial styloid. This is an important orientation point for palpation of the wrist. Tenderness to palpation over this area can suggest tendinitis at the insertion of the brachioradialis as can occasionally occur in athletes whose sport involves backhand motions. Isometric muscle tensing increases the pain.

Anatomical snuffbox and scaphoid. The anatomical snuffbox is located on the dorsum of the wrist, distal to the radial styloid. It is readily discernible with the wrist in slight ulnar deviation and the thumb extended and abducted. This hollow is bounded by the tendons of the abductor pollicis longus and the extensor pollicis brevis on the radial aspect, and the tendon of the extensor pollicis longus on the ulnar aspect. The scaphoid is palpable on the floor of the hollow (Fig. 3.**7**). Pain to palpation in this area, together with pain during radial deviation, suggests injury to the scaphoid. Due to the strong forces acting on it, this is the most frequently fractured carpal bone.

Trapezium and base of the first metacarpal. Together with the base of the first metacarpal, the trapezium forms the joint of the base of the thumb. The trapezium is distal to the snuffbox and is palpable with the thumb in flexion and extension (Fig. 3.**8**). The joint of the base of the thumb has a slight degree of physiologic dorsopalmar mobility. Traumatic changes such as Bennett or Rolando fractures and degenerative changes such as osteoarthritis will be painful to palpation in this area. A rupture of the palmar capsule of the joint results in abnormal motion with respect to the base of the second metacarpal.

Capitate and base of the second metacarpal. The capitate is palpable proximal to the largest and most important of all metacarpal bases, the third metacarpal.

Lunate and Lister's tubercle. The lunate is palpable in flexion and extension immediately distal to Lister's

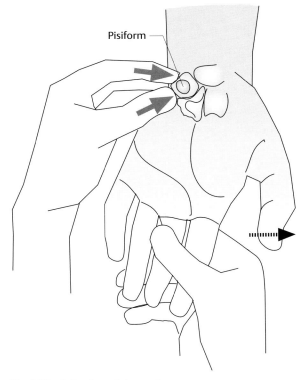

Fig. 3.**9** Linear alignment of Lister's tubercle, lunate and capitate bones, and third metacarpal.

Fig. 3.**10** Palpation of the pisiform.

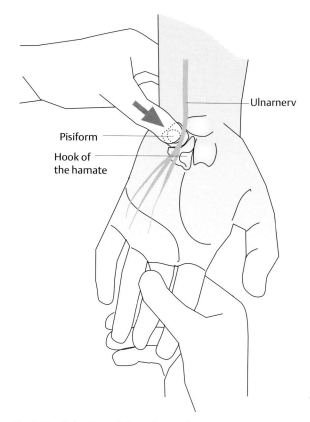

Fig. 3.**11** Palpation of Guyon's canal.

tubercle, which lies on the dorsal aspect of the distal radius directly in line with the third metacarpal (Fig. 3.**9**). The lunate can be damaged by dislocation, avascular necrosis, and fractures. In these cases, palpation will usually reveal localized tenderness, and moving the wrist will be painful. The tendon of the extensor carpi radialis brevis covers the lunate together with the capitate and the base of the third metacarpal.

Ulnar styloid. The ulnar styloid is another important landmark for palpation of the wrist. Pain in this area can be attributable to tendinitis at the insertion of the flexor carpi ulnaris. The tendon of this muscle is ulnar to the tendon of the palmaris longus and palpable if the wrist is extended or dorsiflexed against resistance with the fist clenched. In rheumatoid arthritis, painful swelling can occasionally be demonstrated here. The ulnar styloid is frequently injured in falls and crush injuries.

Triquetrum and pisiform. The triquetrum lies distal to the styloid. It is palpable under the pisiform when the wrist is in radial deviation. The pisiform is palpable as a sesamoid bone on the distal flexor carpi ulnaris (Fig. 3.**10**). The flexor retinaculum, the extensor retinaculum, the tendons of the abductor digiti minimi, and the fibrous complex of the ulnocarpal compartment insert on the pisiform.

Fig. 3.**12**   Anatomy of Guyon's canal.

Hamate and Guyon's Canal. The hamate may be difficult to palpate because it lies in a deep plane and is
covered by a cushion of soft tissue. The prominent
hook of the hamate and the pisiform form the lateral
boundary of Guyon's canal, through which the ulnar
artery and nerve pass (Fig. 3.**11**). The canal becomes
clinically significant with compression of the nerve in
acute and chronic trauma. Tumors can also cause
nerve compression. Specific symptoms can vary significantly; complete or partial compression may be
present depending on the cause, the anatomical position, and the pattern of the nerve branches. (Fig. 3.**12**.)

Palmaris longus. The tendon of the palmaris longus
is best palpated with the wrist slightly flexed and the
thumb and small finger opposed (Fig. 3.**13**). The tendon appears prominently on the palmar aspect of the
wrist. It is distal and marks the palmar surface of the
carpal tunnel. The palmaris longus is among those
muscles that show the greatest variations and form,
attachment, and bilateral symmetry. In approximately 12% of the population, the palmaris longus is
absent. The tendon of this muscle is important as a
graft for replacing injured finger flexor tendons.

Carpal tunnel. The hook of the hamate on the ulnar
side, the scaphoid tuberosity, and the trapezium on
the radial side define the carpal tunnel. This tunnel
contains the median nerve and the flexor tendons of
the fingers that extend from the forearm into the
hand. The transverse carpal ligament covers the tunnel. As in Guyon's canal, various factors such as
connective-tissue disorders with synovialitis, systemic diseases, trauma, and tumors can compress the
nerve in the tunnel and affect sensory and motor
function. Opposition of the thumb can be impaired by
loss of function of the opponens when the thenar
branch is affected. (Fig. 3.**14**).

Flexor carpi radialis. The tendon of the flexor carpi
radialis is radial to the tendon of the palmaris longus
and palpable in flexion with the fist clenched and the
wrist in radial deviation (Fig. 3.**15**). This tendon
crosses the scaphoid and inserts at the base of the
second metacarpal.

Fig. 3.**13**   Palpation of the palmaris longus.

- **Extrinsic extensor tendons**

First dorsal compartment. This compartment forms
the palmar margin of the anatomical snuffbox. It contains the tendons of the abductor pollicis longus and
the extensor pollicis brevis. These tendons can be distinguished as they leave the compartment by having
the patient extend or abduct the thumb (Fig. 3.**16**).
This region is affected in stenosing tenosynovitis (De
Quervain) and because of the close proximity of the
superficial branch of the radial nerve. De Quervain is
caused by inflammatory swelling of the synovial lining of the compartment, which narrows the tunnel
and causes pain during movement. Repetitive rotational motions in the wrist can contribute to this disorder. Paddlers and canoeists are among those frequently afflicted with the disorder. Pain in this region
can also be caused by radial styloiditis, generally a
tendon disorder involving the insertion of the brachioradialis.

Second dorsal compartment. This compartment
contains the tendons of the extensor carpi radialis
longus and brevis. These tendons are palpable when
the patient makes a fist. This causes the tendons to
stand out on the radial side of the Lister tubercle
(Fig. 3.**17**).

Fig. 3.**14** Schematic cross-sectional anatomy of the carpal tunnel.

a Axial section at the inlet at the level of the pisiform.

b Axial section at the outlet at the level of the hook of the hamate. Abbrevations: FR = flexor retinaculum, FDS and FDP = tendons of the flexor digitorum superficialis and flexor digitorum profundus, FCR = flexor carpi radialis tendon, FPL = flexor pollicis longus tendon, MN = median nerve.

c Diagram for measuring the volar deviation (VD) of the flexor retinaculum. This is defined as the distance between the maximum protrusion of the flexor retinaculum and a line drawn between the trapezial tuberosity and the hook of the hamate.

Fig. 3.**15** Palpation of the flexor carpi radialis tendon.

Extensor pollicis brevis
and abductor pollicis
longus

Fig. 3.**16**   Palpation of the first dorsal compartment.

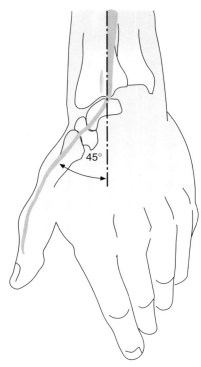

45°

Fig. 3.**18**   Palpation of the third dorsal compartment.

Second dorsal compartment:
extensor carpi radialis
longus and brevis

Lister's tubercle

Third dorsal compartment:
extensor pollicis longus

Fig. 3.**17**   Palpation of the second dorsal compartment.

Third dorsal compartment. The tendon of the extensor pollicis longus can be palpated on the ulnar side of the Lister tubercle in the third dorsal compartment.

This tendon forms a 45° angle (Fig. 3.**18**). It continues on to the thumb, crossing the tendons of the extensor carpi radialis longus and brevis.

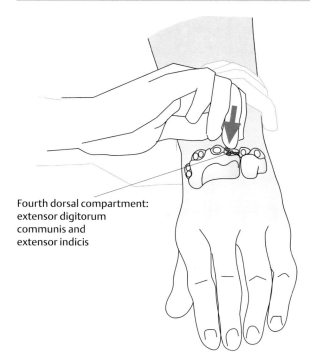

Fourth dorsal compartment: extensor digitorum communis and extensor indicis

Fig. 3.**19**   Palpation of the fourth dorsal compartment.

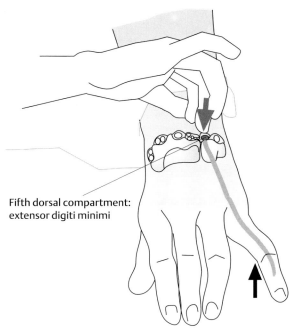

Fifth dorsal compartment: extensor digiti minimi

Fig. 3.**20**   Palpation of the fifth dorsal compartment.

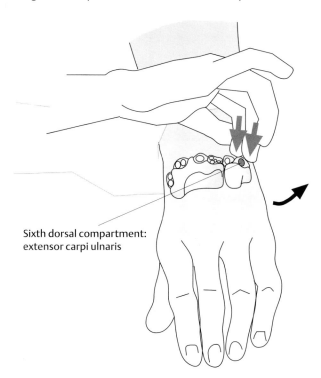

Sixth dorsal compartment: extensor carpi ulnaris

Fig. 3.**21**   Palpation of the sixth dorsal compartment.

Fourth dorsal compartment. The tendons of the extensor digitorum communis and extensor indicis lie in this compartment. They are not as accessible as the other extensor tendons, but each tendon should be palpated individually (Fig. 3.**19**). The tendon of the

extensor muscle lies deeper; in rare cases it will have its own separate tunnel.

Fifth dorsal compartment. The extensor digiti minimi tendon will be palpable immediately lateral to the ulnar styloid when the patient rests the hand on the table and raises the little finger (Fig. 3.**20**). As with the extensor indicis tendon, the extensor tendon of the little finger can move independently of the other extensor tendons; this can be demonstrated by having the patient extend the little finger and index finger while flexing the other fingers. Because of its location immediately adjacent to the radioulnar joint, the extensor digiti minimi tendon can be injured in a posterior dislocation of the ulnar head.

Sixth dorsal compartment. This compartment contains the tendon of the extensor carpi ulnaris. This tendon is palpable between the tip of the ulnar styloid and the base of the fifth metacarpal with the wrist extended and in ulnar deviation (Fig. 3.**21**). If the ulnar styloid is avulsed in a radial fracture, the tunnel can also tear, causing the tendon to dislocate over the ulnar styloid with an audible snapping noise when the wrist is pronated.

● **Intrinsic extensor tendons**
The tendons of the intrinsic muscles of the hand (the interossei and lumbricals) are difficult to palpate. They form a complex extensor apparatus of the finger (Fig. 3.**22**).

Thenar and hypothenar eminences. Palpate the ball of the thumb and little finger, and evaluate their size

Fig. 3.**22**   Anatomy of the extensor tendons of the fingers: (1) tendon of the extensor digitorum, (2) lumbrical, (3) interosseus, (4) deep transverse metacarpal ligament, (5) transverse part of the superficial intertendinous lamina, (6) intertendinous lamina (hood of the extensor expansion), (7) medial part of the interosseus tendon, (8) medial part of the extensor digitorum, (9) lateral part of the interosseus tendon, (10) intermediate band, (11) lateral band, (12) triangular ligament, (13) terminal tendon of the dorsal aponeurosis.

Fig. 3.**23**   Tear of the palmar plate.

and consistency. Prolonged compression of the median nerve in the carpal tunnel can lead to atrophy of the thenar musculature. Compression of the ulnar nerve in or proximal to Guyon's canal can lead to atrophy of the hypothenar eminence. Findings should always be compared with the contralateral hand.

Palm. Structures within the palm are difficult to palpate because of the soft tissue covering them. In Dupuytren's contracture, areas of knotty or cord-like thickening will be palpable in the palmar aponeurosis, particularly on the ulnar side over the fourth and fifth metacarpals. These areas can extend into the fingers. In addition to thin, tendon-like strands that do not show significant adhesions to the skin, thick cord-like and knotty structures with adhesions to subcutaneous tissue will be present. Pitting may also be present. Flexion contractures of the metacarpophalangeal and proximal interphalangeal joints with limited abduction of the fingers can occur.

Dorsum. In contrast to the flexor tendons, the extensor tendons on the dorsum of the hand are readily palpable, particularly at the heads of the metacarpals. The fourth and fifth metacarpals can be passively moved relatively easily, while the second and third metacarpals are securely anchored in the carpal region and allow little motion. Metacarpal fractures

often occur in the neck region. Primary symptoms include swelling and tenderness to palpation. The fifth metacarpal is the most frequently fractured.

Phalanges. The thinner soft-tissue envelope of the phalanges makes them more accessible to palpation. Document any deformities, swelling, or tenderness to palpation, especially in the joints. Swelling in the proximal interphalangeal joints that is tender to palpation is often a sign of disruption of the capsular ligaments, particularly in athletes (Fig. 3.**23**). Delayed or incorrect diagnosis and treatment of these injuries can lead to chronic swelling and impairment of function.

Fingertips. Infections of the hand can arise from minor injuries to the fingers and fingertips that are left untreated. Thorough palpation is required where infection is suspected. Even minor, apparently superficial, infections can progress proximally along the tendon sheaths. An infection in the little finger can spread through the tendon sheaths and the synovial lining of the wrist to the thumb, or vice versa, in a U-shaped pattern of inflammation. Palpation of the infected tendon is intensely painful. Chronic infections can lead to permanent loss of function in the hand and, under certain conditions, to life-threatening situations. Paronychia is the most frequent infection of the hand and usually occurs at the base of the fingernail. A distinction is made between a periungual felon (along the nail fold), a subungual felon (beneath the nail), and a subcutaneous felon that is very painful because of the tight connective tissue.

Assessing Range of Motion

To obtain an overview of hand function, evaluate various forms of grasping, the clenched fist, extension of all the fingers, abduction and adduction of the fingers, and opposition of the thumb. The patient should be able to touch each fingertip with the tip of the thumb. Always compare both hands. These simple tests can often provide important information about possible injuries, which can then be evaluated in more specific examinations. The precise active and passive ranges of motion of the hand and finger joints are determined separately for each joint; the respective measured arcs are recorded in degrees. These initial findings are documented and used as the basis of subsequent studies. The ranges of motion of the elbow, shoulder, and cervical spine should also be determined in preliminary tests.

The patient should be able to perform active motion without pain. The following ranges of motion are regarded as normal:

- **Wrist**
- — Dorsal extension and palmar flexion   35°–60°/0°/ 50°–60°
- — Radial deviation and ulnar deviation   20°/0°/40°
- — Supination and pronation   90°/0°/90°

- **Finger joints**
- — Metacarpophalangeal extension and flexion   10°–30°/0°/90°
- — Proximal interphalangeal extension and flexion   0°/0°/100°
- — Distal interphalangeal extension and flexion   0°/0°/90°
- — Abduction and adduction   20°/0°/20°

- **Thumbs**
- — Metacarpophalangeal extension and flexion   0°/0°/50°
- — Interphalangeal extension and flexion   20°/0°/90°
- — Abduction and adduction   45°/0°/0°
- — Anteversion and retroversion   45°/0°/0°

Mobility of the wrist will vary according to the patient's occupation, age, and sex. Factors influencing the range of motion include the joint contour, the capsular ligaments, and the musculature acting on the joint. Joint motion can be limited in active motion, passive motion, or both. Reversible limitations of normal wrist and finger motion are often the result of acute or chronic tenosynovitis and fibrous proliferation with intra-articular or periarticular adhesions. Permanent limitations result from destruction of the articular surface, fractures, and shortening of the capsular ligaments or tendons.

Fig. 3.**24** Evaluation of the flexor digitorum superficialis tendon.

Differences in active and passive ranges of motion, and changes in the range of motion according to the position of the joint, narrow the differential diagnosis. For example, equal limitations in the active and passive ranges of motion of a joint, regardless of the position of the joint, are a sign of shortening of the surrounding capsule and ligaments. An extension deficit in a proximal interphalangeal joint that does not change as the metacarpophalangeal joint moves is a sign of adhesion of a tendon at the level of the metacarpophalangeal joint. With an adhesion in the palm region, you can neutralize the resulting flexion of the proximal interphalangeal joint by passively flexing the metacarpophalangeal joint. Adhesions of the flexor tendons in the carpal tunnel only permit extension of the fingers when the wrist is in flexion. Adhesions of the extensor tendons in the forearm prevent flexion in the wrist when the patient makes a fist; adhesions of the flexor tendons prevent extension with the fingers extended. Impairment of active movement of only one finger is a sign of a tendon rupture or a neurologic lesion.

Specific Tests

Evaluating Flexor Tendon Function

Tendon injury must be excluded in any wound on the flexor side of the hand and finger. Always evaluate tendon function against resistance to distinguish partial tears from complete tears.

Flexor digitorum superficialis. The tendon of the superficial flexor of the finger inserts at the base of the middle phalanx. To test its function in isolation (flexion of the proximal interphalangeal joint), hold all of the patient's fingers in extension except for the one you want to test (Fig. 3.**24**). This draws all the deep flexor tendons distally and locks them. In an isolated complete tear of the flexor digitorum superficia-

Fig. 3.**25**   Evaluation of the flexor digitorum profundus tendon.

lis, flexion in the proximal interphalangeal joint will be significantly impaired. Since muscle tension proximally displaces the stump of the tendon in any injury to a flexor tendon, you should attempt to palpate the precise position of the proximal end preoperatively. The stump can also appear as a painful thickened area in the region of the proximal phalanx. The superficial flexor tendon can be absent; always compare both hands.

Flexor digitorum profundus. The tendon of the deep flexor of the finger inserts at the base of the distal phalanx. To evaluate its function (flexion in the distal interphalangeal joint), instruct the patient to actively flex the distal interphalangeal joint while you immoblize the proximal interphalangeal joint in passive extension (Fig. 3.**25**). An acute tear of the flexor digitorum profundus tendon renders active flexion in the distal interphalangeal joint immpossible; in an older tear, flexion will be significantly limited. Normal flexion in the proximal interphalangeal and metacarpophalangeal joints will still be possible. If both flexor tendons are served, flexion will only be possible in the metacarpophalangeal joint using the interossei. When the patient places the hand with the dorsum flat on the examining table, the injured finger will be completely extended.

Flexor pollicis longus. Evaluate the function of the flexor pollicis longus tendon with the metacarpophalangeal joint immobilized in passive extension. If the distal interphalangeal joint cannot be flexed, then a tendon tear or paralysis of the muscle is present. Some flexion in the metacarpophalangeal joint may be possible if the thenar musculature is intact.

Evaluating Extensor Tendon Function

Clinical evaluation of extensor tendon lesions is more difficult than that of flexor tendon lesions because of the unique anatomy of the dorsum of the hand. Open injuries occur far more frequently than closed injuries, which are often accompanied by ligament tears with bony avulsion fractures. Function may still be present in partial tears of the extensors. Testing against resistance is required to distinguish partial tears from normal ligaments.

Fingers with three phalanges are extended using the extensor digitorum communis and the intrinsic muscles (interossei and lumbricals). The index and little finger also have their own extensor muscle. To test the function of the extensor digitorum tendon in isolation, have the patient extend the metacarpophalangeal joint against resistance with the interphalangeal joints flexed. When evaluating extension, remember that the extensor tendons influence each other through the juncture in the dorsum of the hand. An isolated lesion proximal to this connection will only result in a slight extension deficit as the affected finger can be extended via the extensor tendons of the adjacent fingers.

If active extension of the distal phalanx of a finger is not possible and the distal phalanx hangs flaccid ("drop finger"), this may be due to an intrasubstance tear in the extensor tendon, avulsion of the tendon from the distal phalanx, or a ligament tear with a bony avulsion fracture (mallet fracture).

Another frequent injury is a tear of the central slip of extensor tendon over the proximal interphalangeal joints. Swelling, hematoma, and tenderness to palpation over the dorsal aspect of this joint may be the only evidence of a tear of the central slip in an acute injury, unless a true lateral radiograph demonstrates an avulsion fracture over the extensor side at the base of the middle phalanx. Active flexion of the distal phalanx in the affected finger should be evaluated with the proximal interphalangeal joint immobilized in extension. Painful reduction of the active flexion in the distal interphalangeal joint can be an important sign of a tear of the central slip.

Stability Tests with Ligament Tears and Dislocations

• Interphalangeal joints

The interphalangeal joints are very stable although ligament injuries regularly occur, particularly in sports. These injuries most often involve the proximal interphalangeal joints. Injuries (tears) of the ligaments usually present as localized swelling and tenderness to palpation; signs of instability with passive hyperextension and lateral displacement are encountered less frequently. Test radial and ulnar opening at the proximal interphalangeal joints with the finger extended. If the palmar capsular plate is torn in addition to the collateral ligament, the middle phalanx will be displaced and tilted toward the uninjured side. Rotational instability will also be present.

Tears of the palmar plate. The palmar plate can tear as a result of dorsally directed force. Comparison of both hands is required to demonstrate abnormal hyperextension. The ligament tears many involve avulsion fractures of the bone.

Collateral ligament tears. Collateral ligament tears result from lateral forces, usually from the radial side. A clinically measured joint opening of less than 20° is regarded as a sign of an incomplete tear; a joint opening of more than 20° is regarded as a sign of a complete tear.

• **Dislocations**
Dislocations of the interphalangeal joints are immediately apparent from the resulting deformity in the dislocated joint. Evaluate stability after closed reduction.

Dorsal dislocation. Dorsal dislocation results from axial stresses with hyperextension. The distal palmar plate tears. This can be accompanied by a torn collateral ligament.

Palmar dislocation. Dorsal stresses and rotation of the flexed middle phalanx will result in palmar dislocation.

Lateral dislocation. The dislocation results from lateral forces. The respective collateral ligament and the volar plate tear.

• **Metacarpophalangeal joints of the long fingers and thumb**
The metacarpophalangel joints of the long fingers are ball-and-socket joints. They allow abduction and adduction in addition to flexion and extension. Collateral ligament tears are rare in these joints. In dislocations, the palmar plate tears as a result of strong hyperextension stresses. Dislocations can be complete or incomplete and dorsal or palmar. Complete dorsal dislocations occur more frequently. Here, the head of the phalanx will be palpable in the palm of the hand. Closed reduction is seldom possible because the palmar plate or tendons are interposed in the joint space.

Stability test for an ulnar collateral ligament tear at the metacarpophalangeal joint of the thumb. Also known as gamekeeper's thumb, this injury to the ulnar collateral ligament at the metacarpophalangeal joint of the thumb occurs as a result of forced radial deviation of the extended thumb. This injury is often sustained in a fall on the hand. Evaluate stability with the thumb flexed 20°–30°; otherwise the accessory collateral ligament (if intact) can mask the tear of the collateral ligament in extension (Fig. 3.**26**). A joint

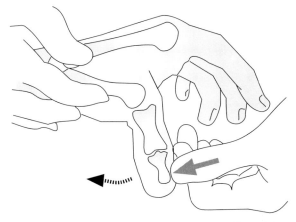

Fig. 3.**26** Stress test in a tear of the ulnar collateral ligament at the metacarpophalangeal joint.

that can also be opened in extension is the sign of a complex capsular ligament injury. Forceful stability testing can itself produce a surgical indication; abducting the thumb causes the collateral ligament to irretrievably slip beneath the extensor aponeurosis of the thumb, which precludes normal healing. Comparative examination of both hands is important as generalized ligament laxity can simulate a ski thumb.

• **Carpometacarpal joints**
Crush injuries and falls on the hand can produce dorsal dislocation of the fourth and fifth carpometacarpal joints as these are less stable. However, fracture dislocations in this region are encountered more frequently. These may present as a bayonet deformity of the hand, which can occasionally be masked by massive swelling. The carpometacarpal joint of the thumb is a very mobile joint. Complete dislocations are rare in comparison to Bennett fracture dislocations.

Tests for Nerve Compression

• **Median nerve**
Carpal tunnel syndrome
Tinel's sign. With compression of the median nerve in the carpal tunnel (carpal tunnel syndrome), you can elicit paresthesia by tapping the nerve at the site of compression (Fig. 3.**27**). This test will produce false negative results in cases where chronic compression has been present and nerve conduction significantly reduced for a long period of time.

Phalen's test. Maximum flexion or extension of the wrist can also lead to significant paresthesias in the distribution of the nerve in carpal tunnel syndrome (Figs. 3.**28a, b**). As with the Tinel's sign, false negative results are possible in chronic cases.

• **Radial nerve**
Wartenberg syndrome
Tinel's sign. When the margin of the brachioradialis

Fig. 3.**27**   Tinel's sign. Eliciting paresthesia by tapping the median nerve when carpal tunnel syndrome is present.

Figs. 3.**28a, b**   Phalen's test. Eliciting paresthesia by compression of the median nerve, at the end of the range of flexion and extension of the wrist, to evaluate carpal tunnel syndrome.

Fig. 3.**29**   Finkelstein test for evaluation of stenosing tenosynovitis (De Quervain disease).

compresses the superficial branch of the radial nerve in the distal forearm, tapping here can elicit tingling sensations.

- **Ulnar nerve**

Distal ulnar nerve compression syndrome

Tinel's sign. This is sometimes negative. Distal ulnar nerve compressive neuropathy presents as a motor paresis of the ulnar nerve without loss of sensation.

Tests to Evaluate Vascular Supply

Allen test. This test is suitable for evaluating the radial and ulnar arteries in the hand. With the thumb, index finger, and middle finger, compress both arteries on the patient's distal forearm. Then instruct the patient to open and close the fist so that the venous blood is pressed out of the hand through the dorsal veins. When the patient opens the fist, the palm of the hand will be pale. Removing compression from

one artery while maintaining it on the other should normally cause the hand to rapidly flush pink as it is perfused. If the released artery is partially or completely occluded, this reaction will not be seen; the hand will only regain its normal color slowly. Test the second artery in the same manner, and repeat the test in the contralateral hand for comparison. If the hand does not become pale, even with increased pressure on both forearm arteries, a "median artery" or other arterial variant may be present. The Allen test can also be used to test vascular supply to a finger.

Other Tests

Finkelstein test. This test can be used to distinguish between simple radial styloiditis and stenosing tenosynovitis (De Quervain disease), a painful irritation of the synovial lining of the first dorsal compartment. Instruct the patient to adduct the thumb into the palm and make a fist. Immobilize the forearm and place the wrist in ulnar deviation. In a positive test, the patient will report pain in the tunnel (Fig. 3.**29**). This test will be false positive in patients with STT-arthrosis.

Neurologic Examination

Examination of both motor and sensory function is required. Muscular strength is evaluated according to Table 1.**8** (see p. 24).

Motor Function Testing

It is important to test motor function with direct muscle or tendon injuries and with central or peripheral nerve lesions. Electrodiagnostic studies are helpful and complement unusual clinical findings. To evaluate complete or partial motor paralysis, it is only necessary to test a few muscles. Complex nerve lesions, particularly peripheral lesions, require a standardized systematic evaluation of the musculature of the forearm and hand. Compensatory movements by muscles other than those being examined should be neutralized to avoid inaccurate diagnoses when testing the function of individual muscles. For example, failure of the dorsal interossei and the abductor digiti minimi can be masked by the function of the finger extensors if the test is done with the metacarpophalangeal joints in hyperextension. Similarly, the finger flexors can simulate movements of the palmar interossei if these muscles are tested with the long fingers flexed at the metacarpophalangeal joints. Other causes of inaccurate diagnoses include anomalies of innervation. These primarily affect the thenar region.

Wrist extension. The primary extensors of the wrist are the extensor carpi radialis longus and brevis (radial nerve, C6–C7), and the extensor carpi ulnaris (radial nerve, C7). Secondary extensors include the extensor digitorum, extensor digiti minimi, and extensor indicis proprius. Immobilize the patient's forearm with one hand and instruct the patient to extend the wrist with the fist clenched against the resistance of your other hand.

Wrist flexion. The primary flexors of the wrist are the flexor carpi radialis (median nerve, C6–C8), and the flexor carpi ulnaris (ulnar nerve, C8–T1). Secondary flexors include the palmaris longus, the flexor pollicis longus, and the deep superficial finger flexors. The strongest flexor is the flexor carpi ulnaris. Flexion is best evaluated with a clenched fist against resistance because the clenched fist neutralizes the function of the finger flexors.

Ulnar deviation of the wrist. This is primarily due to the action of the flexor carpi ulnaris (ulnar nerve, C8–T1). Immobilize the patient's forearm with one hand and instruct the patient to move the wrist into ulnar deviation against the resistance of the thumb of your same hand.

Radial deviation of the wrist. The main muscle effecting radial deviation in the wrist is the flexor carpi radialis (median nerve, C6–C8). The procedure is similar to that of the ulnar deviation test.

Fig. 3.**30**   Evaluation of finger extension.

Finger extension. The primary extensors include the extensor digitorum communis (radial nerve, C7–C8), extensor indicis proprius (radial nerve, C7–C8), and the extensor digiti minimi (radial nerve, C7). Test these muscles at the metacarpophalangeal joint with the wrist immobilized in a neutral position and the interphalangeal joints flexed. Flexion in the proximal interphalangeal and metacarpophalangeal joints is necessary to prevent the intrinsic muscles and secondary extensors from contributing to the extension. (Fig. 3.**30**). Extension in the proximal and distal interphalangeal joints can be tested with a flicking movement of the fingers (Fig. 3.**31**). This test evaluates the function of the interossei and lumbricals (ulnar nerve, C8–T1).

Finger flexion. The primary flexors are the flexor digitorum profundus in the distal interphalangeal joint (ulnar part of the ulnar nerve, C8–T1, and radial part of the median nerve, C7–C8), the flexor digitorum superficialis in the proximal interphalangeal joint (median nerve, C7–C8), and the lumbricals in the metacarpophalangeal joint (median nerve, C7, for the medial lumbricals and ulnar nerve; C8 for the lateral lumbricals). For a preliminary test of the strength of the finger flexors, instruct the patient to flex the fingers. Interlock your fingers with the patient's and try to pull them open. Differentiation between the superficialis and profundus is discussed in the previous section.

Finger abduction. The dorsal interossei (ulnar nerve, C8–T1), and the abductor digiti minimi (ulnar nerve, C8–T1) are the primary abductors. The long extensors of the fingers are secondary abductors. Abduction may be tested in all fingers simultaneously by applying resistance to the second and fifth finger (Fig. 3.**32**), or by testing the middle finger in isolation (Fig. 3.**33**).

Finger adduction. The primary adductors are the palmar interossei (ulnar nerve, C8–T1). The long flexors

Fig. 3.**32**   Evaluation of finger abduction.

Fig. 3.**31**   Evaluation of the interossei and lumbricals with a flicking movement.

Fig. 3.**33**   Evaluation of the abduction and adduction of the middle finger in isolation.

Fig. 3.**34**   Evaluation of finger adduction.

of the fingers act as secondary adductors. To test finger adduction, try to pull the patient's extended adducted phalanges apart. It is best to examine two fingers at the same time (i. e., index and middle finger, middle and ring finger, and ring and little finger). An alternative test is to try to pull a piece of paper from between the patient's extended fingers while the patient attempts to maintain a grip on the paper. Compare the strength of this grip with the strength of the contralateral hand (Fig. 3.**34**).

Thumb extension. The primary extensors are the extensor pollicis brevis at the metacarpophalangeal

joint (radial nerve, C7), and the extensor pollicis longus at the interphalangeal joint (radial nerve, C7). When the thumb extensors are weak, extension can be effected at the metacarpophalangeal joint by the abductor pollicis.

Thumb flexion. The primary flexors are the flexor pollicis brevis at the metacarpophalangeal joint (deep part of the ulnar nerve, C8, and superficial part of the median nerve, C6–C7), and the flexor pollicis longus at the interphalangeal joint (median nerve, C8–T1). To test flexion, instruct the patient to flex the thumb toward the hypothenar eminence against the resistance of your thumb hooked into the patient's.

Figs. 3.**35a, b**   Evaluation of the abduction of the thumb perpendicular to the palm; observation of the abductor pollicis brevis (**a**). Palpation of the tendon of the abductor pollicis longus adjacent to the tendon of the extensor pollicis brevis (**b**).

Fig. 3.**37**   Froment sign

Fig. 3.**36**   Lüthy bottle sign.

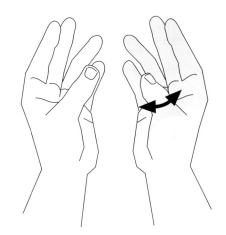

Fig. 3.**38**   Nail sign. Limited pronation of the thumb due to failure of the opponens pollicis. The thumbnail of the affected side is not completely visible.

Thumb abduction. The primary abductors include the abductor pollicis longus (radial nerve, C7) and the abductor pollicis brevis (median nerve, C6–C7). Evaluate these muscles with the thumbs abducted perpendicular to the palm (Figs. 3.**35a, b**). With paralysis of the abductor pollicis brevis, the patient cannot bring the web between thumb and index finger into contact with a bottle when grasping it, as shown. This is known as the Lüthy bottle sign (Fig. 3.**36**).

Thumb adduction. The adductor pollicis with its oblique and transverse heads is the primary adductor (ulnar nerve, C8). To evaluate adduction, first immo-

bilize the ulnar side of the patient's hand. Instruct the patient to attempt to place the extended thumb in a palmar-abducted position with the nail perpendicular to the palm of the hand. Now instruct the patient to adduct the thumb toward the index finger against resistance on the ulnar side of the thumb. Weakness of the adductor pollicis can be detected when the patient attempts to hold a piece of paper between the thumb and index finger. The flexor pollicis longus will compensate, producing forced flexion of the distal phalanx of the thumb known as Froment's sign (Fig. 3.**37**).

Opposition of the thumb and little finger. The primary muscles of opposition are the opponens pollicis (median nerve, C6–C7), and the opponens digiti minimi (ulnar nerve, C8). Evaluate opposition by instructing the patient to oppose the thumb and the tip of the little finger. Then grasp the thenar and hypothenar eminences with one hand each. Try to separate the fingers by pressing on the metacarpophalangeal joints. If the opponens pollicis is paralyzed, the thumb will be weakly pronated compared with the contralateral side (Fig. 3.**38**).

Fig. 3.**39** "O" test. Patients with failure of the flexor pollicis longus and the second flexor digitorum profundus cannot form an "O" with the thumb and index finger.

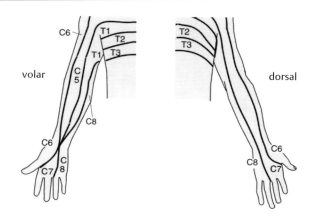

Fig. 3.**40** Sensory supply to the hand.

Pinch mechanism. The pinch mechanism is a combined motion involving several muscles. Normally, the thumb and index finger will form an "O". With normal muscle function you will be unable to change the shape of the "O", even with a strong pull, when you hook your index finger in the circle created by the two fingers. In an anterior interosseous nerve syndrome, the index flexor digitorum profundus and the flexor pollicis longus are paralyzed. The distal phalanx of the thumb and index finger will remain extended and the patient will be unable to form an "O" (Fig. 3.**39**).

Examining Sensation

Examining sensation in the upper extremities is generally limited to evaluating pain and sense of touch. Usually tests for other qualities (temperature sensation and proprioception) are unnecessary. The history will often provide the first important signs of disturbed sensation. One should inquire in particular, about paresthesia and dysesthesia in the hand region. In addition to the location and the time of occurrence of pain, situations that can elicit pain symptoms are also of interest. Often one only needs to apply brief, focused tactile and algesic stimuli to confirm the tentative diagnosis. Insofar as they are not caused by cerebral or spinal lesions or disorders, sensory disorders follow the innervation pattern of the spinal nerve roots, plexus, and peripheral nerves. Knowledge of the segmental (radicular) and peripheral innervation pattern is crucial to making an accurate diagnosis. Overlapping between regions of sensory supply and variations in the pattern of sensory supply must also be taken into consideration. For example, the ring finger can be completely supplied by either the median nerve or the ulnar nerve. Figure 3.**40** shows the segmental sensory supply to the hand.

Peripheral sensory innervation is supplied by the following nerves:

- Radial nerve: this nerve supplies two and a half fingers on the radial side of the dorsum of the hand up to the distal phalanges of the index and middle finger. It also supplies the radial side of the dorsum. The skin area between the thumb and index finger is an autonomous area.
- Median nerve: this nerve supplies the palmar aspect of three and a half fingers and the adjacent areas of skin on the hand. The distal phalanges of the index and middle fingers are autonomous areas.
- Ulnar nerve: this nerve supplies the palmar aspect of one and a half fingers, the dorsal aspect of two and a half fingers, and adjacent areas of skin on the hand.

Tactile sensation is best examined using a cotton swab or the tip of your finger. Test pain using the rounded point of a wooden stick.

The entire upper extremity is best tested for tactile and pain sensation. This includes the medial and lateral aspects of the upper arm, the dorsum of the hand, and the finger pads. Nerves should also be palpated at circumscribed pressure points such as the carpal tunnel and Guyon's canal. A U-shaped piece of wire or bent paper clip can be used to test two-point discrimination. The ends of the wire should be only applied lightly. Pain and tactile tests are also performed on the trunk and lower extremities to avoid overlooking any dissociated disturbances.

Reflex Testing

Intrinsic and extrinsic reflexes can be tested in the hand. Muscle stretch reflexes include:

Trömner reflex. Tap your fingertips against the tips of the patient's slightly flexed fingers. This can cause reflexive contraction of the fingers and thumb. Only a difference between the two sides, or an extremely forceful reaction, is regarded as abnormal since this reaction can also be elicited in normal patients and in patients with autonomous nervous disorders.

Snapping reflex. The snapping reflex is a modification of the Trömner reflex. Perceptible snapping at the end of the nails on the middle and index fingers elicits sudden flexion of the fingers and thumb. Here too, only a difference between the two sides is regarded as abnormal.

The **Mayer metacarpophalangeal reflex** is an extrinsic reflex. Pressing the proximal phalanx of the fourth and fifth fingers into maximum flexion elicits a flexion reflex in the thumb. Since this reflex is extremely variable, only a one-sided reaction is regarded as abnormal. This suggests damage to the pyramidal tract, the median nerve, or ulnar nerve. The thumb reflex is a physiologic reflex. Tapping the long flexor tendon of the thumb produces flexion at the metacarpophalangeal joint of the thumb. This reaction will be absent if the median nerve is compressed.

3.3 Radiology

Indications, Diagnostic Value, and Clinical Relevance

Conventional radiography is still the most important imaging modality to supplement clinical examination in diagnosing hand injuries. Plain radiographs and stress views provide important information about the integrity of bony and ligamentous structures. These radiographic examinations provide the basis for further diagnostic studies. Because of the wide variety of shapes and varying intrinsic mobility of the individual skeletal elements, the position and contour of imaged structures will vary with the position of the hand and elbow and with forearm rotation. Pathologic changes can only be clearly distinguished from normal findings through the use of standardized examination techniques and standardized positioning of the entire upper extremity.

Occasionally, pain associated with acute injuries will make it difficult to achieve optimal positioning, particularly when other injuries to the same extremity are present. In these cases, the patient should be positioned carefully to minimize pain. Comparative radiographs of the contralateral side are helpful in interpreting inconclusive findings.

Standard Views of the Wrist

The PA and lateral views are routinely used for evaluating wrist structures (Figs. 3.41 a, b). The metacarpophalangeal joint and the distal forearm should be included in every view, and the hand should be in a neutral position. The central ray should be aimed at the lunate.

a   b

Figs. 3.**41 a, b**   Standard views of the wrist. PA view (**a**) and lateral view (**b**).

DP view. The patient is seated with the upper arm on the examining table, the shoulder abducted, and the elbow flexed 90°. The wrist is placed in a neutral position by precisely aligning the middle finger so that it forms a continuation of the axis of the forearm. An additional wedge may be placed under the extended fingers to prevent wrist flexion (Fig. 3.42).

Lateral view. In the lateral view, the patient's upper arm is adducted. The elbow is flexed 90° as for the DP view, and the ulnar edge of the hand lies on the examining table. The extended middle finger forms a continuation of the axis of the forearm in a neutral position (Fig. 3.**43**). Often it is helpful to use a supporting board on the extensor side of the hand and forearm. The X-ray tube is tilted 10° caudocranially for the view. This provides better exposure of the wrist.

These standard projections allow sufficient evaluation of most bony details under normal conditions (Table 3.**1**). Anatomical anomalies such as ossicles and fusion of individual carpal bones should be noted as these can influence carpal cinematics.

Standard radiographs also provide parameters for evaluation of the integrity of the wrist. These include:

- **Width of the intercarpal joint spaces.** The width of the intercarpal joint spaces varies only slightly between individuals; its maximum value is 2 mm. An increase beyond 2 mm is a sign of a tear of the intrin-

Fig. 3.**42**   Positioning for the standard PA radiograph of the wrist.

Fig. 3.**43**   Positioning for the standard lateral radiograph of the wrist.

sic ligaments as can occur in scapholunate dissociation.

- **Gilula arcs** (Fig. 3.**44**). According to Gilula (1979), three carpal arcs can be distinguished on the PA radiograph of the wrist. The first arc runs along the proximal convex articular surfaces of the first row of carpals, and the second arc along their distal concave articular surfaces. The last arc is formed by the proximal contours of the capitate and hamate. Discontinuity in the symmetry of these arcs is a sign of carpal instability.

- **Radial inclination** (Fig. 3.**45**). To measure the angle of the distal radius in the coronal plane, examine the PA film. Construct a line that intersects the most distal aspect of the radial styloid and the most proximal aspect of the ulnar side of the distal radius. Draw a line parallel to the longitudinal axis of the radius. Construct a perpendicular to the longitudinal line. The intersection of the perpendicular to the longitudinal and the line intersecting the most distal points on the radial and ulnar sides of the distal radius defines the radial inclination. Its normal value is 15°–20°. The angle is relevant for determining deformity, localizing dislocated fragments, and calculating the correction after a radial fracture.

- **Ratio of radial length to ulnar length** (Fig. 3.**46**). The radioulnar index provides information about anatomical anomalies (positive and negative ulnar variance) and about the extent of subluxation of the distal radioulnar joint after radial fractures. This index is defined by the distance between the two lines perpendicular to the respective longitudinal axes of the radius and ulna. On the radius, the perpendicular line is drawn midway between the most distal point on the dorsal aspect and the most distal and ulnar point on the palmar aspect. On the ulna, the perpendicular line is drawn along the articular surface of the distal ulna.

Table 3.**1**   Structures and abnormal findings that can be evaluated in the standard projections

PA view	
Structure visualized	Abnormal findings
Carpal bones	Fractures, arthritis
Radiocarpal joint	Avascular necrosis of:
Distal radioulnar joint	Radius, ulna, scaphoid, lunate
Carpometacarpal joints	Capitate, metacarpals
Metacarpals	Scapholunate dissociation
Metacarpophalangeal joint	Infections
Lateral view	
Structure visualized	Abnormal findings
Longitudinal view of:	Fractures of:
Radius	Radius, ulna, triquetrum
Scaphoid	Metacarpals
Lunate	Dislocation of the lunate
Capitate	Perilunate dislocations
Third metacarpal	Intercarpal dislocations
	Metacarpal dislocations

Fig. 3.**44** Gilula arcs.

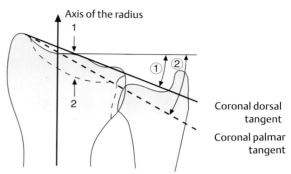

Fig. 3.**45** Angle of inclination of the distal radius in the coronal plane.
① Coronal dorsal angle. ② Coronal palmar angle. 1 Dorsal margin of the radius. 2 palmar margin of the radius.

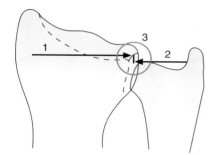

Fig. 3.**46** Radioulnar index. 1 Radial measuring point. 2 Ulnar measuring point. 3 Radioulnar index.

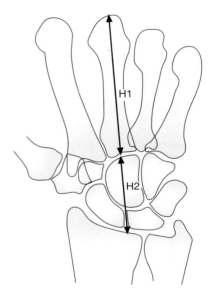

Fig. 3.**47** Carpal height index.

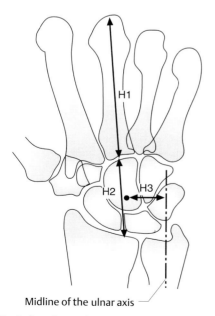

Fig. 3.**48** Index of carpal deviation (ulnar translocation).

• **Carpal height index** (Fig. 3.**47**). This can be determined from the quotient of the height of the midcarpal column (H2) and the length of the metacarpal (H1). The index is reduced in fractures, ligament lesions, arthritis, and carpal collapse. Its normal value according to Sennwald (1987) is 0.54±0.003.

• **Index of carpal deviation and ulnar translocation** (Fig. 3.**48**). The index of carpal deviation is determined by the quotient of H3/H1. H3 represents the distance between the straight line H2 and the midline of the ulnar axis to be measured at the level of the capitate head. Its normal value according to Seenwald (1987) is 0.30±0.03. The convex can be changed by a tear or elongation of the extrinsic ligaments with resulting ulnar translocation of the carpus.

• **Angle of inclination of the distal radial articular surface in the sagittal plane** (Fig. 3.**49**). Together

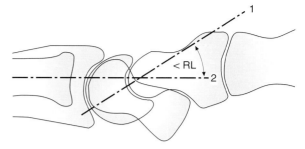

Fig. 3.**49**   Angle of inclination of the distal radial articular surface in the sagittal plane.

Fig. 3.**50**   Radiolunate angle (average value –5°). 1 Axis of the lunate. 2 Axis of the radius.

Fig. 3.**51**   Capitolunate angle (average value –5°). 1 Axis of the lunate. 2 Axis of the capitate.

Fig. 3.**52**   Scapholunate angle (average value <70°). 1 Axis of the lunate. 2 Axis of the scaphoid.

with the coronal radioulnar angle, this angle has practical significance in the evaluation of radius fractures. Its normal value ranges from 15°–25°.

● **Radiolunate angle** (Fig. 3.**50**). This is the angle between the lateral longitudinal axis of the radius and the central axis of the lunate. Its average value is –5°; the angle becomes positive if the lunate is angled toward the dorsal side. A change in this angle is a sign of carpal ligament damage with associated instability. Dorsal intercalated segment instability (DISI), with a radiolunate angle exceeding +15°, is differentiated from palmar intercallated segment instability (PISI) with a radiolunate angle of less than –20° (according to Linscheid et al., 1972).

● **Capitolunate angle** (Fig. 3.**51**). This is created by the intersection of the longitudinal axes of the capitate and lunate. The average value is –5°. In instablility, the capitolunate angle is affected similarly to the radiolunate angle. However, it is less accurate than the radiolunate angle because the axis of the capitate is more difficult to determine than that of the radius.

● **Scapholunate angle** (Fig. 3.**52**). This angle is created by the intersection of the longitudinal axes of the scaphoid and lunate. Its average value is 47°, but it can vary between 30° and 70°. Values exceeding 70° are regarded as abnormal and suggest a lesion of the

scapholunate ligaments or the ligament complex between the scaphoid and the trapezium and trapezoid. Values under 30° suggest a palmar instability.

● **Longitudinal axes of the radius, capitate, and third metacarpal.** The longitudinal axes of the radius, capitate, and metacarpals normally correlate.

● **Tangent of the hamate and longitudinal axis of the radius.** The tangent on the metacarpal articular line of the hamate should intersect the longitudinal axis of the radius at a right angle.

Special Views of the Wrist

The standard views described in the previous section can be inadequate for certain clinical settings and for a more precise determination of the extent of injury to individual carpal bones. Additional projections are often required. The most common ones are briefly described in the following section.

● **PD (palmar-dorsal) view.** Compared with the PA view, the width of the carpal joint spaces is demonstrated more clearly. This can be significant in evaluating a scapholunate dissociation. The ulnar styloid is projected in the middle, as opposed to the edge, of the ulna in the DP view. This feature can be used to distinguish the two projections.

- **PA view with the ulnar side of the hand elevated 20°.** This view is helpful in better demonstrating the articular surfaces between the scaphoid and lunate because the articular surfaces are parallel to the central ray in this projection.

- **Forty-five-degree oblique view in pronation.** This view is helpful primarily for imaging the dorsal aspect of the triquetrum, the radiopalmar part of the scaphoid, and the hamate. It also allows better evaluation of the radial styloid and the articulations between the scaphoid and trapezium and trapezium and trapezoid. The hand and forearm are positioned on a 45° wedge of foam rubber. As in the DP view, the shoulder is abducted 90° and the elbow flexed 90°.

- **Thirty-five-degree oblique view in supination.** This view illustrates the pisiform and the articulation between the pisiform and triquetrum. The ulnar edge of the hand rests on the film cassette. A wedge of foam rubber is used to stabilize the dorsal aspect.

- **Views in ulnar and radial deviation.** Abnormally increased intrinsic mobility of individual bones appears in various wrist radiographs as changes in the width of the intercarpal joint spaces. These findings can provide information about the integrity of the carpal ligament system. The DP view in ulnar deviation also more clearly demonstrates the scaphoid that appears foreshortened in the routine DP view because of its palmar tilt. The view in radial deviation improves exposure of the ulnar compartment. A suspected scapholunate dissociation can be accentuated in a radiograph obtained in ulnar deviation with the fist clenched.

- **Views in flexion and extension.** These projections can also be helpful in the evaluation of carpal instability. However, as with the other special views they only provide a static image of the momentary carpal configuration and do not provide information about dynamic aspects.

- **Clenched-fist DP views.** This is a useful additional view for evaluating suspected intercarpal ligament damage. Muscle tension can demonstrate widening of the joint space (>2 mm).

- **Stress views.** These views can also demonstrate the integrity of the carpal ligaments.

- **Carpal tunnel view.** This view is useful for demonstrating the hook of the hamate, the pisiform, and the palmar surface of the trapezium. A radiograph in this projection should be obtained when evaluating carpal tunnel syndrome involving a suspected bony mass. If there is stenosis of the carpal tunnel due to bony structures, endoscopic transection of the roof of the carpal tunnel is contraindicated. Various techniques may be used for obtaining the carpal tunnel radio-

Figs. 3.**53a–c** Positioning techniques for the carpal tunnel view. (**a**) The forearm and hand in ulnar deviation are held in supination at an angle of 135° on a wedge of foam rubber. (**b**) The affected hand is held in maximum flexion with a strap or the other hand. (**c**) The heel of the hand is pressed flat on the film cassette with the wrist hyperextended.

graph, although the radiographs obtained using the positioning schemes described are not identical. Choose the technique that is least painful for the patient (Figs. 3.**53a–c**).

- **Scaphoid series** (Figs. 3.**54a–d**). A scaphoid series can be helpful to better visualize the scaphoid and other carpal bones where clinical evidence suggests a scaphoid fracture. This series improves exposure of the intercarpal joint spaces. The scaphoid series consists of a sequence of the following four radiographs, each obtained with the hand in a different position:

— Wrist hyperextended and in ulnar deviation with the fist clenched and the thumb extended.
— 15° supination view.
— 15° pronation view.
— Lateral view in a neutral position.

For the PA view, the upper arm is abducted 90° in the shoulder and the elbow is flexed 90°. The hand is in ulnar deviation with the fist clenched and the thumb is extended along the axis of the radius. A 15° foam-rubber wedge is used to stabilize the wrist in supination and pronation. The lateral view is identical to the standard lateral projection except that it images a smaller area.

Figs. 3.**54a–d**   Scaphoid series

examination. Depending on the indication, the motion may be performed actively by the patient or passively by the examiner. Comparison with the contralateral side is recommended when findings are inconclusive. Disadvantages of this method include the relatively high cost of the technology and increased radiation exposure. Cinefluoroscopy with full slow-motion capabilities is currently only available at a few centers.

Standard Views of the Metacarpal Region and the Entire Hand

In contrast to standard views of the wrist, the PA projection is usually supplemented with a standard oblique view in 45° pronation when imaging the metacarpal region or the entire hand. This is because the metacarpals and phalanges are superimposed in a true lateral view. To image the hand, the central ray is aimed at the head of the third metacarpal in the PA view and at the head of the second metacarpal in the oblique view. To image the metacarpal region, the central ray is aimed at the base of the metacarpals. The arm is positioned for the standard view with the shoulder abducted 90° and the elbow in 90° flexion. For the oblique view the fingers are slightly abducted, and the hand and forearm are supported with a 45° wedge of foam rubber. A true lateral view may also be obtained to evaluate the angles between the longitudinal axes of the radius, scaphoid, lunate, and capitate.

Dynamic Examination of the Wrist

Often, static radiographs obtained using standard views will fail to demonstrate instability of the wrist. Instability may only be apparent when the wrist is in motion. Where there is clinical suspicion of a ligament injury, such as a snapping or clicking phenomenon, a dynamic radiographic examination of the wrist (cinefluoroscopy) can be performed. Cinefluoroscopy makes it possible to document the complex motion of the carpus in adduction and abduction and flexion and extension on videotape. The motion sequence can then be precisely analyzed in slow motion after the

Standard and Special Views of the Fingers and Thumb

The standard projections of the fingers and thumb are identical to those used for the wrist. Complete evaluation of bony structures also requires both a PA view and a true lateral view. The central ray is aimed at the respective proximal interphalangeal joint of a finger (Figs. 3.**55a–c**) or at the metacarpophalangeal joint of the thumb (Figs. 3.**56a, b**). Damage to the capsular ligaments of the fingers with collateral ligament tears is often encountered in addition to injuries to the bones. Stress views have proven effective in routine

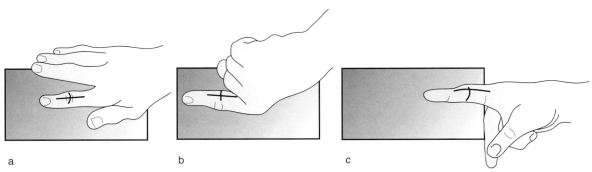

a   b   c

Figs. 3.**55a–c**   Positioning for the PA and lateral views of the index finger.

Figs. 3.**56a, b** Positioning for the PA and lateral views of the thumb.

use in evaluating suspected ligament tears and supplementing inconclusive clinical findings. These views may require a nerve block to eliminate pain. Always obtain views of both sides for comparison. Ligament injuries in this region most frequently involve the ulnar collateral ligament in the metacarpophalangeal joint of the thumb. As in clinical examination, stress views should be prepared with the thumb in 20°–30° flexion (a jig may be used if necessary) because a complete tear of the actual collateral ligament can be overlooked in extension if the accessory collateral ligament remains intact. A difference between the two sides exceeding 10° also suggests a ligament tear.

For detailed views of the interphalangeal joints and phalanges, consider the use of dental bitewing films. These high-quality small films (1 in × 1.5 in) can be obtained in conjunction with a cooperative dentist and have the additional advantage of being able to be included in the patient's chart.

Tomography

Conventional tomography has largely been supplanted by CT and MRI because of the superior quality of image provided by these modalities. However, conventional tomography remains a low-cost modality that is useful for demonstrating fractures or pseudarthroses.

Abnormal Findings

Fractures

- **Distal forearm**
The most frequent cause of such fractures is a fall on the extended hand or, less frequently, the flexed hand. The resulting fracture is influenced by the degree of pronation or supination and by the radial or ulnar

deviation of the hand. Other factors that influence pathophysiology include the magnitude of the forces, the impact zone, counteracting forces, and bone mineralization. The following classic forms of fractures are described in the literature but more common usage is to avoid the eponyms, using descriptions instead.

- **Hyperextension**
Colles fracture (Figs. 3.**57a–e**). The most frequent fracture of the distal forearm occurs as a result of a fall on the outstretched extended hand with the forearm in pronation. Generally, the distal fragment of the radius is impacted and displaced radially and dorsally, or angled in that direction. This produces a typical bayonet deformity. The classic fracture line is extra-articular, generally located 2–3 cm from the articular surface of the distal radius. Often this is accompanied by an avulsion of the ulnar styloid.

Barton fracture. (Fig. 3.**59**) This intra-articular fracture involves the dorsal margin of the distal radius. Occasionally it will be accompanied by a dislocation of the radiocarpal joint. In a volar Barton fracture (Fig. 3.**60**), the fracture line runs through the palmar margin of the distal radius.

- **Hyperflexion**
Smith fracture (Figs. 3.**58a–c**). This is a less frequently encountered fracture of the distal radius that occurs as a result of a fall on the dorsum of the hand or from a direct blow to the dorsum of the hand in flexion. The distal fragment is displaced and angled toward the palmar aspect. The fracture gap can occasionally extend as far as the radiocarpal joint. Smith fractures are divided into three types according to the obliquity of the fracture gap.

Figs. 3.**57a–e**   Variations of the Colles fracture.

Figs. 3.**58a–c**   Variations of the Smith fracture.
(**a**) Fracture gap extends transversely from the dorsal cortex to the palmar cortex of the radius.
(**b**) Oblique fracture-line from the dorsal lip of the radius to the palmar cortex.
(**c**) Intra-articular fracture extending to the palmar cortex of the distal radius.

Fig. 3.**59**   Dorsal Barton fracture.   Fig. 3.**60**   Volar Barton fracture.   Fig. 3.**61**   Hutchinson fracture

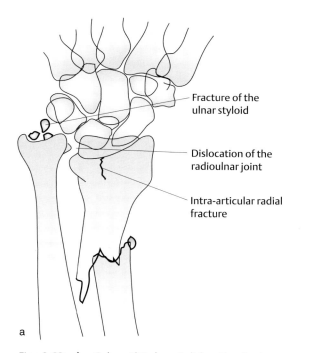

Fracture of the
ulnar styloid

Dislocation of the
radioulnar joint

Intra-articular radial
fracture

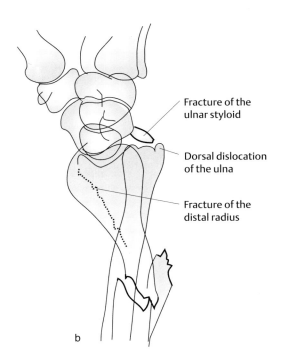

Fracture of the
ulnar styloid

Dorsal dislocation
of the ulna

Fracture of the
distal radius

a   b

Figs. 3.**62a, b**   Galeazzi/Piedmont dislocation fracture.

Palmar Barton fracture. Avulsion of the palmar margin of the distal radius.

- **Axial impacted fractures**

Chauffeur fracture. In the chauffeur fracture, the fracture gap extends obliquely through the base of the radial styloid. This type of fracture is frequently associated with carpal fractures.

Hutchinson fracture (Fig. 3.**61**). This intra-articular fracture involves the radial aspect of the distal radius.

Punch fracture. A punch fracture occurs when the lunate fossa of the radius is impacted.

- **Direct trauma to the radius**

Galeazzi/Piedmont fracture dislocation (Figs. 3.**62a, b**). This is a fracture of the distal radial shaft that can extend into the radiocarpal joint with accompanying dislocation of the ulna in the distal radioulnar joint. Typically, the proximal end of the distal fragment is dorsally displaced and palmarly angled. This type of fracture results from a fall on the outstretched arm with the forearm in extreme pronation.

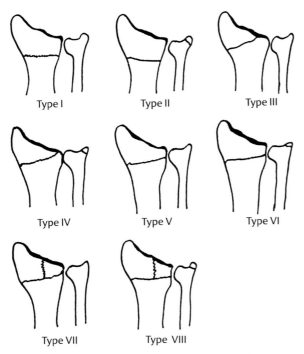

Type I   Type II   Type III

Type IV   Type V   Type VI

Type VII   Type VIII

Fig. 3.63   Frykman's classification of distal radial fractures.
Type I   Extra-articular fracture without a fracture of the
          ulnar styloid.
Type II   Extra-articular fracture with a fracture of the ulnar
          styloid.
Type III Radiocarpal joint fracture without a fracture of
          the ulnar styloid.
Type IV   Radiocarpal joint fracture with a fracture of the
          ulnar styloid.
Type V   Radioulnar joint fracture without a fracture of the
          ulnar styloid.
Type VI   Radioulnar joint fracture with a fracture of the
          ulnar styloid.
Type VII Radiocarpal and radioulnar joint fracture without
          a fracture of the ulnar styloid.
Type VIII Radiocarpal and radioulnar joint fracture with a
          fracture of the ulnar styloid.

• Fractures in children

Slipped epiphyses and epiphyseal and metaphyseal fractures. These fractures are classified using the Salter and Harris criteria, modified by Rang, set out in Table 3.2.

There are many other fracture classification systems in the literature. The most common of these, the classifications of Frykman (1967) and Müller et al. (AO/ASIF classification 1987), are briefly described in the following section.

Frykman's classification distinguishes between extra-articular and intra-articular fractures. The system views the radiocarpal and radioulnar joints separately, and distinguishes fractures with involvement of the ulnar styloid from those without (Fig. 3.63). A disadvantage of this categorization is that it fails to consider dorsal and ulnar dislocation or soft-tissue

Table 3.2   Classification of epiphyseal and metaphyseal fractures

	Salter-Harris modified by Rang
Simple slipped epiphysis	I
Slipped epiphysis with metaphyseal fragment	II
Fracture through the physis and epiphysis	III
Combined epiphyseal and metaphyseal fracture	IV
Crush injury of physis	V
Perichondral ring injury	VI

injuries in the wrist that frequently accompany these fractures (lesions to the capsule ligament and triangular fibrocartilage).

The AO/ASIF classification addresses the respective displacement of the fragments, although it also does not consider accompanying soft-tissue injuries.

Type A refers to strictly extra-articular fractures:

A 1:   ulnar fracture with the radius intact.
A 2:   radial fracture without a metaphyseal zone of comminution or impaction.
A 3:   radial fracture with metaphyseal zone of comminution or impaction.

Type B refers to a simple intra-articular fracture:

B 1:   fracture of the radial styloid.
B 2:   fracture with dorsal displacement of the fragments.
B 3:   fracture with palmar displacement of the fragments.

Type C refers to a multiple-fragment intra-articular fracture:

C 1:   congruity of the articular surfaces is intact.
C 2:   congruity of the articular surfaces is destroyed, but with a simple metaphyseal fracture.
C 3:   congruity of the articular surfaces is destroyed and a compound metaphyseal fracture is present.

An additional index (1–3) describes the respective severity of the fracture or the direction of dislocation of the fragments (Fig. 3.64).

Carpal bones. Carpal fractures occur frequently, although acute nondisplaced fractures can be difficult to diagnose. As a general rule, plain radiographs of the wrist in four planes should be obtained. CT, nuclear medicine studies, or MRI can be helpful where findings are inconclusive but clinical suspicion of a fracture persists. Table 3.3 shows an overview of the incidence of various carpal fractures.

A = Extra-articular

–A1 Isolated ulna

–A2 Colles fracture without metaphyseal comminution zone or impaction

–A3 Colles fracture with metaphyseal comminution zone or impaction

B = Simple intra-articular radial fracture (epiphysis and metaphysis intact)

–B1 Styloid

–B2 Fragment dorsal (Barton fracture)

–B3 Fragment palmar (volar Barton fracture, Smith fracture II)

C = Multiple fragment intra-articular radial fracture

–C1 Congruity of the articular surfaces is intact; simple metaphyseal fracture

–C2 Congruity of the articular surfaces is destroyed; simple metaphyseal fracture (ulnar fracture disregarded)

–C3 Complex metaphyseal fracture

Fig. 3.**64**   AO/ASIF classification of distal radial fractures.

Table 3.**3**   Incidence of carpal fractures

Fracture	Incidence	Fracture	Incidence
Scaphoid	78.8%	Lunate	1.4%
Triquetrum	13.8%	Pisiform	1.0%
Trapezium	2.3%	Capitate	1.0%
Hamate	1.5%	Trapezoid	0.2%

• **Scaphoid.** Fractures of the scaphoid are the second most frequent fracture in the upper extremity (Fig. 3.**65**). Young men are most frequently affected. The cause is usually a fall on an ulnarly deviated, outstretched hand. The acronym FOSH or FOOSH (fall on outstretched hand) is often seen in reports. Scaphoid fractures can be categorized in various fracture types according to the fracture line, stability of the fragments, and location of the fracture (Fig. 3.**66a–d**, Table 3.**4**). Classification according to location has prognostic significance as it considers the blood supply to the scaphoid. Fractures in the middle and distal third of the scaphoid heal relatively easily due to the good vascular supply to the fragments. Healing tends to be protracted in proximal fractures due to the comparatively poor vascularization; pseudarthrosis and

Fig. 3.**65**   Scaphoid fracture.

Figs. 3.**66a–d** Classification of scaphoid fractures.

Fig. 3.**67** Scaphoid pseudarthrosis and avascular necrosis of the proximal fragment.

avascular necrosis of the proximal fragment occur frequently (Fig. 3.**67**). Vertical fractures have a poorer prognosis than transverse fractures. Shear forces acting across the fracture result in a relatively high incidence of pseudarthrosis.

Scaphoid fractures are often difficult to diagnose. The symptoms are often minimal, and routine radiographs can be normal, particularly if there is minimal fracture fragment displacement. Where there is clinical suspicion of a fracture but a scaphoid series fails to clearly demonstrate fracture gaps, we recommend a short arm-thumb spica and follow-up radiographic examination 2 weeks later. If radiographic findings are again negative and clinical suspicion persists, CT examination of the hand in two planes is indicated.

Radiographic features that influence treatment include:

– Dislocated fragments.
– Demonstration of a third fragment.
– Fracture gap wider than 1 mm.
– Ligament instability.

Delayed diagnosis of a scaphoid fracture can lead to complications such as pseudarthrosis, avascular necrosis with subsequent early carpal arthritis, and carpal collapse. Scaphoid pseudarthrosis is observed in 1.3–10% of all diagnosed scaphoid fractures (Monsivais et al. 1986). Pseudarthrosis may be stable or unstable and may show degenerative changes.

SLAC wrist (scapholunate advanced collapse, described by Watson and Ryu 1986) (Table 3.**5**):

Table 3.**4**   Herbert's classification of scaphoid fractures

Type	Description
A1	Tubercle fracture
A2	Nondislocated fracture in the midscaphoid
B1	Oblique fracture
B2	Dislocated (unstable) fracture in the midscaphoid
B3	Fracture of the proximal scaphoid
B4	Fracture with extreme dislocation

Table 3.**5**   Stages of carpal collapse according to Watson and Ryn 1986

Stage	Scaphoid pseudarthrosis
1	Radial styloid and scaphoid
2	Radioscaphoid articulation
3	Capitolunate ± scaphocapitate joint
4	Scapholunate dissociation and migration of the capitate proximally

Fig. 3.**68**   Fracture of the triquetrum.

Fig. 3.**69**   Avulsion fracture of the trapezium.

— Stage 1: arthritis is limited to the radial styloid and scaphoid.
— Stage 2: radioscaphoid articulation.
— Stage 3: capitolunate ± scaphocapitate joint.
— Stage 4: scapholunate dissociation and migration of the capitate proximally.

Radiographic signs of scaphoid pseudarthrosis include resorption zones, resorption cysts, sclerotic halos and superficial areas of sclerosis, periscaphoid arthritis, widening of the pseudarthrosis gap, sclerosis of the proximal fragment, osteoporosis due to inactivity, rotation of the fragments, and axial carpal deformities.

● **Lunate.** Fractures of the lunate are rare and are difficult to diagnose with plain radiographs. Generally the palmar aspect is affected. The cause of the fracture is usually a fall on the hyperextended hand or a blow to the palm of the hand. These fractures also occur as sequelae of Kienböck disease or in association with a perilunar dislocation. CT examination is recommended where there is clinical suspicion of a lunate fracture and radiographic findings are normal. Nuclear medicine and MR studies can be helpful in diagnosing these fractures.

● **Triquetrum.** The cause of a fracture of the triquetrum is either a fall on the hand with the wrist in maximum extension or flexion, or rotation against acute forceful resistance. A differentiation is made between the benign chip fractures, dorsal avulsion of one or more fragments that account for approximately 90% of all fractures, and fractures of the body of the bone itself that are far less frequent (Fig. 3.**68**). The fracture gap is best evaluated in the lateral projection and in an oblique view with the wrist in pronation. Radiographic diagnosis of these fractures is often difficult due to overlapping structures.

● **Pisiform.** Pisiform fractures occur as the result of direct or indirect trauma to the ulnar edge of the hand

and forceful contraction of the flexor carpi ulnaris. Pisiform fractures are occasionally overlooked in routine radiographs. These fractures are best evaluated in radiographs obtained with the wrist in ulnar deviation and the ulnar edge of the hand raised 10°, and in oblique radiographs. A carpal tunnel view may also be useful.

● **Trapezium.** In addition to avulsion fractures (Fig. 3.**69**) of the radial and dorsoulnar tubercles, longitudinal and comminuted fractures of the trapezium are observed. The cause is either direct trauma to the carpal region or the abducted thumb, or a fall on the hand with the wrist extended and in radial deviation. In the latter case, the trapezium is compressed at the base of the first metacarpal and the radial styloid. Trapezium fractures frequently occur in conjunction with an oblique fracture at the base of the first metacarpal and subluxation in the first carpometacarpal joint (Bennett fracture dislocation). On the whole, such fractures of the wrist are rare and can be difficult to diagnose in radiographs. Where a bony fragment can be demonstrated radial to the carpometacarpal joint and a fracture of the trapezium is excluded, an ossicle should be considered. This can usually be visualized in a 45° oblique radiograph with the wrist in supination and ulnar deviation.

● **Trapezoid.** Fractures of the trapezoid are rare. They may occur with a longitudinal impact on the second metacarpal or with direct trauma with the wrist in extreme extension. Dislocations are best demonstrated in the routine radiographs.

● **Capitate.** Fractures of the capitate often occur in combination with injuries to the scaphoid and other carpal bones in a perilunar dislocation (this is known as a scaphocapitate fracture syndrome). Isolated fractures are rare. A differentiation is made between transverse fractures of the body and intra-articular dorsal avulsion fractures, possibly combined with dorsal dislocation of the third metacarpal. There are no radiographic projections of these injuries. CT examinations can be helpful if there is clinical evidence of a fracture.

Fig. 3.**70**   Special view for imaging the hook of the hamate.

a   b

Figs. 3.**71a, b**   De Quervain fracture dislocation.

• **Hamate.** Fractures of the hamate, while rare, are among the most frequent injuries to the distal row of carpal bones. In addition to avulsion fractures of the hook of the hamate, fractures of the body of the hamate also occur. Hypothenar pain on palpation is characteristic. Where a fracture is suspected, a carpal tunnel view should be obtained in addition to the routine radiographs to better image the hook of the hamate. Another useful projection is the view shown in Figure 3.**70** in which the hand is held in a semi-oblique position in maximum radial deviation. Fractures of the hook of the hamate can also occur in sports such as baseball, ice hockey, or golf, when a piece of athletic equipment is forcefully pressed against the tubercle, as can occur in golf when the club inadvertently strikes the ground. Fractures of the body of the hamate usually result from longitudinal impact on the fifth metacarpal in a fall on the hand. This occasionally occurs in tennis players.

Dislocations and Fracture Dislocations of the Carpal Bones

In addition to fracture dislocations, dislocations and subluxations in the carpal bones can also be evaluated when the examiner is thoroughly familiar with the radiographic anatomy of the hand. The normal carpal arcs (Gilula arcs) are helpful as landmarks in the dorsopalmar projection. The physiologic angle of the carpal bones in the lateral plane should be known. Instability, particularly in the mobile proximal row of carpals, can appear as a radiographic abnormality with minimal symptoms. However, the radiographic abnormality can be associated with significant clinical symptoms.

Carpal dislocation injuries are classified as follows:

— Perilunar and lunate dislocations.
— Perilunar and lunate fracture dislocation.

— Scaphocapitate fracture syndrome (Fenton syndrome).
— Axial dislocations and fracture dislocation.

The most common dislocation is the perilunar dislocation which is associated with severe ligamentous injury. Occasionally it occurs in isolation, although more often in combination with fractures of the scaphoid (De Quervain fracture dislocation or trans-scaphoid perilunar dislocation, Figs. 3.**71a, b**, capitate, triquetrum, and the radial or ulnar styloid. The severity and location of injury depend on the magnitude, direction, and velocity of the traumatic forces, and on the position of the wrist at the time of the accident. As in the majority of carpal injuries, the cause of peri-lunate dislocation is a fall on the extended hand in ulnar deviation and supination.

In plain radiographs, the dorsal perilunar dislocation is most readily discernible as a disruption of the normally straight line of the central axis of the radius, lunate, capitate, and the third metacarpal. The capitate is dorsally displaced with respect to the lunate and radius and crosses the dorsal line of the radius. The proximal surface of the lunate and radius retain their articular connection, although the lunate can be slightly tilted because of the perilunar dislocation. In the DP view, the dislocation appears as a disruption of the contour of Gilula arcs II and III with overlapping of the capitate and lunate (Figs. 3.**72,a, b**). The diagnosis is easier to make when additional radiographs in two planes are obtained, with strong longitudinal traction. This will require a regional anesthetic.

Mayfield et al. (1980) describes four stages of perilunar dislocation:

• In stage I, the scapholunate and radioscaphoid ligament connections tear. The radiocapitate ligament is overstretched. This results in scapholunate disso-

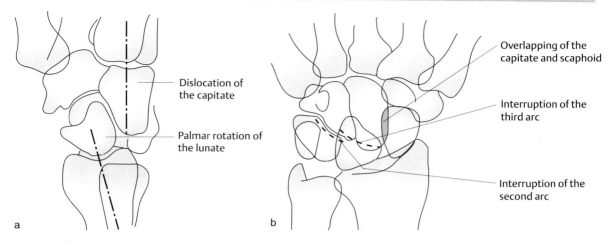

Figs. 3.**72a, b** Dorsal perilunate dislocation in the PA view (**a**) and lateral view (**b**).

ciation with simultaneous rotational subluxation of the scaphoid. This dissociation can generally be demonstrated on PA function radiographs with the wrist in radial and/or ulnar deviation and the fist clenched. Widening of the joint space exceeding 2 mm is regarded as abnormal (Terry-Thomas sign). Additional radiographic characteristics include foreshortening of the scaphoid due to rotation about its transverse axis. Contrary to normal findings, this foreshortening will also be seen in ulnar deviation. Another characteristic sign is the ring-like thickening of the distal scaphoid as the head is imaged parallel to the plane of projection. This is known as the ring sign.

- Stage II is a perilunar dislocation. The capitolunate ligaments are damaged. The lunate and capitate move apart. There is insufficiency of the radiocapitate and radial collateral ligaments.
- Stage III is characterized by divergence of the lunate and triquetrum. The carpal ligaments between the triquetrum and lunate, the radius and

triquetrum, and the ulna and triquetrum are torn or avulsed; occasionally the triquetrum is fractured. Dorsal perilunar dislocation occurs.
- In stage IV the dorsal radiocarpal ligament tears. The capitate displaces the lunate, now only attached to the radiolunate and ulnolunate ligaments, toward the palmar aspect of the wrist out of the proximal row of carpal bones. A palmar lunate dislocation occurs.

In palmar lunate dislocation, the lunate tilts over the palmar margin of the distal articular surface of the radius while the capitate and radius remain in their normal positions. The palmar rotation and dislocation of the lunate are readily discernible in the lateral radiograph. In the DP view, the dislocated lunate typically appears triangular or wedge-shaped. Gilula arcs are disrupted, and the radial contour of the lunate overlaps with that of the scaphoid (Figs. 3.**73a,b**).

Occasionally it will be difficult to precisely classify a dislocation in spite of the relative positions of the axis of the capitate, lunate, and radius. The capi-

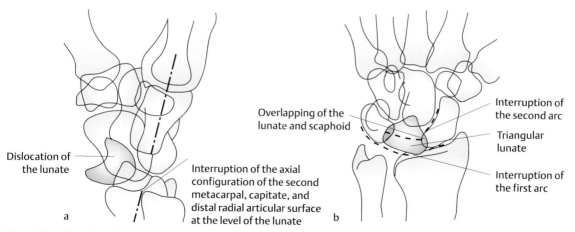

Figs. 3.**73a, b** Palmar lunate dislocation.

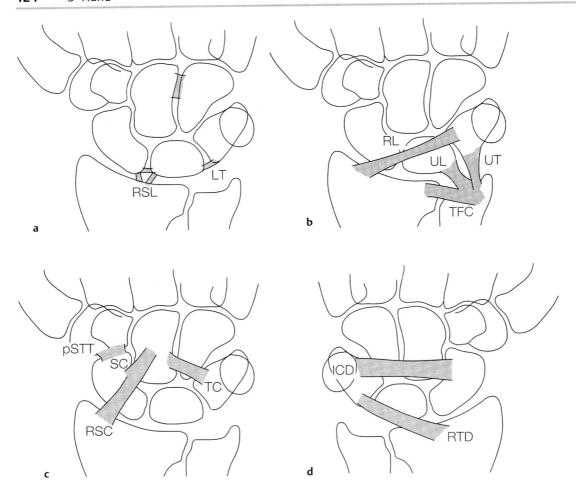

Figs. 3.**74a–d** Diagram of the most important carpal ligaments.
a Interosseous ligaments. Abbreviations: CH = capitohamate ligament, LT = lunotriquetral ligament, RSF = radiolunotriquetral ligament, SL = scapholunate ligament.
b Volar proximal V ligaments. Abbreviations: RLT = radiolunotriquetral ligament, TFC = triangular fibrocartilage, UL = ulnolunate branch of the ulnolunatotriquetral ligament, UT = ulnotriquetral branch of the ulnolunatotriquetral ligament.
c Volar distal V ligaments. Abbreviations: pSST = palmar scaphotrapeziotrapezoid ligament, RSC = radioscaphocapitate ligament.
d Dorsal V ligaments. Abbreviations: DIC = dorsal intercarpal ligament, DRT = dorsal radiotriquetral ligament.

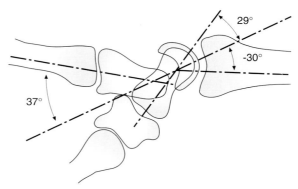

Fig. 3.75 Dorsal instability with a scapholunate angle of 105° (normal value is 60°), positive radiolunate angle (49°), and negative capitolunate angle (–48°). Dorsal rotation of the lunate and palmar rotation of the scaphoid.

Fig. 3.76 Palmar instability with a scapholunate angle of 29°, negative radiolunate angle (–30°), and positive capitolunate angle (37°). Palmar rotation of the lunate and dorsal rotation of the capitate.

a   b

Figs. 3.77 a, b   Scapholunate dissociation.

tate can cross the dorsal line of the radius and the lunate can cross the palmar line of the radius in the radiograph, and the relationship of both carpal bones to the distal radius may be disrupted.

Carpal Instability

The integrity of the carpal bones is crucial to the function of the wrist. Although instability, particularly in the proximal row of carpal bones, can be asymptomatic and only demonstrated by radiographic examination, it is usually very symptomatic. The term carpal instability describes a disturbance in the physiologic connection among the carpal bones themselves and between these bones and the radius. The cause can be either traumatic or degenerative. Injuries to the scaphoid in particular, which is thought to contribute significantly to the stability of the wrist, can lead to instability (Figs. 3.74 a–d).

Other causes of instability include carpal fractures, ligament injuries, congenital ligament laxity, radial fracture malunion, avascular necrosis of the lunate, inflammatory conditions, and degenerative joint disease. Forms of carpal instability are differentiated as follows.

- **Carpal instability defined according to the dorsal or palmar tilt of the lunate**
  - Dorsal intercallated segment instability (DISI) (Fig. 3.75).
  - Palmar intercallated segment instability (PISI) (Fig. 3.76).

Dorsal flexion instability is more common. This involves insufficiency or a tear of the scapholunate ligament connections that causes the scaphoid and lunate to tilt. The distal articular surface of the lunate tilts dorsally, while the scaphoid moves toward the palmar aspect of the wrist. Dorsal instability frequently occurs with scapholunate dissociation (Figs. 3.77 a, b), an unstable fracture of the scaphoid, and perilunar dislocation.

The following radiographic signs indicate **dorsal flexion instability**.

- **In the AP projection:**
  - Overlapping of the lunate and scaphoid.
  - Foreshortening of the scaphoid.
  - Ring sign in the scaphoid as the cortex of the distal scaphoid is imaged parallel to the plane of projection.
  - Triangular shape of the lunate resulting from the dorsal tilt. Normal shape is trapezoidal.

- **In the true lateral projection:**
  - Lunate tilted in dorsal extension.
  - Scapholunate angle exceeds 70°.
  - Positive radiolunate angle exceeds +15° (usually +20°–+50°) (average value –5°).
  - Negative capitolunate angle (usually –20°––50°) (average value –5°).

Palmar flexion instability is encountered less frequently, primarily occurring where the integrity of the carpal region is compromised. This may be the case in avasvular necrosis of the lunate resulting in extensive loss of substance or in congenital or posttraumatic carpal ligament insufficiency. Weakness of the intercarpal ulnar ligaments produces a palmar tilt in the articular surface of the lunate, while the distal portion of the capitate deviates dorsally.

The following radiographic signs indicate **palmar flexion instability**.

- **In the AP projection:**
— Foreshortening of the scaphoid.
— Overlapping of the lunate and capitate.

- **In the true lateral projection:**
— Lunate tilted in palmar flexion.
— Scapholunate angle is reduced to less than 30°.
— Negative radiolunate angle (less than –20°).
— Positive capitolunate angle (greater than 30°).

- **Carpal instability defined according to location**
Radial (lateral) instability between the scaphoid and the adjacent carpals (lunate, trapezium, trapezoid, and capitate). The most common form is the scapholunate dissociation with or without dorsal instability.

Ulnar (medial) instability between the triquetrum, lunate, and hamate. This is further differentiated as triquetrolunate instability or triquetrohamate dissociation. Complete triquetrolunate dissociation occurs in the radiographic syndrome of PISI. Triquetrohamate dissociation can occur in the form of palmar or dorsal flexion instability and can be differentiated from the triquetrolunate form under fluoroscopy.

Proximal instability in the radiocarpal joint. This instability can occur in isolation, as a result of a ligament tear or distal radial fracture healing deformity, or in combination with radial or ulnar carpal instability. A differentiation is made between dorsal and palmar carpal subluxation with a permanent subluxation deformity of the entire wrist region relative to the longitudinal axis of the radius.

- **Other forms of instability**
What is known as ulnar translocation generally occurs as a sequela of rheumatoid arthritis. The entire wrist is displaced relative to the radius and ulnar so that the distance between the radial styloid and the scaphoid is increased. There is also another form of translocation in which the scaphoid remains in its normal position while the rest of the carpal bones are displaced.

Proximal midcarpal instability represents a combination of medial and proximal carpal instability. This is a form of dorsal flexion instability that occasionally occurs as a result of a healing deformity of a distal radial fracture.

Static and dynamic forms should be distinguished in all of these forms of carpal instability. Static instability will usually be recognizable in routine radiographs as a fixed deformity, such as can occur after perilunar fracture dislocations or other damage to bony structures. Dynamic instability is often difficult to diagnose and may only be detectable

in speed views or by analyzing wrist motion under fluoroscopy (cinefluoroscopy).

Dislocation of the Ulna

Isolated dislocation of the ulna in the distal radioulnar joint without a radial fracture is rare. Either the articular disk must avulse from the ulnar styloid or the styloid itself must fracture. Rheumatoid arthritis is the cause of a traumatic dislocation. Lateral dislocations with diastasis of the distal ulna and radius and dorsopalmar dislocations are possible. Widening of the radioulnar joint space in the PA projection is a sign of a lateral dislocation. A joint space of up to 3 mm is normal. In the lateral radiograph, the ulnar will be dorsal or palmar to the radius in a dorsal or palmar dislocation. Comparative radiographs of both sides are recommended where there is clinical suspicion of dislocation or subluxation and where radiographic findings are equivocal. Dislocations of the ulnar head occur more frequently in combination with fractures of the radial shaft (Galeazzi fracture) than in isolation.

Avascular Necrosis

Kienböck disease. This is among the most frequent forms of avascular necrosis. In addition to negative ulnar anomalies and vascular anomalies, acute and chronic injuries that impair circulation have been discussed as possible causes. Decoulx et al. (1957) and Lichtman et al. (1981) distinguish four stages of lunate necrosis in plain radiographs:

— A reversible early stage (stage I) in which sclerosis is evident.
— A second stage involving fragmentation (stage II).
— A transitional stage with collapse of the lunate (stage III).
— A final stage with arthritic changes in the mediocarpal and intercarpal joints (stage IV). The instability in the final stage results in displacement of the neighboring carpal bones and, finally, carpal collapse (Figs. 3.**78 a, b**).

Data on the time frame for the spontaneous course of Kienböck disease vary considerably, ranging from several months to as long as 20 years. Remissions have been described for stages I and II.

The problem with conventional radiographic examination is that initial ischemic changes cannot be detected. The density and cancellous structure of the affected bones does not differ from that of vital bones. Additional imaging modalities such as nuclear medicine studies or MR studies are required to confirm the diagnosis.

Avascular necrosis of the scaphoid. This can be the result of an undiagnosed or untreated scaphoid fracture. Proximal fragments in particular tend to become necrotic because of the poor vascular supply. As in

a   b

Figs. 3.**78a, b**   Kienböck disease (stage IV).

Fig. 3.**79**   Bennett fracture dislocation.

Fig. 3.**80**   Rolando fracture.

Kienböck disease, radiographs will initially show thickening in the bone structure. As the disorder progresses, osteolytic changes will appear. The disintegration of the affected fragment severely compromises the stability and physiologic kinematics of the wrist. Radiographic classification is the same as for Kienböck disease.

Fractures and Dislocations of the Metacarpals

Standard projections for imaging the metacarpals include the DP and oblique views. A true lateral view can be used if necessary. Occasionally it will be difficult to accurately determine axial deviations, shortening, and rotational malalignment when evaluating fractures. In the first carpometacarpal joint, the PD view has proven effective for better visualization of the joint space and the bases of the first and second metacarpals.

The following forms of fractures are differentiated according to location, joint involvement, and the course of the fracture gap:

- **Fractures close to the base of the first metacarpal**
Bennett fracture dislocation (Fig. 3.**79**). Frequently occurring intra-articular fracture dislocation in which the larger shaft fragment dislocates dorsally and radially due to force or action of the abductor pollicis longus, while the smaller ulnar fragment usually remains in its original position on the trapezium. A special view may be useful for better imaging the fracture; the palm is placed on the cassette in 15°–20° pronation with the central ray aimed at the carpometacarpal joint and the tube tilted proximally 15°.

Rolando fracture (Fig. 3.**80**). Intra-articular Y or T-shaped fracture dislocation or comminuted fracture of the base. The ulnar fragment usually remains in its

Fig. 3.**81**   Winterstein fracture.

anatomical position while the metacarpal shaft is dorsally subluxed.

Winterstein fracture (Fig. 3.**81**). Extra-articular oblique fracture close to the base.

- **Fractures close to the base of the second through fifth metacarpals**
As in fractures of the first metacarpal, muscle force or action can result in proximal and dorsal subluxation of the entire metacarpal, particularly in the fifth metacarpal.

- **Shaft fractures** (Fig. 3.**86**)
Shaft fractures of the second and fifth metacarpals, particularly long oblique fractures, tend to produce shortening, axial deviation, and rotational malalignment. The third and fourth metacarpals tend to remain stable, even in a more severe dislocation, because of their strong muscular and ligamentous connections (deep transverse metacarpal ligament).

- **Subcapital fractures**
In subcapital fractures, the force or action of the interosseous and flexor tendons typically causes palmar tilting of the head fragment and radial rotation of the distal fragments, particularly in the fourth and fifth metacarpals. For example, palmar tilting of 50° can often be found in the fifth metacarpal.

- **Metacarpal head fractures**
The integrity of the articular surface is crucial to a

good outcome. Conservative therapy is indicated only if the articular surface is intact.

Isolated dislocations without injury to bony structures are rare in the metacarpals. This particularly applies to dislocations of the second through fourth metacarpals.

Fractures, Dislocations, and Injuries to the Ligaments of the Phalanges

As with metacarpal fractures, fractures of the phalanges are categorized according to their location and course. A distinction is also made between extra-articular and intra-articular fractures (Fig. 3.**84**). Radiographs in true lateral and dorsopalmar projections are required for diagnosing small avulsion fractures. Intra-articular condylar fractures and impaction fractures of the base of the middle phalanx cause particular problems since significant impairment of join function can occur. Lateral fractures of the base of the proximal phalanx lead to avulsion of the collateral ligaments; dorsal fractures of the base are rare.

Pechlaner (1988) divides intra-articular fractures into four different groups. The varying degrees of damage provide a basis for evaluating the necessity and type of surgical treatment.

– Intra-articular fractures without subluxation or articular incongruity.
– Intra-articular fractures without comminution but with subluxation or articular incongruity.
– Intra-articular fractures with comminution and subluxation or articular incongruity.
– Intra-articular fractures with defects in significant portions of the articular surface.

Dislocation in the fingers and thumb (Fig. 3.**82**) frequently leads to a tear of the joint capsule and to damage of the ligaments stabilizing the joint. Where there is clinical suspicion of a ligament tear, comparative stress radiographs of both sides have proven effective. However, this examination can itself exacerbate the injury and change a partial tear into a complete tear. This particularly applies to the relatively frequent injuries to the ulnar collateral ligament of the metacarpophalangeal joint of the thumb (Fig. 3.**83**), known as ski thumb (see also p. 103). The radiographic stability test often results in what is known as a Stener lesion in which the distal portion of the collateral ligament is displaced over the adductor aponeurosis, preventing it from healing in an anatomical position.

Ligament injuries of the **metacarpophalangeal joints of the fingers** are rare and often overlooked. Clinical symptoms alone (swelling, tenderness to palpation, and opening of the joint) should arouse suspicion. In an avulsion of the palmar plate, the patient will complain of pain with every movement without any apparent instability. Dislocations are generally dorsal with a capsule tear. If the palmar plate is interposed into the joint, closed reduction will be impossible.

Fig. 3.**82** Palmar dislocation of the metacarpophalangeal joint of the thumb.

Fig. 3.**83** Tear of the ulnar collateral ligament in the metacarpophalangeal joint of the thumb. Stability test of the thumb in 20°–30° flexion.

Fig. 3.**84** Rare case of an axial fracture gap in the distal phalanx.

Fig. 3.**85** Mallet fracture

Clinical examination is the principal method of diagnosing **dislocations and ligament injuries of the middle phalanx**. Dislocations are always associated with an injury to the palmar plate; often the collateral ligaments are also involved. Ligament tears may involve avulsion fractures, and severe dislocations will require surgical intervention.

In the **region of the distal phalanx**, the dorsal bony insertion of the extensor tendon is important. Fracture dislocations involving avulsion of the extensor tendon from the bone occur relatively frequently in sports and are referred to as mallet fractures. The size of the fragments determines the therapeutic procedure. Large dorsal fragments with more than 40% joint involvement require surgical intervention (Fig. 3.**85**).

Fig. 3.**86**   Metacarpal shaft fracture

Fractures of the underlying bone of the nail bed are treated conservatively, even if severe dislocation is present. Ascertain whether the nail matrix is unjured. Repair of the nail matrix may be required.

Degenerative Joint Disease

There are many causes for arthritis. Abnormal stresses in a normal joint or normal stresses in a previously damaged joint or articular cartilage can lead to degenerative changes. Other causes include metabolic diseases such as acromegaly or hyperparathyroidism. Degenerative joint disease always involves initial cartilage damage. Often genetic disposition is the only identifiable cause for the wear.

Arthritis can be identified by the following general signs in plain radiographs:

— Narrowing of the joint space.
— Subchondral sclerotic zones.
— Osteophytes.
— Subchondral bone cysts.
— Complete or incomplete joint destruction in advanced arthritis.

Deformities that have caused the degeneration can be determined in plain radiographs. Radiography is also used for follow-up examinations in addition to primary diagnosis of joint findings.

Arthritis of the finger joints. Isolated arthritis of the finger is rare. Often there are also generative changes in the first carpometacarpal joint or at the base of the thumb and the triquetrum. Soft-tissue changes on the extensor side are frequently encountered, often in the form of mucoid cysts. Arthritis of proximal and distal interphalangeal joints is referred to as Bouchard and Heberden nodes, respectively, after the authors who first described these findings. Primarily, the index and small fingers are affected. In the fingers, it is primarily the metacarpophalangeal joints of the second and third digits that show degenerative changes (Fig. 3.**87**).

Arthritis of the carpal joints. The first carpometacarpal joint is a frequent location. Often this disorder is a sequela of trauma. Usually women above the age of 40 are affected. The second through fifth carpometacarpal joints are involved far less frequently.

Intercarpal arthritis. Arthritis of the scaphoid-trapezium-trapezoid joint is often without clinical symptoms. Radiographs frequently concave a pattern of wear on the articular surface of the trapezium, while osteophytes are rarely encountered. The most frequent causes of ulnar wrist symptoms are degenerative changes of the pisotriquetral joint. **Pisotriquetral** arthritis is best evaluated in oblique views, with the hand in 70° supination, and in carpal tunnel views.

Arthritis of the radiocarpal joint. In 90% of all cases, the radioscaphoid articular surface is affected. Distal radial fractures and scaphoid pseudarthroses are among the most common causes, although other types of ligament instability such as scapholunate dissociation can also cause wear in this joint. When the degenerative changes above occur together, the clinical syndrome of carpal collapse may be encountered. This may involve a SLAC (scapholunate advanced collapse) wrist (see Table 3.**5**).

Fig. 3.**87** Arthritis of the first carpometacarpal joint.

Arthritis of the distal radiolunate joint. In addition to the general signs of arthritis, one often finds signs of abrasion in the ulnar notch of the radius and on the lunate, together with intra-articular loose bodies.

Rheumatoid Arthritis

The hand is frequently the site of initial manifestation of rheumatoid arthritis. Early radiographic symptoms are found in the periarticular soft tissue of the meta-carpophalangeal and proximal interphalangeal joints. Tenosynovitis and synovial proliferation with accompanying effusion produce spindle-shaped swelling in these joints. The small joints of the wrist are also typically affected. Initial bony changes include osteoporosis close to the joint. Later, a generalized loss of substance is observed. Further on in the disorder, an infiltrative pannus results in increasing cartilage and bone destruction with concentric narrowing of the joint space. Cysts and wear lesions occur (Fig. 3.**88**). The erosive changes may be central or peripheral. The metacarpophalangeal joints frequently demonstrate a "cup and saucer" deformity. Evidence of repair processes is usually minimal, or entirely absent, so that subchondral sclerosis or osteophyte formation will only be seen when secondary arthritic changes are superimposed on the underlying disorder. The most frequent late changes include subluxation and dislocation of the joints as a result of destruction of the capsule and ligaments. This produces typical finger and hand deformities. Tendon ruptures and ankylosis in connective tissue and bone are also occasionally observed.

Larsen et al. (1977) have described a system of clinical and radiologic staging (Table 3.**6**).

Fig. 3.**88**   Radiographic changes in advanced rheumatoid arthritis with narrowing of the joint spaces, cysts, periosteal reaction, and onset of ulnar deviation of the long fingers, particularly the index finger. Destructive changes are also visible in the carpal region.

Table 3.**6** Larsen classification. Radiographic stages of rheumatoid arthritis

Larsen stage 0:	Normal joint.
Larsen stage I:	Slight changes such as periarticular soft-tissue swelling, periarticular osteoporosis, or a slight decrease in the width of the joint space. This decrease is usually apparent only when compared with an older image or with the unaffected contralateral side.
Larsen stage II:	Distinct early changes, erosion (may not be present in weight-bearing joints), and changes in the width of the joint space that are obvious without having to compare them with other images.
Larsen stage III:	Moderate joint destruction with erosion and advanced narrowing of the joint space.
Larsen stage IV:	Severe joint destruction with erosion, subtotal collapse of the joint space, and bony deformities in weight-bearing joints.
Larsen stage V:	Mutilating changes with total collapse of the joint space and gross bony deformities especially in weight-bearing joints. Subluxations and dislocations are usually included in stage V.

Reflex Sympathetic Dystrophy

Reflex sympathetic dystrophy can be encountered in the hand. Given the often protacted clinical course of the disorder, early diagnosis is crucial to initiating appropriate therapy. Initial radiographic examination will usually reveal normal findings in the early stages of reflex sympathetic dystrophy. Only as the disorder progresses will simultaneous radiographs of both hands demonstrate nodular areas of demineralization of bone matrix in comparison with the contralateral side. The cortex will appear splintered, and the contours of individual bones may be indistinct. In the late stage, diffuse increased radiolucency with a coarsely filamentous internal structure will be apparent and the outer contours will become more sharply defined.

3.4 Ultrasound in the Hand

Ultrasonography in the hand is of less utility compared to other imaging modalities. Its diagnostic value is limited. In daily clinical practice it is suitable for differentiating and imaging cysts, ganglia, and determining if a palpable nodule is solid or cystic. Occasionally it may be used to identify a tendon rupture.

Ganglia or cysts generally appear as a hypoechoic mass, while solid nodules have an ectogenic internal structure bounded by a capsule. In a tendon tear the contour of the tendon will be interrupted. Acute tears may show a hematoma at the stump as a hyperechoic area. A cloudy appearance suggests that a clot has formed.

3.5 Arthrography

Indications, Diagnostic Value, and Clinical Relevance

For many years, arthrography was the standard method for radiographic diagnosis of carpal-ligament and disk lesions, and for changes in the joint capsule and articular cartilage. When imaging structures indirectly, it is often difficult to evaluate the size and character of pathologic changes. Since the 1980s, the importance of arthrography has decreased relative to MRI, which offers the additional advantage of being noninvasive. Arthrography is primarily used where MRI is not available and where a simple low-cost imaging modality is required as an adjunctive diagnostic procedure to routine plain radiography. Arthrography is performed in one or more compartments with sequential injections of a water-soluble contrast medium into the radiocarpal, midcarpal, and distal radioulnar joints. The distribution of the contrast medium in the individual articular spaces is observed under fluoroscopy and documented in serial radiographs. The thickness and surface contour of the cartilage are evaluated and any signs of the changes in the articular capsule are noted. Some authors recommend performing arthrography in preparation for arthroscopy to be better prepared to intraoperatively address pathologic conditions revealed during initial arthrography. If, for example, leakage of contrast medium from the proximal wrist into the distal radioulnar joint is demonstrated, the leakage site should be inspected closely with a hooked probe to distinguish degenerative disk perforations from tears.

Technique, Instrumentation, and Examination Procedure

As in any invasive procedure, sterile conditions must be maintained for arthrography of the hand and finger joints.

For arthrography of the radiocarpal joint, the hand is placed on a sterile transparent support in pronation, slight flexion, and ulnar deviation to expand the joint for needle placement. The joint is usually aspirated dorsoradially under fluoroscopic control between the middle third of the scaphoid and the radial styloid. A 20/22 G aspiration cannula is used, through which 2 mL of water-soluble contrast medium is injected. Fluoroscopic control during injection is important to ascertain the order in which joint compartments are filled and where there is possible pathologic joint communication. This is necessary to localize capsule and ligament injuries to document them in spot views. When radiographs of the entire wrist are subsequently in three planes (dorsopalmar, lateral, and oblique), it may no longer be possible to determine the exact sites of the leaks. These and other lesions may already be obscured by contrast medium, with the result that pathologic changes may go undetected. Since the static views do not provide any information about the relevance of a lesion, it is best to observe the flow of contrast medium during careful passive and active joint motion after removing the cannula. This is known as a dynamic arthrogram.

The midcarpal joint is usually aspirated between the scaphoid, trapezoid, and capitate. As for arthrography of the radiocarpal joint, the hand is in pronation, slight flexion, and ulnar deviation on a sterile support. Water-soluble contrast medium (1.5–2.0 mL) is injected under fluoroscopic control. The main focus of interest is whether there is a contrast-medium leak between the midcarpal and radiocarpal joint at the level of the connection between the scaphoid and lunate and the lunate and triquetrum. An alternative approach to the midcarpal joint is between the lunate, capitate, triquetrum, and hamate. However, this approach entails a risk of injuring the dorsal branch of the ulnar nerve.

For arthrography of the radioulnar joint, the hand is placed flat on the examining table. The aspiration cannula is advanced into the joint at an angle of 20°–30° to the surface of the radius. Approximately 1.5–2.0 mL of water-soluble contrast medium is injected under fluoroscopic control. If the articular disk is torn or there are degenerative changes, the contrast medium will leak into the radiocarpal joint. However, some patients will show evidence of contrast-medium leakage even without trauma or degeneration. This is generally the result of a cogenital central perforation of the disk.

Normal Findings

Normal findings in a wrist arthrogram can vary greatly due to individual differences in the flexor, extensor, and ulnar recesses. This occasionally makes it difficult to evaluate findings. The recess on the volar and dorsal aspects in particular show a wide range of variation in the distribution of contrast medium. Even the ulnar recess surrounding the ulnar styloid can vary depending on the length of the ulnar styloid. If an ulnar lesion of the articular disk is suspected, it should be inspected to distinguish anatomical anomalies from abnormal findings with ulnar contrast-medium leakage into the distal radioulnar joint. In arthrography of the radiocarpal joint, the joint between the pisiform and triquetrum is often also imaged in the arthrogram. The intercarpal and carpometacarpal joint spaces are usually finely contrasted at the midcarpal joint. The dorsal recess appears next to this joint; the other recesses are small

Fig. 3.**89** Schematic diagram of normal findings in wrist arthrography.

and barely visible. The distal radioulnar joint appears in the AP arthrogram almost as a right angle. It is surrounded by a flaccid joint capsule that forms the sacciform recess. Normal findings at rest can change significantly when the wrist is moved. In arthrography the joint should be moved actively and passively in every direction.

False negative findings can be caused by inflammatory adhesions and fibrous covering of a defect at the time of the examination. Figure 3.**89** shows a schematic diagram of normal findings.

Abnormal Findings

Distinguishing physiologic anomalies from abnormal findings in arthrography can occasionally be difficult. Contrast-medium leakage from the radiocarpal joint to the distal radioulnar joint at the level of the articular disk alone is not sufficient to confirm a triangular fibrocartilage tear. Congenital communication through a central triangular fibrocartilage perforation will produce contrast-medium leakage in a disk that is otherwise normal for the patient's age. Fissures and perforations due to degenerative changes can appear, especially after longer periods of asymmetric stress. These changes may be age-related or may result from altered stress patterns in negative ulnar anomalies. Some authors recommend comparative arthrography of the left and right wrists to help confirm findings. However, since triangular fibrocartilage anatomy is by no means always identical in the left and right wrists, the value of such findings would hardly seem to justify the additional risk of infection from an invasive procedure in the contralateral wrist. Arthrography alone is not sufficient for differential diagnosis of posttraumatic and degenerative changes. The diagnostic value of these studies, particularly in older patients, is doubtful.

Demonstrated leakage of contrast medium into the interacarpal space is also not sufficient to confirm a ligament lesion and intercarpal instability. Some

Fig. 3.**90** Arthrography of the proximal wrist showing contrast-medium leakage from the midcarpal to the radio-carpal joint.

leakage of contrast medium into the joint spaces may be visible, even when ligaments are stable. For this reason, communication between radiocarpal and midcarpal joints demonstrated during arthrography should only be regarded as abnormal in the presence of clinical suspicion. The most frequent sites of damage are the scapholunate and lunotriquetral ligaments (Fig. 3.**90**). Contrast-medium filling of the metacarpal joints in addition to the intercarpal joints is a sign of additional ligament injuries. Occasionally a CT examination is performed after arthrography.

In addition to ligament damage, arthrography can also demonstrate inflammatory synovial changes and cartilage lesions before visible soft-tissue changes and bone destruction are visible in plain radiographs. Arthrographic signs of inflammatory processes can be distinguished according to location. These include:

— Inflammatory ligament and cartilage changes (surface irregularities and joint space narrowing.
— Inflammatory capsular changes (irregular villous structure with gaps in the contrast medium).
— Soft-tissue reactions (contrast-medium leakage into adjacent structures such as tendon sheaths, muscle, fatty tissue, and lymph vessels).

Arthrography can demonstrate ganglia and postoperative fistulas. Intra-articular loose bodies can be located and intracapsular bodies distinguished from extracapsular bodies by evaluating the distribution of contrast medium on the articular surfaces. Midcarpal arthrography can demonstrate the pseudarthrosis gap in scaphoid pseudarthrosis.

Complications

Few complications of wrist arthrography have been described to date. However, infections and complications involving contrast medium are possible. A disadvantage is that the examination itself is often painful, even when performed under anesthesia.

3.6 Nuclear Medicine Studies

See chapter 1 (Shoulder, p. 54) for a general discussion on the utility of nuclear medicine studies.

3.7 Computed Tomography

Indications, Diagnostic Value, and Clinical Relevance

As a cross-sectional imaging process, CT is superior to conventional radiography in that it can visualize individual structures in three dimensions, unobscured by superimposed shadows. It is suitable as an adjunctive procedure for diagnosing traumatic and degenerative bony lesions that cannot be reliably evaluated in the image of a plain radiograph. The extent of tumors, including soft-tissue reactions, can be more reliably determined. CT is useful in the following settings:

— Diagnosis of acute hand injuries, such as dislocations and fractures of the carpal bones, that are difficult to demonstrate in plain radiographs.
— Diagnosis of initial degenerative changes of post-traumatic or inflammatory origin, particularly in the radiocarpal and distal radioulnar joints.
— Visualization of bone tumors and soft-tissue masses.
— Demonstration of distal radioulnar joint instability.
— Demonstration of pathologic rotation in pronation or supination following a distal radial fracture.
— Demonstration of intra-articular loose bodies of cartilage or bone.
— Postoperative follow-up examination to evaluate bony union following surgery for scaphoid pseudarthrosis.

Technique, Instrumentation, and Examination Procedure

The patient is prone or supine on the examining table, or seated next to it. The upper arm is abducted 90° in the shoulder as for routine radiographs, and the elbow is flexed 90°. Position the hand and forearm parallel to the axis of the table for axial planes, and perpendicular to it for sagittal longitudinal planes.

Fig. 3.**91** CT image in the transverse plane showing an older scaphoid fracture with multiple fragmentation of the body of the bone.

Fig. 3.**92** Hamate fracture

Fig. 3.**93** Three-dimensional reconstruction of a hamate fracture.

The hand is pronated and in neutral radial/ulnar deviation. Views with the wrist in maximum radial and ulnar deviation or maximum extension and flexion, similar to those used in conventional radiography, may be useful where carpal instability is suspected. Plastic bands are used to fix the hand in the desired position throughout the examination. Scaphoid fractures or pseudarthroses can be visualized using special imaging planes parallel to the longitudinal axis of the scaphoid. Position the forearm and hand in maximum supination on a 45° wedge for these views. Axial examination of both hands is performed with the patient prone and the elbows and forearms resting on the examining table. Fine cuts are recommended to maximally evaluate the detailed structures.

Abnormal Findings

Scaphoid Fracture and Scaphoid Pseudarthrosis

In a scaphoid fracture, CT examinations can often provide important additional information about associated injuries that are not visible in conventional radiographs. Longitudinal imaging planes or imaging planes parallel to the axis of the scaphoid are usually able to provide unobscured visualization that unequivocally demonstrates the fracture line and the direction of fragment displacement or rotational subluxation. CT scans often show a more severe degree of injury than is apparent in conventional radiographs. Knowledge of these additional findings can significantly influence the decision as to whether surgical intervention is indicated. The onset of fragment avascular necrosis can be diagnosed from initial sclerosis in the cancellous bone. The otherwise difficult evaluation of fragment size and the nature of the tissue bridging the gap in scaphoid pseudarthrosis is made easier by CT (Fig. 3.**91**). The structure of interest should be visualized in longitudinal plane, parallel to the imaging plane (parallel to the axis of the third finger), with a slice thickness of 1.5 mm.

Avulsions with sclerosis of the fragment margins and small resorption cysts are detected more thoroughly and with greater sensitivity.

Circumscribed radiocarpal arthritis between the radial styloid and the palmar-tilted peripheral scaphoid fragment are detected earlier in CT scans, as is mediocarpal arthritis in the capitoscaphoid and capitolunar compartment. Postoperative CT scans can be used to evaluate the union of corticocancellous grafts. Even fine bony bridges will be visible.

Postoperative healing is significantly easier to evaluate in CT images.

Fractures of the Other Carpal Bones

The sensitivity of CT studies is also helpful in evaluating fractures of the other carpal bones. For example, oblique fractures of the pisiform or small fissured fractures of the capitate can be better visualized.

Carpal Dislocations and Dislocation Fractures

Determining the extent of a dislocation and classifying complex dislocation fractures in conventional radiographs can be difficult, even when the methods described in section 3.3 are followed meticulously. Individual carpal bones and fragments can overlap and make it impossible to precisely identify the dislocation and dislocation fragments in plain films.

In these cases, the unobscured visualization of individual bones and fragments provided by CT makes it possible to reliably evaluate the severity of trauma. Unusual carpal lesions and additional fractures can also be diagnosed (Figs. 3.**92**, 3.**93**). Structures preventing reduction can be readily located, particularly in the sagittal slices. This provides a basis for deciding whether open reduction is indicated. After reduction, the result can be easily evaluated and precisely quantified with the patient relaxed in a comfortable position. CT can also supplement the information provided by conventional radiographs where older dislocations with chronic deformities of the carpal bones and resulting degenerative changes are to be evaluated.

Carpal Instability

CT permits a greater degree of precision in diagnosing forms of carpal instability that are difficult to classify. It provides information about secondary arthritis in cases of chronic dissociation; this can decisively influence the choice of therapeutic procedure. In the framework of a flexible diagnostic program, consisting of conventional radiographs in two planes, stress views in the four directions of motion, and cinefluoroscopy, CT has proven effective in evaluating ulnar carpal instability and lesions of the distal radioulnar joint in particular.

Pathologic Rotation

Where limited motion or other symptoms persist after a distal radius fracture, CT examination can provide information about possible pathologic rotation in pronation or supination. The degree of rotational deformity can be determined relatively easily by addition of the image slices of the radial epiphysis and metaphysis.

Subluxation and Dislocation of the Ulna

Where posttraumatic symptoms are present in the distal radioulnar joint, one must occasionally consider the possibility of instability. These changes are also easier to diagnose in CT images than in conventional radiographs.

Intra-articular Loose Bodies

Intra-articular loose bodies can rarely be demonstrated in conventional radiographs. However, even small cartilage fragments can be demonstrated in plain CT images or after intra-articular injection of air.

Carpal Tunnel Syndrome

CT is not used to diagnose carpal tunnel syndrome. However, it can provide information about the cause (trauma, arthritis, inflammation, or tumor), location, and size of a stenosing process in the nonidiopathic forms of the disorder.

Cystic Bone Processes

Cystic changes in bone detected in conventional radiographs should be more closely evaluated in the absence of arthritic changes in the joint to exclude an intraosseous ganglion. An intraosseous ganglion can often be demonstrated in CT scans as a disruption of the cortex at a circumscribed location through which the intraosseous portion of the ganglion communicates with the extraosseous portion.

Tumors

In the hand, suspicious findings can be more precisely localized and size evaluated in CT examination. Important information about the type of tumor can be obtained using special criteria such as density behavior, calcifications, contrast-medium enhancement, location, and infiltration of surrounding tissue. This information is essential for preoperative planning. CT is superior to MRI, a competing modality, in detecting bone destruction and tumor calcifications. However, the higher contrast of MRI studies often makes it easier to define the borders of the tumor.

3.8 Magnetic Resonance Imaging

Indications (Table 3.**7**)

The three-dimensional imaging techniques and the ability to select any plane render MRI particularly suitable for tracing carpal and radioulnar instabilities in various axial movements. Other indications are suspected lesions of the triangular fibrocartilage, fractures, avascular osteonecrosis, arthritis, ganglia,

Table 3.**7**   Possible indications for MRI in the hand and fingers

- Triangular fibrocartilage complex injuries
- Ligament injuries
- Kienböck disease
- Scaphoid pseudarthrosis and avascular necrosis
- Cartilage damage
- Carpal tunnel syndrome
- Subluxations
- Tumors
- Osteomyelitis
- Rheumatoid arthritis

Rupture of the radioulnar joint

Tear of the triangular fibro-cartilage

Fig. 3.**94** Sagittal oblique image (GRE 500/10 out of phase after application of intravenous gadolinium contrast medium) showing a tear of the triangular fibrocartilage with rupture of the radioulnar joint.

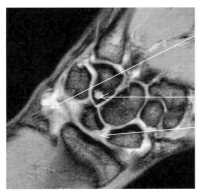

Tear of the triangular fibro-cartilage

Subchondral cyst

Tear of the scapholunate ligament

Fig. 3.**96** Coronal image (GRE 350/11 out of phase after application of intravenous gadolinium contrast medium) showing a tear of the scapholunate ligament, tear of the triangular fibrocartilage, and subchondral cyst in the hamate.

tenosynovitis, and osteomyelitis, as well as tumors. A less frequent indication is investigation of carpal tunnel syndrome.

Technique and Examination Protocol

Depending on the equipment and the patient's constitution, the examination is performed with the patient supine and the hand placed alongside the body, or with the patient prone and the hand elevated above the head. To avoid motion artifacts, hand and coil should be immobilized. Even for dynamic examinations, immobilization in the selected position is recommended. The echo sequences are determined by the clinical questions to be answered. Anatomical changes are best appreciated on the T1-weighted sequences. Dynamic examinations demand short gradient echo (GRE) sequences. T2-weighted and short-time inversion recovery (STIR) sequences reveal pathologic fluid accumulations or edematous changes.

Minute ligamentous lesions are often better delineated after intravenous administration of gadolinium-based contrast medium. This also allows assessment of the vascularity of the process.

Tear of the triangular fibro-cartilage

Rupture of the radioulnar joint

Fig. 3.**95** Coronal image (SE 500/20) showing a tear of the triangular fibrocartilage with rupture of the radioulnar joint.

Pathologic Findings

Triangular Fibrocartilage Complex
(Figs. 3.**94**–3.**96**)

The most frequent pathologic changes are degenerative in nature and occur with increasing frequency after the third decade of life. In all sequences, they are characterized by increased signal intensity in the central area of the disk. In the advanced stage, discontinuities can appear mostly at the site of the radial fixation, creating a communication between radioulnar and radiocarpal articulation. This is best documented on T2-weighted or STIR sequences. Traumatic lesions more often involve the ulnar fixation and the meniscus-homologous ulnar component, frequently with coexisting torn ligaments of the fibrocartilaginous complex. The tear is generally horizontal and exhibits an increased signal intensity on T2-weighted and STIR images owing to accumulation of fluid from the surrounding tissues. In contrast to degenerative changes, fresh injuries show a perifocal enhancement after intravenous administration of gadolinium-containing contrast medium.

Ligamentous Lesions (Fig. 3.**96**)

Tears of the interosseous ligaments are difficult to detect directly by MRI. The scapholunate ligament is most frequently involved. A ligamentous tear can be inferred from the communication between otherwise separated joint spaces. This is most impressive on T2-weighted and STIR sequences. Dislocations of neighboring carpal bones indicate a ligamentous tear. The sagittal images disclose any associated dorsal or volar tilt of the lunate.

Avascular Osteonecroses

This condition most frequently affects the lunate, followed by the scaphoid. Etiologically, it is an intraosseous ischemia secondary to stress, which can be caused by malpositioned carpal bones owing to a short ulna, or by microtraumas (for example, vibra-

Fig. 3.**97** Coronal image (SE 600/20) showing stage II Kienböck's disease.

Fig. 3.**99** Coronal image (GRE 350/11 out of phase) showing osteoarthritis of the scaphotrapezoidal joint.

Fig. 3.**98** Coronal image (GRE 350/11 out of phase after application of intravenous gadolinium contrast medium) showing fracture of the scaphoid with pseudarthrosis and avascular necrosis in the distal fragment and a tear of the triangular fibrocartilage.

tion traumas caused by working with a jackhammer). It can also follow fractures of the lunate or scaphoid.

Avascular necrosis of the lunate. Based on the progression of the disease, three stages of the avascular necrosis of the lunate are distinguished by MRI.

— Stage I: Shape and size of the lunate are maintained. Spot-like area of decreased signal intensity on the T1-weighted image with corresponding increased signal intensity on the T2-weighted or STIR image. The area of abnormal signal is indistinct in outline and shows subtle peripheral contrast enhancement. If fissures are present, they appear as sharp lines of intense contrast enhancement.
— Stage II (Fig. 3.**97**): Larger spot-like area of decreased signal intensity on the T1-weighted images and increased signal intensity on the T2-weighted or STIR image. Cysts with homogeneous signal alteration appear. Marked contrast enhancement.
— Stage III: Collapse of the lunate and migration of the capitate. The signal alteration involves the entire bone, but is usually heterogeneous corre-

sponding to the osseous fragmentation. Heterogeneous but distinct contrast enhancement.
— Stage IV: Collapse and destruction of the bone. The initially high signal intensity on the T2-weighted and STIR image decreases. Only slight and occasional contrast enhancement.

Avascular necrosis of the scaphoid and pseudoarthrosis (Fig. 3.**98**). Avascular necrosis of the scaphoid is usually caused by a fracture. It frequently affects the proximal pole. On MRI, it is characterized by a high signal intensity on the T2-weighted or STIR image with decreased signal intensity on the T1-weighted image. Marked contrast enhancement is almost always present.

The fracture line is best seen on the GRE sequences with phase contrast. These sequences show pseudoarthrosis as a persistent transcortical band of high signal intensity.

Damaged Cartilage (Fig. 3.**99**)

T1-weighted GRE sequences with high-resolution matrix are most suitable for evaluation of the cartilaginous structures. Chondromalacia is seen as fusiform thickening with centrally decreased signal intensity. Defects are well visualized on high-resolution images. On the T2-weighted or STIR image, the defect is seen as punctate area of high signal intensity within the weak signal intensity of the healthy cartilage. An irregular outline of the cartilaginous layer with loss of height and a subchondral zone of decreased signal intensity in all sequences are the MR findings of degenerative osteoarthritis.

Carpal Tunnel Syndrome (Fig. 3.**100**)

Any process that narrows the carpal tunnel can damage the median nerve. These are some of the most common causes fractures and dislocations of the car-

Fig. 3.100   Coronal image (GRE 500/10 out of phase after application of intravenous gadolinium contrast medium) showing tenosynovitis of the flexor tendons in carpal tunnel syndrome.

Tenosynovitis of the flexor tendons

Fig. 3.101   Transverse image (SE 500/20) showing a lipoma of the palm enveloping the flexor tendons.

Lipoma

Fig. 3.102   Coronal image (GRE 500/10 out of phase after application of intravenous gadolinium contrast medium) showing a ganglion arising from the flexor digiti minimi tendon sheath.

Ganglion

Fig. 3.103   Coronal image (SE 500/20) showing osteomyelitis of the wrist and metacarpals.

Osteomyelitis with bone destruction

pal bones; tenosynovitis of flexor tendons; tumors of the nerve itself or of adjacent structures, such as ganglion cysts, lipomas, and hemangiomas; and post-traumatic and postsurgical fibroses and hematomas. These processes can be visualized by MRI. If they induce inflammatory changes in the nerve, it shows an increased signal intensity on the T2-weighted images. The tendon sheath can also show contrast enhancement.

Tumors (Fig. 3.**101**)

Osteogenic tumors of the wrist are very rare. Neurinomas are well delineated by MRI since they show marked contrast enhancement. The morphologic connection with the corresponding nerve is generally well displayed. Furthermore, lipomas are clearly characterized by high signal intensity on T1-weighted and T2-weighted images. Hemangiomas show a characteristic spongioid structure in which small thromboses are visualized as high signal intensities on the T1-weighted image. In general, MRI primarily serves to

delineate the extension of the tumor and its relationship to adjacent structures.

Ganglions Cysts (Fig. 3.**102**)

Ganglion cysts have a characteristic MR feature. They are homogeneously bright on T2-weighted images. A delicate stripe of high signal intensity extends to the joint or tendon sheath from which the ganglion cyst originates. After intravenous administration of gadolinium-based contrast medium, the T1-weighted phase contrast images display the enveloping synovial membrane with high signal intensity, with the content of the ganglion cyst appearing darker.

Infections (Fig. 3.**103**)

Osteomyelitis shows increased signal intensity in the affected carpal bone on the STIR image. Cortical destructions are frequently found. Effusion is observed in the adjacent joint spaces. The adjacent bones and soft tissue show an inflammatory reaction, recognized by the increased signal intensity on the STIR image. The inflammation-induced increased permeability of the vascular system leads to pronounced

Osteomalacia

Effusion

Fig. 3.**104**   Coronal image (STIR 1900/125) showing rheumatoid osteoarthritis with effusion, osteomalacia, and synovitis.

Pannus

Fig. 3.**105**   Sagittal image (STIR 1900/125): Rheumatoid osteoarthritis with pannus and synovitis.

contrast enhancement, best appreciated on the T1-weighted phase contrast image. The reactive changes induced in structures neighboring the affected bone are relevant for the differentiation from osteonecrosis. Infections in the soft tissues can spread diffusely and are difficult to distinguish from nonspecific inflammatory processes. Frequently, they follow the tendons and form abscesses in the tendon sheaths or, more proximal, between the pronator quadratus and flexor tendons (Parona space). The extent of the inflammatory changes is also best appreciated on STIR images. The abscess border shows distinct contrast enhancement.

Rheumatoid Arthritis (Figs. 3.**104**, 3.**105**)

Generally, all carpal joints are involved, with corresponding edematous swelling of the capsule and tendon sheaths and joint effusion. The ligamentous destruction is followed by subluxation of the carpal bones. With progressing synovial hypertrophy, osseous and cartilaginous erosions develop. Subchondral cysts appear in large numbers. The morphologic changes are well visualized on T1-weighted and proton-density images. The inflammatory changes are better appreciated on T2-weighted and STIR images.

Synovial hypertrophy and pannus formation are best shown after intravenous administration of gadolinium-based contrast medium, which will also reveal any reactive osseous hyperemia.

References

Buck-Gramcko D. Instabilitäten der Handwurzel. *Orthopäde.* 1986; 15: 88–94

Buck-Gramcko D, ed. *Frakturen am distalen Radiusende.* Stuttgart: Hippokrates; 1987

Buck-Gramcko D, Hoffmann R, Neumann R. *Der Handchirurgische Notfall.* Stuttgart: Hippokrates; 1989

Brunelli G, Saffar P, eds. *Wrist Imaging.* Berlin–Heidelberg–New York: Springer; 1992

Calleja Conacho E, Schawe-Calleja M, Milbradt H, Galanski M. Sonoanatomie und Untersuchungstechnik des normalen Karpaltunnels und des distalen Nervus medianus. *Fortschr Geb Rontgenstr Nuklearmed.* 1989; 151: 414–418

Decoulx P, Marchand M, Minet P, Razemon JP. La maladie de Kienböck chez le mineur. *Lille Chir.* 1957; 12: 65

Dobyns JH, Linscheid RL, Chao EYS, Weber ER, Swanson GE. Traumatic instability of the wrist. *AAOS Instr Course Lect 24.* St. Louis: Mosby; 1975: 182–199

Fisk GR. Carpal instability and the fractured scaphoid. Hunteriam Lecture; 1968. *Ann R Coll Surg Engl.* 1970; 46: 63–76

Fornage BD, Schernberg FL, Rifkin MD. Ultrasound Examination of the Hand. *Radiology.* 1985; 155: 785–788

Frykman G. Fracture of the distal radius including sequelae-shoulder-hand-finger-syndrome. Disturbance in the distal radio-ulnar joint and impairment of nerve function. A clinical and experimental study. *Acta Orthop Scand Suppl.* 1967; 108: 1–153

Gilula LA. Carpal injuries: analytic approach and case exercises. *AJR.* 1979; 133: 503–517

Gilula LA, Weeks PA. Posttraumatic ligamentous instabilities of the wrist. *Radiology.* 1978; 129: 641–651

Hardy DC, Totty WG, Reinns WR, Gilula LA. Posteroanterior wrist radiography: Importance of arm postioning. *J Hand Surg.* 1987; 12A: 504–508

Imaeda T, Nakamura R, Miura T, Makino N. Magnetic Resonance Imaging in Kienböck's disease. *J Hand Surg.* 1992; 17B: 12–19

Jerosch J, Marquardt M. *Sonographie des Bewegungsapparates.* Zülpich: Biermann; 1993: 101–111

Kuderna H. Frakturen und Luxationsfrakturen der Handwurzel. *Orthopäde.* 1986; 15: 95–108

Larsen A, Dale K, Eck M. Radiographic evaluation of rheumatoid arthritis and related conditions by standard reference films. *Acta Radiol.* 1977; 18: 481–491

Larsen CF, Stigsby B, Mathiesen FK, Lindequist S. Radiography of the wrist. A new device for standardized radiographs. *Acta Radiol.* 1990; 31: 459–462

Lichtman DM, Schneider JR, Swafford AR, Mack GR. Ulnar midcarpal instability – Clinical and laboratory analysis. *J Hand Surg.* 1981; 6: 515–523

Lindscheid RL, Dobyns JH, Beabout JW, Bryan RS. Traumatic instability of the wrist. Diagnosis, classifications and pathomechanics. *J Bone Joint Surg.* 1972; 54A: 1612–1632

Martini AK. Der spontane Verlauf der Lunatummalzie. *Handchir Mikrordt Plast Chir.* 1989; 22: 14–19

Mayfield JK, Johnson RP, Kilcoyne RK. Carpal dislocations: Pathomechanics and progressive perilunar instability. *J Hand Surg.* 1980; 5: 226–241

Milbradt H, Calleja Cancho E, Quiyumi SAA, Galanski M. Sonographie des Handgelenks und der Hand. *Radiologe.* 1990; 30: 360–365

Monsivais JJ, Nitz PA, Scully TJ. The role of carpal instability in scaphoid nonunion: casual or causal? *J Hand Surg [Br].* 1986; 11(2): 201–206

Müller ME, Nazariam S, Koch P. *Classification AO des fractures.* Berlin–Heidelberg–New York: Springer; 1987

Nägele M, Wilhelm K, Kugelstatter W, Hahn D. Kienböck'sche Erkrankung: Kernspintomographische und röntgenologische Vergleichsstudie. *Handchir Mikrochir Plast Chir.* 1990: 23–27

Nigst H, ed. *Frakturen, Luxationen und Dissoziationen der Karpalknochen* (Bibliothek für Handchirurgie). Stuttgart: Hippokrates; 1982

Nigst H, Buck-Gramcko D, Millesi H. *Handchirurgie.* 2 vols. Stuttgart–New York: Thieme; 1981/83

Palmer AK, Dobyns FH, Linscheid RL. Management of the posttraumatic instability of the wrist. Secondary to ligament rupture. *J Hand Surg.* 1978; 3: 507–532

Pechlaner S. Die operative Versorgung intraartikulärer Daumen- und Fingerfrakturen. In: Nigst G, ed. *Frakturen der Hand und des Handgelenkes* (Bibliothek für Handchirurgie). Stuttgart: Hippokrates; 1988

Sennwald G. *Das Handgelenk.* Berlin–Heidelberg–New York: Springer; 1987

Taleisnik J. Classification of carpal instability. *Bull Hosp Jt Dis Orthop Inst.* 1984; 44: 511–531

Taleisnik J. *The wrist.* New York: Churchill Livingstone; 1985.

Watson HK, Ryu J. Evolution of arthritis of the wrist. *Clin Orthop.* 1986; 202: 57–67

Weissmann BNW, Sledge CB. *Orthopedic Radiology.* Philadelphie: Saunders; 1986: 111–167

4 Hip

4.1 Introduction

In contrast to the other major joints of the body, particularly the shoulder and knee, hip disorders are mostly the result of degenerative or inflammatory changes. Isolated injuries to the capsule and ligaments are only rarely encountered and will occur in combination with fractures of the femoral neck or acetabulum as the result of high-energy trauma.

Congenital disorders of the acetabulum and femoral epiphysis represent a further large group of hip disorders.

4.2 Clinical Examination

Standard Examination

Obtaining the patient's history is the first step of the examination. This will provide significant insight into the nature of disorder. It is particularly important to enquire about the type, location, and time of occurrence of complaints.

The clinical examination consists of measuring leg length (see p. 144), observing gait, measuring the circumference of the muscles at standardized measuring points, and assessing the active and passive ranges of motion. Functional tests provide further information in certain lines of inquiry.

In newborns and infants, provocative tests (Ortolani and Barlow) can be also performed in the presence of suspected hip instability. The dynamic ultrasound examination complements these tests.

Patient History

The patient's history can provide valuable information about the presence and causes of a hip disorder. The patient's age is the first clue that the history provides. In newborns and infants, the disorders encountered are most often due to abnormal development such as developmental hip dysplasia. Risk factors for developmental hip dysplasia in newborns may include:

— Positive family history
— First pregnancy
— Breech presentation
— Female sex
— Other anomalies such as club feet or torticollis
— Subsidence of spontaneous kicking toward the end of pregnancy

Children and adolescents with a disturbed gait may have Legg–Calvé–Perthes disease or a slipped capital femoral epiphysis. Symptoms of degenerative diseases such as idiopathic chondrolysis or degenerative joint disease are more prevalent in adults and older patients.

Questions to ask the patient include:

● **Location of pain**
Pain is usually felt in the groin or in a retrotrochanteric location, occasionally radiating to the inner thigh and extending as far as the knee. This means, especially in children, that a hip disorder can masquerade as knee pain. The differential diagnosis should consider pathology in the adductor insertions and involvement of the lumbar spine, particularly the sacroiliac joints.

● **Onset of pain**
Acute pain is indicative of inflammation, infection, or involvement of the femoral head as in an acute slipped capital femoral epiphysis, a subchondral collapse in Legg–Calvé–Perthes disease, or pathologic fractures. Pain that develops slowly suggests a degenerative disorder or tumor.

● **Time and duration of pain**
Transient morning pain that subsides after the patient has taken a few steps, but which reappears with exercise such as walking longer distances or climbing stairs (exercise pain), is typical of degenerative hip disorders.

The differential diagnosis should consider neurogenic claudication (in the presence of stenosis of the spinal canal) and vascular claudication (in the presence of peripheral vascular disease). With neurogenic claudication, the patient feels no pain when beginning exercise, and bending forward in a sitting position lessens the pain. Generally, the pain radiates symmetrically into both the front and back of the thigh. With vascular claudication, the patient reports more rapid onset with exercise, and distal rather than proximal pain. This will be accompanied by alterations in perfusion, and occasionally by murmurs detectable by auscultation over the femoral arteries.

Fig. 4.**1**   Adduction contracture

Fig. 4.**2**   Abduction contracture

- **Pain provocation**

If a hip disorder is present, pain can usually be provoked by exercise (standing up from a sitting position, climbing stairs) or detected during the examination (pain felt upon forced internal rotation). In contrast to disorders of the lumbar spine, advanced hip disease will not allow extension of the affected leg; active flexion may only be possible at the hip, causing pain.

- **Pain intensity**

To help determine the appropriate therapeutic measures, the physician should ask the patient about the intensity of the pain and the resulting impairment of patient well-being. A number of scoring systems have been developed for assessing this impairment (Harris, Hospital for Special Surgery, and Iowa).

Observation

Observation with the Patient Standing

The patient is observed standing. The following items can provide important information about the cause of the disorder:

- Orientation of the pelvis (pelvic obliquity, flexion contracture of the hip)
- Deviation of the axis of the legs (genu valgum, genu varum)
- Rotation of the legs

- Foot deformities
- In women, the shape of the Michaelis rhomboid (visible rhomboid-shaped depression over the sacral area)
- Structure of the spinal column (scoliosis, tilt)
- Muscle contour (asymmetry)
- Leg length
- Muscle atrophy
- Swelling or erythema

Leg length is best evaluated indirectly by observing the position of the pelvis. Sit behind the standing patient so that the patient's iliac crests are at about the level of your eyes. The patient's knees are fully extended. While palpating the iliac crests, place shims under the shortened extremity until the pelvis is level. Leg-length differences can be measured quite accurately using this method.

This method can produce inaccurate information if:

- In the presence of acetabular dysplasia, corresponding deformities of the iliac wing also occur. The pelvis obliquity palpated in such a situation can be misinterpreted as a difference in leg length.
- Pelvic obliquity is the result of functional leg shortening due to contracture of the adductors or abductors in the hip (Figs. 4.**1** and 4.**2**).

In an adduction contracture of the hip, the affected leg will appear shorter because the patient must raise the pelvis on the affected side when trying to place the foot of the affected side beside that of the nonaffected side. Conversely, an abduction contracture requires the patient to raise the contralateral side to place both feet together parallel to each other.

Radiographic techniques are available for more exact measurements and should be considered for more precise measurement. Radiographs with a ruler (the "Scanogram") or using the CT Scanner with a few cuts at the hips, knees, and ankles yields the most accurate information.

Gait Analysis

After observing the patient standing, inspect his or her gait. Gait irregularities may be due to:

— Pain
— Muscular weakness (Trendelenburg sign)
— Leg shortening (compensatory limp)
— Arthrodesis of the hip (compensation for a fused joint)

Antalgic gait (Duchenne). The patient attempts to reduce stress on the painful hip with an antalgic gait. There are essentially two mechanisms for achieving this:

When the affected leg is in the stance phase, the patient shifts the upper body, and thus the body's center of gravity, over the affected joint. This shortens the lever arm, with which the body weight acts on the hip, and reduces the tension in the gluteal musculature, relieving the stress on the joint as a whole. The second mechanism is for reducing the duration of stress on the joint, i.e., the stance phase. This leads to a typically truncated gait.

Trendelenburg gait due to weakness. In the Trendelenburg gait (Fig. 4.**3**), weakness of the hip abductors, primarily the gluteal musculature, causes the pelvis to dip toward the unaffected side in the stance phase. Again, the patient attempts to relieve the weakened gluteal musculature by shifting the upper body over the affected side. However, the stance phase is not as sharply truncated as in an antalgic gait, and motion is more uniform. A bilateral Trendelenburg gait produces typical waddling. Testing for the Trendelenburg sign will determine whether such a gait is a true Trendelenburg gait.

Compensatory limp with leg shortening. The upper body is shifted slightly over the leg in the stance phase. Otherwise, the gait is relatively smooth.

Compensation for hip fusion. Arthrodesis of the hip does not produce a true limp in the sense that the pelvis dips in the stance phase. Rather the increased tilt of the pelvis in the sagittal plane, as it moves from hyperlordosis into lumbar kyphosis, produces femoral anteversion in the swing phase. Since most hip fusions result in some degree of femoral shortening, the post hip fusion gait may demonstrate upper body

Fig. 4.**3** Trendelenburg limp

shift to the affected side in the stance phase as well as femoral anteversion in the swing phase.

A number of computerized methods have been developed to supplement clinical examination of gait. These methods, some of which are used in combination with electromyographic studies, may allow the examiner to define the anatomical and functional cause of gait irregularities with far greater precision.

Palpation

To palpate the hip, first locate the origins and insertions of the hip muscles to evaluate tendon disorders involving the muscular insertions (Table 4.1). Muscle pulls in the iliopsoas often occur in athletes (Fig. 4.4).

It is almost impossible to palpate the joint capsule in adults. Ultrasound studies should be performed if an effusion is suspected. Further palpation should attempt to exclude disorders such as inguinal and femoral hernias, varicoceles, and lymph node disorders. Palpate the femoral arteries and listen to them through a stethoscope to exclude arterial peripheral vascular disease.

Assessing the Range of Motion in Adults

In the initial position, the patient is supine with the hip fully extended. The medial aspects of both knees are barely touching, and both feet are parallel. The legs are correctly positioned when the axes of support (the straight lines connecting the midpoints of

Table 4.1   Important palpation points for hip disorders

• Iliac spines and sacrum	Origin of the gluteal musculature and the erector spinae
• Anterior superior iliac spine	Origin of the sartorius
• Anterior inferior iliac spine	Origin of the rectus femoris
• Branches of the pubic bone	Origin of the gracilis and abductors
• Ischial tuberosity	Origin of the hamstrings
• Lesser trochanter	Insertion of the iliopsoas
• Greater trochanter	Insertion of the gluteal musculature
• Pes anserinus	Insertion of the sartorius, gracilis, and semitendinosus
• Fibular head	Insertion of the biceps femoris
• Lateral tibial epicondyle	Insertion of the iliotibial tract

Fig. 4.4   Palpating the lesser trochanter at the insertion of the iliopsoas while rotating the leg.

the hip, knee, and ankle) are parallel. The pelvis is horizontal when the straight line connecting the anterior superior and anterior inferior iliac spine is at an angle of approximately 12° from horizontal. In the neutral position, the pelvis is tilted slightly anteriorly by the lumbar lordosis.

Flexion and Extension

Perform the examination with the patient supine on a stable surface. Ensure that the pelvis is in a neutral position by placing your hand under the sacrum. Now flex the contralateral leg at the hip until the lumbar lordosis is neutralized and the sacrum touches your hand. In this position, the patient holds his or her own leg (Thomas grip; Fig. 4.5). Now flex the leg to be examined until the pelvis begins to move. Immobilize the pelvis with your hand on the sacrum. The angle between the thigh and the examining table corresponds to the angle of flexion. Evaluate extension

with the patient supine by flexing the contralateral leg past the position in the Thomas grip until the leg being examined is lifted off the table (Fig. 4.6).

The difference in the angle between both femurs corresponds to extension.

Hip flexion and extension can also be evaluated in the lateral position. Place the patient on the contralateral side while immobilizing the pelvis in the neutral position of 12° anterior tilt with one hand. To evaluate flexion, flex the leg until the pelvis begins to move. To evaluate extension, place the patient supine, immobilize the contralateral leg with the Thomas grip, and extend the hip until the pelvis begins to move.

Make sure that the knee is flexed when evaluating hip flexion so that the hamstrings are relaxed. The knee should be extended to relax the rectus when extension is evaluated. Contractures in the knee can simulate limited hip motion.

Normal values in adults:
Extension: 10°–15°
Flexion: 130°–140°

Fig. 4.5   Evaluating flexion using the Thomas grip.

Fig. 4.**6** Evaluating hip extension.

Fig. 4.**7** Evaluating abduction in extension (one hand holds the anterior superior iliac spine).

Fig. 4.**8** Evaluating adduction in flexion (with slight flexion so that the leg may be lifted over the contralateral leg).

Fig. 4.**9** Evaluating rotation in 90° flexion with the patient supine.

Abduction and Adduction

Abduction and adduction are also evaluated with the patient supine. In children, this examination is performed with the hip extended; in adults, the hip is usually flexed 90°. Two lines are used for orientation in the neutral position. The first is the line connecting the two anterior superior iliac spines, which should be perpendicular to the axis of the body. The second is the line connecting the midpoints of the hip, knee, and ankle joints. This line should be parallel to the axis of the body.

Examination in extension. Immobilize the pelvis with one hand so that your thumb and small finger palpate the anterior superior and inferior iliac spines. With this action, compensatory movement of the pelvis is readily detectable. The extended leg is abducted until passive motion of the pelvis is detected (Fig. 4.**7**). To test adduction, place the leg being examined in slight flexion and lift it over the contralateral leg. Another option is to immobilize the contralateral leg with the Thomas grip. This makes it possible to adduct the leg even in full extension (Fig. 4.**8**).

Normal values in adults:
Abduction: 30°–45°
Adduction: 20°–30°
Examination in 90° flexion

This examination can be used in adults in addition to the examination in extension. In newborns, it is the only way to measure abduction and adduction because of physiologic flexion contracture. As in the examination in extension, immobilize the two anterior superior iliac spines with one hand while abducting the flexed leg from the vertical position until the pelvis begins to tilt in the transverse plane. Proceed similarly to evaluate adduction.

Normal values in adults:
Abduction: 60°–70°
Adduction: 20°–30°

Internal Rotation and External Rotation

Hip rotation is usually evaluated in children with the patient prone and the hip extended (Fig. 4.**9**). In adults, the examination may also be performed with

Fig. 4.**10** Drehmann test in a child. The thigh moves into compensatory external rotation as flexion increases.

the heel with the hip extended and pressing down on the midfemur will elicit groin pain.

Clinical Examination of Newborns and Infants

When examining the hip in children and newborns, obtaining a precise history is essential (see also Patient History). Inquire about a history of hip dysplasia in the family, whether the child is the first born, about breech presentation, details of delivery, the size of the child, the presence of other position anomalies, and differences in kicking motions. The type of pain can also be a sign because small children especially will present with referred pain into the knee. Even temporary pain with exercise can be an early sign of hip dysplasia. Sometimes "start-up" pain will be present, which children may barely notice. In some cases, the only sign will be gait irregularity. Other causes of such symptoms aside from hip dysplasia include an undiagnosed neurologic disorder, spasticity, or flaccid paralysis. Limps are categorized in various forms as discussed above. The Trendelenburg gait, Duchenne antalgic gait, leg shortening, and a fused joint should be distinguished. Examination of leg length can provide crucial information, particularly in the case of unilateral hip dislocation, where the affected leg appears shortened. Leg length is best evaluated with the child supine and the hips and knees flexed 90°. If this type of apparent leg shortening is present, one could estimate the difference between the legs by the level of the knees. The appearance of the soft tissue would also alter in a fully dislocated hip. Additional skin folds would be present.

the patient supine and the hip flexed 90°. When performing the examination with the patient supine, make sure that the axis through the two iliac spines is perpendicular to the axis of the body. Move the hip while monitoring the movement of the iliac spines until passive motion of the pelvis is detected. When performing the examination with the patient prone and the knee flexed, place your hand on the sacrum to immobilize the pelvis.

Normal values in adults (in extension):
External rotation: 40°–50°
Internal Rotation: 30°–40°

Normal values in adults (in flexion):
External rotation: 40°–50°
Internal rotation: 40°–45°

Specific Tests for Adolescents and Adults

Drehmann Test

In a slipped capital femoral epiphysis, the thigh will move into compensatory external rotation as hip flexion increases (Fig. 4.**10**).

Ludloff–Hohmann Test

The knee can be completely extended when the hip is in flexion and adduction because the relative shortening of the thigh relaxes the hamstrings. Positive results are a sign of hip dysplasia.

Fulcrun or Stinchfield Test

In the presence of proximal femur, femor neck, or subcapital pathology such as stress fractures, holding

Assessing Range of Motion

The differences in technique in the examination of newborns are due primarily to the physiologic flexion contracture in newborns, which precludes evaluation of hip abduction and rotation in extension. The examination is performed with the baby supine with hips and knees in 90° flexion. Make sure that the axis through the two superior iliac spines is horizontal to the examining table and perpendicular to the axis of the baby's body. Estimate the flexion contracture before performing the examination. It can vary, but will generally be about 20°–35°.

Normal values for abduction and rotation in newborns fluctuate and are difficult to specify. Haas' studies cite the following ranges of motion:

Normal values in newborns:
Internal rotation: 50°–70°
External Rotation: 75°–105°
Abduction: 65°–90°

According to studies by Harris, the range of abduction decreases in the first 9 months of life to 60°–70°. A range of abduction of less than 50° at birth can be regarded as abnormal. It is important to compare

Fig. 4.**11** Congenital hip dysplasia can simulate a shortened leg with asymmetric skin folds.

Table 4.**2** Associations and signs of hip dysplasia

Associations:
— Positive family history
— Abnormalities during pregnancy (breech presentation)
— Other deformities (clubfeet)
— Asymmetric skin folds in the glutei

Signs:
— Range of abduction less than 50°
— Positive snapping phenomenon (Ortolani, Barlow)

Fig. 4.**12** Ortolani test in examination of the hip in newborns.

findings with the contralateral side in each case. Tönnis cites a difference between sides of 10°–30° for hip dysplasia and 30°–40° for dislocation. Differences between the sides in the range of abduction can also be the result of a deformity with pelvic obliquity. Symmetric bilateral limited abduction occurs in bilateral hip dysplasia or dislocation.

Range-of-motion testing can include **estimation of femoral anteversion.**

With the child supine, hold the leg to be examined with the hip and knee flexed 90° in 0° rotation. Palpate the greater trochanter with the other hand. Now internally rotate the leg to maximize lateral displacement of the greater trochanter. Internal rotation now corresponds to anteversion. The angle of anteversion is 30°–40° at birth and decreases to values of 10°–15° in adults.

Specific Examinations for Hip Dysplasia

• Inspection

Two anomalies consistent with hip dysplasia may occasionally be detected by inspection. One of these is the decrease in leg length resulting from subluxation of the femoral head; the other is asymmetry in skin folds. Leg shortening is most readily recognizable when you hold the child supine with the hips and

knees flexed 90°. Sit in front of the child so that the child's knees are at the level of your eyes.

Asymmetric skin folds in the adductor and buttocks region are the result of superior protrusion of the femoral head on the affected side; the soft tissue of the thigh is too long for this pathologic anatomical configuration and forms folds (Fig. 4.**11**). However, this is not a specific sign (Table 4.**2**) as it can occur in up to 30% of children with normal hips. Asymmetrical folds may also be observed in scoliosis.

• Palpation

There are three situations in developmental dysplasia of the hip. The first is a dislocated hip, the second a dislocatable hip, and the third a subluxatable hip.

• Ortolani Test

A snapping sound in the first few days and weeks of life suggests an unstable hip (Fig. 4.**12**). Sit in front of the supine newborn. With one hand, grasp the leg to be examined by the flexed knee so that your thumb is touching the medial thigh and your second finger and ring finger are touching the greater trochanter. Bring the contralateral hip into maximum flexion with your other hand by grasping the knee so that the pelvis is immobilized. Now flex and slightly adduct the leg to be examined. In this position, apply slight anteropos-

Fig. 4.**13**   Barlow dislocation test.

Fig. 4.**14**   Evaluating the iliopsoas.

terior (AP) pressure to the knee you are holding with your hand. This will cause posterior subluxation of the femoral head. Abduct the hip under slight pressure. Apply slight pressure to the greater trochanter. In a positive test, you will hear a characteristic snapping sound during the abduction motion as the femoral head reduces into the acetabulum.

- **Barlow test**

In this examination, the hips are brought into intermediate abduction, and pressure is applied to the greater trochanter to evaluate reduction (Fig. 4.**13**). Then try to dislocate the hip by applying posterior and lateral pressure to the femoral head.

Neurologic Examination

Examining the Muscles

Not every nerve root has a specific corresponding muscle.

To maximize clinical information, examining the muscles according to their function is recommended. They are then evaluated according to the muscle grading chart.

Flexors

Primary flexor: iliopsoas (femoral nerve, L1, 2, and 3).

The iliopsoas is the primary flexor. To test it, have the patient sit and let his or her legs dangle over the side of the examining table. Stabilize the pelvis by placing your hand on the iliac crest and having the patient lift the thigh off the table. Press on the distal portion of the thigh with your other hand to determine maximum resistance. Use both hands with strong patients (Fig. 4.**14**). Repeat the test on the contralateral side for comparison.

Extensors

Primary extensor: gluteus maximus (inferior gluteal nerve, S1).

To test the gluteus maximus in isolation, have the patient lie prone with the knee flexed. Place your arm over the patient's iliac crest to stabilize the pelvis before instructing the patient to lift the leg. Provide resistance to this motion by pressing against the distal thigh with your other hand. Palpate the muscle tone during this examination. Repeat the test for the contralateral side.

Abductors

Primary abductor: gluteus medius (superior gluteal nerve, L5).

To evaluate abduction, place the patient in a lateral position and stabilize the pelvis at the iliac crest. Have the patient abduct the leg against your resistance. Another option is to examine the patient supine with the leg abducted about 20°. Again, instruct the patient to abduct the leg against your resistance.

Adductors

Primary adductor: adductor longus (obturator nerve, L2, 3, and 4).

To evaluate adduction, have the patient adduct the abducted leg against your resistance (Fig. 4.**15**). Another option is to examine the patient supine. Again, instruct the patient to adduct the abducted leg against your resistance.

Examining Sensation

Findings on sensation testing are easier to evaluate than muscular findings because the sensory supply is divided into demarcated dermatomes (Fig. 4.**16**) that are relatively similar among all patients.

Dermatome L1 covers a transverse band along the anterior aspect of the proximal thigh directly distal to the inguinal ligament.

Dermatome L3 extends in an oblique band proximal to the knee.

Dermatome L2 lies precisely between these two. Dermatome L4 includes the area of skin on the medial thigh; dermatome L5 supplies the lateral calf including the dorsum and medial edge of the foot.

Dermatome S2 supplies a long strip along the posterior aspect of the thigh from the fold of the buttocks to the popliteal fossa.
Dermatome S3, often clinically significant because of the lateral femoral cutaneous nerve, is a wide oval area located on the lateral aspect of the thigh.

Dermatomes S3 through S5 are arranged in three concentric rings around the anus, from medial to lateral.

4.3 Radiology

Standard Views

Standard views of the hip include the AP radiograph of the hip and lateral radiograph of the hip.

The AP radiograph is used to determine the neck-shaft angle and assess possible varus or valgus deformity. It can be used for detecting fractures of the ipsilateral anterior pelvic ring, acetabulum, and femoral head and neck; for confirming dislocations of the hip; and for preoperative evaluation of the vertical origin of the lumbar spine where it exits the sacrum. It may be used in preoperative planning for leg-length operations.

The lateral radiograph demonstrates the anteversion of the femoral neck, the anterior and posterior cortex of the femoral neck, the ischial tuberosity, and rotation and displacement of the femoral head in fractures.

The AP radiograph is prepared with the patient supine with the legs in slight internal rotation to compensate for anteversion of the femoral necks. If the entire pelvis is to be imaged, the ray is centered on the middle of the pelvis; if a hip is to be imaged, it is centered on the respective femoral head.

The lateral radiograph is taken with the patient supine. The affected leg is extended, and the opposite

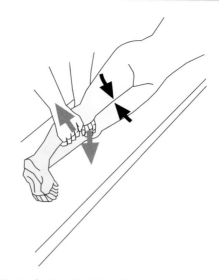

Fig. 4.**15**   Evaluating the hip adductors.

Fig. 4.**16**   Sensory dermatomes of the lower extremity.

Fig. 4.**17**   Positioning for the lateral radiograph of the hip.

Fig. 4.**18**   Technique of the anterior oblique radiograph (obturator view).

Fig. 4.**19**   Obtaining the posterior oblique radiograph (iliac wing view).

leg is lifted and abducted (Fig. 4.**17**). The cassette is placed along the side of the affected hip with the ray centered on the groin and inclined 20° cranially from horizontal. This permits calculating the angle of anteversion as described by Dunn, Müller, and Rippstein (see section Hip Dyplasia, p. 153).

Special Views

Special views include inlet and outlet views of the pelvis, variations of the lateral radiographs, various oblique views, Lauenstein views, AP radiographs with altered settings, views for preoperative planning, and special views for precise evaluation of the acetabulum and the femoral neck.

In a trauma setting, inlet and outlet views of the pelvis can be helpful in defining a fracture detected in the AP radiograph. The patient is supine with the legs extended for both views. For the **inlet view** (Fig. 9.**37**), the central ray is angled 40° caudad and enters the midline at the level of the anterior superior iliac spine. For the **outlet view** (Fig. 9.**39**), the central ray is angled 40° cephalad and enters at the inferior aspect of the pubic symphysis.

The **lateral radiographs** mentioned in the previous section can be varied by altering the projection. Epiphyseal dislocation can be documented precisely in a straight lateral projection. A vertical projection, i.e., inclining the projection 20° cranially from horizontal (see above), is especially suitable for documenting anteversion and a slipped epiphysis. A horizontal projection (Sven Johnson) is useful as a second imaging plane if fractures of the femoral neck are to be internally fixed.

The **oblique radiographs (Judet views** see also p. 434) include anterior (internally rotated) and posterior (externally rotated) views. These views are most suitable for diagnostic purposes and preoperative planning for treatment of acetabular fractures. The anterior oblique view shows fractures of the anterior column or posterior acetabular margin, and the linea terminalis. The posterior view shows fractures of the posterior column or anterior acetabular margin, and the quadrilateral plate.

The **anterior oblique radiograph (obturator view)** is prepared with the patient positioned supine and rolled 45° onto the healthy contralateral hip (Fig. 4.**18**). The ray is centered vertically on the affected hip.

The **posterior oblique radiograph (iliac wing view)** is also prepared with the patient supine, but rolled 45° onto the affected side (Fig. 4.**19**). Here too, the ray is centered vertically on the affected hip.

The **Lauenstein view** is particularly suited for visualizing fractures of the femoral head or neck and

Fig. 4.**20** Preparing a Ferguson view as a modified AP radiograph to better evaluate the pubic and ischial rami.

Fig. 4.**21** Technique of the Faux profile view for evaluation of the roof of the acetabulum.

of the greater or lesser trochanter. For a Lauenstein radiograph, the patient is positioned supine with the knees flexed, pressing the soles of the feet together at maximum abduction. If both hips are to be imaged, the ray must be centered vertically or inclined about 10° cranially and centered on a point slightly superior to the pubic symphysis. If one of the hips is to be imaged, the ray is centered directly on that hip.

The **Ferguson** view and **Letournel** view represent modifications of AP radiographs in which the X-ray tube is inclined 30°–40° cranially or caudally (Fig. 4.**20**) The cranially inclined view visualizes fractures of the pubic rami, sacral fractures, and ruptures of the pubic symphysis and sacroiliac joint. The caudally inclined view permits the surgeon to assess the pelvic ring and the sacroiliac joints.

Preoperative planning studies are prepared if a varus or valgus correction in abduction or adduction is planned. The surgeon may often elect views in flexion or hyperextension for preoperative planning in the presence of defects in the femoral head.

The **Faux profile** view is recommended for precise evaluation of the anterior acetabulum. The patient stands with the pelvis against a diagonal wall fixed at an angle of 65° to the X-ray plate (Fig. 4.**21**). The leg bears the patient's weight during the exposure and must remain strictly parallel to the X-ray plate. The center of the film plate is positioned behind the patient's hip. When using this technique, it should be noted that increased anteversion may increase the anterior inclination of the roof of the acetabulum.

Abnormal Findings

Hip Dysplasia

Developmental dysplasia of the hip can only be imaged in AP views, which can be altered by placing the hips in abduction or internal rotation. However, a variety of reference lines can be used to quantify this disorder.

The initial purpose of the radiograph is to demonstrate the relationship between the femoral head and the acetabulum. Determining reference angles, lines, etc. can provide more precise information about the severity of the dysplasia. Evaluation of the ossification center in the femoral capital epiphysis will provide clear signs of delayed development even during the first years of life.

When evaluating radiographs of newborns and children, always bear in mind that about a quarter of all girls and about half of all boys do not yet have an ossified core in the femoral head. Differences in shape and size often represent physiologic rather than pathologic findings. At age three or four, the ossified core of the femoral head will usually be recognizable as a hemispheric shape. The epiphysis between the femoral neck and head courses obliquely from superior and lateral to inferior and medial. Its physiologic appearance is slightly wavy. The younger the child, the wider the joint will be, opening at the margins. By the age of 18, the head fuses completely with the femoral neck.

As there is a wide variety of reference lines, we will limit our discussion to a selected few in the interests of clarity. Proper positioning of the child's pelvis is crucial to all of these methods as unreliable findings might otherwise result.

Hilgenreiner's line is also known as the triradiate cartilage line since it connects these two structures (Fig. 4.**22**). This line is tangent to the most distal points of the iliac wings, at the distal margins of the acetabula.

Perkins' line intersects Hilgenreiner's line since it is drawn down to Hilgenreiner's line from the most lateral point of the acetabulum. It forms four quadrants used to determine the degree of hip dislocation.

Perkin's Line

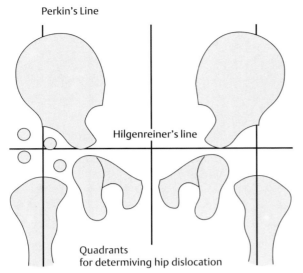

Hilgenreiner's line

Quadrants
for determiving hip dislocation

Fig. 4.**22**   Lines of Perkins for evaluating hip dysplasia.

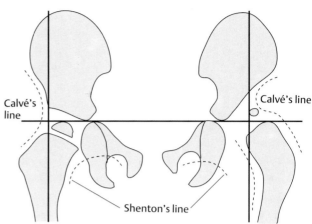

Calvé's
line

Calvé's line

Shenton's line

Fig. 4.**23**   Shenton's line (medial) and Calvé's line (lateral).

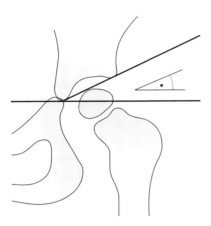

Fig. 4.**24**   Hilgenreiner's acetabular index.

In a normal hip, the core of the femoral head will be located in the inferior medial quadrant. In subluxation, it will be more in the superior medial quadrant. In a dislocation it will be in the inferior lateral quadrant; in a high dislocation, in the superior lateral quadrant.

Shenton's line follows the superior curve of the obturator foramen and continues in a curve along the inferior margin of the femoral neck (Fig. 4.**23**). This line is interrupted in early dislocations and in Legg–Calvé–Perthes disease.

Calvé's line (Fig. 4.**23**) extends the lateral margin of the iliac wing from the acetabular convexity to the femoral neck. Normally it should touch the lateral margin of the femoral neck.

Hilgenreiner's acetabular index can be influenced by patient positioning (Fig. 4.**24**). A proven technique is to place the patient with the legs extended in a strict neutral position. The angle is obtained by marking a point in the triradiate cartilage

at the lowest lateral corner of the ilium on both sides and connecting these points with a horizontal line. A second line is drawn from this point on the ilium to the lateral acetabular convexity. This point should lie within the sclerotic area.

If the angle of pelvic inclination is great, the anterior and posterior margins of the acetabulum may project separately. In this case, the tangent extending to the acetabular convexity should not be drawn at the inferior projection line but should be drawn directly to the intersection of the two projection lines at the acetabular convexity. The desired angle is located between the triradiate cartilage and the line to the acetabular convexity.

Defining normal values in the first few months of life is difficult. Hilgenreiner defined a value of 35°, although fluctuation occurs within a wide range. In practice, a system of classification according to one or two standard deviations was introduced, which determines how observation of the hip should continue. It became apparent that hips ranging between both values (20°–25° and 35°–40°) can remain normal or become abnormal, whereas hips with values exceeding the standard deviation should generally be regarded as pathologic.

Wiberg's center/corner angle can be used to evaluate the position of the femoral head relative to the acetabulum (Fig. 4.**25**).

This angle is measured between a line drawn parallel to the longitudinal axis of the body and a line connecting the midpoint of the femoral head and the lateral apex of the superior acetabular margin. This angle increases as the depth of the acetabulum increases, and decreases in a shallow acetabulum.

Normal values are 25° between the ages of five and eight, 30° between the ages of nine and 12, and 35° above that age.

The neck-shaft angle described by M. E. Müller as the collum-center-diaphysis or CCD angle is an

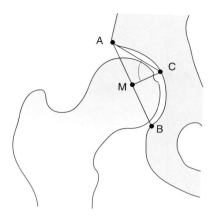

Fig. 4.**25** Wiberg's center/corner angle.

Fig. 4.**26** Neck-shaft angle described by M. E. Müller.

Fig. 4.**27** Radiographic image of Legg–Calvé–Perthes disease in the condensation and fragmentation stage.

important angle in the femoral neck (Fig. 4.**26**). This angle is formed by an arc intersecting the most lateral point of the epiphysis and the diaphyseal "spine" as the medial reference point on the section of the femoral neck that forms the head. Another lateral point, which lies on the arc around the midpoint of the femoral head in the narrowest part of the femoral neck, is marked and included. The points of intersection are then connected with the cortex of the femoral neck. A line drawn form the center of the head perpendicular to this line represents the axis of the femoral neck. The axis of the femur is the midline between the margins of the shaft. The neck-shaft angle is measured medially between the femoral neck and the axis of the femur. Since the physiologic anteversion of the femur will result in an excessively high value, the measured value should be converted using Müller's tables to determine the actual value.

Legg–Calvé–Perthes Disease

The radiologic diagnosis of Legg–Calvé–Perthes disease is usually made with an AP pelvic radiograph and with a Lauenstein view of both hips.

If indicated, these views can be supplemented with anteversion or lateral radiographs.

For documenting early stages of the disease, we recommend a radiograph with the hip flexed 30° and in neutral rotation, with the tube centered if necessary.

Throughout the course of the disease, the radiologic diagnosis is made on the basis of a few features that may be very unspecific, particularly in the initial stages of the disease. Upon initial presentation it may be difficult, except in retrospect, to identify at which stage of the disease process a patient is.

A soft-tissue shadow can be an early sign of the disorder.

Widening of the joint space or lateralization of the femoral epiphysis may be a further sign.

Changes in the epiphysis become increasingly apparent as the disorder progresses; the epiphysis shrinks and loses its sphericity. These changes affect the anterolateral quadrant in particular and can be seen in a Lauenstein view.

Kite and French described the flattening of the lateral and medial epiphyseal dome as a **roof sign.**

Köhler referred to the enlargement of the acetabular teardrop with an increase in the width of the anterior acetabular margin.

In the early stages of the disorder, the Lauenstein view can reveal a transient subchondral radiolucent line, which has been described as a fracture line, resorption zone, or crescent sign.

The **condensation and fragmentation stage** (Fig. 4.**27**) is usually characterized by compression of the core of the head and loss of roundness, later by a chaotic nodular structure and collapse of the epiphysis.

Lateralization (sometimes referred to as decentralization) also occurs as the femoral head enlarges and subluxes. At this time, the epiphysis is insufficiently covered. Decentralization results in disturbed anterolateral growth and creates a rounded recess inferior to the roof of the acetabulum. At times the epiphysis

Fig. 4.**28**   Radiographic image of Legg–Calvé–Perthes disease in the reossification stage.

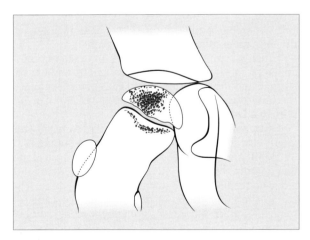

Fig. 4.**30**   Catterall, group II.

will appear to have sunk laterally in the shape of a saddle. Later, this will be accompanied by calcification-like image fogging and bony islands in the lateral aspect.

Small cystic structural irregularities, radiolucent bands, and large cysts form in the metaphysis. Here, too, the changes affect primarily the anterolateral aspect.

Fig. 4.**29**   Catterall, group I.

Increased density and ongoing repair processes give the femoral neck an increasingly broad and solid appearance.

The **reossification stage** is characterized by the formation of new trabeculae, reossification of the cartilaginous mantle, growth of anterolateral bone islands, and fusion of the epiphysis (Fig. 4.**28**).

The final stage is usually characterized by a flattened, broadened, enlarged, and lateralized femoral head. Particularly in young children, restoration of joint integrity is sometimes possible. The femoral neck is shortened and widened, and sometimes the trochanter protrudes superiorly. This form is collectively referred to as coxa plana.

The so-called **"sagging rope sign"** has been described by Apley and Weintroub. This sign gets its name from the dense, inferiorly concave line at the upper femoral metaphysis, which is reminiscent of a sagging rope.

Catterall has suggested classifying radiologic findings into the four groups according to their prognosis:

Group 1: The anterior aspect of the epiphysis is only slightly affected; no metaphyseal changes are present, and the prognosis is good (Fig. 4.**29**).

Group 2: The anterior aspect of the epiphysis is significantly affected, with profound involvement of the medial and lateral aspects (Fig. 4.**30**); small cystic changes are present in the metaphysis. A subchondral fracture line is present, but does not extend beyond the tip of the epiphysis and lies in the anterior half. The prognosis is still good, especially in a younger child.

Group 3: The entire epiphysis is involved, and the condition is most acute in the anterior lateral aspect (Fig. 4.**31**). A long, prominent fracture line is present that covers the tip of the epiphysis on the AP radiograph. The AP radiograph in particular reveals the head-within-a-head phenomenon; the femoral neck is widened. The prognosis is considerably worse.

Fig. 4.**31** Catterall, group III.

Fig. 4.**32** Catterall, group IV.

Fig. 4.**33** Schematic diagram of the Gage sign.

Group 4: The entire epiphysis is necrotic, and the head is mushroom shaped. A triangular shape is discernible medially and laterally, and there is generalized metaphyseal involvement. The prognosis is very poor (Fig. 4.**32**).

Salter and Thompson have described another similar classification system that emphasizes the significance of the subchondral fracture line.

Catterall has supplemented his classification system with risk factors, the four "head-at-risk signs" visible on the AP radiograph. Their presence denotes a substantially worse prognosis, and they are more significant than the extent of epiphyseal necrosis.

One of these signs is the **Gage sign** (Fig. 4.**33**), that represents an area of lysis in the lateral epiphyseal margin and the adjoining metaphysis. According to Catterall, this sign is indicative of a lateral deformation of the femoral head.

Lateral calcification is another sign. Lateral subluxation is regarded as an important criterion and is almost always indicative of an unfavorable outcome.

Metaphyseal changes should also be regarded as indicative of an extremely unfavorable development.

Additional risk factors can only be determined by measurement. These include containment of the femoral head, increase in radius or hypertrophy of the femoral head in the early fragmentation stage, coxa magna and coxa brevis, early epiphyseal closure, and lateral closure of the epiphysis of the femoral head.

Obtaining objective results from radiographic studies requires the use of indices that are partly specific to Legg–Calvé–Perthes disease and partly unspecific. We will discuss only the most common indices.

The **epiphyseal index** described by Eyre-Brook specifies a measure for epiphyseal flattening in terms of the ratio of the height of the epiphysis to the width of the epiphyseal line. This index is calculated from the quotients of the height and width of the epiphysis. In children below the age of seven, values between 45% and 55% are normal; in older children, values between 35% and 45% are normal.

The **epiphyseal quotient** described by Sjövall compares the healthy side with the affected side. The quotient is calculated by division, using the indices of the affected side and the healthy side. Normal values range from 90% to 100%.

The **head–neck quotient** represents a measure for the compaction of the femoral neck. It is the percentage quotient of the head–neck index of the affected and healthy sides. The head-neck index itself consists of the quotient of the length and shortest width of the femoral neck multiplied by 100. Normal values lie between 190 and 150.

The **acetabulum–head index** is a measure for the disproportion between head and acetabulum, particularly for the completeness of coverage. The index is calculated from the quotient of the horizontal diameter of the covered section of the head (i.e., from the medial epiphysis to the perpendicular of the acetabular convexity) and the horizontal diameter of the entire head. Normal values lie between 90% and 70%.

The comprehensive index according to Heyman and Herndon is an additional index for Legg–Calvé–

Fig. 4.**34** Radiographic image of slipped capital femoral epiphysis.

Perthes disease that covers the shape of the head, neck, and acetabulum. Results from 100% to 90% are regarded as having an excellent prognosis, from 90% to 80% good, from 80% to 70% satisfactory, from 70% to 60% poor, and below 60% very poor.

Infection and Inflammation

Hip inflammation or infection can be purulent or nonpurulent.

Early signs of purulent inflammation include an effusion and periarticular osteoporosis. Occasionally a shadow consistent with soft-tissue swelling will be visible.

As the disease progresses, articular cartilage is destroyed. This is visible in subchondral changes, particularly in narrowing of the joint space.

A nonpurulent arthritis such as tuberculous arthritis will characteristically exhibit **Phemister's triad:** periarticular osteoporosis, peripheral bone erosion, and gradual narrowing of the joint space. Occasionally, wedge-shaped necrotic areas known as kissing lesions will be detected in the radiograph on both sides of the joint.

The late stage of the disorder is characterized by complete destruction of the joint with significant sclerotic areas.

Slipped Capital Femoral Epiphysis

Early diagnosis of this disorder is often only possible in radiographic examinations.

Lauenstein views of both hips are required in addition to an AP view of the pelvis for diagnosing this disorder.

Early radiographic evidence prior to dislocation may include an irregularly bounded epiphyseal line and broadening of the epiphysis, thinned-out structure, localized atrophy of the metaphyseal bone structures, increased thickness of the boundary of the femoral head, and slight atrophy of the head and neck area. In mild cases, loss of the lateral overhang of the

femoral ossific nucleus (Klein's line) and blurring of the proximal femoral metaphysis may be all that is seen on the AP film.

Capener's **triangle sign** in the AP radiograph is early evidence of a slipped capital femoral epiphysis. The medial side of the femoral neck will be seen to overlap the posterior wall of the acetabulum, forming a triangle. In addition to this, the cranial S-shaped line marking the boundary of the femoral neck and head is flattened. Occasionally, proliferations of bone will be seen at the inferior posterior angle between the neck and epiphysis. The height of the epiphysis may be reduced as it begins to slip posteriorly (Fig. 4.**34**). The lines of the epiphysis may close prematurely.

The lateral projection can show increased bone resorption in the posterior metaphysis of the femoral neck. The contour of the head and neck may also be flattened. A common radiographic finding is loss of the smooth curve from the obturator foramen along the inferior femoral neck— a break in Shenton's line.

The late stages of the disorder are characterized by convex deformation of the head, widening and shortening of the femoral neck, and structural changes in the metaphysis of the femoral neck. Bone remodeling and formation of osteophytes can occur in the femoral neck.

Osteoarthritis of the Hip

Osteoarthritis of the hip is diagnosed by narrowing of the joint space, increased sclerosis, formation of osteophytes at non-weight-bearing sites (i.e., usually at the edge of the joint), and formation of cysts or pseudocysts as a sign of microfractures and penetration of synovial fluid into the cancellous bone (Fig. 4.**35**). Acetabular cysts of this sort are referred to as **Egger cysts.**

Special craniolateral oblique views are essential for evaluating osteophytes on the anterior circumference of the acetabulum and femoral head. Posterior or medial cysts can only be imaged in Faux profile views.

Appositions of osteophytes on the medial contour femoral neck (which Lequesne refers to as a "hammock") show a double contour with a convex outer layer of ossification.

The Faux profile view will show a circular area of cartilage necrosis with a tendency to dislocate anteriorly, or primarily inferior and posterior cartilage necrosis with ossification of the interacetabular ligament.

In addition to these signs of arthritis, migration of the femoral head will be observed: the direction is generally superolateral.

The type of deformation and the displacement of the head relative to the acetabulum provide further information. Views in adduction and abduction, Faux profile views (see section Special Views, p. 152), and views in internal and external rotation may be helpful.

Fig. 4.**35** Degenerative changes in the hip.

Table 4.**3** Ficat's stages of osteonecrosis

Stage	Films	Bone scan	MRI
0	NL	NL	NL
1	NL	Nondiagnostic	Early changes
2	Porosis/sclerosis	+	+
3	Flat/crescent sign	+	+
4	Acetabular changes	+	+

Hip dysplasia with osteoarthritis is a special case. In its early stages, it is characterized by an excessively small roof of the acetabulum, a center/corner angle of less than 25°, a pathologic acetabular index, an excessively large neck-shaft angle, and pathologic anteversion (see section Hip Dysplasia, p. 153). The femoral head may show flattening around the fovea, an abnormal position in the acetabulum, or the beginning of cartilage necrosis with congruity of the femoral head and acetabulum.

The late stage is characterized by arthritis and subluxation. Shenton's line (see section Hip Dysplasia, p. 153) is disrupted, and there is increased sclerosis of the acetabular convexity, joint-space narrowing, and deformation of the femoral head.

Avascular Necrosis of the Femoral Head

Early signs of this disease that have been described include thickening and loss of roundness or subsidence of the anterosuperior contour of the femoral head.

Occasionally these discrete changes will only be visible in **Schneider tangential views** as these views visualized the largest part of the circumference.

Four radiographs should be obtained: a 30° oblique view demonstrating the posterosuperior sec-

tor, an AP view for the superior sector, and views in 30° and 60° flexion to demonstrate the anterosuperior portions.

Arlet and Ficat have developed a standard system for classifying the entire course of the disorder (Table 4.**3**).

— Stage 1 describes a normal radiograph while MRI reveals early changes.
— Stage 2 describes nodular changes in the cancellous bone with porous or sclerotic areas. At this time the joint space and the contour of the femoral head are still normal.
— Stage 3: the contour of the femoral head is interrupted. Sequestration as a result of collapse is observed while the joint space remains unchanged.
— Stage 4 represents the complete clinical syndrome. The joint space appears narrow and shallow. Massive joint destruction is present.

Rheumatoid Disease

Radiologic characteristics of rheumatoid hip disease include erosion, osteoporosis, and soft-tissue swelling. In contrast to degenerative hip disease, sclerosis or osteophytes can rarely be demonstrated.

Osteoporosis is a significant characteristic of the disorder. Initially it is localized; later, generalized osteoporosis can be demonstrated.

Narrowing of the joint space usually causes the femoral head to migrate axially, occasionally medially. In some cases, protrusion of the acetabulum will occur (Fig. 4.**36**).

This is a synovial-based process. Areas of joint erosion occur on both sides of the joint at the synovial insertions. These areas destroy the joint without any repair processes such as formation of osteophytes or sclerosis.

Synovial cysts and pseudocysts can be demonstrated in the immediate vicinity of the joint. Occasionally there will be radiographic evidence of an effusion.

Fig. 4.**36**   Radiographic image of protrusion of the acetabulum.

Fig. 4.**37**   Radiographic image of pigmented villonodular synovitis.

Pigmented Villonodular Synovitis

This rheumatic disorder is characterized by a lack of joint changes. Only in a few cases can small diffuse cysts be demonstrated (Fig. 4.**37**).

Femoral Neck Fractures

Fractures of the femoral neck are generally visible in the plain pelvic radiograph, although some can only be demonstrated in Lauenstein or lateral axial views. Extracapsular, intracapsular, and articular fractures are differentiated. Fractures can be described using the AO/ASIF classification system (Fig. 4.**38**).

The first step in diagnosing a fracture is to differentiate between intracapsular and extracapsular fractures. **Intracapsular fractures** show a fracture line in the femoral neck, occasionally involving the femoral head or the base of the femoral neck.

Intracapsular fractures can be classified according to the system defined by Garden.

Garden's classification system is based on the position of the main medial weight-bearing trabecula. This system differentiates four degrees of severity (Fig. 4.**39a–d**).

— Type 1: describes an incomplete subcapital non-dislocated fracture. The distal fragment is externally rotated, and the proximal fragment is in a valgus position. The trabeculae of the medial femoral head and those of the medial femoral neck form an angle of 180°. The prognosis is good.
— Type 2: defined as a complete subcapital fracture without deformity. The distal fragment is in a normal position with respect to the proximal fragment. The trabeculae of the medial femoral head form an angle of 160° with those of the medial femoral neck. The prognosis for these fractures is also good.
— Type 3: involves a complete subcapital fracture with a certain degree of deformity. The proximal fragment is twisted, abducted, and tilted into a varus position. This form of fracture is regarded as unstable, and the prognosis is unfavorable.
— Type 4: involves a complete subcapital fracture with pronounced deformity. In these fractures, the distal fragment is externally rotated, superiorly displaced, and lies anterior to the proximal fragment. However, the medial fragment is in a correct position in the acetabulum. The prognosis is least favorable for these fractures.

Extracapsular fractures are either intertrochanteric or subtrochanteric. Usually the fracture line can be followed from the lesser trochanter to the greater trochanter.

Intertrochanteric fractures can be described according to the AO/ASIF classification as simple fractures with respect to the number of fragments, according to the Boyd-Griffin classification or the classification of Fielding and Zickel.

The **Boyd-Griffin classification** shows a linear intertrochanteric fracture line in type 1, a comminuted fracture in the trochanter region with type 2, a comminuted fracture including a subtrochanteric component in type 3, and an oblique fracture extending into the subtrochanteric region in type 4 (Figs. 4.**40a–d**).

Subtrochanteric fractures are divided into five types according to **Seinsheimer's classification** as shown in Table 4.**4** and Figure 4.**41**.

Fig. 4.**38**   AO/ASIF classification of proximal femoral fractures.

Table 4.**4**   Seinsheimer's classification of subtrochanteric fractures (from Seinsheimer, F., III: Subtrochanteric fractures of the femur. *J Bone Joint Surg* 1978; 60-A: 302)

Type I	Non or minimally displaced
Type II	Two part
Type III	Three part
Type IV	Comminuted
Type V	Subtrochanteric–intertrochanteric

4.4 Ultrasound

Indications

Ultrasound has become popular as a method of early diagnosis of hip dysplasia in newborns.

Other indications include suspicion of a joint effusion, Legg–Calvé–Perthes disease, and slipped capital femoral epiphysis.

In adults, ultrasound can be used to demonstrate synovitis, a joint effusion, and trochanteric bursitis.

Examination Technique

Positioning for ultrasound examination of the hip depends on the patient's age. Newborns are examined in the lateral position in special examination tubs. The examiner stands to the right of the baby so that the acetabular region is imaged on the right and the trochanter region is imaged on the left (Fig. 4.**42**). High-contrast image settings should be used to better demonstrate cartilage and bone structures.

Older children or adults are positioned supine, rarely laterally. At this age, ultrasound examination can only provide information about periarticular

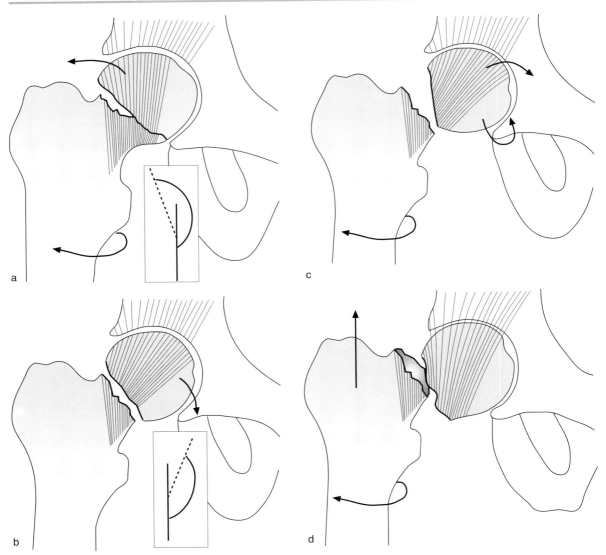

Figs. 4.**39a–d** Femoral neck fracture, stages 1–4 according to Garden.
a Type 1, **b** Type 2, **c** Type 3, **d** Type 4.

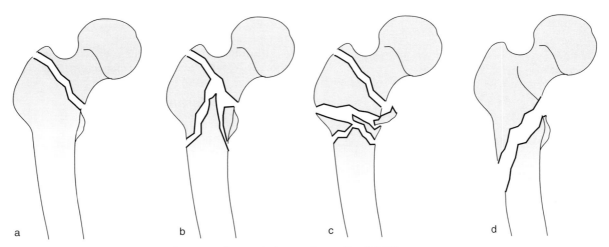

Figs. 4.**40a–d** Intertrochanteric fractures of types 1–4 according to Boyd-Griffin.
a Type 1, **b** Type 2, **c** Type 3, **d** Type 4.

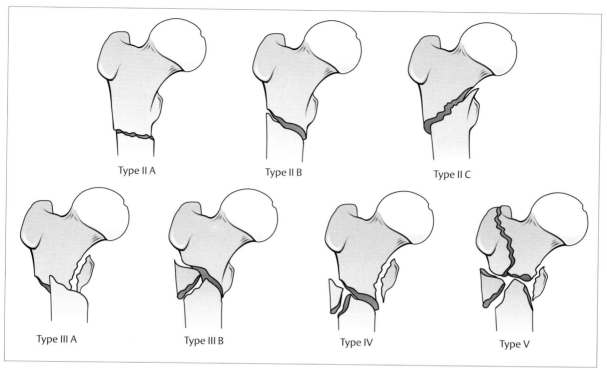

Fig. 4.**41** Classification of subtrochanteric fractures (from Seinsheimer, F., III: Subtrochanteric fractures of the femur. *J Bone Joint Surg* 1978; 60-A: 302).

Fig. 4.**42** Positioning for ultrasound examination of the hip in a newborn.

structures so that softer image settings should also be preferred in these patients.

A distinction is made between the anterior and lateral imaging planes.

In the anterior imaging plane, the patient is supine and the transducer is placed on the region of the femoral neck perpendicular to the axis of the body. In the lateral imaging plane, the patient is positioned laterally and the transducer is placed perpendicular to the hip in a strictly coronal plane.

Normal Findings

Ultrasound examination of the **hip in newborns** follows the studies of Graf and Schuler.

The examiner attempts to image hyaline cartilage structures. These appear as hypoechoic or anechoic in the sonogram. If the core of the femoral head has formed completely, this examination will no longer be possible because the bone will completely eliminate sound reflection and produce what is known as an acoustic shadow. This will occur within the first year of life (Fig. 4.**43**).

In **healthy adults** the hip appears in the sonogram as a hyperechoic triangular acetabular labrum, a sharp-edged hyperechoic acetabular convexity, and a hyperechoic band representing the joint capsule. The femoral head also appears as a hyperechoic structure. Occasionally, pseudolesions will be visible on the femoral neck.

Fig. 4.**43** Sonogram of a 3-month-old infant.
1 Gluteus maximus
2 Gluteus medius
3 Gluteus minimus
4 Acetabular labrum
5 Joint capsule
6 Femoral head
7 Epiphyseal center of the femoral head
8 Chondro-osseous boundary in the femoral neck
9 Inferior margin of the ilium
10 Bony acetabular convexity
11 Proximal perichondrium (rectus tendon)
12 Silhoutte of the ilium

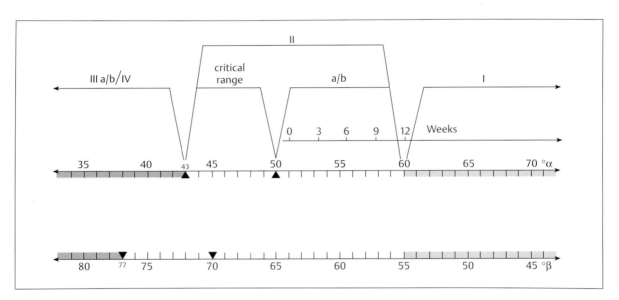

Fig. 4.**44** Sonometer. The alpha and beta angles are graphed so that alpha values increase linearly from left to right, whereas beta values decrease. Classification of sonographic hip types: type I hips are on the right side and dislocated hips (types IIIa, IIIb, and IV) are on the left. The center section shows type II hips, which include subclassifications type IIa, type IIb, and type IIc. Time scale for newborns: Birth (zero) corresponds to an alpha angle of 50–51°. The twelfth week of life corresponds to an alpha angle of 60°.

Abnormal Findings

Developmental Hip Dislocation

This clinical syndrome is diagnosed with the aid of ultrasound studies in infants, i.e., from birth until the end of the first year of life (Figs. 4.**44**–4.**50**). Developmental hip dislocation is a congenital disorder of the hip involving disturbed maturity, delayed development, or underdevelopment of the elements forming the hip. Subluxation or dislocation of the hip will usually occur in the first 6 months of life as a result. Rarely, a genuine congenital dislocation will be present; frequently this disorder will occur in combina-

tion with other deformities. Genetic and geographic factors influence etiology, as do exogenous factors such as breech presentation.

Legg–Calvé–Perthes Disease

Ultrasound examination of Legg–Calvé–Perthes disease is based on observation of the effusion (Fig. 4.**51**). This distends the joint capsule in the superior middle section of the femoral neck. The capsule distension is less than for infections, and can be detected for a significantly longer period of time.

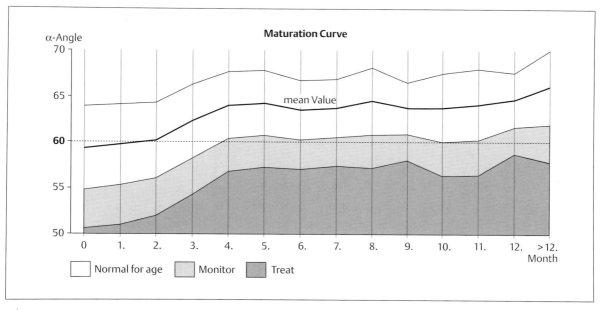

Fig. 4.**45** The alpha value is obtained from images in the longitudinal plane in a normal infant. The control range lies within the standard deviation; the therapeutic range lies within twice the standard deviation.

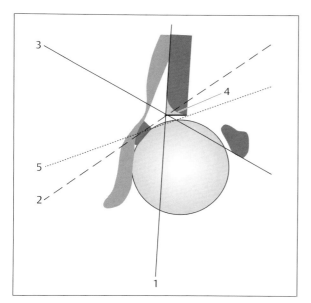

Fig. 4.**46a** Schematic diagram of a type I hip. The acetabular convexity is either angular or slightly rounded.
1 Baseline
2 Line of the cartilage roof
3 Line of the roof of the acetabulum
4 Rounded bony acetabular convexity
5 Line of the cartilage roof with a blunted acetabular convexity

Fig. 4.**46b** Type I hip with an acetabular convexity.

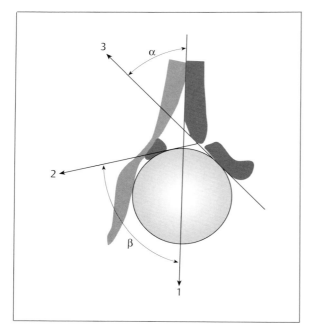

Fig. 4.**47a** Schematic diagram of sonographic type II hip. Total joint coverage is insufficient; relationship between the bony and cartilaginous parts of the acetabular roof shifted in favor of the cartilage.
1 Baseline   **2** Line of the cartilage roof
3 Line of the roof of the acetabulum
    α: Bone angle
    β: Cartilage angle

Fig. 4.**47b** Sonogram of the left hip in a 9-month-old infant. The bony acetabular convexity is rounded, and the bony molding is insufficient. A broad rim of cartilage still covers the femoral head (type II). The plane of the image visualizes the bony defect of the acetabular convexity.
1 Transition point   **2** Cartilaginous acetabular convexity
3 Acetabular labrum

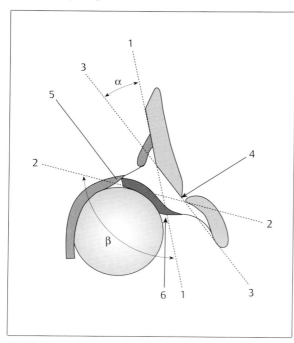

Fig. 4.**48a** Schematic diagram of a type IIIa eccentric hip without histologic change. The hyaline cartilage of the roof of the acetabulum is hypoechoic.
1 Baseline   **4** Transition point
2 Line of the cartilage roof **5** Superiorly elongated labrum
3 Bony roof line   **6** Fulcrum
    α: Bone angle
    β: Cartilage angle

Fig. 4.**48b** Hip in an 8-week-old infant. Bony acetabular molding is poor and the acetabular convexitiy is flattened. The cartilaginous rim of the roof of the acetabulum is superiorly displaced cranially (type IIIa).
1 Acetabular labrum   **2** Bony acetabular convexity
Note: The inferior margin of the ilium cannot be clearly visualized as the femoral head no longer lies within the standard imaging plane.

Fig. 4.**49a** Schematic diagram of a type IIIb hip. Pressure on the cartilage roof alters its histologic structure, causing increased echogenicity.

1 Baseline
2 Line of the cartilage roof
3 Bony roof line
   α: Bone angle
   β: Cartilage angle
4 Transition point
5 Superiorly elongated labrum
6 Fulcrum

Fig. 4.**49b** Sonogram of right hip in a 6-month-old infant. The cartilaginous roof is clearly echogenic (3). Bony molding is extremely poor, and the acetabular convexity (2) is flattened. The cartilaginous portion of the acetabular convexity roof (3) is hypoechoic, widened, and displaced along with the acetabular labrum (1). The inferior margin of the ilium lies outside the standard imaging plane and is not visible.

Fig. 4.**50a** Schematic diagram of a type IV hip. The hyaline portion of the acetabular roof with the elongated labrum is compressed between the femoral head and the acetabulum.

1 Joint capsule
2 Elongated compressed labrum
3 Medially and inferiorly displaced, compressed portions of the cartilaginous roof of the acetabulum. This tissues acts as a fulcrum for the dislocated femoral head.

Fig. 4.**50b** Type IV hip in a 4-week-old infant. The sonogram corresponds with Figure 4.**50a**. The femoral head is significantly eccentric; it is displaced farther laterally than superiorly. The cartilaginous roof of the acetabulum is compressed between the femoral head and the bone (1). There is no cartilaginous roof superior to the femoral head and outside the strip of capsule and perichondrium. There is increased echogenicity in the acetabular fossa indicative of tissue filling the vacant space (2).

Fig. 4.**51**   Ultrasound image of Legg–Calvé–Perthes disease.

Fig. 4.**52**   Ultrasound image of slipped capital femoral epiphysis.

Fig. 4.**53**   Hip effusion demonstrated in a sonogram.

Slipped Capital Femoral Epiphysis

This disorder is demonstrated in the sonogram by a reduction in the height of the epiphysis, and especially by slippage (Fig. 4.**52**). An effusion may be present in acute cases.

Effusion

A hip effusion is characterized by hypoechoic widening of the intra-articular space with separation of the joint capsule from the femoral neck (Fig. 4.**53**). In children, the cartilaginous portion of the joint and the iliopsoas may also appear hypoechoic. This can be misinterpreted as an effusion. Comparison of both hips is recommended.

Trochanteric Bursitis

The lateral imaging plane demonstrates the trochanter. In this disorder, a widened hypoechoic bursa will be seen to extend far distally.

Problems and Sources of Error

In adults, but particularly in infants, imaging planes must be painstakingly followed to permit precise evaluation of the images and accurate measurements. Topographic structures must be clearly identified, and the images should be evaluated immediately so that the examination can be repeated if necessary. High image quality is particularly important in adults. This can require the use of a low-frequency transducer.

4.5 Arthrography

Indications and Contraindications

Arthrography of the hip is used primarily in children and rarely in adults.

The main indication of arthrography in children is to identify impediments to reduction in a dysplastic hip.

Arthrography can also provide information about the position of the femoral head and acetabulum in Legg–Calvé–Perthes disease, and can provide information about the articular surfaces. It is used to confirm needle placement in aspiration arthrograms for suspected septic arthritis in children.

Contrast-medium allergy is a contraindication. One must also consider the relatively high degree of radiation exposure and, especially in children, the risks of anesthesia. However, tolerance of a single application of anesthesia represents a minor risk in light of the definitive information arthrography provides for further therapy. The use of arthrography for other indications has decreased with the advent of CT and MRI. However, arthrography continues to offer the advantages of a low-cost method that is easy to use and permits dynamic examination.

Technique, Instrumentation, and Examination Procedure

Arthrography involves injection of a negative contrast medium, such as air or some other gas, or a positive contrast medium. Occasionally, one may elect to use a double-contrast method using air and a positive contrast medium.

The contrast medium is usually injected from an inferior approach (Fig. 4.**54**). Other possible approaches are from a superior, anterior, or medial approach, and via the greater trochanter.

The inferior approach is obtained by positioning the anesthetized child with the hip flexed 110° and abducted approximately 40°. The needle is inserted lateral and anterior to the ischial tuberosity, and is aimed at the acetabulum. Leakage of the injected

Fig. 4.**54**   Arthrography

Fig. 4.**55**   Intraoperative arthrogram

Fig. 4.**56**   Arthrogram of Legg–Calvé–Perthes disease.

Ringer solution shows that the proper position has been achieved before contrast medium is injected. Fluoroscopic control images are then obtained in the initial position and after reduction (Fig. 4.**55**).

Normal Findings

Arthrography in infants should permit evaluation of articular cartilage. The acetabular labrum appears as a pointed gap in the contrast medium in the joint. Adjacent to the labrum lies a small recess, and inferior to the gap in the contrast medium lies a recess caused by the transverse acetabular ligament. This ligament can be found on the inferior margin of the acetabulum as the continuation of the acetabular labrum. This gap bridges the acetabular fossa, which is visible above the transverse ligament as a widened area of contrast medium. Contrast medium on the floor of the acetabulum should only be visible as a fine line.

Abnormal Findings

Legg–Calvé–Perthes Disease

With the aid of arthrography, the surgeon can assess the position of the femoral head, surface texture, and width of the joint cavity (Fig. 4.**56**). Images that can demonstrate containment are recommended for preoperative planning.

Osteoarthritis of the Hip

The surface of the femoral head can also be demonstrated in various imaging planes. This is useful for preoperative diagnosis.

Hip Dysplasia (Fig. 4.**57**)

The primary indication for arthrography is to identify an impediment to reduction. The femoral head is increasingly displaced superiorly and laterally. There may be a fold in the acetabular labrum that prevents the femoral head from entering the acetabulum.

Implant Loosening

In cases of implant loosening, contrast medium can penetrate between the implant and the surrounding bone. This can provide a clear visual image of implant loosening.

Problems and Sources of Error

The primary sources of error in arthrography lie in inaccurate interpretation of the images. This is

Fig. 4.**57**   Completely dislocated hip.

internus as an axial slice. The bony structures appear light, and the soft-tissue structures appear in various shades of gray.

Abnormal Findings

Abnormal Version of the Femoral Neck

To measure the **angle of anteversion** of the femoral neck and head with respect to the coronal plane, the angle of relative anteversion and the angle of internal or external rotation are determined to obtain the true angle of anteversion.

The patient is supine with the legs placed firmly together.

First define a straight line through the femoral neck in a slice through the femoral neck using the femoral head and the trochanter as landmarks. The angle between this line and the level of the table or horizontal is referred to as the angle of relative anteversion.

The angle of internal or external rotation is measured between the horizontal and a tangent along the posterior margins of the condyles.

In internal rotation, the true angle of anteversion is measured as the sum of the angle of internal rotation and the angle of relative anteversion. In external rotation, this angle is subtracted from the angle of relative anteversion.

because structures are often difficult to identify. Another source of error is the evaluation of images obtained in inaccurately positioned imaging planes. Periarticular injection of contrast medium should be avoidable using the technique described.

4.6 Nuclear Medicine Studies

See chapter 1 (Shoulder, p. 54) for a general discussion on the utility of nuclear medicine studies.

4.7 Computed Tomography

Indications

Indications for CT of the hip include diagnosis of fractures or dislocations, tumors, inflammatory or rheumatoid arthritis, and destructive changes. CT can demonstrate the relative positions of hip structures and image joint effusions. Changes to bony structures and soft tissue can be imaged.

Technique and Examination Procedure

The patient is supine in the CT gantry. In contrast to MRI, the examiner can only choose between horizontal and three-dimensional CT, although different slice thicknesses may be selected.

Normal Findings

The image demonstrates the acetabulum, the femoral head, the neck of the femur, and the obturatorius

Osteoarthritis of the Hip

In osteoarthritis with hip dysplasia, the major advantage of CT is its ability to faithfully reproduce three-dimensional relationships in a manner suitable for preoperative planning. One may also obtain measurements for designing total hip implants.

CT can image osteophytes and the extent of cartilage destruction and accompanying synovitis in degenerative or traumatic osteoarthritis of the hip.

Fractures

Fractures about the hip are divided into fractures of the pelvis, femoral head, and femoral neck.

CT studies can determine whether pelvic fractures are stable (i.e., when the pelvic ring is not compromised) or unstable. The acetabulum in particular can be readily visualized. Thinner slice thickness may be used where required to visualize fractures in this region that are otherwise difficult to image. It is important to identify intra-articular fragments or structures that block a concentric reduction of an acetabular fracture or hip dislocation.

A change in the width of the joint space at the anterior or posterior margin of the acetabulum can suggest a dislocation.

Intramuscular changes such as hematomas may be indirect signs of a fracture.

Three-Dimensional Reconstruction for Preoperative Planning

Three-dimensional images of bony surfaces (Fig. 4.**58**) are obtained by processing adjacent CT slices using image-processing equipment and software.

The image can be observed from any perspective. For clinical purposes, horizontal perspectives in 45° increments are standard.

However, any direction may be chosen if warranted by the specific line of inquiry. It is also possible to break the image of the joint down into its individual components and view them separately.

Three-dimensional reconstruction in the hip and pelvis is suitable for visualization of changes in osteoarthritis of the hip, acetabular dysplasia, and axial deformities. Acetabular imaging is helpful in preoperative planning for treatment of acetabular fractures, corrective osteotomies, or total hip arthroplasty. It also permits custom design of hip implants.

Fig. 4.**58** Three-dimensional reconstruction of the hip and pelvis.

4.8 Magnetic Resonance Imaging

Indications

The most frequent indication to perform an MRI is the avascular necrosis of the femoral head in adults, and Legg–Calvé–Perthes disease in children. MRI discovers pathologic changes earlier than other imaging modalities. Septic arthritis can be distinguished from aseptic arthritis. Soft-tissue injuries associated with fractures can be visualized. Furthermore, MRI can detect so-called occult osseous injuries. Osteoarthritis is an indication whenever the evaluation of the cartilage is needed to determine the therapeutic approach. Tumors of the hip region are primarily examined to assess size and location, less often to obtain a tissue diagnosis.

Examination Protocol

The examination is generally performed with the body coil, though the head coil is preferable for children. As for other joints, proton density weighted sequences are used for delineating the morphology, and T1-weighted and T2-weighted sequences, including fat suppression sequences, for displaying the pathology.

Pathologic Findings

Arthritis (Fig. 4.**59**)

Transient synovitis (irritable hip) is a painful condition occurring in the pediatric age-group (Fig. 4.**59**). It resolves spontaneously with rest. MRI reveals an effusion and synovial thickening, best seen on the STIR image and on the T1-weighted phase-contrast image after intravenous administration of gadolinium-based contrast medium. This condition must reliably be separated from septic arthritis, which, in addition to a joint effusion, shows involvement of the osseous structures and periarticular soft tissue. The STIR image reveals linear areas of high signal intensity, which are close to the cortex and indistinctly demarcated from the bone marrow. They are mostly in the transition zone between femoral head and neck, but can also be found in the acetabulum. The periarticular soft tissues also show a high signal intensity that frequently spreads along the muscle fibers. The synovial

Fig. 4.**59** Coronal image (GRE 280/6.8 out of phase after application of intravenous gadolinium contrast medium) showing transient synovitis with a hypertrophic synovial membrane.

Synovitis

Transient
osteoporosis

Fig. 4.**60a**   Coronal image
(GRE 280/6.8 out of phase)
showing transient osteoporosis with medullary edema in
the right femoral head with
low signal intensity.

Transient
osteoporosis
with contrast-
medium
enhancement

Fig. 4.**60b**   Coronal image
(GRE 280/6.8 out of phase
after administration of intravenous gadolinium contrast
medium) showing transient
osteoporosis with contrast-
medium enhancement in the
femoral head and neck
accompanied by synovitis.

membrane as well as the affected soft tissues and
osseous areas show intense contrast enhancement,
usually less extensive than the area of increased signal intensity seen on the STIR image.

Transient osteoporosis of the hip is a condition
found in adults (Figs. 4.**60a, b**). MRI shows striking
edema of the femoral head and neck with increased
signal intensity on the STIR and T2-weighted images
and decreased signal intensity on the T1-weighted
image, accompanied by a small effusion.

Perthes Disease (Fig. 4.**61**)

This is an infarction of the femoral head in childhood
and MRI shows a circumscribed zone of decreased
signal intensity on the T1-weighted image. The
infarcted area is in the center of the epiphysis. In the
early stage, the femoral head keeps its spherical
shape and the articular cartilage is unremarkable. The
T2-weighted and STIR images show the infarcted area
as a central increase in signal intensity. Enhancement

is very strong. A small effusion is usually encountered. With progression of the disease, edema spreads
through the femoral head and can extend into the
neck. An enhancing demarcating zone can be recognized. The epiphysis collapses, with resultant epiphyseal extrusion and flattening. A cartilaginous lesion is
generally not found. A subchondral zone of decreased
signal intensity is seen in all sequences as a sign of
increased sclerosis. The peak incidence of this condition is between the ages 5 and 8. Its diagnosis is difficult before the fatty conversion of the epiphysis, since
the epiphysis still has a low signal intensity on the T1-
weighted and a high signal intensity on the T2-
weighted image.

Avascular Necrosis of the Femoral Head
(Figs. 4.**62a, b**)

This is an infarction of the femoral head in adulthood.
In the early stages, the infarcted area is best seen as
decreased signal intensity on the T1-weighted image.

Avascular
epiphyseal
necrosis

Fig. 4.**61**   Coronal image
(SE 650/14) showing necrosis
of the epiphysis with low
signal intensity.

Subchondral infarction

Beginning avascular necrosis

Fig. 4.**62a** Coronal image (SE 650/14) showing avascular necrosis in the left femoral head with subchondral infarction. Beginning avascular necrosis may be seen in the right femoral head with diffuse subchondral edema.

Infarction zone with contrast-medium enhancement

Beginning avascular necrosis with slight contrast-medium enhancement

Synovitis

Fig. 4.**62b** Coronal image (GRE 380/6.8 out of phase after administration of intravenous gadolinium contrast medium) showing avascular necrosis in the left femoral head. Significant contrast-medium enhancement indicative of vital tissue is present, as is synovitis. Beginning avascular necrosis may be seen in the right femoral head with slight contrast-medium enhancement and synovitis.

Cartilage defects

Cysts associated with synovitis

Fig. 4.**63** Coronal image (GRE 280/6.8 out of phase after application of intravenous gadolinium contrast medium) showing bilateral osteoarthritis with cartilage defects and synovitis.

The STIR image shows the edema and its spread toward the femoral neck. The lesion shows a marked contrast enhancement. After several weeks, the focus becomes demarcated and is seen as a relatively well demarcated band of high signal intensity on the STIR image. This band enhances strongly and can be interpreted as a zone of increased vascularity. An effusion is always present. In the late stages, the T2-weighted and STIR images as well as the T1-weighted phase contrast images reveal a markedly heterogeneous structure, with areas of high signal intensity intermixed with areas of low signal intensity. The femoral head is generally collapsed, and the cartilage shows fissures as well as large defects. This variegated picture reflects the concurring processes of necrosis, sclerosis, and revascularization with hyperemia and local edema. Since the disease is frequently bilateral, though it often differs in severity, both hips should always be examined. Avascular necrosis confined to the femoral head should be distinguished from a bone infarct, which shows sharply demarcated areas along the vascular supply in the femoral head, neck, and trochanteric region. These areas have a low signal intensity on T1-weighted images and a high signal intensity on STIR and T2-weighted images.

Osteoarthritis (Fig. 4.**63**)

Osteoarthritis is caused by cartilage degeneration and induces subchondral sclerosis and osteophyte formation along the acetabulum and also around the circumference of the femoral head, associated with more or less severe reactive synovitis. Initially, the cartilage is slightly thickened, followed by thinning and the formation of defects. These changes are best observed on high resolution T2*-weighted sequences. Osteophytes are easily seen on the T1-weighted image. The accompanying inflammatory changes are best seen on the STIR image or after intravenous administration of gadolinium-based contrast medium on the T1-weighted phase contrast image, with the synovial changes exceptionally well discernible.

Fractures (Fig. 4.**64**)

MRI is not the primary modality for diagnosing fractures. It contributes to the detection and evaluation of pseudoarthroses since the non-ossified tissue is well demarcated from the osseous structures on the phase contrast image. Occult fractures, however, are a domain of MRI. They are characterized on the STIR image as indistinct zones of high signal intensity in the trabecular bone.

Fracture line

Fig. 4.**64**   Coronal image (GRE 500/10 out of phase after application of intravenous gadolinium contrast medium). The hyperemia causes the contrast medium to enhance the fracture line in the femoral neck.

Muscle fiber tear

Fig. 4.**65**   Coronal image (STIR 2200/125) showing a muscle fiber tear in the quadratus femoris.

Muscular Injuries (Fig. 4.**65**)

They are primarily sport injuries ranging from sprains, usually involving the adductors, to tears. In sprains, the STIR or heavy T2-weighted sequences show a high signal intensity along the fascicular orientation of the muscle. The same sequences show the muscular fascicles to be interrupted with more or less severe hemorrhage in the created gap. After about 4 days, high signals relative to the low signal musculature are seen on the T1-weighted image. Intramuscular abscesses, usually appearing after intramuscular injections, have a homogeneously high signal intensity on the STIR and T2-weighted images. After intravenous administration of a gadolinium-based contrast medium, strong peripheral enhancement is seen on the T1-weighted image.

References

Catteral A. *Legg Calve Perthes disease.* New York–Edinburgh: Churchill Livingstone; 1982

Endler F, Fochem K, Weil KH. *Orthopädische Röntgendiagnostik.* Stuttgart–New York: Thieme; 1984

Feine U, Müller-Schauenburg W. *Szintigraphie.* Nürnberg: Wachholz; 1989

Fries G, Tönnis D. *Hüftluxation und -dysplasie im Kindesalter.* Uelzen: ML Verlag; 1981

Gage HC. A possible early sign of Perthes Disease. *Br J Radiol.* 1933; 4: 925

Geleker J. *Die Hüftepiphysenlösung. Radiometrie und Korrekturplanung* (Bücherei des Orthopäden, Vol 19). Stuttgart: Enke; 1977

Graf R. *Sonographie der Säuglingshüfte und therapeutische Konsequenz. Ein Kompendium.* 4th ed. Stuttgart: Enke; 1993

Graf R, Schuler P. *Sonographie am Stütz- und Bewegungsapparat bei Erwachsenen und Kindern.* 2nd ed. Weinheim: Chapman & Hall; 1994

Greenspan A. *Skelettradiologie.* 2nd ed. Weinheim: Chapman & Hall; 1993

Hilgenreiner H. Zur Frühdiagnose- und -behandlung der angeborenen Hüftgelenkverrenkung. *Med Klin.* 1925; 21: 1385,1425

Hoppenfeld S. *Orthopädische Neurologie.* Stuttgart: Enke; 1980

Hoppenfeld S. *Klinische Untersuchung der Wirbelsäule und der unteren Extremitäten.* Stuttgart–New York: G Fischer; 1992

Jerosch J, Marquardt M. *Sonographie des Bewegungsapparates.* Zülpich: Biermann; 1993

Matin P. Bone Scanning of Trauma and Benign Conditions. In: Freeman M, Weissman S, eds. *Nuclear Medicine.* New York: Raven Press; 1982: 81

McRae R. *Klinisch-orthopädische Untersuchung.* Stuttgart–New York: G Fischer; 1989

Mitchell MD, Kundel HL, Steinberg MEL, Kressel HY, Alavi A, Axel L. *Avascular Necrosis of the Hip: Comparison of MR, CT and scintigraphy.* AJR. 1986; 147: 67–71

Müller ME. *Die hüftnahen Femurosteotomien.* Stuttgart: Thieme; 1957

Perthes GC. Über Osteochondritis deformans oder Legg's disease. *Zentralbl Chir.* 1920; 6: 123

Rütt A, Küsswetter W, ed. *Gelenknahe Osteotomien bei der Dysplasiehüfte des Adoleszenten und jungen Erwachsenen.* Stuttgart–New York: Thieme; 1983

Salter RB. Legg Perthes disease. The scientific basis for methods of treatment and their indications. *Clin Orthop.* 1980; 150: 8

Schlegel KF. Die angeborene Hüftluxation. In: Hohmann G, Hackenbroch M, Lindemann K (eds). *Handbuch der Orthopädie.* Vol 4, pt 1. Stuttgart: Thieme; 1961

Schulitz KP, Dustmann HO. *Morbus Perthes.* Berlin–Heidelberg–New York: Springer; 1991

Sciuk J, Schober O. Nuklearmedizinische Diagnostik von Hüftgelenkerkrankungen im Erwachsenenalter. *Radiologe.* 1989; 29: 492

Tönnis D. *Die angeborene Hüftdysplasie und Hüftluxation im Kindes- und Erwachsenenalter. Grundlagen, Diagnostik, konservative und operative Behandlung.* Berlin–Heidelberg–New York: Springer; 1984

5 Knee

5.1 Introduction

The knee accounts for approximately 7% of all traumatic joint injuries. Recreational sports activities can lead to events that exceed the tolerance of stabilizing structures. There is a relative increase in the incidence of knee injuries due in part to an increasing participation in highly demanding recreational activities and a rising level of performance in these sports. At the same time, patients' expectations have increased to the point where complete restoration of knee function is often expected. The physician must promptly determine whether conservative or surgical management is indicated.

The anterior cruciate ligament is frequently involved in knee trauma. This ligament plays a key role in the function of the knee. The importance of diagnosing damage to this ligament is obvious.

The sensitivity of diagnostic studies varies according to the examiner. Only 7–48% of initial examiners diagnose a tear in the anterior cruciate ligament upon clinical examination. Even a bloody effusion is not conclusive. Effusions occur in 23–65% of all meniscus injuries, but in over 60% of anterior cruciate tears.

Diagnosing degenerative changes in the knee is equally difficult. One is unlikely to assume the presence of "wear and tear" symptoms, particularly in young patients. In the absence of a history of trauma or occupational overuse, degenerative meniscus damage or cartilage changes are usually thought to be of secondary importance, and their sequelae are minimized.

In older patients precise diagnostic information is also crucial. The decision to perform total knee arthroplasty in the case of severe arthritis decisively impacts the patient's life.

5.2 Clinical Examination

Standard Examination

The standard examination begins with taking the patient's history. This permits differentiation between acute injury and possible degenerative changes, and provides initial clues as to the possible involvement of certain joint structures.

Inspect both knees from the front (contours, axes, position of the patella, muscular contour, and skin), from the side (leg axes for extension deficit, genu recurvatum, and position of the patella and fibular head), and from behind with the patient standing (swelling, muscular contour, and leg axes).

The rest of the examination should be performed with the patient supine. After a preliminary examination of the hip and ankle joints, palpate the patella and joint capsule. Watch for signs of inflammation such as warmth, swelling, and erythema. Next look for effusion, then palpate the medial and lateral joint space, fibular head, insertion of the patellar tendon, and the popliteal fossa.

Palpation is followed by range of motion tests (flexion/extension, external rotation/internal rotation with the knee extended and flexed). This can provide initial signs of locking and impingement syndromes. Document any crepitus, evaluate the rolling and gliding mechanism, and check the play of the patella. Observing the rotational motion can provide initial evidence of instability of the knee.

Continue the examination by assessing tenderness to palpation and evaluating the meniscus. Several tests should be used closely examine the patella, its adjacent structures, and the patellofemoral articulation. Pay careful attention to subluxation and retropatellar findings.

Next test stability. The anterior cruciate ligament is tested at 30° flexion (Lachman test) and at 90° (anterior drawer). This is followed by the pivot-shift test to evaluate the rolling and gliding mechanism. The posterior cruciate ligament is tested in a similar way.

The next step in the procedure is the evaluation of the collateral ligaments. This is done with the knee extended and flexed 20°–30°. Additional special tests should be used if signs of instability of the anterior cruciate ligament are detected. The examination is completed by assessing vascular supply and sensation in the affected leg.

Patient History

Every examination begins with taking the patient's history. This provides information and helps establish a relationship of trust between examiner and patient. You should devote just as much attention to the

Table 5.**1**   Schematic diagram of relevant questions for patient history

"Twelve commandments" for taking patient history	
1	Brief description of accident by patient
2	Time of accident
3	Precise mechanism of injury and specifics of type of sport
4	Tentative diagnosis specifying pattern of injury
5	Previous trauma or first injury?
6	Estimation of magnitude and direction of traumatic force
7	Behavior after trauma (ability to walk or participate in sports, feeling of instability, incarceration symptoms, swelling)
8	Previous therapy
9	Character of pain (time, duration, location)
10	Present pattern of symptoms (ability to walk or participate in sports, "giving-way" phenomenon, locking, swelling tendency, limited motion, signs of inflammation)
11	Estimation of patient's expectations regarding diagnosis and treatment
12	Estimation of psychosocial background (personal need for bodily function, sense of responsibility, compliance, occupational situation)

Table 5.**2**   Mechanisms of injury in the knee

- Hyperflexion or hyperextension
- Varus or valgus stress
- Internal or external rotation
- Valgus stress in external rotation
- Varus stress in internal rotation
- Lateral and/or anterior impact

patient in this initial conversation as in the subsequent physical examination. For very young and very old patients, information supplied by family members can be important.

The patient will often find it difficult to describe the key aspects of his or her knee disorder in chronological order, therefore some structure will have to be provided. It is essential to record the therapy performed; when inquiring about previous therapy, one should ask about measures undertaken by the patient (cooling, dressings, immobilization, and pain medication) as well as about previous treatments (injections, aspiration, medications prescribed, physical modalities, therapeutic exercise, and, if applicable, surgical intervention).

When taking the patient's history, one should be alert to an accident or the sudden onset of atraumatic symptoms and should attempt to determine their chronological order. In acute trauma, one must differentiate between blunt and sharp external trauma and trauma without "action by an opponent."

The history should be taken according to a scheme that follows the "twelve commandments" with respect to detail and documentation (Table 5.**1**). A differentiation should be made between sports, leisure, occupational, and traffic accidents. The elapsed time between the injury and the examination will decisively influence the findings. After the first 6–8 hours, expect to encounter reflexive splinting of the muscles during specific tests, which will make exami-

nation more difficult. Rarely, examination under anesthesia may be required.

Precise reconstruction of the mechanism of injury is extremely important. Generally, it will consist of a combination of rotation and abduction or adduction of the knee in flexion with the thigh or calf immobilized. The most frequent mechanisms of injury are valgus flexion with external rotation or varus flexion with internal rotation. Other mechanisms of injury can occur in isolation or in combination (Table 5.**2**).

Instability of the knee is classified according to the direction of motion of the tibia with respect to the femur. Nicholas (1973) classifies injuries to the capsular ligaments of the knee as: 1 simple, 2 complex, or 3 combined instability.

Information about the duration of symptoms and mechanism of injury (including the specific sport when applicable) will usually be sufficient for an accurate tentative diagnosis. Additional information about prior injuries and immediate post-injury events should be obtained.

The character, duration, and location of pain will provide helpful information. Displaced menisci can cause focal pain in addition to snapping or locking. A meniscus with degenerative changes and a small longitudinal or transverse tear will tend to cause deep, dull pain. A bucket-handle tear may cause pain at the end of the range of motion in flexion and extension. A partially torn cruciate in the acute phase can cause stabbing pain at rest, an isolated tear of the anterior cruciate ligament will tend to cause pain during exercise. Additional acute injuries may then cloud the picture.

An acute tear of the anterior cruciate ligament may show massive swelling that occurs immediately after trauma, persisting for up to 12 hours. Hemarthrosis may or may not be present. This massive swelling may not be present if the synovial membrane investing the anterior cruciate ligament is intact, if the anterior cruciate ligament had preexisting degenerative cruciate changes, or if the hemarthrosis drained through a capsular rupture. A useful piece of information from the history is the patient's description of the "pop." Many patients report a sound or sensation of some structure breaking, often heard by teammates and spectators in sporting events.

Table 5.**3** Typical knee disorders according to age group

Newborns Infants	Adolescents Young adults	Older patients
Congenital knee dislocation	Osgood–Schlatter disease	Quadriceps tendon tear
Discoid meniscus	Osteochondritis dissecans	Patellar tendon tear
Septic arthritis	Prepatellar bursitis	Degenerative bucket-handle tear
Osteomyelitis	Acute meniscus tear	Osteoarthritis of the knee
Slipped epiphysis	Cruciate tear: ligamentous/bony	Synovitis
	Chondrocalcinosis	Retropatellar arthritis
	Tendon disorders/tenosynovitis at the muscular insertions	Meniscus ganglia
	Osteosarcoma	Chondromatosis
	Recurrent patella dislocation	Baker cyst
	Sinding–Larsen–Johansson syndrome	Aseptic osteonecrosis
	Patellar chondrosis	Patellar degenerative joint disease
	Jumper's knee	
	Runner's knee	

The capability of the acutely injured knee can vary greatly. Some patients will immediately refrain from placing weight on the injured knee. Ambitious athletes, often influenced by their coach and teammates, will continue to participate and initially ignore the "giving-way" symptom that can occur with an anterior cruciate tear.

Personal impressions of the patient should not be underestimated. The patient's description of all events will be colored by the situation in which the injury occurred. Patients with high demands, whether with respect to their occupation or sport, may minimize symptoms and expect a rapid return to the previous level of performance after minimal therapy.

In an acute exacerbation of a chronic problem or pain without specific trauma, it is important to inquire about occupational exposures and sports activities. Bent-knee activities can lead to early meniscus degeneration in association with cartilage damage. Overuse in track and field events, weight lifting, and martial arts may also lead to early symptoms that can occur during exercise and at rest. Inquiries should be made about previous treatments and partial successes.

Repetitive microtrauma causes characteristic symptoms in adolescents and older patients. Adolescents will complain of pain at the tibial tubercle during jumping in school sports. This may be a sign of Osgood–Schlatter disease or, in older adolescents, of "jumper's knee." Runners complaining of symptoms across the lateral side of the knee should be questioned for signs of tenosynovitis at the muscular insertions (biceps femoris and iliotibial tract) and overuse syndrome of the lateral collateral ligaments ("runner's knee"). Changes in footwear and malalignment at the knee and ankle provide important information (Table 5.**3**).

Even in young adults, degeneration of previous meniscal injuries can produce sudden meniscus symptoms in the absence of a specific triggering event. This condition may improve within a few hours of its onset. Often, arthroscopy will demonstrate a bucket-handle tear of the medial meniscus or a lesion of the posterior horn of the meniscus. So-called "snapping phenomena" may be encountered. These can be caused by intra-articular loose bodies or patellar subluxation. The semitendinosus tendons can cause such phenomenon medially, and the biceps tendon and iliotibial tract laterally. Bursal hypertrophy can exacerbate the snapping.

In older patients diffuse knee pain without trauma is almost always a sign of meniscus degeneration. Occasionally, minimal swelling and warmth will confirm the tentative diagnosis. Accompanying synovitis will almost always be present.

When retropatellar arthrosis is present, the patient will complain of pain when climbing stairs and walking downhill. In contrast, advanced osteoarthritis of the knee can lead to a feeling of instability with sudden episodes of the knee giving way for no apparent reason. The patient may then experience a stabbing pain as opposed to a dull, deep pain.

Patellar pain in young patients often occurs when climbing stairs or sitting for long periods. The "theater sign" (selecting an aisle seat to allow for knee extension) may be elicited.

Pain in the popliteal fossa is reported by patients with Baker cysts or posterior ganglia of the menisci. The patient experiences a sensation of tension with the knee extended, which may lessen with drainage of the cyst. This feeling of relief is temporary and is reduced as the cyst reforms.

Any uncharacteristic pain reported by the patient should be carefully investigated. Consider disorders of adjacent joints. Hip arthritis, for example, can produce thigh pains that radiate into the knee. Changes in the sacroiliac joint and lumbar spine can cause knee pain, as can limb-length inequalities and ankle deformities.

The history should include questions about vascular supply and sensation.

Figs. 5.**1a, b**   Knee deformities: (**a**) genu varum, (**b**) genu valgum.

Finally, inquire about disorders of other organ systems to exclude causes of knee symptoms related to systemic diseases, such as diabetes mellitus, hemochromatosis, gout, hemophilia, hyperparathyroidism, thyroid condition, rickets, and psychogenic causes. The history should also explore benign tumors such as exostosis, enchondromas, fibromas, osteomas, and bone cysts. It should explore the possibility of malignant tumors, neuropathic joint diseases such as poliomyelitis, tabes dorsalis, and syringomyelia, and the wide variety of rheumatic and infectious diseases.

If you suspect chronic rheumatic disease, inquire about involvement of multiple joints, symmetric distribution, and chronicity. The knee is affected in over 60% of rheumatic disorders. Further diagnostic studies should include various laboratory tests such as antinuclear antibodies or HLA-B27.

The different diagnosis in monarthritis causes is broad (Table 5.**4**). Prior history is important; inquire about travel to foreign countries, the patient's social environment, venereal diseases, previous injections, surgery, and injuries. Acute inflammatory knee diseases require immediate diagnostic studies and treatment.

The information obtained from a thorough patient history provides a guideline for subsequent diagnostic procedures.

Observation

Always be present to observe how the patient enters the examination room. If you wait until the patient has undressed and is lying on the examining table, you will miss important information about the patient's gait, exertional ability, walking aids, single-leg stands, and knee flexion while undressing and getting on to the examining table. Information during this informal testing may be different from the information obtained during formal testing. This may be crucial in situations where disability, compensation, or litigation are involved.

Table 5.**4**   Differential diagnosis of monarthritis

- Inflammatory rheumatic joint disorders
- Collagen vascular disease
- Chronic inflammatory gastroenteritis with joint involvement
- Metabolic arthropathy
- Infectious arthritis
- Arthropathy resulting from coagulatory disorders
- Malignant tumors
- Arthritis

Fig. 5.**2** Infrapatellar swelling indicative of prepatellar or infrapatellar bursitis.

Fig. 5.**3** Injury patterns of knee extensor mechanism. **1** evulsion of tibial tubercle; **2** intraligamentous rupture of the patella ligament; **3** proximal rupture of the patella ligament; **4** patella fracture; **5** rupture of the quadriceps tendon.

Initial inspection should detect any external signs of injury that may indicate associated injuries. The presence of a traumatic arthrotomy is a surgical emergency. Watch for signs of contusion, hematomas, and open skin wounds.

Inspect the knee for contusion of the prepatellar bursa, even if the skin is intact, since it may require surgical excision.

Always inspect both knees for comparison. With the patient standing, inspect the anterior aspect of the knee (Figs. 5.**1 a, b**) for varus, valgus, internal rotation, and external rotation deformities. Also check for any scoliotic changes in the spine, and evaluate muscle contour of the thigh and calf and changes in the popliteal fossa.

Inspection of the knee from the side with the patient standing will reveal flexion contractures of the hip and knee and ankle deformities.

Note any compensatory postures with pelvic obliquity, scoliotic curvatures, and abduction or adduction contractures of the hip. Document the position of the patellar and changes in the popliteal fossa.

With the patient supine, inspect the normal joint contour of the unaffected side in the absence of a bilateral disorder. This will serve as a reference for locating swelling in the superior recess (synovitis and exostosis), the parapatellar region (hemarthrosis or dislocation injuries), the medial or lateral joint space (meniscal ganglia or osteophytes), and the prepatellar region, patella tendon, tibial tubercle, pes anserinus, and fibular head (Fig. 5.**2**). Document any erythema and skin changes. Thickening of the retropatellar fat pad can produce a second prominence in the lateral aspect distal to the patella, known as the camel sign.

The position of the patella can indicate the presence of changes or previous trauma. Lateral displacement is a sign of patellar hypermobility and possible subluxation. An indentation proximal to the superior pole of the patella suggests a tear in the quadriceps tendon; extreme proximal displacement of the patella is indicative of a tear in the patella tendon. A transverse patellar fracture with a gap between the fragments can produce an indentation in the patella (Fig. 5.**3**). Patella dislocation with an abnormal prominence and an indentation between the femoral condyles is another diagnosis that can be made by inspection (Table 5.**5**).

Measurement of the Q angle permits estimation of the lateral patellar displacement (Fig. 5.**4**). Measure

Table 5.**5** Knee diagnoses that can be made by inspection

- Quadriceps tendon tear
- Patella tendon tear
- Patella dislocation
- Transverse patellar fracture
- Complete dislocation
- Prepatellar bursitis
- Baker cyst
- Spontaneous posterior drawer with posterior cruciate ligament tear

Fig. 5.**4** The Q angle is measured by pointing the proximal arm of the goniometer toward the anterior iliac spine and the distal arm along the patellar tendon to the tibial tuberosity. The angle is measured with the quadriceps tendon contracted.

Fig. 5.**5** The bayonet sign shows distal malalignment of the patella.

Fig. 5.**6** **A**: Normal position of the patella with the knee flexed over the side of the examination table with the front of the patella facing straight ahead. **B**: In patella alta the patella is facing the ceiling.

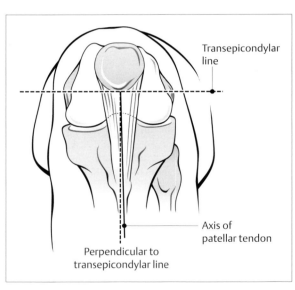

Transepicondylar line

Axis of patellar tendon

Perpendicular to transepicondylar line

Fig. 5.**7** In 90° of knee flexion the transepicondylar line is assessed. The axis of the patellar tendon is compared to this line.

this angle with the patient supine, placing a goniometer on the patella. The proximal arm points toward the anterior superior iliac spine and the distal arm points toward the tibial tubercle. A Q angle of up to 10° in males and up to 15° in females is normal. A wide pelvis, increased femoral anteversion, increased tibial external rotation, and genu valgum lead to an increased Q angle.

Pathologic internal rotation of the femur and external rotation of the tibia produce a particularly unfavorable deformity known as a bayonet sign (Fig. 5.**5**). This may be found in "malignant malalignment syndromes."

A superiorly displaced patella (patella alta) will be apparent when the patient is sitting (Fig. 5.**6**). The tubercle sulcus angle can also be documented in the sitting position (Fig. 5.**7**). The patient flexes the knee 90°, forming an angle between the horizontal transepicondylar line and the axis of the patella ligament.

This angle should be 0°; an angle exceeding 10° is regarded as pathologic.

Muscular imbalance between the vastus medialis and vastus lateralis can be detected by inspection. There may be noticeable atrophy of the vastus medialis. Patella tracking is readily discernible at about 45° of flexion. If there is evidence of muscular imbalance, this will be coupled with lateral displacement and patella tilt (Fig. 5.**8**). In such a case the patient will often exhibit a positive J sign in the dynamic examination. As the knee is extended from a flexed position, the patella forms a reverse J indicative of the predominance of lateral forces (Fig. 5.**9**).

Next inspect the musculature of the knee at rest and with isometric contracture. This can reveal new or older muscle fiber tears. Atrophy can be documented by comparing both knees. Generalized atrophy of a quadriceps leads to a visible decrease in the circumference of the thigh. This may be found in the presence of cruciate ligament insufficiency, meniscus injury, and retropatellar pain syndrome. Atrophy of the vastus medialis is typical of anterior cruciate ligament insufficiency. Irreversible muscle atrophy often occurs following arthrotomy with partial dissection of the quadriceps.

Additional information can be obtained by instructing the patient to demonstrate certain movements. For example with a tear in the quadriceps tendon the patient will be unable to lift the leg from a supine position. The active pain-free range of motion should be documented. This can deviate considerably from the passive range of motion. Evaluate the motion of the patella during tests. Impaired extension and, less frequently, impaired flexion can indicate injury to the meniscus and/or cruciate ligament with impingement. This should be differentiated from injuries to the soft-tissue envelope accompanied by swelling, intra-articular effusion, and loose bodies.

Finally, test for a spontaneous posterior drawer when the anterior margin of the tibia "sinks" back after an injury to the posterior cruciate ligament.

Fig. 5.**8** Lateral tilting secondary to tightness in the lateral structures when looking from the front and below the right knee.

Preliminary Examination of the Thigh, Calf, and Adjacent Joints

Evaluation of knee function requires the examination of adjacent structures and joint because the pattern of stress acting on the knee depends on hip and ankle function. Abnormal stresses on the knee occur when the function of adjacent joints is impaired or their motion is limited. Abduction and adduction contractures of the hip place additional stresses on the medial and lateral compartments of the knee. Knee flexion contractures are often sequelae of hip flexion contractures or spine pathology.

If knee flexion contractures of unclear cause are present, the patient should be evaluated for neurologic disorders (spina bifida, cerebral palsy, and polio-

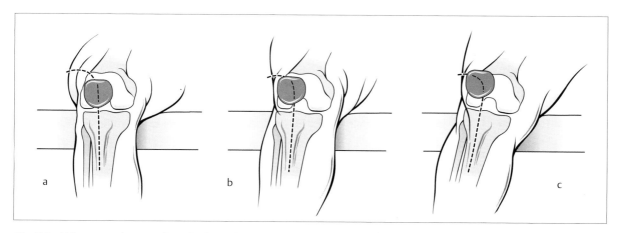

Fig. 5.**9** When actively extending the knee from a 90° flexed position (**A**) to full extension (**C**) the patella describes an exaggerated inverted J-shaped course, which indicates predominance of laterally directed forces.

Fig. 5.**10** Ballottable patella is indicative of an intra-articular effusion.

myelitis) and congenital disorders and symptoms (arthrogryposis and Larsen syndrome).

The function of the calf musculature should be examined and contractures evaluated. Initially muscular dystrophy may be present with calf muscle abnormalities.

Finally, the preliminary examination should include a vascular evaluation including arterial pulse, capillary refill, and venous drainage, as well as sensory examination in the lower extremity.

Palpation

Initial bodily contact with the patient is through palpation. We recommend palpating the unaffected knee first. Maintain eye contact with the patient when performing all manual testing. This will allow early detection of painful sensations.

First check the skin temperature, comparing both knees. Palpate swelling from proximal to distal. Palpation of the suprapatellar recess can reveal the presence of an intra-articular effusion, and swelling may be differentiated as synovitis, inflammation, or infection.

Palpating a ballottable patella is a further step in diagnosing an effusion. The synovial fluid is pressed from the recess under the patella. Experienced examiners can estimate the volume of the effusion to within 10–20 mL (Fig. 5.**10**).

Patellofemoral joint. Palpate the patella facets and check for tenderness. Evaluate the medial and lateral excursion of the patella. Tenderness at the medial facet of the patella is a sign of previous patellar dislocation. After tilting the patella, palpate the retropatellar aspects to obtain information about chondrosis. Evaluate the medial and lateral tilts of the patella. The femoral condyles should be palpated at the same time. Often this examination will reveal signs of avulsed fragments at the lateral condyles with local tenderness and crater formation and corresponding findings on the medial patella facet.

Local tenderness at the distal end of the patella can suggest "jumper's knee." Palpable hypertrophy of the retropatellar fat pad and a corresponding history will support this suspicion (Fig. 5.**11**).

Fig. 5.**11**   Palpating the tip of the patella and the proximal patellar tendon.

After palpating the patella tendon for swelling, thickening, and hardening, continue in the region of the tibial tubercle. In patients with occupational exposure, prepatellar bursitis and bursitis at the insertion of the patella tendon may be present.

Evaluate the continuity of the insertion of the quadriceps tendon when palpating the proximal end of the patella. A gap here suggests a tear in the tendon.

Document possible patellar hypermobility by comparing both knees. Perform this examination with the knees extended. With the palm of your hand on the knee, listen for audible and palpable crepitus when the patient flexes the knee.

Posterior aspects of the knee. With the knee extended, palpate the contours of the gastrocnemius and hamstrings. Palpate the pulse of the popliteal arteries in both knees. Tenderness in the popliteal fossa suggests a lesion of the posterior horn of the meniscus. Look for a Baker cyst that will usually be located posterolaterally. In rare cases, bursitis at the insertion of the biceps femoris or tumors in the surrounding soft tissue may produce palpable bulges in the popliteal fossa.

Tibiofibular joint. There are no characteristic findings upon palpation. The anatomical proximity of many structures renders diagnosis difficult. Tenosynovitis at the insertion of the iliotibial tract (runner's knee) can make the tract appear hardened and tender. Differential diagnosis should include overuse of the lateral collateral ligament and tenosynovitis at the insertion of the biceps femoris, although this will usually cause localized tenderness above the fibular head.

Rotational stability should be evaluated in addition to tenderness to exclude a dislocation of the fibular head. A hematoma at the fibular head can be a sign of a tendon tear or proximal fibular fracture. In

Fig. 5.**12** Palpating the fibular head and the tibiofibular joint.

this case, damage to the peroneal nerve should be excluded (Fig. 5.**12**).

Medial aspect of the knee. Palpate the medial collateral ligament from proximal to distal. Tenderness at the medial femoral condyle is a sign of a lesion of the collateral ligament that is most frequently found proximally. Hardening from an older injury may also be palpable. Tenderness further distally suggests distal ligament lesions. To differentiate these from meniscus lesions, palpate further posteriorly.

In slender patients a palpable cord on the medial femoral condyle may correspond to a medial patellar plica.

To evaluate the cartilage, palpate the medial femoral condyle in maximum flexion. Focal soft spots will often be tender. Osteochondritis dissecans can appear as a crater.

Carefully palpate the joint space from anterior to posterior. Meniscal lesions are often detected as tenderness in the joint space. Degenerative changes such as osteophytes, cartilage lesions, or synovitis produce similar symptoms that duplicate meniscal lesion pain. Degenerative lesions of the posterior horn of the medial meniscus can produce tenderness at the posteromedial corner of the capsule.

Hypertrophy of the retropatellar fat pad will be palpable at the anterior medial joint space. A displaced meniscus will rarely project prominently; reduction will initially relieve the symptoms.

In the posteromedial area of the joint, tears of the posterior oblique ligament and tendinitis or bursitis of the semimembranosus may be palpable as swelling or fluctuation.

Distal to the medial joint space, examine the insertion of the collateral ligament for lesions. Further anteriorly, bursitis at the insertion of the pes anserinus may be seen as swelling.

Lateral aspect of the knee. Lesions of the proximal insertion of the lateral collateral ligament are rare. Despite this, the lateral condyle should be palpated to exclude such lesions.

The anterior sections of the lateral joint space should be examined for lesions of the lateral meniscus. These lesions will produce tenderness much less often then medial meniscus lesions. A palpable swell-

ing not necessarily accompanied by meniscal symptoms is a characteristic finding with a lateral meniscal ganglion.

Next, palpate the posterior portions of the joint space. Injuries of the popliteus tendon are associated with complex injuries of the knee ligaments. Bursitis and tendinitis of the popliteus tendon are palpable as tender hardened areas on the distal posterior aspect of the lateral collateral ligament, and should be differential from corresponding changes to the biceps femoris tendon.

A lateral plica may also be palpated. A history of snapping phenomena will provide important information.

Continue the examination by palpating the lateral tibial plateau. Tenderness here could be an injury of the distal collateral ligament, iliotibial tract, popliteus muscle, or peroneal nerve, or irritation of the periosteum.

Assessing Range of Motion

Instructing the patient to move the knee provides information about the tolerated range of motion, as a patient will rarely exceed the discomfort threshold. Function of the muscles, specifically the quadriceps, in active motion can also be evaluated.

When evaluating passive range of motion, be alert to crepitus. Audible grinding sounds should be localized. Retropatellar friction suggests a cartilage lesion or patellar dysfunction in the trochlear groove. With advanced arthritis, "gear phenomenon" can often be documented by placing the palm of the hand on the knee. Severe cartilage destruction in the joint will produce visible steps in the pattern of motion.

The active and passive ranges of motion are documented. Individual differences, such as are to be expected between ballet dancers and bodybuilders, should be observed. Soft-tissue contractures may reduce the range of motion.

The patient will rarely be able to actively overcome a locked joint. A snapping phenomenon can occur when testing passive range of motion, for example in adolescents with osteochondritis dissecans and intra-articular loose bodies. These conditions can cause locking of the joint. Other cause of a snapping phenomenon in adolescents include subluxing patella and discoid lateral meniscus. In addition, meniscal and cruciate ligament tears can cause snapping or locking phenomena.

Locking phenomena in older patients tend to be caused by degenerative tears in the menisci, intra-articular loose bodies in arthritis and chondromatosis, and hypertrophic synovial tissue.

Pain at the end of the range of motion in flexion and maximum extension suggests a meniscal lesion.

Active and passive ranges of motion in external and internal rotation are assessed at various degrees of flexion. Thirty degrees of external rotation and 15° of internal rotation should be achieved. Excessive or

Figs. 5.**13a, b** Quadriceps contracture test. When attempting to press the heel against the buttocks (**a**) a gap may remain if the musculature is well developed and the quadriceps shortened (**b**).

Figs. 5.**14a, b**   Rectus contracture test. Normal knee flexion of 90° (**a**) cannot be achieved if the rectus femoris is shortened (**b**).

restricted rotation requires examination of the lateral capsular ligaments and menisci. However, painfully restricted motion after injury is not specific to any single cause.

As the joint is moved through its range of motion, a pivot shift can occur in the presence of severe instability. This phenomenon refers to anterior subluxation of the lateral tibial plateau as the joint nears extension. If the iliotibial tract and medial collateral ligament are intact, a pivot-shift phenomenon consistent with injury of the anterior cruciate will only occur when provoked by the examiner. In complex instability, pivot shift may be observed during the normal range-of-motion tests.

Muscle Elasticity Tests

The muscle are evaluated in conjunction with range-of-motion tests. In addition to evaluating individual muscle groups, note any shortening or contractures of the calf and thigh. Often adolescent patients will complain about patellofemoral pain during sports. Tightness in the quadriceps and hamstrings will increase patellar contact pressure and should be considered as a possible cause of such pain.

Evaluate the quadriceps with the patient prone. Passively flex the knee until the heel is positioned against the buttocks. This should be possible with both legs (Figs. 5.**13 a, b**).

If the quadriceps musculature is tight, it will not be possible to press the heel against the buttock and a gap will remain.

Test the rectus femoris and the hamstrings with the patient supine. To test the rectus, instruct the patient to hold the unaffected leg in maximum flexion. With the affected leg hanging over the edge of the examining table, passively flex the affected knee (Figs. 5.**14 a, b**). Normally, the knee can be flexed slightly more than 90°, allowing for hip extension. Shortening of the rectus femoris will result in flexion less than 90°. To test the hamstrings, lift the patient's extended leg and document the degree of hip flexion attainable with lordosis of the lumbar spine neutralized. Angles less than 90° are regarded as abnormal. If the hamstrings are shortened, further hip flexion can only be achieved by bending the knee (Figs. 5.**15 a, b**).

Specific Tests

Systematically performing specific tests can verify tentative diagnoses. However, results of specific tests may also conflict with all previous findings (Table 5.**6**).

Table 5.**6**   Specific tests

Patella	Meniscus	Medial and lateral collateral ligaments	Anterior cruciate ligament	Posterior cruciate ligament
Facet test	Hyperflexion test	Valgus/varus test at:	Anterior drawer at:	Active posterior
Compression test	Hyperextension test	0°, 20°	0°	drawer
Zohlen's sign	Payr's sign	Internal rotation	Internal rotation	Passive posterior
Crepitus test	Steinmann signs I and	External rotation	External rotation	drawer
Apprehension test	II		Lachman test	Reversed Lachman
	Apley distraction test		— active	test
	Apley compression test		— passive	Godfrey test
	Böhler's sign		— prone passive	Reversed pivot-shift
	McMurray test		— stable	test
	Fouché's sign		Pivot-shift test	Dynamic posterior
	Bragard's sign		— active	shift test
	Merkel's sign		— passive	External rotation
			Slocum test	recurvatum test
			Losee test	
			Noyes test	
			Giving-way test	

Figs. 5.**15a, b**   Hamstring contracture test. If the hamstring muscles are shortened, the extended leg cannot be flexed 90° at the hip (**a**); this is only possible by flexing the knee (**b**).

Figs. 5.**16a, b**   Evaluating lateral (**a**) and medial (**b**) patellar mobility.

Specific Tests for Patellar Disorders

Patellar tracking. The motion of the patella in the trochlear groove provides information about the ligaments and muscles guiding it. Grasp the patella with your thumb and index finger, and instruct the patient to slowly flex the knee from an extended position. Watch for patellar shift (lateral displacement) and tilt (vertical tilting). The test corresponds to radiographic positioning at 30°, 60°, and 90° of flexion for evaluating a lateral displacement tendency. Then observe patella tracking from the front during active flexion.

Patellar mobility. With the knee extended, evaluate the medial and lateral mobility of the patella (Figs. 5.**16 a, b**). This test should compare both legs in evaluating hypermobility as a possible cause of sub-

Fig. 5.**17**   Facet test. Elevating the lateral patellar facet.

Fig. 5.**18**   Zohlen's sign (patellar inhibition). The patella is displaced distally and the patient is instructed to tense the quadriceps.

Fig. 5.**19**   Payr's sign. The cross-legged position produces pain at the medial joint space indicative of an medial meniscus lesion.

luxation. Hypomobility is a sign of degenerative changes. Quadriceps contracture must also be considered when evaluating patellar mobility.

Facet test (Fig. 5.**17**). This test can detect retropatellar cartilage irritation. Tilt the patella to palpate beneath it. A painful reaction can often be provoked in chondromalacia or with a history of patella dislocation.

Compression test. A retropatellar cartilage lesion in the trochlear groove or synovial hypertrophy will cause a sensation of pain when pressure is applied to the patella.

Zohlen sign/patellar inhibition (Fig. 5.**18**). Grasp the proximal end of the patella with your thumb and index finger so that the web of skin in between is in contact with the patella. Move the patella distally while the patient actively tenses the quadriceps, pressing the patella onto the femoral condyles. This will be painful if cartilage pathology is present. This pain must be differentiated from pain that can be provoked in the manner described in a normal knee when the patient's leg is lifted with the patella displaced distally.

Crepitus. Audible grinding phenomena occurring when the patient dynamically assumes a squatting

position suggest advanced cartilage damage. This crepitus must be distinguished from medial and lateral compartment pathology.

Apprehension test for patella dislocation and subluxation. As with the apprehension test for anterior instability, this test is intended to reproduce patellar dislocation. Patient distress provides important diagnostic information. Previously described by Fairbank (1948), this test consists of attempting to dislocate the patella laterally with the knee extended, and progressively increasing flexion. Patients who have experienced previous dislocations will show apprehension and pain in their facial expression.

Specific Tests for Meniscus Disorders

Degenerative meniscus disorders often present with increasing pain in response to exercise. Minor trauma can often produce a tear in a chronically damaged meniscus. These specific tests are designed to determine the location, extent, and type of meniscus lesion.

Meniscus pain on pressure. Palpating the medial and lateral joint space with the patient's knee flexed is very useful for evaluating a meniscus lesion. Often the only positive finding with a meniscus injury will be pain to palpation.

Pain at the end of the range of motion. Pain in the popliteal fossa at the end of the range of flexion suggests involvement of the posterior horn of meniscus. Hyperextension with stress applied to the anterior horns can produce corresponding pain; rubbery resistance to motion in partial flexion is a sign of displaced meniscus fragments.

Payr's sign. In a cross-legged position, pressing down on the thigh produces pain at the medial joint space with a medial meniscus lesion (Fig. 5.**19**).

Fig. 5.**20**   Apley distraction test. Traction is applied to the calf while rotating the tibia on the femur. Meniscal and chondral injuries will cause pain.

Fig. 5.**21**   Apley compression test. Axial compression is applied in a grinding motion. Meniscal and chondral injuries will cause pain.

Fig. 5.**22**   McMurray test. The knee is extended from flexion and external rotation. Patients with injuries to the medial meniscus or medial ligaments will experience pain at the medial joint space.

Steinmann's sign. Grasp the patient's heel with one hand while fixing the knee against lateral motion with the other hand. For Steinmann's sign I, perform forced external or internal rotation at various degrees of flexion. Pain at the medial or lateral joint space suggests involvement of the inner or lateral meniscus.

Steinmann's sign II involves a painful pressure point that migrates posteriorly as flexion is increased.

Apley distraction test. With the patient supine and the knee flexed 90°, apply axial traction to the calf while rotating it (Fig. 5.**20**). This unspecific test will produce pain if injuries to the meniscus or capsular ligaments are present.

Apley compression test. With the patient in the same position, apply axial compression while rotating the calf in a grinding motion (Fig. 5.**21**). Pain experienced in the medial or lateral joint compartment is relatively specific for medial or lateral meniscus lesions.

Böhler's sign. Like the sign, this test opens the joint space by applying a valgus or varus stress while compressing the opposite compartment. This can also be performed as an additional dynamic test (from extension to flexion).

McMurray test. The calf is in external rotation and maximum flexion. Grasp the calf as for Steinmann's sign I test. Maintaining external rotation, extend the knee to assess the medial meniscus and the medial capsular ligaments (Fig. 5.**22**). Test the lateral structures in a similar manner with the calf in internal rotation. A snapping phenomenon is characteristic of injured meniscus structure impinging on the femoral condyle.

Fouché's sign. In contrast to the McMurray test, the medial meniscus is evaluated with the calf in internal rotation. With increasing extension, a palpable snapping phenomenon can occur due to the medial meniscus retracting from between the femur and tibia to avoid impingement. The lateral meniscus is tested similarly, with the calf in external rotation.

Bragard's sign. With the patient's foot in external rotation, compress the medial portions of the meniscus with your palpating finger. In internal rotation, these portions of the meniscus will be inaccessible to this finger and the patient will experience less pain.

Merke's Sign. Patients typically experience a similarly pain to that experienced in this test in corresponding situations in daily life. With the foot immobilized, the knee is rotated, producing pain in the medial or lateral joint compartment. A capsular ligament injury should be considered if this sign is positive in a trauma patient.

Specific Tests for Instability

Nicholas (1973) classifies capsular ligament injuries of the knee according their pattern of instability with respect to an axis or plane. These include:

— Simple instability
— Complex instability
— Combined instability

Simple instability. Pathologic ability is present in one axis or plane:

— Anterior instability
— Posterior stability
— Medial instability
— Lateral instability

Complex instability (rotational instability). Complex instability comprises pathologic patterns of motion around one axis and one plane. Since clinical testing can provoke pivoting motions of the calf, this is also referred to as rotation instability. Four forms of complex instability are differentiated according to the direction of pathologic ability:

● **Anteromedial rotational instability:** Here, the medial tibial plateau rotates too far anteriorly, and the joint space opens medially. Injured structures in order of increasing severity include:

— Posterior oblique ligament
— Medial collateral ligament
— Anterior cruciate ligament

● **Anterolateral rotational instability:** Here, the lateral tibial plateau rotates too for anteriorly, and the joint space opens laterally. Injured structures in order of increasing severity include:

— Lateral capsule
— Anterior cruciate ligament
— Arcuate complex

● **Posterolateral rotational instability:** Here, the lateral tibial plateau rotates too far posteriorly, and the joint space opens laterally. Injured structures in order of increasing severity include:

— Posterolateral capsule
— Arcuate complex
— Posterior cruciate ligament

● **Posteromedial instability:** If the posterior cruciate ligament is still stable, rotational instability with one central axis of rotation may occur. With a tear in a ligament, this axis migrates to the lateral periphery. The tibial plateau rotates medially and posteriorly, and the joint space opens medially. Injured structures in order of increasing severity include:

— Semimembranosus corner
— Medial collateral ligament
— Anterior cruciate ligament
— Overstretched posterior cruciate ligament

Posteromedial instability is present with a tear in the posterior cruciate ligament and the anterior cruciate ligament intact. The term "rotational instability" is not used in the strict sense when describing this injury. The migration of the tibial plateau in a tear of the posterior cruciate ligament will produce severe instability in and of itself even without involvement of the other structures. For this reason, Gradinger (1989) proposes a change in terminology: rotational instability is a translational change in all three dimensions.

Combined instability. Complex patterns of injury can occur in more extensive injuries. The following combinations have been described:

● **Combined anterolateral/anteromedial rotational instability:** This is the most frequently encountered combination. It is characterized clinically by an anterior drawer in neutral, anterior, and exterior rotation, and by a pivot-shift phenomenon. The posterior cruciate ligament is intact.

● **Anteromedial/posteromedial rotational instability:** As a result of damage to medial and posterior structures, including both cruciate ligaments, an anterior drawer is present in neutral and external rotation, a posterior drawer is present in neutral and internal rotation, and the joint can be widely opened medially.

The most severe form, **complete dislocation** with complete tear of the capsular ligaments, is associated with instability in every plane.

Fig. 5.**23**   Evaluating medial stability.

Anteromedial rotational instability is the most frequently encountered form of instability, both in acute and chronic injuries of the knees. Instability increases with the severity of injury to the respective structures. Severity is proportional to the magnitude of the valgus stress in flexion and external rotation.

In evaluating the unstable knee, use a systematic approach that incorporates the tests mentioned above and examine both knees. The wide variety of injuries to the capsular ligaments makes it impossible for the less experienced examiner to identify injuries to isolated knee ligaments and combinations of ligaments without a structured approach.

Always compare the affected knee with the uninjured knee to allow for laxity in the ligaments which can vary between individual patients. The following ranges can be taken as normal values in uninjured patients (Müller 1982):

— Medial gap at 30° flexion: 5.8–12.1 mm in men, 5.2–9.8 mm in women.
— Lateral gap at 30° flexion: 9.2–16.9 mm in both sexes.
— Anterior drawer at 90° flexion: 0–5 mm in both sexes.
— Posterior drawer at 90° flexion: 0–5 mm in both sexes.

Note the quality of the endpoint of motion in all tests. A hard endpoint is consistent with an intact ligament. A soft endpoint is typical of a partial tear or chronic severe instability. Assessing the quality of the endpoint of motion often requires repeating the test. This may be difficult with acute injury since pain will lead to voluntary tensing of the muscles, which can obscure the degree of instability. The results of the initial test should be carefully documented in patients with acute trauma, and should be repeated over time.

Complete ligament tears may be less painful upon examination than partial tears. If a patient has an acute injury and is resting in a comfortable position, proceed with the tests that can be performed without causing pain. It may be necessary to defer specific tests and the diagnosis until a complete examination can be performed.

The following sequence is recommended:

— Medial and lateral stability (gap test)

a

b

Figs. 5.**24a, b**   Evaluating lateral stability with the knee extended (**a**) and slightly flexed (**b**).

— Active and passive drawer tests
— Dynamic subluxation tests

Gap test. Evaluate the stability of the collateral ligaments with the knee in full extension and 30° of flexion. Slightly flexing the knee relaxes the structures that provide lateral stability in addition to the collateral ligaments. This allows test of the stability of the collateral ligaments in isolation.

The medial collateral ligament is examined with the calf in internal rotation. The posteromedial portions of the capsule are relaxed, and the anterior cruciate ligament is under tension. If a wide gap is present, the possibility of injury to the cruciate ligament must be considered. Hertel and Schweiberer (1975) postulate that a gap of more than 25 mm is always associated with injury to the anterior cruciate ligament. Involvement of the posteromedial portions of the capsule can be evaluated with increasing external rotation.

When examining the supine patient, grasp the patient's ankle with your hand nearest the patient while placing your other hand slightly above the lateral joint space and using it as a fulcrum (Fig. 5.**23**). To evaluate the lateral collateral ligament, place your hand beneath the patient's knee, using its as a medial fulcrum (Figs. 5.**24 a, b**).

Evaluate the degree of valgus or varus displacement by palpating the joint space with your index and middle fingers (Fig. 5.**25**). Grasp the knee from both sides while supporting the calf. As in evaluating the gap, perform the test with the knee in full extension and 30° of flexion. The test in extension and external rotation will reveal signs of posterolateral instability and possible involvement of the posterior cruciate ligament as well as, in rare cases, the anterior cruciate ligament. As a rule of thumb, an increase in

Fig. 5.**25** Evaluating medial laxity by palpating the joint space.

Fig. 5.**27** Performing the Lachman test while grasping the tibia with both hands.

the medial or lateral gap in flexion or extension usually corresponds to an increase in the number of injured structures (posterior capsule, semimembranosus corner, arcuate ligaments, iliotibial tract, and anterior column).

Injuries to the medial collateral ligament are divided into four categories. The same grading system is often applied to the lateral collateral ligament as well:

Grade I: opening of 0–5 mm, minimal tears, with no instability.
Grade II: opening of 5–10 mm, partial tears, with some instability.
Grade III: opening of 10–15 mm, significant tears, with moderate instability.
Grade IV: opening exceeding 15 mm, complete tears, with gross instability.

Active and passive drawer tests. Since the cruciate ligaments are inaccessible to palpation, they must be evaluated in special tests. The Lachman test is regarded as the most sensitive test for demonstrating isolated anterior cruciate ligament tears. The Harvard Community for Health cites the reliability of this test as over 90%. Some authors regard it as the only useful test.

Fig. 5.**26** Lachman test. The tibia is translated anteriorly with the knee flexed 20°–30°.

Anterior instability is most reliably evaluated with the knee near full extension, and posterior instability at close to 90° flexion. One source of error in the Lachman test can occur with posterior instability that can produce a false positive anterior drawer. A hard anterior and soft posterior endpoint suggest a posterior cruciate ligament tear.

Passive Lachman test. The advantage of this test lies in its high specificity for the anterior cruciate ligament, the minimal pain it causes in the presence of acute trauma, and the more obvious anterior motion than is seen with the knee in 90° flexion.

The patient is supine and relaxed with the leg flexed approximately 45° at the hip and 20°–30° at the knee. Grasp the thigh with one hand while pulling the tibia anteriorly with the other (Fig. 5.**26**). Grasping the tibial plateau with both hands simplifies the examination in muscular patients (Fig. 5.**27**). In addition to evaluating the tibial plateau in the neutral position, evaluate anterior translation of the tibia from the side. The depressions between the patella tendon and the anterior joint spaces are important anatomical landmarks for this test.

Prone passive Lachman test. Occasionally the extremely large patient may be difficult to examine, especially if the physician is small. In this case, the prone Lachman is a useful test. The patient is prone and the knee is flexed 20°–30°. Place the patient's heel in your axilla, your thumbs on the medial and lateral heads of the gastrocnemius, and your index fingers on the medial and lateral joint lines. Control the proximal tibia with the long, ring, and small fingers. Apply anterior and posterior forces with the thumbs or long, ring, and small fingers, respectively. The index fingers should sense the translation of the medial and lateral aspects of the tibial plateau.

In this position, the examination table supports the patient's thigh and the examiner's upper arm and axilla support the patient's calf. This allows a small physician to easily examine a large patient.

Fig. 5.**28** Passive Lachman test. Stabilize the patient's knee by placing it on your thigh.

Figs. 5.**29a, b** Active Lachman test. The tibial plateau is actively translated anteriorly by tensing the quadriceps musculature with the knee flexed (**a**) and extended (**b**).

Fig. 5.**30** Active Lachman test. The patient tenses the quadriceps musculature while the examiner immobilizes the foot.

Fig. 5.**31** Passive anterior drawer test. The tibia is translated anteriorly with the knee flexed 90°.

Stable passive Lachman test. Use your thigh as an additional fulcrum. Resting the patient's thigh on yours, immobilize it with one hand while grasping the tibial plateau with the other and pulling it anteriorly (Fig. 5.**28**). Translation is usually easily achieved by modifying the test in this manner.

Passive Lachman test in rotation. Rotating the calf places tension on neighboring capsular ligament structures if they are intact. Translation in internal rotation (up to 30°) and external rotation (up to 20°) provides information about possible injury to these structures.

Active Lachman test. With the patient supine, lift the patient's leg while he or she tenses the quadriceps. This translates the tibia anteriorly and produces a lateral step in the plane of the patella and tibial tubercle (Figs. 5.**29 a, b**). You can help by supporting the patient's calf on your forearm while immobilizing the foot of the affected leg on the examining table (Fig. 5.**30**).

Passive drawer test at 90° flexion. This test corresponds to the Lachman test at 90° flexion. However, the braking effect of the medial meniscus makes it more difficult to provoke translation of the tibial head at 90° flexion, and the stabilizing function of the anterior ligament is also reduced in this position. These aspects make the test less specific than the Lachman test for evaluating an isolated tear of the anterior cruciate ligament.

Perform the examination with the patient's knee flexed 90° and the sole of the foot flat on the examining table. Place your thigh over the patient's foot to immobilize it. To perform the test, grasp the tibial head with both hands (Fig. 5.**31**), or place your forearm behind it, and evaluate the translation from the side.

Passive drawer in rotation. Fix the calf in rotation with your thigh or buttocks. Increased translation in internal rotation suggests involvement of the lateral capsular ligaments and vice versa (Figs. 5.**32 a, b**).

Active anterior drawer or quadriceps active test. To assess the stability of the posterior cruciate ligament,

a

b

Figs. 5.**32a, b**   Passive anterior drawer test with the calf in internal (**a**) and external (**b**) rotation.

Fig. 5.**34**   Reversed Lachman test. Posterior translation of the tibia with insufficiency of the posterior cruciate ligament.

c

Figs. 5.**33a–c**   Active drawer test in 90° flexion. With posterior cruciate ligament insufficiency, a posterior drawer will be detectable (**a**). This is enhanced by tensing the hamstrings (**b**) and neutralized by tensing the quadriceps musculature, which translates the tibia anteriorly (**c**).

evaluate the plane of the patella and tibial tubercle at 90° flexion. If the tibial head sinks back, injury to the ligament must be considered. This phenomenon can be enhanced by having the patient tense the hamstrings, which is further evidence of injury to posterior structures. This posterior drawer is equalized when the patient tenses the quadriceps, restoring the plane of the patella and tibial tubercle (Figs. 5.**33 a-c**).

Passive posterior drawer. This examination is performed in a similar manner to the anterior drawer test and provokes posterior translation of the tibial head. Make sure that femur and tibia are in a neutral position. This test can be negative with a posterior

cruciate ligament tear if the arcuate ligaments are intact.

Reversed Lachman test. This for a drawer near full extension evaluates the translation of the tibia with the patient prone. Grasp the tibial head with both hands, palpating the posteromedial and posterolateral corners of the capsule with your thumbs and the femoral condyles with your index fingers. With the hamstrings relaxed, this test provokes posterior movement of the tibial head (Fig. 5.**34**). A positive reversed Lachman test suggests injury to the posterior cruciate ligament; it is more specific than the posterior drawer test.

Godfrey test. The patient is supine with the hip and knee flexed 90°. Supporting the ankle, apply anterior

Figs. 5.**35a, b**   Passive pivot-shift test. The lateral portion of the tibia subluxes anteriorly near full extension (**a**). As flexion is increased, the lateral tibia is visibly reduced (**b**) with anterior cruciate ligament insufficiency.

pressure to the tibia. With posterior cruciate ligament insufficiencies, the calf will move posteriorly.

With cruciate ligament injuries, the displacement between tibia and femur is estimated in millimeters in the Lachman test. Results are categorized using the following values (Müller 1982):

Normal: 0–3 mm
Grade I: 3–5 mm
Grade II: 5–10 mm
Grade III: more than 10 mm

Dynamic subluxation tests. Pure anterior and posterior drawer phenomena are rare. This is due to the higher incidence of rotational instability following knee trauma. In a positive rotational drawer, the tibial plateau can pivot out of its normal position under the injured structures. The pivot point of the knee will move toward the side of the uninjured structures. In a cruciate ligament injury, the rolling and gliding mechanism is destroyed. The rolling motion gives way to a sudden slipping of the femur across the tibia, which may cause a snapping phenomenon. Patients find this unpleasant and contract their hamstrings to prevent the motion (splinting or apprehension).

Passive pivot-shift test. This test is difficult to interpret in the presence of injuries to the iliotibial tract, medial collateral ligament, menisci, and articular cartilage. The patient is supine with the leg extended. Grasp the patient's heel and lift the calf, rotating it internally. With your other hand, apply a valgus stress by pressing on the thigh proximal to the knee (Figs. 5.**35 a, b**). A snap, clunk, or pop that occurs at approximately 30° while slowly flexing the knee is a sign of injury to the anterior cruciate ligament. The pivot-shift test will more often be positive in the presence of an older injury than a fresh one.

Active pivot-shift test. With the knee flexed 80°, instruct the patient to tense the quadriceps. Lateral subluxation of the tibial plateau can be provoked if the anterior cruciate ligament is torn.

Reversed pivot-shift test. Described by Jakob, this test suggest posterolateral instability when positive. The patient is supine with the knee flexed. Grasp the ankle and hold the calf in external rotation with one hand while applying a valgus stress to the knee as in the passive pivot-shift test (Figs. 5.**36 a, b**). This will

Figs. 5.**36a, b**   Reversed pivot-shift test. With the calf externally rotated and a valgus stress applied (**a**), the posteriorly subluxed tibial plateau will be anteriorly reduced into its original position as extension is increased (**b**).

Figs. 5.**37a, b**   (**a**) In the external rotation recurvatum test both legs are rested on the examining table with the patient in a supine position. With relaxed quadriceps musculature the examiner grasps the great toes of both sides and lifts the feet. In PLRI (posterolateral rotatory instability) the knee shifts into a hyperextension varus position with the tibia rotating externally and the tibial tubercle moving laterally.
(**b**) A modification of this test is performed with the examiner holding the heel of the foot in his hand while gradually extending the knee from 30° of flexion. The opposite hand palpates the posterolateral aspect of the knee to detect hyperextension.

cause the tibial plateau to sublux posteriorly. There will be palpable and visible snapping as the knee flexion is increased and the tibial plateau is reduced anteriorly.

Dynamic posterior shift test. This test also involves reduction of the subluxed tibial plateau near full extension in posterior instability. As in the Godfrey test, the patient's hip and knee are flexed 90°. The knee is passively extended. In a positive test, this will provoke a reduction phenomenon with an anterior snap, clunk, or pop with movement of the tibia.

External rotation recurvatum test. This test demonstrates the relationship between the tibia and femur in extension, revealing posterolateral instability. It may be performed in two ways.

With the patient relaxed and supine on the examining table, grasp the patient's toes and lift the legs. The patient's quadriceps should be relaxed. In posterolateral rotational instability, a hyperextension varus deformity with external rotation of the tibia and lateral displacement of the tibial tubercle will be observed (Fig. 5.**37 a**). Alternatively, slowly extend the patient's knee from 30° flexion. To do this, grasp the sole of the patient's foot with one hand while palpating the posterolateral aspect of the knee with the other hand to evaluate hyperextension (Fig. 5.**37 b**).

Jerk test. After a positive pivot-shift test, the jerk test is performed to reduce the tibial plateau. As the internally rotated calf is returned from flexion to extension, the lateral tibial plateau will snap into reduction at 20°–30° of flexion.

Losee test. The knee is flexed with the calf slightly externally rotated. Apply a valgus stress to the knee while pressing on the fibular head with your thumb. In anterolateral instability, the tibial plateau will sublux as the knee is extended.

Slocum test. The patient is in an oblique lateral position resting on the contralateral side. The contralateral knee and hip are slightly flexed, and the leg is extended parallel with the heel resting on the examination table. The weight of the affected leg places it in internal rotation with a slight valgus stress (Figs. 5.**38 a, b**). Increase the valgus stress and slowly flex the patient's knee. At about 30°, the lateral tibial plateau will snap into a reduced position.

Noyes test. This test combines dynamic subluxation and the Lachman test. With the patient's knee slightly flexed, apply an anterior stress. As flexion is increased, the knee will be seen to reduce in internal rotation.

Giving way test. Like the Merkel meniscus test, this test is performed with the aid of the patient who is standing. Instruct the patient to assume a squatting position as you apply a valgus stress. As knee flexion increases, the patient will describe a snapping phenomenon that is occasionally audible and visible to the examiner.

Additional Examinations for Specific Disorders

Use of Diagnostic Instruments

Instrumentation may be used where quantifiable measurement is desired. This is often necessary

Figs. 5.**38a, b** Slocum test for anterolateral rotational instability. The test is performed with the patient in an oblique lateral position with the knee extended (**a**) and flexed (**b**).

where information must be presented to third parties, such as in litigation or insurance cases. The instrumentation may include:

— Instruments for measuring the medial or lateral opening (gap)
— Instruments for measuring rotation
— Instruments for quantifying drawer
— Goniometer
— Complex instrumentation

These instruments do not negate or neutralize muscle tensing by the patient. Remember that the instruments can accurately record inaccurate or misleading results. They do not substitute or replace clinical testing.

Static and dynamic methods are possible, though most tests involve static methods.

Most injuries encountered are complex injuries. There are few commonly used instruments for evaluating the lateral gap. Quantifying rotation is subject to many sources of error because of the innumerable variables in pathophysiology and anatomy. Clinical use of instrument-measured rotation is unusual.

Evaluating a drawer movement involves the problem of ascertaining the neutral position. This is not easy to determine. Daniel's KT arthrometer has gained acceptance for clinical use. At defined knee flexion and calf rotation, the anterior translation of the tibia can be determined with specified forces. The

most commonly mentioned instrument is the KT 1000 arthrometer.

Devices measuring several axes of instability include the goniometer, the knee analysis system (Genucom), and the knee signature system (Acufex). These time-consuming highly technical measuring methods are useful in research settings much more than in clinical orthopedics.

Laboratory Studies

Routine laboratory studies are important in chronic conditions and acute atraumatic conditions. Inflammatory, rheumatic, infectious, and metabolic syndromes must be excluded.

In addition to a white-cell count, erythrocyte sedimentation rate, serologic tests for virus, bacteria, and autoimmune diseases should be performed. HLA-B27 typing is also important (Table 5.**7**).

Arthrocentesis of the Knee

With recurrent effusions, arthrocentesis of the knee provides quick additional diagnostic information and in some cases can be therapeutic.

In patients with a history of acute trauma, the hemarthrosis should be aspirated only if the effusion threatens to damage other structures and surgical intervention is not planned.

The knee is aspirated under sterile conditions. A lateral approach is easiest. Prior application of local anesthesia permits painless use of large-diameter aspiration cannulae suitable for draining viscous effusions. Aspiration is performed slightly superior to the proximal end of the patella in the superior lateral recess. Press the effusion toward the needle from medial to lateral while tilting the patella.

After evaluating and documenting the quantity, color, degree of opacity, and viscosity (Table 5.**8**), the aspirate is sent for further studies including a cell count, glucose measurement, gram stain, and culture.

Neurologic Examination

Testing sensation, motor response, and vascular supply comprises the final phase of clinical examination.

Both knees are compared in sensation testing (see also Fig. 4.**16**, p. 151). Due to exposed location, special attention should be paid to possible lesions of the peroneal nerve. These can result in sensory changes and muscle weakness. Damage to the medial meniscus can produce hypesthesia of the infrapatellar branch of the saphenous nerve (Turner's sign).

Muscular strength is evaluated in complex motions performed against resistance (see Table 1.**8**, p. 24). The two sides are compared. The following patterns of movement are evaluated:

Flexion. Instruct the supine patient to attempt to flex the knee against resistance. Evaluate the hamstrings,

Table 5.**7** Laboratory studies for differential diagnosis of knee disorders

Routine		
ESR	Blood count	Differential blood count
Na$^+$, K$^+$	Ca^{++}, phosphate	Iron
Creatine	Uric acid	Total bilirubin
Cholesterol	Triglycerides	Creatine Kinase (CK)
GOT, GPT, GT	Alkali phosphates	Lactic dehydrogenase (LDH)
Amylase	Coagulation	Blood sugar
IgB, IgA, IgM	C-reactive protein (CRP)	Ferritin
Electrophoresis	Rheumatism factor	Urine status
Virus serology		
Rubella	Ebstein-Barr virus (EBV)	Mumps
Hepatitis	Coxsackie	HIV
Bacteria		
Borrelia	Yersinias	Salmonellas
Shigella	Brucellas	Chlamydias
Mycoplasmata	Treponema (TPHA)	Mycoplasmata
Antistreptolysin (ASL)	Campylobacter	Legionellas
Rheumatism serology		
RF	Antinuclear antibodies (ANA)	HLA-B27
C3, C4	HeP2 cell test	ENA antibodies
DNA antibodies	C3d	

Table 5.**8** Knee aspiration

	Normal	Noninflammatory	Inflammatory	Septic
Volume (knee, in mL)	<3.5	>3.5	>3.5	>3.5
Viscosity	Very high	High	Low	Variable
Color	Clear	Xanthochromic	Xanthochromic to opalescent	Varies with organisms
Clarity	Transparent	Transparent	Translucent. Opaque at times	Opaque
WBC/mm	200	200–2 000	2 000–100 000	Usually >100 000
PMN%	<25	<25	>50	>75
Culture	Negative	Negative	Negative	Usually positive

the semimembranosus, the pes anserinus muscle group, and the gastrocnemius.

Extension. Instruct the sitting patient to extend the knee against resistance. Evaluate the strength of the quadriceps.

Rotation. The sitting patient rotates the internally or externally rotated foot in the opposite direction against resistance. Evaluate the strength of the biceps femoris, vastus lateralis, semimembranosus, popliteus, and pes anserinus group, respectively. The tendon reflexes of the leg should be examined (see Fig. 8.**49**, p. 314).

The final part of the examination includes checking the arterial pulse in the femoral, popliteal, dorsalis pedis, and posterior tibial arteries and evaluating the veins for varices and postthrombotic syndrome.

b

Figs. 5.**39a, b**   For the AP radiograph, the leg is extended in neutral rotation on the film cassette (**a**). The radiograph (**b**) shows both femoral condyles, patella, tibial head with intercondylar tubercle, and fibular head.

5.3 Radiographs

Indications, Diagnostic Value, and Clinical Relevance

Radiographic evaluation of clinical findings is part of the routine examination. Radiographs are used to confirm clinical diagnoses but they can also reveal quiescent degenerative or posttraumatic changes.

Knee radiographs are obtained in the two classic planes. Tangential views of the patella and the tunnel view are also used where indicated. Stress may be needed to evaluate instability and to document the injury. In most cases, radiographic examination of the affected side is sufficient. Radiographs of the contralateral knee in children can provide information about the normal state of the epiphyseal growth-plates and bone development, which can aid in diagnosing the affected knee. In degenerative and dysplastic changes, do not underestimate the value of comparative radiographs of both knees in supplementing the patient's history and clinical findings.

Radiographs are not only useful for arriving at a diagnosis. With regard to follow-up examinations they are important for assessing fracture healing, for postoperative documentation, and for evaluating internal fixation.

Comparative radiographs of both sides are also helpful in evaluating bone density.

Standard View

The AP view. This view provides the most diagnostic information and can detect many changes in the articular surfaces of the femur and tibia. The patella is difficult to evaluate because it appears superimposed on the femur, although longitudinal patellar fractures are better visualized in the AP view than in the lateral view.

The patient is supine with the knee extended and the leg in a neutral position on the table. Since the femoral condyles interfere with visualization when the central ray is perpendicular to the axis of the leg, the X-ray tube is angled approximately 6° cranially (Figs. 5.**39 a, b**).

This view images the femoral condyles, the tibial plateau with the spinous processes, the fibular head, and the patella. The standard AP radiograph will demonstrate arthritic changes (Fig. 5.**40**), intra-articular loose bodies, fractures, deformities, osteonecrosis, osteochondritis dissecans (Fig. 5.**41**), patellar anomalies, and tumors. Axes and joint incongruities can be quantified. The values obtained should be compared with the normal values for the axial knee angle (170°–175°) and the width of the joint space (3–5 mm).

A common site for osteochondritis dissecans is the non-weight-bearing lateral aspect of the medial femoral condyle (Fig. 5.**42**).

A small bony fragment at the lateral tibial plateau is seen with injury to the anterior cruciate ligaments (Fig. 5.**43**). A full-leg radiograph, including the hip, knee, and ankle and obtained with the patient stand-

Fig. 5.**40**   Standard AP radiograph showing medial arthritis with joint-space narrowing.

Fig. 5.**41**   Standard AP radiograph showing osteochondritis dissecans of the medial femoral condyle.

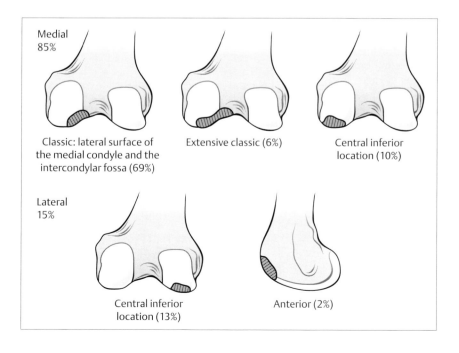

Medial 85%

Classic: lateral surface of the medial condyle and the intercondylar fossa (69%)

Extensive classic (6%)

Central inferior location (10%)

Lateral 15%

Central inferior location (13%)

Anterior (2%)

Fig. 5.**42**   Common sites of osteochondritis dissecans.

Fig. 5.**44**   Varus and valgus malalignment in the X-ray. ML: Mikuliz line; FA: femur axis; TA: tibia axis; BA: body axis; KJL: knee joint line.

Fig. 5.**43**   Segond fracture of the tibia in a patient with a traumatic tear of the anterior cruciate ligament.

Figs. 5.**45a, b**   For the lateral radiograph, the knee is placed on the film cassette slightly flexed (**a**). The radiograph (**b**) shows the two overlapping femoral condyles, patella, proximal tibia, and adjacent portions of the fibular head in profile.

Fig. 5.**46**   Lateral radiograph showing retropatellar arthritis with narrowing of the patellofemoral articulation (arrow) and increased sclerosis and formation of cysts (arrowheads) on the posterior surface of the patella.

Fig. 5.**47**   Lateral radiograph showing patella alta.

Fig. 5.**48**   Assessment of patella alta (technique of Insall and Salvati). The ratio of the longest diagonal of the patella to the length of the patellar tendon should be 1.0, plus or minus 20%.

Fig. 5.**49**   Assessment of patella alta (technique of Blackburn and Peel). The normal ratio of the articular length of the patella (**B**) to the height of the inferior margin of the articular cartilage above the tibial plateau (**A**) lies between 0.54 and 1.06.

a

b

Figs. 5.**50a, b** Tunnel view. This view can be obtained with the patient supine (**a**) and the knee flexed 40°–50°. Visible are the posterior femoral condyles, intercondylar fossa, and intercondylar eminence of the tibia (**b**).

ing, is required to evaluate the weight-bearing axis of the leg (Fig. 5.**44**).

Lateral view. The patient lies with the affected side on the table with the hip and knee slightly flexed. The X-ray tube is inclined about 6° cranially. This view visualizes the femoral condyles, which appear superimposed, the profile of the tibial head and patella, and the adjacent portions of the fibular head (Figs. 5.**45 a, b**).

With the lateral radiograph, fracture lines and arthritic changes are imaged in a second plane. The patellofemoral joint (Fig. 5.**46**) and the position of the patella (patella alta or patella baja; Fig. 5.**47**) can be evaluated and intra-articular loose bodies can be located.

The position of the patella is generally measured using the method described by Insall and Salvati or Blackburn and Peel. According to Insall and Salvati, the ratio of the longest diagonal of the patella to the length of the patellar tendon should he between 0.8 and 1.2 (Fig. 5.**48**). According to Blackburn and Peel, the ratio of the articular length of the patella to the distance between the inferior margin of the patella and the tibial plateau normally lies between 0.54 and 1.06 (Fig. 5.**49**).

The lateral radiograph can also document the patellofemoral joint space, which should be a maximum of 5 mm.

Tunnel view. The patient is supine with the knee flexed 35°–45°. The central ray enters the posterior region of the knee at a caudal angle of about 40° (Figs. 5.**50 a, b**).

This special view visualizes the posterior femoral condyles, the intercondylar fossa, the intercondylar eminences, and the tibial plateau. It also permits evaluation of the articulation and congruity of the articular surfaces. This projection is helpful for locating intra-articular loose bodies and evaluating a suspect cruciate tear with bony avulsion fracture.

Axial patella projection. The axial patella projection is routine for retropatellar symptoms. It allows evaluation of the shape of the patella and its articulation in the trochlear groove, and of the femoral condyles.

The patient is supine with the calf supported on a bolster and the knee flexed 45°. The central ray passes through the patella at an angle of 60° to perpendicular (Figs. 5.**51 a, b**). Where indicated, additional views at 30°, 60°, and 90° of flexion may be obtained to assess patella travel.

This axial patella projection can measure the angle of congruity, the trochlear angle, and the patellofemoral angle.

The trochlear angle, the angle between the femoral condyles with its apex at the deepest point of the trochlear groove, is normally approximately 138° (Fig. 5.**52**).

Figs. 5.**51a, b**   Axial (tangential) view of the patella. The patient is supine with the knee flexed 45° (**a**). The central ray enters from an inferior anterior position. The radiographs show the articular surfaces of the patella and femur (**b**).

Fig. 5.**52**   Trochlear angle. The angle between the femoral condyles with its apex at the lowest point of the trochlear groove.

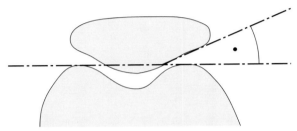

Fig. 5.**53**   Lateral patellofemoral angle. The angle between the line connecting the femoral condyles and the tangents of the lateral facet of the patella. This angle should open laterally and is used to measure the tilt of the patella (rotation around the vertical axis).

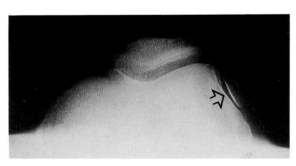

Fig. 5.**54**   Axial patella projection showing osteochondral shear fracture (arrow) following patella dislocation.

The angle of congruity is the angle between the line drawn from the apex of the femoropatellar articular surface to the anterior patella apex and the line connecting the apex to the deepest point of the articular surface of the patella. Angles exceeding 16° on both sides should be regarded as abnormal.

The lateral patellofemoral angle is formed by a line between the femoral condyles and a tangent to the lateral patellar facet (Fig. 5.**53**). This angle may be used to evaluate patellar tilt with subluxation.

Examining the axial projection of the patella with the aid of these parameters permits evaluation of the

patella facets (Fig. 5.**54**), patellar dysplasia, fracture (Fig. 5.**55**), patella dislocation or subluxation, patellar arthritis, and changes in the femoropatellar articular surface (Fig. 5.**56**).

Full-leg views for evaluating the axis of the leg. Full-leg views are obtained in two planes to measure the anatomical and biomechanical axes and to evaluate the femoral and tibial shafts. Axis views are essential for preoperative planning for osteotomies near the knee or total knee replacement. Differences in leg length can be measured.

Oblique views. The radiographs obtained in the AP projection at 45° are routinely used to evaluate fractures of the tibial plateau.

Special views for degenerative changes

The width and contour of the joint space, the shape of the articulating surfaces of the femur and tibia, and marginal osteophytes can be evaluated in the AP radiograph. The lateral radiographs provide additional information, particularly about the condition of the posterior joint compartment and the patellofemoral joint with respect to retropatellar arthritis. The severity of arthritis can be ascertained from the width

Fig. 5.**55** Axial patella projection showing a longitudinal fracture of the patella with a wide fracture gap and articular involvement (arrow).

Fig. 5.**56** Axial patella projection showing chondrocalcinosis in the patellofemoral joint space (arrows).

Figs. 5.**57a, b** Implant loosening in the AP and lateral radiographs. In addition to periprosthetic radiolucency, the radiograph demonstrates a severe generalized reduction in bone density.

of the joint space and the size and number of osteophytes.

In addition to the standard radiographs, special views are used in diagnosing degenerative changes.

Knee radiographs with the patient standing. In radiographs in which the patient stands and the knee bears weight, arthritic changes, particularly narrowing of the joint space, can be better visualized.

Rosenberg view. This view in the PA projection with

the patient kneeling and the knees flexed 45° is used for verifying cartilage lesions. It permits visualization of joint space narrowing.

Tunnel view. Frik's technique described above can be used to demonstrate degenerative changes in the intercondylar fossa, intra-articular loose bodies, and medial foci of osteochondritis.

Radiographs following total knee replacement. Prior to surgery ensure that the available radiographs adequately image the shaft of the femur and tibia. Sufficiently long radiographs in at least two planes are required postoperatively to evaluate implant position (Figs. 5.**57 a, b**).

Special Views for Instability

Stress radiographs permit quantitative evaluation and documentation of instability after acute trauma or with chronic instability following an older ligament injury. Anterior and posterior instability and medial and lateral instability are differentiated. Stress radiographs should be obtained using appropriate jigs. Manual stresses are discouraged since they do not offer the same precision, and subject the examiner to unnecessary radiation. Active test procedures using the patient's volitional muscle contraction can be inaccurate.

Procedures with instrumentation. Jigs are used to measure medial or lateral opening and tibial translation. The calf is held in a specified rotation, and the force applied to the knee is adjusted to 147–245 N.

The medial or lateral opening is documented in comparative AP radiographs of both sides with the knee flexed approximately 20°. Figure 5.**58** shows leg positioning in the jig. Where indicated, such as with injuries of posteromedial and posterolateral capsular ligaments, radiographs may be obtained with the knee in full extension.

Fig. 5.**59** Stress view with the patient's leg held in position for evaluating posterior tibial translation. The knee is flexed 90°, and the jig is in contact with the anterior surface of the proximal tibia.

Fig. 5.**58** Stress view for a evaluating medial or lateral laxity. Typically, films are taken in full extension and slight flexion (20°–30°).

Figs. 5.**60a, b** Anterior cruciate ligament tear with avulsion of a bone fragment (arrow) from the tibia, which is visible in both AP and lateral projections.

Fig. 5.**61**   Bone avulsion of the posterior cruciate ligament.

Fig. 5.**62**   Conventional tomogram of a compression fracture of the tibial plateau.

fragment, can be readily visualized in the lateral projection (Fig. 5.**61**).

Older cruciate ligament tears may be suspected if prominence of the tibial spines is seen in the intracondylar notch.

Special Views for Trauma

In addition to the standard radiographs in two planes, oblique views are helpful in evaluating and classifying supracondylar femoral, tibial, and patellar fractures. Tomography may also be used for evaluating fractures of the tibial plateau (Fig. 5.**62**), although CT scans with reconstructions in the AP and sagittal planes are often used in place of plain tomography.

Fractures of the distal femur are classified according to the AO/ASIF system as extraarticular, partial, and complete articular fractures, depending on the location and extent of the fracture line.

Fractures of the tibial plateau are classified as follows by Schatzker (Fig. 5.**63**):

— Type I: pure cleavage fracture. The lateral femoral condyle is driven into the articular surface of the tibial plateau. This results in a typical wedge-shaped fragment that is split off and displaced outward and downward.
— Type II: cleavage combined with depression. A lateral wedge is split, as in type 1, but in addition varying portions of the remaining lateral tibial plateau and articular surface are comminuted.
— Type III: pure central depression. The articular surface of the lateral plateau is depressed and driven into the lateral tibial condyle. There is no lateral wedge and the lateral cortex is intact.
— Type IV: fractures of the medial condyle. Two subtypes. The medial plateau is either (a) split off as a wedge fragment, or (b) depressed and comminuted. Either (a) or (b) may be combined with fractures of the tibial spines.

For radiographic documentation of an anterior or posterior drawer, lateral radiographs are obtained in 30° or 90° of flexion. The jig exerts translation forces on the joint (Fig. 5.**59**).

Radiographs of both sides are required to minimize error in interpreting the findings. A difference between the sides of more than 3 mm, measured using a reference line, is regarded as significant. Particularly after acute trauma, the examination should be performed with anesthesia to reduce false negative results and eliminate "splinting" by the patient.

The following radiographic changes suggest ligament damage:

Radiodense shadows along the medial femoral condyle can be a sign of a medial collateral ligament tear with avulsion of a bone fragment or periosteal new bone formation in an older medial collateral ligament injury.

Epiphyseal injuries in children can clinically simulate a collateral ligament injury.

Usually, it is not possible to identify an intrasubstance injury to the anterior cruciate ligament in the plain radiograph. However, avulsion, which often occurs distally at the tibial plateau, can be visualized in the standard radiograph (Figs. 5.**60 a, b**). Posterior cruciate ligament tears, involving avulsion of a bone

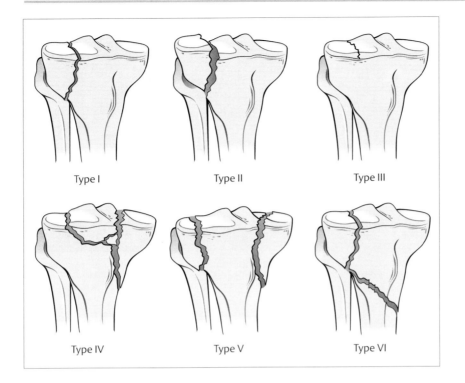

Fig. 5.**63** Classification of tibial plateau fractures according to Schatzker. Type I, pure cleavage fracture; type II, cleavage combined with depression; type III, pure central depression; type IV, fractures of the medial condyle; type V, bicondylar fractures; type VI, tibial plateau fractures with dissociation of the tibial metaphysis and diaphysis.

Fig. 5.**64** Epiphyseal fracture of the proximal tibia.

— Type V: bicondylar fractures. Both tibial plateau are fractured. The fracture line often has the appearance of an inverted Y. An associated fracture of the intercondylar eminence may be present. The distinguishing feature is the fact the metaphysis and diaphysis retain continuity.
— Type VI: tibial plateau fractures with dissociation of metaphysis from the diaphysis. In addition, there are varying degrees of communication of one or both tibial condyles and articular surface.

In adolescents with open physes, always consider the possibility of injuries to the epiphysis (Fig. 5.**64**).

Patellar fractures are best imaged in the AP, lateral, or axial patellar view, depending on the type of fracture. The non-displaced transverse fracture can be reliably imaged only in the lateral view (Fig. 5.**65**). A transverse fracture in which the fragments are displaced can be detected in the AP radiograph, although the lateral view is better (Fig. 5.**66**). Comminution zones are also easier to evaluate in the lateral view (Fig. 5.**67**). Longitudinal fractures show up better in the AP and axial patellar projections (Fig. 5.**68**) than in the lateral view. A differential diagnosis must include accessory ossification centers. These are usually located in the upper outer patellar quadrant; in contrast to a fracture, the fragments fit together to form a normally shaped patella. The incidence of a bipartite patella is between 0.2% and 6.0%. It is primarily encountered in adolescent males, occurring nine times as frequently in males than in females, and is unilateral in 57% of all cases.

Fig. 5.**65**   Non-displaced transverse fracture of the patella.

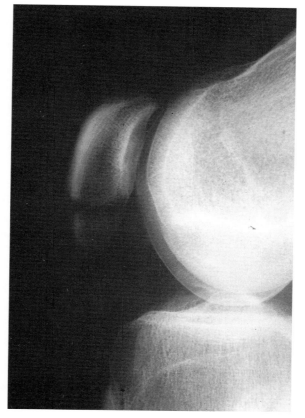

Fig. 5.**66**   Displaced transverse fracture of the patella.

Fig. 5.**67**   Comminuted fracture of the patella.

Fig. 5.**68**   Frik view of a longitudinal patellar fracture.

Table 5.**9**   Indications and clinical value of knee ultrasound

Baker cyst	+++
Meniscal cyst	+++
Quadriceps tendon	+++
Patellar ligament	+++
Effusion	+++
Bursitis	+++
Soft-tissue tumors	++
Synovitis	++
Meniscus	+
Collateral ligaments	+
Trochlear groove	+/–
Cruciate ligaments	+/–

Patellar fractures are classified as vertical fractures, transverse fractures, comminuted fractures, and avulsion of bone fragments by the quadriceps tendon (Fig. 5.**69**).

5.4 Ultrasound

Indications, Diagnostic Value, and Clinical Relevance

Ultrasonography of the knee is of lesser importance compared with more recent imaging modalities. Its diagnostic value is limited, particularly with respect to changes in the menisci and cruciate ligaments. Despite improvements in ultrasound technology that have focused on improving ultrasound propagation in the joint space and on minimizing artifacts, extensive clinical experience and skill on the part of the examiner are essential for reliable ultrasound diagnosis.

In a day-to-day clinical setting, ultrasound is suitable for imaging an effusion, bursitis, meniscal cysts (Fig. 5.**71**), baker cysts (Fig. 5.**72**), or ganglia. In addi-

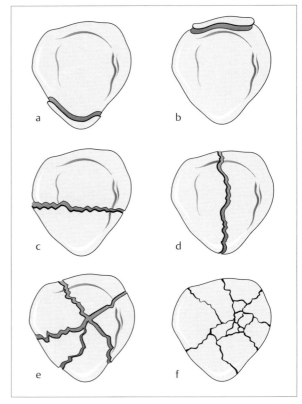

Fig. 5.**69**   Different types of patella fractures. **a**: inferior pole fracture; **b**: superior pole fracture; **c**: transverse fracture; **d**: longitudinal fracture; **e**: star fracture; **f**: comminuted fracture.

tion to defining the affected structures, the position and size of the lesions can be determined. Ultrasound is also helpful in differentiating cysts from solid masses. Changes in the quadriceps and patella tendons (Fig. 5.**70**) can also be demonstrated with ultrasonography. Follow-up ultrasound examinations for purposes of documentation are quickly performed and easily repeated.

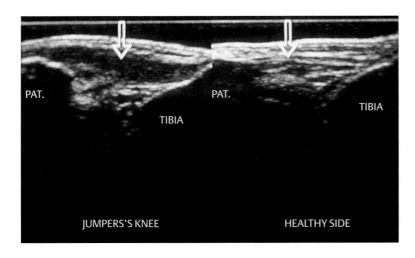

PAT.   PAT.

TIBIA   TIBIA

JUMPERS'S KNEE   HEALTHY SIDE

Fig. 5.**70**   Ultrasound image of chronic "jumper's knee" showing irregular surface with varying echogenicity.

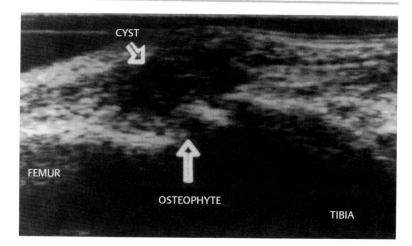

Fig. 5.**71** Ultrasound image of a meniscal cyst. This appears as a hypoechoic sac-like structure lateral to the base of the meniscus above the joint space.

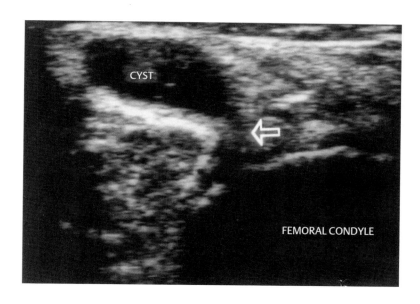

Fig. 5.**72** Ultrasound image of a hypoechoic sac-like structure in the popliteal fossa (Baker cyst). The shaft of the cyst is also demonstrated (arrow).

Table 5.**10** Indications for knee arthrography

- Meniscal lesions
- Discoid meniscus
- Fractures
- Cartilage lesions
- Synovitis and bursitis
- Formation of new cysts
- Cruciate-ligament tear
- Collateral-ligament tear

5.5 Arthrography

Indications, Diagnostic Value, and Clinical Relevance

In the knee, the arthrogram has been almost entirely superseded by MRI studies. Before MRI the knee arthrogram was a useful screening study where clinical findings were equivocal. It was a very accurate method for evaluating most meniscal tears, but it was invasive, and the radiation exposure from the multiple images was considerable. One disadvantage was that cruciate ligament evaluation was less accurate. Cartilage and synovial pathology could be identified. Evaluation of the collateral ligament injury was very difficult.

5.6 Nuclear Medicine Studies

See chapter 1 (Shoulder, p. 54) for a general discussion on the utility of nuclear medicine studies.

5.7 Computed Tomography

Indications, Diagnostic Value, and Clinical Relevance

CT permits unobscured visualization in the axial plane. Bony structures and soft-tissue changes are easily differentiated.

Fractures are the main indication for CT examination of the knee. These include fractures of the tibial plateau and femoral condyles, avulsion fractures, and tendon tears with avulsion from the bone. Plain CT is highly accurate in diagnosing the size and number of fragments, the involvement of adjacent bony structures, and the exact location of the fracture line. Lesions of the cartilage, particularly in the patellofemoral joint, can be evaluated using contrast medium.

Special CT examinations are also helpful for evaluating torsion deformities of the lower extremity and bone density.

Finally, three-dimensional reconstruction of the CT imaging planes is helpful in visualizing complex structures and aids in preoperative planning for open reduction of fractures and correction of axial deformities.

Although CT can be used to evaluate the intra-articular structures (Figs. 5.**73a, b**), MRI has replaced CT to image the cruciates, menisci, collaterals, and extensor mechanisms.

Abnormal Findings

Bony and Cartilaginous Changes

CT is the method of choice for analyzing knee fractures, and is preferable to conventional tomography and MRI. Even plain CT can provide an unobscured image of the fracture line and the relationship of the fragments in the transverse axial plane (Fig. 5.**74**). The image provides precise information about the extent of compression, the fracture line in the cortical bone, and the size of the fragments.

CT arthrography can demonstrate acute and chronic cartilage damage. Cartilage contusions, chondral fractures, and osteochondral fractures can be differentiated. Chondromalacia shows characteristic changes in the CT arthrogram that Fründ (1926) divides into three stages.

– Stage 1: edematous swelling of the articular cartilage produces a circumscribed area of reduced density. The thickness of the cartilage is generally increased in this early phase.

– Stage 2: shows diffuse strips of contrast-medium uptake or circumscribed, superficial entry of contrast medium into the cartilage.

– Stage 3: characterized in the CT arthrogram by broad deposits of contrast medium extending to the bone as a result of ulcerous chondrolysis.

Not every articular surface of interest can be imaged perpendicularly in the axial projection. Often diagnosis of cartilage disorders is limited to the patellofemoral joint.

Subchondral bone necrosis in osteochondritis dissecans can be imaged in CT scans but is better visualized by MRI.

5.8 Magnetic Resonance Imaging

Indications

The primary indications are traumatic and degenerative lesions of the ligaments and menisci, osteonecroses, osteochondritis dissecans, and arthritis (Table 5.**11**).

Table 5.**11** Indications for MRI for diagnosing knee disorders

- Meniscal lesions
- Cruciate ligament tears
- Collateral ligament lesions
- Cartilage lesions: arthritis and osteochondritis dissecans
- Inflammatory changes: synovitis
- Changes in bone: edema, necrosis, fracture
- Cysts: Baker cyst
- Tumors
- Intra-articular loose bodies
- Soft-tissue envelope: tear, hematoma, tumor
- Plica

Examination Procedure (Figs. 5.**75**–5.**78**)

The examination is best performed with a cylindric coil to achieve a homogeneous receiver field. The reference structures for the imaging planes are the femoral condyles and the tibial plateau. The knee is placed in 30° flexion. The transverse sections are parallel to the tibial plateau, and the coronal sections perpendicular to this and the femoral epicondyles. The sagittal sections can be perpendicular to the coronal sections, but must be angled to visualize the anterior cruciate ligament and are then parallel to the medial surface of the lateral condyle.

a

Figs. 5.**73a, b**   CT image of a lesion of the anterior cruciate ligament (**a**), showing discontinuity (arrow) with a visible stump. The second image (**b**) shows a posterior cruciate ligament tear in which the ligament structure is completely missing (double arrow).

b

Fig. 5.**74**   CT image of a fracture of medial and lateral tibial plateau (arrows). The fracture lines and size of the fragments can be evaluated in the transverse plane.

Fig. 5.**75**   MR image in the sagittal plane (SE 500/20) showing the femur, patella, tibia, patella ligament, synovial membrane, and cruciate ligaments.

Fig. 5.**76**   MR image in the transverse plane (GRE 500/11 out of phase) showing the patellofemoral joint and the intercondylar region.

Fig. 5.**77**   MR image in the coronal plane (GRE 500/10 out of phase) showing both menisci, portions of the anterior cruciate ligament, the tibia, femur, and collateral ligaments.

Fig. 5.**78**   Sagittal plane (GRE 500/10 out of phase) showing the anterior and posterior horns of the lateral meniscus. The increase in signal intensity at the posterior horn is due to the popliteus tendon (arrow).

Table 5.**12**   MRI classification of meniscal lesions

Grade I	Uniformly dark meniscus without increase in signal
Grade II	Minimal punctate hyperintense areas, round, oval, or irregularly bounded, without contact with the surface of the meniscus
Grade III	Linear or multiple punctate hyperintense areas without contact with the surface of the meniscus
Grade IV	Longitudinal, diffuse, or complex hyperintense areas that communicate with the surface of the meniscus

Fig. 5.**79a** Sagittal image (SE 500/14) showing grade I meniscus degeneration.

Fig. 5.**79b** Sagittal image (SE 500/14) showing grade II meniscus degeneration.

Fig. 5.**79c** Sagittal image (SE 500/14) showing grade III meniscus degeneration.

Fig. 5.**80** Sagittal image (GRE 300/11 out of phase after application of intravenous gadolinium contrast medium) showing traumatic tear in the posterior horn.

Meniscal Lesions (Table 5.**12**)

The degenerative changes of the meniscus can be classified into three grades according to the severity of the findings.

The grading is based on the signal pattern of the T1-weighted or T2*-weighted images.

Grade 1: Focal intrameniscal increase in signal intensity (Fig. 5.**79a**).

Grade 2: Horizontal, linear intrameniscal areas of increased signal intensity without involvement of the meniscal surface (Fig. 5.**79b**).

Grade 3: Extensive and communicating intrameniscal areas of increased signal intensity with delicate linear extensions to the meniscal surface, usually the undersurface. These delicate lines also frequently show an increase in signal intensity on the T2-weighted image and are then to be interpreted as tears (Fig. 5.**79c**).

Traumatic lesions of the menisci (Fig. 5.**80**) are seen as thin lines of high signal intensity that extend to the meniscal surface. They can be radial, horizontal, or even radial-oblique. In general, they also have a high signal intensity on T2-weighted or STIR images. After intravenous administration of Gadolinium-based contrast medium, intrameniscal enhancement can be observed, usually at the meniscal base. The contrast enhancement decreases with time.

Traumatic lesions as well as degenerative changes of the meniscus can lead to meniscal cysts or ganglion, usually occurring laterally (Fig. 5.**81**). Owing to their mucoid content, they have a high signal intensity on STIR and T2-weighted images. Their synovial lining shows intense enhancement.

The discoid meniscus is a dysplastic, and is susceptible to degeneration and trauma. It is easily recognized on both sagittal and coronal sections.

Ganglion with
reactive synovitis

Fig. 5.81 Coronal image (GRE 500/10 out of phase after administration of intravenous gadolinium contrast medium) showing meniscal ganglion on the medial aspect of the knee.

Cruciate tear with contrast medium enhancement around the torn fibers and in the synovial membrane

Fig. 5.82a Sagittal image (GRE 300/11 out of phase after administration of intravenous gadolinium contrast medium) showing a complete tear of the anterior cruciate ligament.

Some intact fibres, contrast medium enhancement around the torn fibers and in the synovial membrane

Fig. 5.82b Sagittal image (GRE 700/10 out of phase after administration of intravenous gadolinium contrast medium) showing an incomplete tear of the anterior cruciate ligament.

Stump of the avulsed posterior cruciate with perifocal contrast medium enhancement

Fig. 5.83 Sagittal image (GRE 600/11 out of phase after administration of intravenous gadolinium contrast medium) showing a tear of the posterior cruciate.

Pathologic Findings with Instabilities

Lesions of the Anterior Cruciate Ligament
(Figs. 5.82a, b, Table 5.13)

With a complete tear, the sagittal sections through the course of the anterior cruciate ligament show the continuity of the ligament to be lost. The edges of the torn ligament are broadened and frayed, with an increased signal intensity on all sequences. A joint effusion is invariably present. Blood in the joint space appears as increased signal intensity on the T1-weighted images. Gadolinium-based contrast medium early enhances the reactively inflamed synovial membranes. In rare cases, the synovial covering around the anterior cruciate ligament remains intact despite a complete tear, with the synovial covering well delineated after intravenous administration of contrast medium. Furthermore, the ligamentous remnants show enhancement. The resultant instability causes buckling of the posterior cruciate ligament.

Partial tears appear as lines of increased signal intensity in a thickened ligament. This again is associated with definite contrast enhancement, both in the injured ligament and its synovial covering. Occasionally, an intraligamentous hemorrhage is seen as increased signal intensity on T1-weighted images. In rare cases, the trauma causes avulsion of the medial intercondylar tubercle leaving the ligament itself intact. The resultant osseous gap is seen on all sequences.

Table 5.13 MRI signs of anterior cruciate ligament tears

- Interruption in continuity
- Irregular wavy contour of the anterior cruciate ligament
- Loss of normal anatomical position or typical ligament orientation in extension
- High signal intensity in T2-weighted images due to edema or blood
- Curved contour of the posterior cruciate ligament as a sign of anterior tibial displacement
- Intra-articular effusion

Fig. 5.**84a** Coronal image (SE 500/20) showing reconstruction of the anterior cruciate ligament 8 weeks postoperatively.

Normal appearance following reconstruction of the anterior cruciate ligament

Fig. 5.**84b** Coronal image (GRE 500/20 out of phase after administration of intravenous gadolinium contrast medium) showing reconstruction of the anterior cruciate ligament 20 weeks postoperatively. Peripheral zones of tissue remodeling are visible.

Remodeling Zone with slight increase in signal intensity

Fig. 5.**85** Coronal image (GRE 500/11 out of phase after administration of intravenous gadolinium contrast medium) showing a tear of the medial collateral ligament.

Medial collateral ligament tear with contrast medium enhancement around the torn fibres

Fig. 5.**86** Transverse image (GRE 500/11 out of phase after administration of intravenous gadolinium contrast medium) showing a Baker's cyst with contrast-medium enhancement of the synovial membrane.

Communication with joint

Baker's cyst

Lesions of the Posterior Cruciate Ligament (Fig. 5.**83**)

Complete and incomplete tears of the posterior cruciate ligament have the same characterizing findings as tears of the anterior cruciate ligament. Injured meniscofemoral ligaments can mimic a partial tear of the cruciate ligament due to their vicinity to the posterior cruciate ligament.

Lesions of the Reconstructed Anterior Cruciate Ligament (Figs. 5.**84a, b**)

An autologous reconstruction undergoes changes with time. Immediately after the implantation, the autograft is seen as a thick, straight, dark band on T1-weighted images. Over time, remodeling surrounds it with a band of medium signal intensity, with the intensity increasing from the periphery to the center. The remodeled ligament returns to its decreased signal intensity, which decreases from the periphery to the center. The remodeling should be completed by

the 30th to 40th week. Persistent or recurring increases in signal intensity indicate secondary degenerative changes.

Lesions of the Collateral Ligaments (Fig. 5.**85**)

The medial collateral ligament is injured with considerably more frequency than the lateral collateral ligament. Complete and partial tears are easily recognized on coronal T2*-weighted images. T2-weighted and STIR images can visualize the lesions owing to the accompanying effusion, which is bright in contrast to the dark ligamentous structures. So-called ligamentous strains are disclosed by enhancement along the injured ligament.

Baker Cysts (Fig. 5.**86**)

These are frequently associated with traumatic internal derangement of the knee and constitute synovial protrusions between the heads of the gastrocnemius.

Thickened cartilage with aqueous effusion (decreased signal intensity)

Cartilage defect filled with synovial fluid

Fig. 5.**87a** Transverse image (GRE 500/11 out of phase after administration of intravenous gadolinium contrast medium) showing grade I patellar chondropathy.

Fig. 5.**87b** Transverse image (STIR 3800/135) showing grade III patellar chondropathy.

Avascular necrosis

Cartilage thinning

Contrast medium enhancement within and around the tendon

Fig. 5.**88** Transverse image (STIR 300/135) showing osteoarthritis of the patella with multiple necrotic sites and cartilage thinning.

Fig. 5.**89** Sagittal image (GRE 300/11 out of phase after administration of intravenous gadolinium contrast medium) showing tendinitis of the patella tendon.

They form a crescent that surrounds the medial gastrocnemial caput.

Pathologic Findings of the Cartilage and Bone

Femoropatellar Articulation

The chondral and subchondral changes are best evaluated on the transverse sections because of the concave configuration of the articulating surfaces of the patella. The cartilage has a medium signal intensity on T1-gradient-echo (GRE) images. Water accumulation of early chondromalacia leads to swelling of the cartilage and a fusiform central decrease in signal intensity (grade I) (Fig. 5.**87a**). Superficial fissures present as irregularities of the cartilage surface. They are often better recognized on the T2-weighted image because of their high contrast relative to the synovial lining (grade II), in particular if they extend to the cortical surface (grade III) (Fig. 5.**87b**). Fissuring of the underlying subchondral bone induces an osseous reaction, which is best seen as perifocally increased signal intensity on the STIR image (grade IV).

Osteoarthritis of the patella exhibits an irregular contour of the thinned patellar and femoral cartilaginous cover (Fig. 5.**88**). Patellar osteophytes are also identified but are better recognized on the sagittal section.

In athletes, overuse can induce inflammatory degenerative changes of the patellar tendon (Fig. 5.**89**). The lesions are best visualized on the STIR sequence since it also reveals any involvement of the patellar apex as high signal intensity. Tears of the patella almost always occur as osseous avulsions of

Table 5.**14** Gradation of chondromalacia in MR images

Grade 0	Cartilage intact
Grade I	Inhomogeneity in the imaged cartilage covering without a surface defect
Grade II	Irregular surface boundary, subchondral line (cortex) intact
Grade III	Defect extending to subchondral bone
Grade IV	Fissure of the subchondral bone with osseous reaction

Fig. 5.**90** Transverse image (STIR 3000/135 showing the synovial fold.

Fig. 5.**91** Coronal image (GRE 500/10 out of phase after administration of intravenous gadolinium contrast medium) showing osteochondritis dissecans of the medial condyle.

Fig. 5.**92** Coronal image (GRE 500/11 out of phase after administration of intravenous gadolinium contrast medium) showing spontaneous aseptic bone necrosis.

the tibial tuberosity. They are visualized with all sequences on sagittal and transverse planes. Fractures of the patella are visualized on coronal and transverse sections. In contradistinction to a bipartite patella, fracture fragments have a reactive zone of increased signal intensity on the STIR image.

A synovial plica appears as negative contrast relative to a coexisting effusion on the T2-weighted image (Fig. 5.**90**). GRE sequences with phase contrast T1-weighting delineate the plica with high signal intensity after intravenous administration of contrast medium.

Femorotibial Articulation

For the evaluation of chondral lesions, the MR criteria are the same as those used for the femoropatellar articulation. Sagittal and coronal sections are adequate.

Osteochondritis dissecans in juveniles is an avascular necrosis (Fig. 5.**91**). It primarily affects the lateral aspect of the medial femoral condyle. In the early stage, the T1-weighted image delineates a subcortical lentiform decrease in signal intensity, which is bright

on the STIR image. Contrast enhancement as manifestation of reactive hyperemia and local edema is almost always seen and is best appreciated on the T1-weighted phase contrast image. In later stages, the lesion becomes demarcated by a rim-like enhancement. This is accompanied by changes of the underlying cartilage due to progressing chondropathy. Synovial fluid extended into tears within the articular cartilage appears as bright lines on the STIR image. Any contrast enhancement of the lesion indicates viability. It is rather uncommon to find a "mouse bed" created by a detached osteocartilaginous fragment.

Osteonecrosis in adults which characteristically involves the medial femoral condyle, exhibits a similar signal pattern (Ahlbäck disease) (Fig. 5.**92**).

A subchondral signal with increased intensity on the STIR image and decreased intensity on the T1-weighted image is found in one-third of patients with traumatic lesions of the menisci, cruciate ligaments, and collateral ligaments. The medial femoral and tibial compartments are primarily affected. A cortical injury is not encountered in the majority of the patients, and the finding is attributed to accompanying subcortical trabecular fractures.

Arthritis (Fig. 5.**93**)

The most frequent type encountered in the knee is probably rheumatoid arthritis. Its early stages are characterized by synovitis with effusion. The synovitis is most impressively visualized on the T1-weighted phase contrast image after intravenous injection of gadolinium-based contrast medium. The same technique also best delineates any granulation tissue and pannus occurring with progression of the diseases, as well as degeneration of the menisci and cruciate ligaments induced by the chronic inflammation. Involvement of the cartilaginous structures is disclosed on the T2*-weighted images.

Rare bacterial arthritis is marked by early extension into the osseous spaces and involvement of the periarticular soft tissues (STIR or T2-weighted

Pannus

Fig. 5.**93** Coronal image (GRE 500/11 out of phase after administration of intravenous gadolinium contrast medium) showing osteoarthritis of the knee with pannus.

Invasive proliferation of synovial membrane

Synovialoma

Fig. 5.**94** Coronal image (GRE 500/11 out of phase after application of intravenous gadolinium contrast medium) showing a synovialoma.

images), often making its differentiation from primary osteomyelitis difficult.

Tumors (Fig. 5.**94**)

As with other joints, MRI can determine the extent of the tumor, in particular its intra-articular and extra-articular growth.

It is generally accepted that a tissue diagnosis is rarely possible. A medullary enchondroma is hardly distinguishable from a cortical chondrosarcoma. In cortical lesions, extra-osseous extent, periosteal reaction, and contrast enhancement are signs of malignancy. Imaging should be performed in all three planes and with all weightings.

References

Ahrendt E, Frenzel G. Erfahrungen in der Diagnostik, Therapie und Rehabilitation bei Kreuzbandverletzungen. *Medizin und Sport.* 1982; 22: 145–149.

Baumbartl F, Thiemel G. *Untersuchung des Kniegelenks.* Stuttgart–New York: Thieme; 1993

Blauth W, Helm C. Vordere Kreuzbandruptur – ein diagnostisches Problem? *Unfallchirurg* 1988; 91: 358–365

Bradley WG. Normal variations in MR imaging of the knee: appearance and frequency. *AJR.* 1989; 153: 341–344

Fairbank T. Knee joint changes after meniscectomy. *J Bone Joint Surg* 1948; 30-Br: 664

Feagin JA, Curl WW. Isolated tear of the anterior cruciate ligament: 5 year follow up study. *Am J Sports Med* 1976; 4: 95–100

Felsenreich F. Die Röntgendiagnose der veralteten Kreuzbandläsion des Kniegelenkes. *Fortschr Geb Rontgenstr Nuklearmed* 1943; 49: 341

Fründ H. Traumatische Chondropathie der Patella, ein selbständiges Krankheitsbild. *Zentralbl Chir* 1926; 53: 707–710

Gold RH. Meniscal injuries: Detection using MR imaging. *Radiology* 1986; 166: 753–757

Gradinger R. Epidemiologie und Verletzungsmuster der Kniebänder. *Prakt Orthop* 1989; 21: 185–190

Greenspan A. *Skelettradiologie. Orthopädie, Traumatologie, Rheumatologie, Onkologie.* London–Weinheim: Chapman & Hall; 1993

Hertel P, Schweiberer L. Biomechanik und Pathophysiologie des Kniebandapparates. *Hefte zur Unfallheilkunde.* 1975; 125: 1

Hughston JC et al. Classification of knee ligament instabilities; Part I: The medial compartment and cruciate ligament; Part II: The lateral compartment. *J Bone Joint Surg* 1976; 58-A: 159

Jäger M, Wirth CJ. *Kapselbandläsionen.* Stuttgart–New York: Thieme; 1978

Jakob RP, Hassler H, Staubli HU. Observations of rotatory instability of the lateral compartment of the knee – experimental studies on the function anatomy and the pathomechanism of the true and reversed pivot-shift sign. *Acta Orthop Scand (Suppl)* 1982; 191: 1–30

Kennedy JC, Weinberg HW, Wilson AS. The anatomy and function of the anterior cruciate ligament as determined by clinical and morphological studies. *J Bone Joint Surg* 1974; 56-A: 223–235

Kramer J et al. MRT des Kniegelenkes. In: Reiser M, Nägele M, eds. *Aktuelle Gelenkdiagnostik.* Stuttgart–New York: Thieme; 1992

Laurin CA, Dussault R, Levesque HP. The tangential X-ray investigation of the patellofemoral joint: X-ray technique, diagnostic criteria and their interpretation. *Clin Orthop* 1979; 144: 16–26

Lehner K. CT and CT-Arthographie des Kniegelenkes. In: Reiser M, Nägele M, eds. *Aktuelle Gelenkdiagnostik.* Stuttgart–New York: Thieme; 1992

Mahlstedt J, Schümichen C, Biersack HJ. *Skelettszintigraphie. Methoden in der Nuklearmedizin.* Darmstadt: GIT Verlag; 1981

Menke W et al. Nachuntersuchungsergebnisse bei unbehandelter vorderer Kreuzbandruptur. *Sportverletzung, Sportschaden.* 1990; 4: 169–174

Menke W et al. Habituelle Patellaluxation und Operation nach Goldthwait. *Aktuel Traumatol* 1991; 21: 261–264

Müller W. *Das Knie. Form, Funktion und Ligamentäre Wiederherstellungschirurgie.* Berlin–Heidelberg–New York: Springer; 1982

Munk PL, Helms CA. *MRT of the knee.* New York: Aspen; 1992

Nicholas JA. The five-one reconstruction for anteromedial instability of the knee. *J Bone Joint Surg* 1973; 55-A: 899–922

Niethard FU, Pfeil J. *Orthopädie* (MLP Duale Reihe). Stuttgart: Hippokrates; 1992

Pavlov H, Hirschv JC, Torg JS. Computed Tomography of the cruciate ligaments. *Radiology.* 1979; 132: 389–393

Pfannenstiel P, Semmler U. Die diagnostische Bedeutung der Szintigraphie bei entzündlichen Erkrankungen der Gelenke. *Nuklearmediziner.* 1987; 1: 47–57

Reicher MA, Bassett IW, Gold RH. High-resolution magnetic resonance imaging of the knee joint: pathologic correlations. *AJR* 1985; 145: 903–909

Reiser M, Nägele M (ed). *Akutelle Gelenkdiagnostik.* Stuttgart–New York: Thieme; 1992

Reiser M, Rupp N. Computertomographie bei Sportverletzungen. *Radiologie* 1984; 24: 40–45

Reiser M et al. Erfahrungen mit der CT-Arthographie der Kreuzbänder des Kniegelenkes. *Fortschr Geb Röntgenstr Nuklearmed* 1982; 137: 372–379

Reiser M et al. Der retropatellare Knorpelschaden im CT-Arthrogramm. *Röntgenpraxis* 1985; 38: 390–395

Smilie IS. *Injuries of the knee joint.* Edinburgh: Livingstone; 1962

Steinbrich W et al. MR des Kniegelenkes. *Fortschr Geb Röntgenstr Nuklearmed* 1985; 143: 166–172

Strobel M, Stedtfeld W. *Diagnostik des Kniegelenkes.* Berlin–Heidelberg–New York: Springer; 1991

Tapper EM, Hoover NW. Late results after meniscectomy. *J Bone Joint Surg* 1968; 51-A: 517

Wiberg G. Roentgengraphic and anatomical studies on the femoropatellar joint. With special reference to chondromalacia patellae. *Acta Orthop Scand* 1941; 12: 319–323

Wirth LJ, Häfner H. Biomechanische Aspekte und klinische Wertigkeit des Lachman-Testes bei der Diagnostik von Kreuzbandverletzungen. *Orthopädische Praxis* 1988; 11: 904–908

Wirth JW, Jäger M, Kolb M. *Die komplexe vordere Knie-Instabilität.* Stuttgart–New York: Thieme; 1984

Yulish BS et al. Chondromalacia patellae: assessment with MR imaging. *Radiology* 1987; 164: 763–766

6 | Ankle

6.1 Introduction

The ankle is formed by the articular surfaces of the dome of the talus and the distal ends of the fibula and tibia. Motion occurs around the transverse axis through the malleoli.

The ankle is more than a hinge joint that permits motion in only one plane. The primary movements include dorsiflexion (raising the forefoot above the level of the heel) and plantar flexion (lowering the forefoot below the level of the heel).

Average dorsiflexion is 30° and plantar flexion 50°. The working position or neutral position is a right angle (90° angle between foot and calf).

Plantar flexion is important when pushing off in running and jumping activities. It permits standing on the toe in ballet and gymnastics. A contracture with the foot in plantar flexion (an extreme example would be talipes equinus) would interfere with walking and standing. This is why the foot should be immobilized in its 90° working position when applying a cast or taping for various injuries. Dorsiflexion is important for the rolling-off motion.

Ankle motion is guided by the mortise formed by the tibia and fibula, which permits a certain degree of lateral motion in extreme plantar flexion. In this position there is a certain amount of play between the mortise and the talus, whose anterior aspect is wider than its posterior aspect (Fig. 6.1).

Despite this, the talus is in close contact with the articular surface of the mortise, regardless of the position of the foot. This should be taken into account when treating ankle injuries. This close contact surface must be restored for biomechanical reasons; over time, slight incongruities will result in posttraumatic arthritis with degenerative changes.

If the joint remains in extreme plantar flexion for an extended period of time, the syndesmosis and the capsular ligaments contract, narrowing the mortise and contributing to the equinus contracture mentioned above.

In contrast, extreme dorsiflexion expands the mortise formed by the tibia and fibula, placing tension on the ligaments of the tibiofibular syndesmosis. This dorsiflexion stabilizes the joint in the weight-bearing phase.

A tight syndesmosis connects the distal tibia and fibula, giving the mortise a certain degree of elasticity.

Broad ligaments such as the anterior and posterior tibiofibular ligaments lie along the ankle's anterior and posterior surfaces and are stressed in extreme dorsiflexion. These ligaments extend horizontally and anteriorly from the lateral malleolus and posteriorly to the talus.

Another major ligament, the calcaneofibular ligament extends vertically from the lateral malleolus to the calcaneus and provides lateral stability.

Fig. 6.1 Motion of the talus within the mortise in plantar and dorsiflexion.

The strongest medial ligament is the deltoid ligament, extending from the medial malleolus in a fan-shaped pattern to insert on the talus, calcaneus, and the navicular. This ligament has anterior and posterior tibiotalar bands, a tibiocalcaneal band, and a tibionavicular band.

Insufficiency of a ligament resulting from a tear or sprain produces instability in the ankle. This instability can result in joint incongruity. Extended periods of abnormal weight-bearing can produce degenerative symptoms similar to arthritis.

The capsule of the ankle extends from the cartilage-covered surfaces anteriorly as far as the neck of the talus. Here it fuses with the sheaths of the extensor tendons, preventing impingement of these structures in dorsiflexion.

The weakest point of the joint capsule is its posteromedial aspect. This is often the site of dislocation of the talus.

Thirteen tendons traverse the ankle. The Achilles tendon and the anterior tibial tendons are the structures frequently injured. The peroneal tendons can dislocate from their groove posterior to the lateral malleolus. The tendon of the tibialis posterior passes posterior to the medial malleolus. This tendon is often incarcerated between the talus and malleolus in ankle injuries.

Nerves that transverse the ankle include the saphenous nerve anteromedially, the superficial peroneal nerve in the anterolateral region, and the sural nerve in the posterior region.

The ankle is crucial to walking and standing and is essential for athletic activities. In sports, injuries to the ankle such as ligament injuries and fractures occur frequently.

6.2 Clinical Examination

The stability of the ankle depends on the integrity and interaction of bony structures, ligaments, muscles, and tendons.

Patient History

As in other areas of orthopedics, obtaining a history is the initial step in examining the ankle.

In addition to age-related degenerative changes and occupational stresses, sports in general and stresses specific to particular athletic activities are important. Involvement in sports known for a high incidence of ankle injuries should be identified. This is import for making a diagnosis and for counseling the patient about athletic activities. Sports that involve an increased risk of ankle injury include those that require acceleration and deceleration motions such as volleyball, track and field, basketball, badminton, squash, and gymnastics. Knowledge of the mechanism of injury aids in determining which structures are most susceptible to injury.

The most frequent injuries to the capsular ligaments of the ankle occur as a result of pronation and supination trauma. Depending on the mechanism of injury and the magnitude of the stresses involved, the injury may involve isolated damage to the capsular ligaments or may extend to avulsion injuries of the bone.

Malleolar fractures are usually the result of indirect trauma, and some fracture types always occur in combination with certain ligament injuries or avulsion fractures. There are many classification systems. One system classifies according to the height of fibular involvement – the Danis and Weber system. In this system, knowledge of the mechanism of injury and the height of fibular involvement can provide information about ligament injuries. The general rule is, the higher the fibular fracture, the greater the injury to the tibiofibular ligaments and the greater the danger of insufficiency of the mortise.

A transverse fracture of the lateral malleolus distal or at the level of the tibial plafond is caused by supination trauma and is classified as a type A injury. The tibiofibular ligaments remain intact (Fig. 6.**2**). An oblique or spiral fracture of the ankle extending proximally and posteriorly is generally encountered as the result of a pronation eversion injury. At the very least, the ligament injury will include a partial tear of the anterior syndesmosis. This is a type B injury (Fig. 6.**27**).

A fracture of the fibular shaft proximal to the syndesmosis will always be associated with a tear or avulsion fracture of the ligaments including the interosseous membrane. This type C injury usually severely compromises the stability of the ankle (Fig. 6.**3**).

In addition to bone and ligament injuries, the possibility of chondral or osteochondral injuries to the articular surfaces must always be considered.

Injuries sustained while jumping or falling from a great height tend to involve complex compression fractures of the distal tibia, although torsional trauma will more likely produce fractures of the malleoli or ligament injury. Distal tibial fractures involving the articular surface are referred to as "pilon fractures."

Many ankle fractures may be treated with closed methods. The choice of open or closed treatment is less important than the quality of the reduction obtained. A nonanatomical reduction will have a bad outcome, even if it was attained with open methods.

The most favorable time for surgical treatment of malleolar fractures is within the first 6–8 hours after injury. If this time frame is exceeded or if severe swelling is present (possibly including fracture blisters), surgical treatment should be delayed approximately 6–8 days.

The goal of treatment is to restore the anatomy and stability of the articular surface.

Observation

When inspecting the ankle, abnormalities in shape and changes in the contour of the various regions may

Fig. 6.**2**   Type A malleolar fracture according to Weber and Danis.

Fig. 6.**3**   Type C malleolar fracture according to Weber and Danis.

Fig. 6.**4**   Palpation of the tibiofibular syndesmosis.

be distinguished. Causes may include soft-tissue swelling, sequelae of fractures, sequelae of infections, or intra-articular effusion.

If swelling is present, document whether it is diffuse or localized and unilateral or bilateral. Bilateral edema suggests a systemic cause.

Inspection will also reveal any open lesions such as scrapes or open fractures.

Palpation

To palpate the ankle, have the patient sit on the edge of the examining table with the legs dangling. Immobilize the patient's foot and calf with one hand, grasping the calcaneus. Palpation of both bony structures and soft tissue should be documented.

Thickening of the joint capsule medial and lateral to the extensor tendons can be evaluated by palpation. Examine local areas of tenderness such as above the distal syndesmosis (Fig. 6.**4**), the deltoid ligament, and the lateral fibular ligaments. In extreme plantar flexion, part of the talar dome is accessible to palpation on the medial side of the foot proximal to the navicular (Fig. 6.**5**). Tenderness to palpation may be caused by traction osteophytes, osteochondritis dissecans, or degenerative changes. Continue the examination proximally, palpating the medial malleolus (Fig. 6.**6**). The deltoid ligament will be palpable immediately beneath the malleolus (Fig. 6.**7**). This strong, broad ligamentous structure compensates for the short length of the medial malleolus compared with the lateral malleolus. Tenderness to palpation in this region suggests ligament injury.

Localized tenderness to palpation immediately above the joint space and at maximum dorsiflexion of the foot with slight lateral migration of the fibula is the sign of an injury to the anterior talofibular ligament (Fig. 6.**8**). On the posterior aspect of the medial malleolus, several structures can be palpated in a

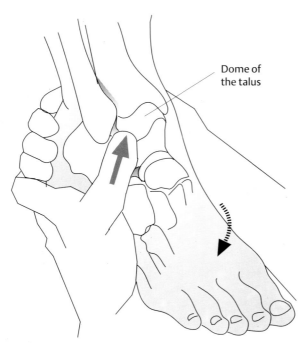

Dome of
the talus

Fig. 6.**5**   Palpation of the talar dome in plantar flexion.

Flexor digitorum longus

Tibialis posterior

Posterior
tibial artery

Tibial nerve

Flexor hallucis
longus

Fig. 6.**7**   Palpation of the deltoid ligament.

Fig. 6.**6**   Palpation of the medial malleolus.

Anterior talofibular
ligament

Fig. 6.**8**   Palpation of the anterior talofibular ligament.

small groove medial to the Achilles tendon. These include, from anterior to posterior, the tendons of the tibialis posterior and flexor digitorum longus muscles, the posterior tibial artery and nerve, and the flexor hallucis longus (Fig. 6.**7**). If tenosynovitis in this region is suspected, check for tenderness to palpation and for swelling along the tendons (Fig. 6.**9**). Another sign of tenosynovitis is pain that occurs when the foot is in plantar flexion and pronation (Fig. 6.**10**). In this position, tenderness to palpation and a palpable defect in the tibialis posterior tendon will be encountered in a tear (Fig. 6.**11**).

The thick cord of the Achilles tendon is located further posteriorly and medially.

To evaluate the Achilles tendon, the patient is prone with the feet extending past the edge of the examining table. Evaluate strength and integrity by having the patient actively bring the feet into plantar flexion against your resistance. Observe and palpate the tensing of the tendons. If a tear is present, a loss of strength and a change in the contour of the tendon will be noticeable on the affected side (Figs. 6.**12a, b**).

If the Achilles tendon is intact, compressing the calf will produce plantar flexion. Absence of plantar flexion in this test is a sign of a tear in the Achilles tendon (Figs. 6.**13a, b**).

The lateral malleolus is palpated at the distal tip of the fibula. The anterior talofibular ligament, calcaneofibular ligament, and the posterior talofibular lig-

Fig. 6.**10** Pain in passive plantar flexion and pronation of the foot with tenosynovitis of the tibialis posterior tendon.

Fig. 6.**9** Palpation of the tendons of the tibialis posterior, flexor digitorum longus, flexor hallucis longus, and posterior tibial artery.

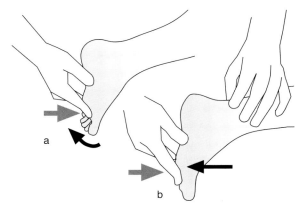

Figs. 6.**12a, b** Palpation of the Achilles tendon and evaluation of active strength in both ankles.

Fig. 6.**11** Palpation of the tibialis posterior tendon for tenderness in tenosynovitis or a palpable defect in a tear.

ament are important stabilizing structures that are palpable in this region. These structures are frequently injured in supination trauma.

The anterior talofibular ligament is tensed in the foot in plantar flexion and supination.

The calcaneofibular ligament inserts on the calcaneus toward the plantar aspect of the foot. Usually,

it is only affected in severe ankle trauma after injury to the anterior talofibular ligament.

The posterior talofibular ligament is the strongest of the lateral ankle ligaments. It stabilizes the ankle as the talus moves anteriorly and is usually only damaged in high-energy injuries.

The peroneal ligaments can be palpated at the lateral malleolus. These will be tender to palpation if tenosynovitis is present. Extreme passive inversion and plantar flexion will also cause pain in the peroneal tendons with tenosynovitis (Fig. 6.**14**).

In dislocation of the peroneal tendons, there will be a palpable snap anterior to the malleolus as the patient actively pronates the foot (Fig. 6.**15**).

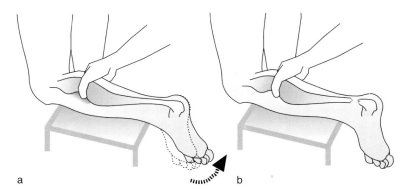

Figs. 6.**13a, b** Evaluating the integrity of the Achilles tendon by compressing the calf.

Fig. 6.**14**   Passive strong plantar flexion and inversion intensifies pain in tenosynovitis of the peroneal tendons.

Fig. 6.**15**   Palpation of the peroneal tendons while the patient actively pronates the foot in peroneal tendon dislocation.

Fig. 6.**16**   Evaluating posterior extension in shortening of the Achilles tendon.

Assessing Range of Motion

As with every joint, range-of-motion testing for the ankle evaluates the active and passive ranges of motion.

Motion is measured around the main axis. This axis connects the medial and lateral malleoli through the talus. It permits lifting of the foot (dorsiflexion) and lowering of the foot (plantar flexion). The range of motion is measured and documented using the neutral-O method.

Assessing Active Range of Motion

To examine plantar flexion, instruct the patient to walk a short distance on tiptoe. Walking on the heels is used for evaluating dorsiflexion.

Assessing Passive Range of Motion

To evaluate the passive range of motion of the ankle, have the patient sit on the examining table with the legs dangling. In this position with the knees flexed 90°, the action of the gastrocnemius is minimized, permitting unimpeded evaluation of dorsiflexion even in the presence of a shortened Achilles tendon (Fig. 6.**16**).

Pressing the foot downward produces plantar flexion. Normally the range of motion according to the neutral-O method will be 30° dorsiflexion and 50° plantar flexion.

Specific Tests

These tests permit a rough estimation of the severity of an injury.

According to the direction of motion, a distinction is made between pronation and supination trauma of the ankle. Supination trauma, i.e., trauma in which the medial aspect of the foot bends upward beyond the patient's control, is more common for anatomic reasons. Since the medial malleolus is shorter than the lateral malleolus, the talus tends to supinate rather than pronate. The lateral ligaments as isolated structures are not as strong as the deltoid ligament.

All specific tests can be performed under local anesthesia to neutralize reflexive muscle tensing by the patient if the pain is too great.

Specific Tests for Instability

Anterior drawer (Figs. 6.**17a**, **b**). Anterior drawer is best evaluated with the patient supine. Immobilize the patient's distal tibia with one hand while holding the back of the foot with the other. Now apply pressure against the back of the foot. Repeat the test for both sides. A positive test is the sign of injury to the anterior and posterior capsular ligaments of the ankle.

In an isolated tear of the talofibular ligament, the talus can be shifted anteriorly against the tibia. This ligament does not allow such mobility when intact. This test may also be documented in radiographic and ultrasound studies.

Figs. 6.**17a, b**   Evaluating the anterior drawer of the talus.

Figs. 6.**18a, b**   Evaluating lateral and medial opening.

Lateral and medial opening (Figs. 6.**18a, b**). This may also be known as talar tilt. It is also best tested with the patient supine and relaxed. Again, examine both sides for comparison. Apply a varus and valgus stress to the ankle to evaluate the lateral and medial capsular ligaments.

Damage to the talofibular and calcaneofibular ligaments produces lateral instability. This can be verified by supination of the calcaneus. If the joint space opens widely compared with the contralateral ankle and there is excessive play between talus and mortise, it is probable that the capsular ligaments, particularly the two mentioned above, are injured.

The posterior talofibular ligament usually only tears in severe injuries involving injuries to other lateral ligaments, such as dislocations.

Evaluate the stability of the medial side (deltoid ligament) by pronating the calcaneus while palpating the joint space.

Joint opening can also be documented in radiographic and ultrasound studies, providing an indirect impression of the stability of the lateral capsular ligaments.

Neurologic Examination

The neurologic examination gives the examiner an overview of the strength of individual muscle groups. Sensation, reflexes, and vascular supply are evaluated.

Muscle Function

Muscular strength is divided into five gradations (see shoulder chapter, Table **1.8**, p. 24).

Fig. 6.**19**   Achilles tendon reflex.

Fig. 6.**20**   Sensory distribution.

• Dorsiflexion

The tibialis anterior, extensor digitorum communis, and extensor hallucis longus effect dorsiflexion. They all receive their sensory supply from the deep peroneal nerve that originates from the common peroneal nerve and sciatic nerve (L4–S3).

A lesion along this nerve path from a mass (tumor, nerve-root compression at any level from L4–S3), trauma, iatrogenic injury to the common peroneal nerve (such as a plaster cast), or damage resulting from a compartment syndrome lead to weakness or paresis of the dorsiflexors. This produces a typical drop-foot or steppage gait.

Muscle function can be evaluated by having the patient actively tense the muscles against your resistance.

• Plantar flexion

Plantar flexion is primarily effected by the triceps surae (gastrocnemius, soleus, and plantaris supplied by the tibial nerve). This becomes particularly apparent in ballet when the dancer balances on the toe. The muscle can only develop its full strength when the knee is extended; with the knee flexed, the gastrocnemius is already contracted.

The peroneal muscles, the flexor digitorum longus and the tibialis posterior, are also involved in plantar flexion and are also supplied by the tibial nerve.

Reflexes

• Physiologic Reflexes

The Achilles tendon reflex and tibialis posterior reflex are the most important ankle reflexes.

Achilles tendon reflex (S1). With the patient supine and the leg flexed, tap the Achilles tendon. Normal response will be plantar flexion of the foot (Fig. 6.**19**).

Tibialis posterior reflex (L4 and L5). With the patient supine, tap beneath the medial malleolus. This results in supination of the foot. This reflex cannot always be elicited; comparison of both sides is clinically relevant.

Examining Sensation

Three dermatomes provide sensation in the ankle, distal calf, and foot (Fig. 6.**20**).

L4: anterior medial edge of the tibia, medial malleolus, and medial sole of the foot.

L5: narrow strip along the anterior edge of the tibia, and posterior and plantar surface.

Fig. 6.**21** Osteochondritis dissecans in the medial talar dome in the AP projection.

Fig. 6.**22** Osteochondroma anterior to the ankle on the lateral projection.

Fig. 6.**23** Intra-articular fracture of the distal tibia involving the epiphysis.

S1: lateral strip along the thigh and calf, posterior distal calf in the Achilles tendon region, sole of the foot, and plantar and posterior surface.

Vascular Supply

Pulsations in the posterior tibial artery can be pal-

pated at the medial malleolus. The other artery is the dorsalis pedis artery on the dorsum. It is palpable between the tendon of the extensor hallucis longus and the tendons of the extensor digitorum longus.

6.3 Radiographs

Standard Views

AP and lateral radiographs are sufficient for evaluating most ankle injuries and disorders. Images in these planes visualize degenerative and traumatic changes such as fractures, osteochondritis dissecans (Fig. 6.**21**), and tumors (Fig. 6.**22**). Whenever clinical symptoms are present, one of the two standard planes should always image proximally to permit visualization of fractures that may also extend to the articular surfaces of the ankle (Fig. 6.**23**).

Twisting forces can fracture the proximal tibia and may injure the peroneal nerve. Damage to the peroneal nerve results in symptoms ranging from altered sensation to complete paresis of the dorsiflexors. A proximal spiral fracture of the fibula ("Maisonneuve fracture") often results from an indirect force applied to the lower leg (Fig. 6.**24**).

AP View (Figs. 6.**25 a, b**)

The AP radiograph can evaluate the configuration of the joint, congruity of the articular surfaces, and inclination of the talus with respect to the tibia (talar tilt).

The patient is supine with the legs extended and the ankle in a neutral position, i.e., with the calf and

Fig. 6.**24**   Malleolar fracture with high proximal fibular fracture (Maisonneuve fracture).

sole of the foot forming a 90° angle. The distal fibula overlaps the lateral portion of the tibia in this view. The central ray is perpendicular to the ankle, entering approximating 1 cm above the tip of the medial malleolus.

In osteochondritis dissecans, there will generally be a defect in the subchondral bone of the talus.

Depending on the extent of the damage to the articular cartilage, this may range from a small osteochondral body in situ to an intra-articular loose body (Fig. 6.**26**).

The so-called "Tillaux fracture" of the anterior tubercle of the tibia can be visualized on the AP radiograph.

This projection eliminates the overlapping mentioned above and visualizes the joint space between the distal fibula, the lateral edge of the tibia, and the talus.

Twisting forces to the calf can involve a fracture of the proximal tibia that may result in injury to the peroneal nerve. Damage to the peroneal nerve results in symptoms ranging from simple altered sensation to complete paresis of the dorsiflexors. This proximal spiral fracture of the fibula ("Maisonneuve fracture") often results from an indirect force applied to the lower leg.

If a fracture is suspected, use a long cassette to image the knee and proximal tibia.

The AP or lateral radiograph can reveal stress fractures in the distal fibula indicative of chronic overuse (Fig. 6.**27**).

Lateral View (Figs. 6.**28 a, b**)

The patient is positioned laterally with the ankle in a neutral position. The malleoli must be precisely aligned one above the other, parallel to the plane of the cassette. Cushions should be used for support if necessary. The contralateral leg is placed in front of the leg being imaged. Here too, the central ray is aimed at the joint space, entering the joint 1 cm cranial to the tip of the medial malleolus. This view images the ankle, talocalcaneonavicular joint, and the calcaneus in a true lateral projection. The anterior and

a

b

Figs. 6.**25a, b**   Normal AP ankle radiograph.

Fig. 6.**26**   Osteochondritis dissecans of the medial surface of the talus.

Fig. 6.**27**   AP radiograph of a stress fracture of the distal fibula.

Figs. 6.**28a, b**   Lateral radiograph of the ankle.

a

b

Fig. 6.**29**   Fracture of the distal posterior margin of the tibia (Volkmann triangle).

Fig. 6.**30**   Lateral radiograph of the ankle showing advanced osteoarthritis.

posterior margins of the distal tibia, the "posterior malleolus," and the talus are demonstrated in profile (Fig. 6.**29**).

Typical signs of arthritis of the ankle in the lateral projection include narrowing of the joint space, sclerotic zones, and marginal osteophytes (Fig. 6.**30**).

Neuropathic arthropathy (Charcot joint) is distinguished by degenerative changes with destruction of articular cartilage, subchondral sclerosis, and severe marginal osteophytes. This leads to dislocation or subluxation with severe joint deformity (Fig. 6.**31**). In chronic instability of the ankle, the lateral projection will frequently demonstrate traction osteophytes on

the talus or anterior margin of the tibia as sequelae of recurrent supination trauma (Fig. 6.**32**).

Special Views for Diagnosing Trauma

Oblique views may be used to supplement standard views to facilitate more precise evaluation of the bony structures in diagnosing ankle fractures.

Oblique radiograph of the ankle in 30° internal rotation with the patient supine. This is also referred to as the "mortise view." The patient is supine with the knees extended and the ankle in a neutral position and internally rotated approximately 15°–20° (Figs. 6.**33a, b**). Supporting cushions may be required.

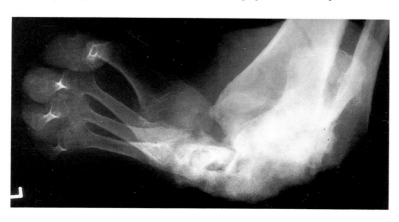

Fig. 6.**31**   Severe joint destruction in neuropathic arthropathy.

Fig. 6.**32**   Traction osteophyte of the anterior tibia.

The mortise view can be used to obtain an image of the ankle without overlapping structures. This view is a variation of the AP projection with the ankle internally rotated 10°–30° (Fig. 6.**34**).

The central ray is aimed at the lateral malleolus. This positioning demonstrates the articular surfaces and the mortise without overlapping structures.

In a simple rupture of the syndesmosis without accompanying bone injuries, this projection will show medial displacement of the distal tibia and an increase in the distance between the fibula and tibia (Fig. 6.**35**).

Radiographs may also be obtained in approximately 30°–35° internal rotation to evaluate the tibiofibular syndesmosis (Fig. 6.**36**).

Oblique radiograph of the ankle in external rotation with the patient supine. The patient is positioned as for the oblique radiograph in internal rotation, except that the leg is placed in 40°–45° external rotation. In this projection, the lateral malleolus, the posterior lip of the tibia (malleolus tertius), and the anterior tibial tubercle are demonstrated.

Dynamic examination with fluoroscopy. In the AP projection in 45° external rotation the anterior tubercle of the tibia is demonstrated, superimposed on the lateral malleolus.

b

a

Figs. 6.**33a, b**   Mortise view. The ankle is imaged in an AP projection at 30° internal rotation.

Fig. 6.**34** Mortise view

Fig. 6.**35** Disrupted syndesmosis in the mortise view.

Fig. 6.**36** Oblique radiograph of the ankle in 30° internal rotation with the patient supine. The mortise joint is demonstrated without overlapping shadows. The arrow indicates a malleolar fracture at the level of the syndesmosis.

In neutral rotation, the medial portion of the joint space will open. As rotation is increased to 45° internal rotation, the joint space also opens laterally. The entire joint space is exposed in this projection.

Stress Views for Evaluating Ligaments

Once an acute fracture is excluded, comparative stress radiographs of both sides may be obtained immediately after injury. Muscular resistance due to pain or extensive swelling can make these studies difficult. In applicable cases, these symptoms can be reduced with a local anesthetic.

AP view with inversion stress (Figs. 6.**37a, b**). The patient is supine with the foot internally rotated 15° for a mortise view. Immobilize the patient's distal calf with one hand while pushing the back of the foot into supination with your other using the same amount of force (22–33 lbf). Wear a protective lead apron and gloves. A jig may also be used.

The central ray is perpendicular to the middle of the ankle. As the varus position is increased, the heel is adducted and the talus tilted. The tilt of the talus is measured as the angle between the tangents of the distal end of the tibia and the talar dome. Measurements of both sides are compared. Abnormal values suggest injury to a lateral ligament. With forced inversion stress angles below 5° are normal, and angles over 15° are probably abnormal.

a

b

Figs. 6.**37a, b**   AP view with inversion stress.

With generalized ligamentous laxity, talar tilt can be as much as 25°. For this reason comparative measurements of both sides are recommended. A relative difference of more than 5° must be demonstrated to confirm a ligament injury.

AP view with eversion stress. This view is used only in rare cases to demonstrate injuries to the medial ligaments or the medial malleolus.

The patient is positioned as for the stress view with inversion stress.

Talar tilt exceeding 10° is regarded as pathologic.

Lateral stress view with anterior displacement of the talus (Figs. 6.**38a, b**). The patient is supine with the foot internally rotated 15° and the heel elevated on a plate so that the calf is not in contact with the tendon table. The ankle is in a lateral position with the foot in slight plantar flexion.

Wearing protective clothing, apply posterior pressure to the calf (22–33 lbf). A jig may also be used.

The central ray is aimed at the middle of the joint space.

Evaluate and measure the posterior mobility of the tibia with respect to the talar dome, comparing both ankles. The anterior displacement of the talus is

a

b

Figs. 6.**38a, b**   Lateral stress view showing anterior displacement of the talus.

Fig. 6.**39**   Posterior longitudinal plane. The left image shows normal findings; the arrow indicates the Achilles tendon. The right image shows a hematoma (arrow) in an Achilles tendon tear.

Fig. 6.**40**   Anterior longitudinal plane showing a hypoechoic cyst. The arrows indicate the stem of the cyst.

measured as the distance between the distal tibia and the talus in the sagittal plane.

This test is regarded as an indirect sign of ligament injury, primarily the anterior talofibular ligament. Anterior displacement less than 5 mm is regarded as normal, and values exceeding 10 mm indicate ligament injury.

6.4 Ultrasound

Ultrasonography is not as useful in the ankle as it is in the shoulder or for the evaluation of hip dysplasia in newborns. However, its greatest utility is in evaluating the Achilles tendon and surrounding structures. As in other areas of the body, ultrasonography can be used to determine if a mass is solid or cystic. Ultrasonography of the ankle may include static and dynamic examinations.

Achilles Tendon Pathology

Tear in the Achilles Tendon (Fig. 6.**39**)

Ultrasound studies are suitable for diagnosing a complete tear of the Achilles tendon, especially when clinical findings are inconclusive. They may also be used to confirm physical examination findings and for follow-up examinations during treatment.

In proximal tears where clinical examination cannot distinguish between injury to the muscle or a tendon tear, an intramuscular hematoma will often be discernible as a hypoechoic mass, and the tendon will be intact. In a tendon tear, the hyperechoic conti-

nuity of the tendon will be interrupted; a hypoechoic zone between the stumps consistent with a hematoma will be visible. Dynamic examination in dorsiflexion permits distraction of the stumps and demonstration of the lack of continuity and tension in the tendon. This examination does not allow measurement of the distance between the stumps.

Achilles Tendinitis

Ultrasound is capable of visualizing tendon changes in acute or chronic Achilles tendinitis and is helpful as follow-up examinations during treatment. The increased fluid content of the tendon makes it appear as a widened hypoechoic structure in the sonogram. In chronic tendinitis, contour irregularities will also be visible on the surface of the tendon. Always compare both ankles in every ultrasound examination.

With lesions of the muscle tendon junction, the insertion region will appear as a widened hypoechoic structure similar to the patellar tendon in "jumper's knee." Here too, both ankles should be compared.

Retrocalcaneal Bursitis

Bursitis beneath the Achilles tendon is often difficult to distinguish from Achilles tendinitis during clinical examination. A hypoechoic mass beneath, and lateral to, the Achilles tendon in the sonogram is a sign of bursitis. Comparison of both sides can confirm the diagnosis if the contralateral ankle lacks a hypoechoic zone and the insertion region of the Achilles tendon appears normal.

Other Abnormal Findings (Cysts and Ganglia)

Ultrasonography is very well suited for visualizing various masses in the ankle. A **ganglion** appears in the sonogram as a hypoechoic mass with isolated hyperechoic internal echoes. These findings require additional imaging studies or intraoperative confirmation; ultrasonography does not provide a pathoanatomical diagnosis.

A **cyst** will appear as a hypoechoic, fluid-filled mass. Occasionally, ultrasound studies can demonstrate a stem that communicates with the intra-articular space (Fig. 6.**40**).

6.5 *Arthrography and Tenography*

Arthrography

Ankle arthrography continues to be valuable for diagnosing ligament lesions in the ankle. The method is easy to learn, may be quickly performed, is well tolerated by the patient, and the risk of complications is minimal.

Indications and Technique

Indications for ankle arthrography include ligament lesions, osteochondritis dissecans, intra-articular loose bodies, talar fractures, capsular abnormalities, and degenerative changes.

Ankle arthrography may be performed using a single-contrast method (contrast medium only) for imaging the ligaments. It may also be performed as a double-contrast method with contrast-medium and air injection. This aids in visualizing articular cartilage.

The double-contrast technique is used for evaluating articular cartilage and the articular surfaces, and to demonstrate loose intra-articular bodies where present. Double-contrast arthrography is preferred for imaging osteochondral lesions.

Used in combination with CT, arthrography provides information for evaluating complex fractures.

The patient is supine and relaxed with the foot in slight plantar flexion. Aspirate the joint under fluoroscopic control between the tendon of the extensor hallucis longus and the tibialis anterior using a local anesthetic. Take care to avoid injuring the dorsalis pedis artery that courses adjacent to these structures.

Immediately after inserting the needle and aspirating a sample of joint fluid, inject a nonionic contrast medium under fluoroscopic control. Then move the joint through its range of motion to distribute the contrast medium. Obtain AP and lateral radiographs, images at 10° internal rotation, and oblique radiographs at 35° and 45° internal and external rotation, respectively. Additional stress views may also be indicated.

Ankle arthrography should be performed within 48 hours of an acute injury to evaluate ligaments. Otherwise, false negative findings may result from adhesions or coagulation.

Only a few **contraindications** to ankle arthrography are described in the literature. **Complications** of this examination include joint infection, swelling after improper injections, and allergic reactions to the contrast medium used.

Normal Findings

Normal fingings show the joint homogeneously filled with contrast medium with a smoothly demarcated anterior and posterior joint recess.

The intra-articular space filled with contrast medium will be seen to extend to the tips of the malleoli. Occasionally, the medial tendon sheaths of the flexor hallucis longus and the flexor digitorum profundus will also fill with contrast medium.

Abnormal Findings

Arthrography cannot image ligaments directly. However, characteristic extra-articular patterns of distribution can provide information about the various ligament structures.

The most frequent mechanism injury is supination, which injures the anterior talofibular ligament. In the arthrogram, injury to this ligament will result in contrast-medium leakage anterior and lateral to the fibula after intra-articular injection. The extent of this leakage is proportional to the size of the lesion and injection pressure.

Areas of contrast medium may also be visible medial to the lateral malleolus. An additional lateral image may be obtained to differentiate between rupture of the syndesmosis and a tear in the anterior talofibular ligament. Broad areas of contrast medium anterior to the syndesmosis will be seen in a ligament tear.

High-contrast visualization of the fibular tendon sheaths (peroneal tendons) is a sign of a tear of the calcaneofibular ligaments.

Tears of the posterior talofibular ligament can only be demonstrated as part of a combined injury involving lesions to the other lateral capsular ligaments.

Complex injuries of the capsular ligaments are rarely diagnosed by arthrography.

Injuries to the medial capsular ligaments will evidence an extra-articular deposit of contrast medium due to leakage at the medial malleolus. Leakage of contrast medium between the tibia and fibula, extending proximally into the mortise, may suggest injury to the syndesmosis (Fig. 6.**41**). The standard lateral view will show contrast medium anterior to the fibula.

Osteochondral lesions of the talus resulting from avulsion injuries or in osteochondritis dissecans are best visualized with the double-contrast technique. Conventional tomography or CT studies are required to determine the exact size and boundaries of the lesions.

In capsulitis of the ankle, the arthrogram will reveal a significantly reduced volume and a reduction in the filling of the anterior and posterior joint recess, together with increased injection pressure.

Tenograms

Ankle tenography can be used to visualize inflammatory or posttraumatic changes in various tendon sheaths by injecting contrast medium. It can be used as an additional procedure in the peroneal tendons to

Fig. 6.**41** Abnormal arthrogram showing contrast-medium leakage defining an injury to the syndesmosis.

Fig. 6.**42** Three-dimensional reconstruction of the ankle.

increase the precision of arthrography in imaging injuries to the calcaneofibular ligament (see below).

Injuries to the Achilles tendon and the tendons of the peroneus, tibialis posterior, flexorum digitorum longus, and flexor hallucis longus are the primary lesions that can be imaged with this modality.

After advancing the injection cannula under fluoroscopic control, inject approximately 15 mL of contrast medium under fluoroscopic control. Contrast-medium stoppage, leakage, and spread into an adjacent joint are signs of a tendon tear.

As mentioned above, tenography may be used to confirm the diagnosis of an injury to the calcaneofibular ligament. Contrast medium injected into the fibular tendon sheaths will be seen to spread into the ankle.

6.6 Nuclear Medicine Studies

See chapter 1 (Shoulder, p. 54) for a general discussion on the utility of nuclear medicine studies.

6.7 Computed Tomography

CT of the ankle in standardized imaging-planes provides important information about the size, extent, position, and type of masses, injuries, or degenerative changes.

Imaging planes in CT follow anatomic structures and are perpendicular to each other. Three standard imaging planes for evaluating the ankle are described in the literature. Slices measuring 1.0–3.0 mm may be used, depending on the region of interest.

CT arthrography with air or contrast medium can visualize intra-articular loose bodies or damage to articular surfaces.

Articular involvement such as talar cysts or fractures can be evaluated. This is important for subsequent therapy. Posttraumatic ligament lesions, tendon pathology, and tendon dislocations can be verified by CT.

Three-dimensional CT reconstruction permits precise preoperative planning. The advantage this method might offer in routine diagnostics is unclear and is currently the subject of scientific studies (Fig. 6.**42**).

6.8 Magnetic Resonance Imaging

Indications

The most frequent indications are traumatic lesions of the ligaments, tendons, and bones, as well as osteochondral lesions and inflammatory changes.

Examination Procedure (Figs. 6.**43a–c**)

With the patient supine and the foot immobilized, imaging is best performed with cylindrical coils. Following the protocol used for the other joints, T1-weighted and T2-weighted spin echo (SE) images, short-time inversion recovery (STIR) images, and various gradient-echo (GRE) images are acquired.

Fig. 6.**43a** Transverse image (GRE 500/11 out of phase) showing a normal ankle.

Medial malleolus

Tendon of the flexor digitorum longus

Posterior tibial artery

Tendon of the flexor hallucis longus

Tendon of the peroneus longus and peroneus brevis

Fig. 6.**43b** Sagittal image (GRE 500/11 out of phase) showing a normal ankle and talocalcaneonavicular joint.

Flexor hallucis longus

Achilles tendon

Ankle

Talonavicular joint

Subtalar joint

Quadratus plantae

Fig. 6.**43c** Coronal image (GRE 500/11 out of phase) showing a normal ankle.

Deltoid ligament

Tendon of the tibialis posterior

Complete tear
of the talofibular
ligament

Sprain of the
posterior talo-
fibular ligament

Fig. 6.**44a**   Transverse image
(GRE 500/11 out of phase
after administration of intravenous gadolinium contrast
medium) showing complete
tear of the anterior talofibular ligament, sprain of the
posterior talofibular ligament,
and contrast medium
enhancement along the
intact fibers.

Partial tear of
the ligament

Fig. 6.**44b**   Coronal image
(GRE 500/11 out of phase
after administration of intravenous gadolinium contrast
medium) showing a partial
tear of the calcaneofibular
ligament, discontinuity in
individual fibers with
contrast-medium enhance-
ment at the tear sites and
along the sprained fibers.

Pathologic Findings

Injuries of the Ligamentous Structures
(Figs. 6.**44a, b**)

Supination trauma most frequently injures the anterior talofibular ligament, ranging from a sprain to a
partial or complete tear. The traumatic changes are
best seen on T2-weighted and STIR images. As with
other ligamentous injuries, intravenous administration of gadolinium-based contrast medium has been
proven advantageous for T1-weighted GRE images
with phase contrast since it visualizes the perifocal
edema at high contrast and delineates the torn ligamentous fibers within it as delicate, partly swollen or
spirally shortened dark structures. With sprains, the
fibers remain discernibly intact and lines of increased
signal intensity are seen along the ligamentous direction. To orient the sections accordingly, they should

be obliquely transverse for the anterior talofibular ligament. The next weaker ligament is the posterior
talofibular ligament, that is also well visualized on
the transverse image. The calcaneofibular ligament is
rarely torn. It is best visualized on the coronal image.
For injuries of the deltoid ligament, transverse and
coronal sections are selected.

Injuries, Degenerations, and Inflammatory
Changes of the Tendons (Figs. 6.**45a, b** and 6.**46**)

The Achilles tendon is most frequently injured with
forced dorsal flexion against the contracted gastrocnemius and soleus musculature. With incomplete
tears, the tendon shows fusiform thickening with
increased signal intensity on the T1-weighted image.
The GRE images reveal fibrous dehiscences. The STIR

Fig. 6.**45a** Sagittal image (SE 700/20) showing a complete tear of the Achilles tendon. The tendon fiber structures that are normally dark in T1-weighted images are interrupted. The medium signal intensity is due to the influx of protein-rich serum components.

Complete tear of the Achilles tendon

Degeneration of the Achilles tendon with a small cyst

Fig. 6.**45b** Sagittal image (STIR 2000/155) showing degeneration of the Achilles tendon with thickening, a strip of increased signal intensity, and a central cyst.

Tenosynovitis of the peroneus longus tendon

Fig. 6.**46** Sagittal image (GRE 500/11 out of phase after administration of intravenous gadolinium contrast medium) showing tenosynovitis of the peroneus longus tendon with contrast-medium enhancement in the tendon sheath and within the tendon itself.

Osteochondritis
dissecans

Fig. 6.**47**   Coronal image
(STIR 3000/150) showing
osteochondritis dissecans
with high signal intensity
along the demarcation line
and perifocal bone edema.

Epiphysis

Growth plate

Epiphyseal fracture
with injury to
the growth plate

Fig. 6.**48**   Coronal image
(GRE 500/11 out of phase after
administration of intravenous
gadolinium contrast medium)
showing an epiphyseal fracture with injury to the
epiphysis and growth plate.

Synovitis
associated with
arthritis.
Enhancement in
the synovial
membrane with
effusion

Fig. 6.**49**   Sagittal image
(GRE 500/11 out of phase after
administration of intravenous
gadolinium contrast medium)
showing arthritis of the ankle
and talocalcaneonavicular
joint.

image shows an increase in signal intensity that is linear within the tendon and usually circular around it. The complete tear is easily recognized on all sequences as a tendinous gap, definite hemorrhage, and considerable edema of the tendon edges. This injury is frequently accompanied by a muscle tear. Degenerative changes, caused by repetitive microtraumas or occurring in a tendon predisposed by rheumatoid arthritis or long-term corticosteroid therapy, frequently display a central fusiform cystic transformation, aside from ligamentous thickening that encloses a linear, moderately increased signal intensity. The sections are obtained sagittally and transversely.

Trauma, but also overuse, can damage the tendon of the flexor hallucis and the tendons of the tibialis posterior and the peroneus muscles. This leads to tenosynovitis and is best seen on STIR or T2-weighted sequences as well as on the phase contrast images after administration of contrast medium. Sagittal and transverse sections are selected here. The tendon and, even more so, the tendon sheath show signal intensity.

Osteochondritis Dissecans (Fig. 6.**47**)

Osteochondritis dissecans of the talar dome is considered a traumatic sequela. Analogous to its manifestation at the knee, the findings range from subchondral foci with a high signal intensity on the STIR images and an intact articular cartilage to detached fragments. Grade II of this condition is characterized by a delicate line of high signal intensity on the STIR image, demarcating the lesion from the uninvolved bone. After intravenous administration of gadolinium-based contrast medium, enhancement reveals the hyperemia of the viable zones. In accordance with the most frequent traumatic mechanism, the medial aspect of the trochlea is usually involved.

Fractures (Fig. 6.**48**)

MRI is rarely used for fractures, with plain films and CT being the preferred imaging modalities. However, a trimalleolar fracture in a skeletally immature patient has to be scrutinized for any extension of the fracture line into the epiphyseal growth plate. Since it is clearly delineated on all weightings, in particular on the T2*-weighted sequences, this can be reliably achieved. Osseous avulsions of the ligamentous attachements are often more difficult to diagnose because of the frequent accessory bones observed at the ankle. Enhancement around the osseous fragment and osseous edema favor an avulsion. Trabecular fractures are found in the calcaneus after compression trauma and are delineated by a markedly increased signal intensity on the STIR image and a decreased signal intensity on the T1-weighted image. These injuries can induce osteonecrosis, particularly if they involve the talus, but osteonecroses are also observed

in the navicular and, rarely, in the cuboid. Strong enhancement is suggestive of osteonecrosis, which narrows to the demarcation zone during the course of the disease.

Arthritis (Fig. 6.**49**)

Inflammatory arthritis of the ankle is rare. It is characterized by a diffuse loss of articular cartilage and small cartilaginous lesions, accompanied by synovitis. The imaging parameters for the cartilaginous structures are T2*-weighted sequences for the cartilaginous structures, T2-weighted or STIR sequences for the effusion, and the T1-weighted phases GRE for any enhancement after administration of contrast medium.

References

Gebing R, Fiedler V. Röntgendiagnostik der Bänderläsionen des oberen Sprunggelenkes. *Radiologe* 1991; 31: 594–600
Hoppenfeld S. *Klinische Untersuchung der Wirbelsäule und der Extremitäten.* Stuttgart–Jena–New York: Fischer; 1992
Jerosch J, Marquardt M. *Sonographie des Bewegungsapparates.* Zülpich: Biermann; 1993
Johnson K. *Surgery of the Foot and Ankle.* New York: Raven Press; 1989
Kerr R, Forrester D, Kingston S. MRI of the foot and ankle. *Orthop Clin North Am* 1990; 21: 591–601
Liou J, Totty W. Magnetic resonance imaging of ankle injuries. *Top Magn Imag* 1991; 1: 1–22
Ludolph E, Hierholzer G, Gretenkord K. Untersuchungen zur Anatomie und Röntgendiagnostik des fibularen Bandapparates am Sprunggelenk. *Unfallchirurgie* 1985; 88: 245–249
McRae R. *Klinisch-orthopädische Untersuchung.* Stuttgart–New York: Fischer; 1989
Mann RA, Coughlin MJ. *Surgery of the Foot and Ankle.* St. Louis: Mosby; 1993
Pavlov H. Imaging of the foot and ankle. *Radiol Clin North Am* 1990; 28: 991–1018
Rijke A et al. Magnetic resonance imaging of the injury to the lateral ankle ligaments. *Am J Sports Med* 1993; 21: 528–534
Rosenberg Z. Current imaging techniques for assessment of ankle tendons. *Bull Hosp Jt Dis Orthop Inst* 1990; 50: 139–148
Rubin G, Witten M. The talar tilt angle and the fibular collateral ligament. *J Bone Joint Surg* 1960; 42-A: 311
Schricker T, Hien NM, Wirth CJ. Klinische Ergebnisse sonographischer Funktionsuntersuchungen bei Kapselbandläsionen am Knie- und Sprunggelenk. *Ultraschall* 1987; 8: 27–31
Striepling E, et al. Die sonographische Beurteilbarkeit des Sprunggelenkes bei Supinationstraumen. *Aktuel Traumatol* 1991; 5: 154–156
Weiss C. Die gehaltene Aufnahme des oberen Sprunggelenkes – eine einfache Routineuntersuchung? *Röntgenpraxis* 1985; 38: 385–389
Winkel D, et al. *Nichtoperative Orthopädie und Manualtherapie* Vol 2. Stuttgart–New York: Fischer; 1990: 317–367
Zwipp H. Verletzungen des OSG aus unfallchirurgischer Sicht. *Radiologe* 1991: 31; 585–593

7 Foot

7.1 Introduction

The foot is the link between the body and the surface that it moves across. Four interrelated requirements permit this everyday feat to occur.

The foot must be stable, allowing weight-bearing at rest, and capable of absorbing the accelerations and decelerations of walking and running. These forces can be up to 5.5 times an individual's body weight.

The foot must be flexible and able to adapt and provide optimum contact with the surface in various positions.

The foot must act as a sensory organ, providing information to the central nervous system about pressure, temperature, vibration, and its position in space.

The foot acts as a propulsion unit, responding to central nervous system inputs to move the body through space.

These four characteristics enable the human body to move with minimal expended energy. As an organic system, the foot is subject to some of the highest mechanical stresses in the body, yet it is an end organ with respect to its vascular supply. The combination of high mechanical stresses and lack of collateral vascular supply predispose the foot to demonstrate disorders early in the disease process.

Most foot disorders fall into three major categories:

— Biomechanical
— Infectious
— Manifestations of systemic disease

The aging process can exacerbate existing foot disorders or create new ones.

The pathophysiology of most foot disorders is complex. Both osseous and soft tissues are involved. Biomechanical factors are related to all foot disorders because of the static and dynamic stresses imposed by the body. Also to be considered is the fact that hip and knee disorders can impose abnormal loads on the foot.

When examining the foot, precise evaluation and documentation of physical characteristics is required. These normal variables are appearance, contour, and mobility. These variables are used to classify the foot.

7.2 Clinical Examination

Clinical examination of the foot should begin with a complete examination to exclude other diseases that might be responsible for the reported symptoms. Examine the patient for gout and rheumatoid arthritis, and for changes in the lumbar or sacral region of the spine.

Pay special attention to axial deviations in the lower extremities. These may influence the structural mechanics of the foot.

Examining the hands often provides useful information, especially in the presence of gout, rheumatoid arthritis, psoriasis, and Dupuytren contracture. Moist warm palms and evidence of nail biting are valuable signs of the patient's autonomous and psychological condition.

Standard Examination

Both feet should be examined and compared. The legs should be bare, from the knees down at least. All deformities such as flatfoot, metatarsus varus, and varicosities are evaluated with the patient standing as they will be more pronounced during weight bearing than when the patient is supine.

The form of the foot including its height, circumference, width, and the relative size of the forefoot and calcaneal region are described. Document the size of both feet. If there are significant deviations between the feet, shoes of different sizes will be required. Identify valgus or varus deformities of the heel and arthropathy or hypertrophy of the calf from behind the standing patient. Then have the patient walk back and forth in a relaxed, natural manner and observe the motion of the foot and ankle.

Toe walking, heel walking, and walking on the lateral edge of the foot are rough indications of muscular control and stabilization of the foot. Difficulty or inability to perform any one of these gaits will require more detailed examination of muscular status.

Document the range of motion of the ankle and midfoot in plantar flexion and dorsiflexion, and in pronation and supination, using the neutral-0 method. It is difficult to completely separate pronation and supination from adduction and abduction of the forefoot. For this reason, inversion is a more suitable term as it refers to a combination of adduction and supination. Similarly, eversion describes the combination of abduction and supination. Document the range of motion in flexion and extension of the metatarsophalangeal joints and the proximal and distal interphalangeal joints. Describe any differences in active and passive ranges of motion, joint crepitus, or painfully limited motion at the end of the range of motion, as well as dislocations, subluxations, or rigid joint deformities.

The examination should also include palpation of the pulse of the dorsalis pedis artery distal to the ankle between the tendons of the flexor hallucis longus and the flexor digitorum longus, and of the posterior tibial artery posterior to the medial malleolus. Palpate the courses of the tendons of the peroneal group, extensors, and flexors. In addition, evaluate the tone of the subcutaneous tissue and bursa.

Patient History

The history should cover four areas:

— Evaluation of systemic disorders.
— Identification of changes with secondary effects on the foot, and occupational and athletic stresses.
— Description of localized foot symptoms.
— Previous injuries and treatments.

Systemic Disorders

Certain systemic disorders tend to involve the foot. Frequently the foot will be the site where systemic disorders are manifested. Such diseases include diabetes mellitus, peripheral vascular disease, gout, psoriasis, collagen diseases, and rheumatoid arthritis.

Peripheral vascular disease can occur with diabetes mellitus. There will be both large and small vessel involvement. The end result is ulcerative lesions of the foot.

Congestive heart failure or impaired venous or lymphatic drainage can cause bilateral edema of the feet.

Inquire in detail about any previous medical or surgical events. The same applies to medication allergies.

The history should be supplemented by laboratory tests, particularly of serum glucose levels. A glucose-tolerance test is indicated in the presence of borderline normal-to-elevated blood glucose levels to exclude latent diabetes mellitus. The uric acid level can be important for identifying foot symptoms.

Document any congenital disorders as they are frequently associated with foot deformities that do not respond to treatment.

For example, arthrogryposis multiplex congenita should be distinguished from true clubfoot. Congenital hip subluxation or dislocation is associated with clubfoot; radiographic or ultrasound examination of the hip is indicated wherever clubfoot is diagnosed.

Neurologic disorders such as peroneal muscular atrophy (Charcot–Marie–Tooth disease), neurofibromatosis, and Friedreich's ataxia frequently affect the foot in young patients. Three-quarters of patients with Friedreich's ataxia have associated pes cavus and scoliosis. In most cases, peroneal muscular atrophy develops into pes cavus. However, in neurofibromatosis, the soft tissue can produce gigantism of the foot or of one or more toes.

Disorders with Foot Manifestations

Axial deviation and abnormal rotation can produce secondary foot symptoms. For example, an internal rotation deformity of the tibia can lead to a flatfoot deformity.

Other disorders of the central nervous system can present with foot pain. These include spina bifida and herniated lumbar disks, which can cause radicular symptoms such as pain in one side of the foot. Back pain is not necessarily always present in herniated lumbar disks.

Also inquire about foot stresses in occupation and advocation. Ballet and other professional dances predispose the patient to sesamoiditis, synovitis, and osteoarthritis because of the stresses caused by tiptoe positions. Be prepared to distinguish sesamoiditis from osteochondritis of the sesamoid. Sports such as volleyball and soccer involve an increased incidence of tendonitis, neuropathy, tenosynovitis, bursitis, and ligament injuries.

Local Foot Symptoms

The type, intensity, duration of symptoms, and causes of local foot symptoms should be described. Gout frequently begins as an acute disorder, associated with heightened sensitivity and pain during motion. Morton's neuroma of the interdigital nerve frequently manifests itself only during exercise or when the patient wears tight shoes. Osteoid osteomas in the foot can be effectively treated with aspirin so that a diagnosis by trial of treatment can be made. Intermittent claudication permits diagnosis of peripheral occlusive vascular disease. Pain while walking on uneven surfaces, such as a broken pavement, suggests subtalar pathology.

The quality of pain is also useful in arriving at a diagnosis. Burning pain under the heads of the metatarsals is typical of anterior metatarsalgia with hyperkeratosis. The pain in heel spur syndrome typically appears with initial weight bearing, such as when taking the first few steps in the morning. This is an intense stabbing pain. However, a heel spur may also be totally asymptomatic (Fig. 7.**1**).

There are patients who, for reasons best known to themselves, describe various symptoms and pains that cannot be objectively demonstrated. These patients frequently describe multiple, varying symptoms that do not have an anatomic basis. Objective findings are absent. Local anesthetics are often ineffective in these patients. Despite this overlay of non-organic pathology, these patients can suffer from actual foot disorders.

Fig. 7.**1** Prominent heel spur in a 68-year old female patient without clinical symptoms (incidental finding during diagnostic studies for a foreign body).

When examining this type of patient, keep in mind that if the symptoms are plausible, can be anatomically localized, and are not associated with multiple somatic symptoms, then treatable pathology is present.

Previous Foot Injuries and Treatments

The history must document any information about previous injuries to the legs and feet and the treatment of these injuries.

Immobilization in a short-leg cast or traction with a Steinmann pin through the calcaneus can lead to pain and stiffness in the subtalar joint, even if the original injury was not in the foot.

Occasionally foreign-body granulomas can be responsible for foot symptoms. These granulomas may be due to injuries from thorns or splinters that the patient no longer remembers.

Ask the patient about all previous foot symptoms and treatments. Even questioning about the type of previous examinations can be helpful. You may want to request examination material from the previous attending physician. Also inquire about orthotics.

Many patients are unable to explain where they hurt, or how they were injured. Often this can give rise to verbal misunderstanding. To avoid confusion, the patient's feet and calves should always be exposed for the examination, and the patient should indicate the points of greatest pain himself or herself. It may be helpful to have the patient demonstrate the mechanism of injury because terms like "twisting to the inside or outside" are often misunderstood. The patient's demonstration of the mechanism of injury is usually more reliable.

Observation

Inspection of the foot includes describing the shape of the foot, its position, and noting vascular changes and skin eruptions.

The shape of the foot may be categorized according to the length of the lesser toes in relation to the great toe. The Egyptian form, in which the great toe exceeds the length of the lesser toes, is distinguished from the Greek form, in which the length of the first digit is less than that of the others, and from the intermediate or square form (Figs. 7.**2a–c**).

Measure the width of the forefoot and hindfoot during weight bearing and at rest. The full extent of splayfoot and metatarsus varus is only apparent

a   b   c

Figs. 7.**2a–c** Foot shapes. (**a**) Square. (**b**) Greek. (**c**) Indifferent or Egyptian.

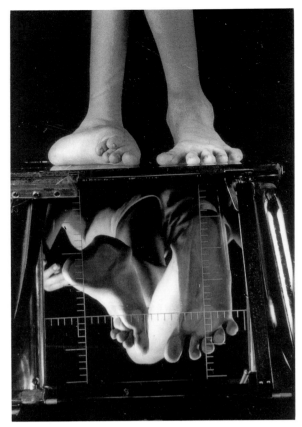

Fig. 7.**3** Image of the foot of a 16-year-old boy with Marfan syndrome and right-sided spastic hemiplegia on a podometer. Disintegration of the ankle and extreme talipes valgus can be seen in the right foot. The sole bears almost no weight and the heel and the head of the first metatarsal are subject to medial weight bearing.

prominences such as swelling, exostoses, or joint effusions. Also document the location and size of any calluses.

Evaluate the alignment of the toes. Document any axial deviation, deformities, subduction, or superduction. Record any joint deformities, contractures, subluxations, or dislocations, proceeding from proximal to distal and from the great toe to the fifth toe. There are four degrees of deformity:

— Grade 0:   no deformity
— Grade I: dynamic deformity
— Grade II: contracted deformity
— Grade III: dislocation

For example, a contracted hammer toe in the proximal interphalangeal joint of the second toe, accompanied by a dynamic deformity in the metatarsophalangeal joint, is documented as follows: hammer toe MTP 2 grade I — PIP 2 grade II — DIP 2 grade 0.

A podometer is outstanding for quickly quantifying foot deformities. The feet are placed on a glass plate illuminated from below. A mirror beneath the glass plate reveals the distribution of weight-bearing surfaces on the sole of the foot. The device is particularly suitable for photographic documentation because the foot is simultaneously visible from the front or back and from the sole with its weight-bearing surfaces (Fig. 7.**3**).

Pes Planus

The term "pes planus" includes all foot deformities involving an extremely low or nonexistent medial longitudinal arch. Normally, the talar head and/or navicular in the inferomedial aspect will be prominent in pes planus. Abduction of the forefoot will be more or less pronounced, and the great toe will be pronated with hallux valgus. Since pes planus is usually associated with an unstable talocalcaneonavicular joint, hammer-toe deformities will frequently develop as a sign of flexor stabilization.

The deformity is often associated with a valgus hindfoot (pes planovalgus; Fig. 7.**4**). The small toes will be visible on the lateral margin of the foot because of the abduction of the forefoot. In contrast, the toes will not be visible next to the heel in a normal foot because of their axial alignment.

Pes Cavus

The generic term "pes cavus" refers to foot deformities with talipes equinus of the forefoot relative to the hindfoot. This significantly increases the height of the medial longitudinal arch. Pes cavus is more frequently associated with a varus deformity of the hindfoot than with a valgus deformity. Prominent calluses under the heads of the metatarsals indicate increased weight bearing in this area, while there will frequently be no calluses in the midsole, even on the lateral aspect. The talipes equinus deformity in the fore-

when the foot is bearing weight with the patient standing.

The position of the hindfoot relative to the horizontal plane or the longitudinal axis of the dorsal distal calf can be measured using a protractor of transparent plastic to document varus or valgus deformities. The degree to which a valgus deformity of the heel may straighten out when the patient stands on tiptoe is an important sign of the flexibility of the deformity.

Deviations in adduction and abduction can be clinically determined by evaluating the axial alignment of the heel and tarsals, as can pronation and supination deformities.

The height of the medial longitudinal arch of the foot is described while bearing weight and at rest. When examining the arch, note the pattern of calluses on the sole, as well as the position of the calcaneal region relative to the metatarsus and the position of the metatarsus relative to the forefoot.

Describe the coloration, consistency, size, location, mobility, temperature, and painfulness of any

Fig. 7.**4** Talipes valgus. The photograph shows a child with pes planovalgus. The valgus position of the hindfoot is conspicuous, as is the phenomenon of "too many toes" on the left side. The right foot has already undergone prior surgery.

Fig. 7.**6** Lateral view of pes cavus. The lateral view of Figure 7.**5** demonstrates the pes cavus deformity.

Fig. 7.**5** Podometer view of pes cavus in a child with spina bifida and pes cavus in the left foot. The podometer image shows the different patterns of weight bearing in the right and left feet. Weight distribution is nearly physiologic in the right foot, whereas in the left foot weight is borne solely by the heel and the medial ball of the foot. Secondary findings include hallux valgus in the left foot with a pronounced pronation deformity.

foot or metatarsus can often simulate superior displacement of the heel. Motion analysis will reveal decreased dorsiflexion. This is because the talocalcaneal complex is in dorsiflexion in the ankle to compensate for the pes cavus deformity in the tarsus.

The varus deformity of the hindfoot can be caused by fixed plantar flexion of the great toe because the supination of the forefoot forces the hindfoot into varus in the standing position. The standing-block test evaluates the flexibility of the varus deformity of the hindfoot. Place a block about 1.0–1.5 in thick under the lateral aspect of the foot. A flexible varus deformity of the hindfoot will straighten out as the lateral column is supported and the medial column hangs freely.

Hammer-toe deformities may develop because of the increased activity of the extensors (Figs. 7.**5**, 7.**6**).

Clubfoot

The term "clubfoot" describes a large complex of symptoms encompassing various types of deformities. The talus plays a key part in this deformity. Inspection will reveal superior displacement of the heel with a varus deformity of the hindfoot. A supination deformity of the metatarsus is present, and there is increased adduction of the forefoot.

Untreated clubfoot can be recognized by a typical callus pattern with increased callusing in the laterodorsal cuboid area. Hammer-toe deformities will also frequently develop with this deformity; in contrast to pes cavus, these involve a flexion deformity.

A clubfoot deformity should be described according to the rigidity of its individual components and the degree to which these are correctable (Figs. 7.**7a, b**). To evaluate correction potential, grasp

a   b

Figs. 7.**7a, b**   Infant with idiopathic clubfoot. The two photographs demonstrate the varus deformity of the hindfoot, talipes equinus component, and supination deformity.

the heel between your middle and index fingers while pressing the cuboid with your thumb. This will move the foot into abduction and pronation. At the same time, try to correct the talipes equinus at the calcaneus.

Elasticity can be ascertained by applying moderate traction in the direction of correction.

Preliminary Examination of the Lower Extremity

Examination of the foot includes a preliminary examination of the lower extremity. Evaluate the range of motion in the hip and knee. Determine the angle of femoral anteversion with the patient supine. Evaluate for tibial torsion with the patient supine and the legs dangling from the examination table.

Determine differences in leg length using clinical methods or by radiographic examination.

Axial deviations such as coxa valga, coxa vara, genu valgum, or genu varum are determined by clinical or radiographic examination.

Instability of the knee involving cruciate or collateral ligament deficiency is also important when evaluating foot symptoms and planning appropriate therapy.

Palpation

Palpation is an important part of the clinical examination because complex deformities make it difficult to document many findings in diagnostic imaging studies. Symptoms involving nerves, tendons, joints, bursae, and vascular supply are also accessible to thorough palpation.

Examine the skin for trophic changes and possible infections. Lymphatic swelling can be distinguished from venous swelling since pressure applied

to the dorsum of the foot will leave a temporary depression in venous engorgement. Examine vascular supply to the foot by palpating the dorsalis pedis artery slightly below the anterior aspect of the ankle between the extensor hallucis longus and extensor digitorum longus, and the posterior tibial artery directly posterior to the medial malleolus. Remember that the dorsalis pedis artery may be absent in 10% of the general population due to normal variants in vascular anatomy.

Palpating the posterior tibial artery may be difficult or impossible in patients with large amounts of adipose tissue in the ankles, or with an edema or synovial thickening posterior to the medial malleolus.

If palpation does not reveal the arteries, Doppler studies are indicated. Where signs of occlusive disease of the arteries is present, vascular supply to the lower extremities should be evaluated in Doppler ultrasound studies prior to any invasive procedure. Preoperative angiography is rarely indicated unless vascular surgery is indicated. The appropriate literature should be consulted for further information on vascular diagnostic methods.

The presence of a palpable pulse does not exclude small-vessel disease that occurs with diabetes or arthrosclerotic disease.

The tendons and peritendinous tissue are palpated to detect synovitis and painful degenerative or traumatic changes. The peroneal tendons can be distinguished from each other at the peroneal tubercle of the calcaneus. The peroneus brevis tendon courses superior to the tubercle and the peroneus longus inferior to it.

The flexor hallucis longus tendon can be readily palpated along its plantar course with the great toe in dorsiflexion (see also Fig. 7.**24**). Stenosing synovitis of the flexor hallucis longus tendon will cause symptoms near the posterior process of the talus.

The tibialis anterior and tibialis posterior tendons are best palpated during muscle strength tests.

Examine the Achilles tendon for thickening, swelling, and palpable defects.

Compression neuropathies of the foot can be divided into three groups:

— Superficial neuromas caused by repetitive trauma
— Interdigital neuromas (Morton neuroma)
— Tarsal tunnel syndrome

Compressive neuropathy syndromes require specific palpation according to the anatomy and symptoms. The examination should also include evaluation of the patient's shoes for possible projections, edges, or ridges that may contribute to the compression neuropathy.

The nerves of the dorsum of the foot are particularly exposed, as are the sensory branches of the superficial peroneal nerve, the sural nerve, and the saphenous nerve at the Achilles tendon. Radiating tingling sensations can be elicited by palpating and tapping the nerves.

Interdigital neuromas usually occur between the heads of the third and fourth metatarsals and can simulate metatarsalgia. Applying dorsal and plantar compression with the thumb and index finger elicits characteristic pain and tingling.

Pain can occur along the course of the posterior tibial nerve where it branches into the tarsal tunnel or in the heel region. This pain can be identified by tapping about 1 cm dorsal and inferior of the medial malleolus. Accompanying tenosynovitis that presents as swelling posterior to the medial malleolus may also contribute to the compression syndrome.

Assessing Range of Motion

Instruct the patient to walk on tiptoe, on the heels, and on the medial and lateral borders of the feet. These maneuvers are a rough but effective way of assessing muscle strength in the foot and ankle and demonstrating the range of motion in the ankles and subtalar joints.

If the Achilles tendon is torn, the patient will be unable to walk on tiptoe. Subtalar injuries and symptoms will make walking on the medial borders, and to a greater degree the lateral border, of the feet difficult and painful.

An internally rotated gait may be due to internal tibial torsion or increased femoral anteversion. Normally, the toes and feet are dorsiflexed with each step. A "drop-foot" gait warrants further investigation. A patient simulating a disorder will often exhibit a drop foot or weak extensor hallucis, but then walk with normal dorsiflexion of the foot and toes.

Examine the foot independent of the gait cycle. The patient should sit on the examining table so that the popliteal fossa of each knee is in contact with the table and the feet dangle freely. Sit on a stool directly in front of the patient. Normally the foot will hang in

Fig. 7.**8** Tibialis anterior test. To test the tibialis anterior, stabilize the calf above the ankle with one hand while exerting pressure in plantar flexion and eversion on the dorsum of the foot with the other hand.

slight plantar flexion and inversion. The spastic flatfoot will typically be involuntarily held in dorsiflexion and eversion.

Evaluate the strength of the dorsiflexors, plantar flexors, evertors, and inverters.

Acute tears of the tibialis posterior are rare. Tears in the tibialis anterior tendon can occur suddenly. Neither tendon can be palpated across the ankle. Injuries of the tibialis posterior tendon result in pes valgus and pes planus. The defect can be palpable across the medial navicular tubercle. Chronic degeneration changes in the posterior tibial tendon may have diffuse tenderness to palpation along its entire course.

Evaluation of the range of motion of the ankle, subtalar joint, and toes should take both age and individual variability into consideration.

Examining the Muscles

Tibialis anterior. The patient is seated with the knees flexed. If severe weakness is present, the patient may be placed in a lateral position. Immobilize the distal calf with one hand while exerting pressure in plantar flexion and eversion with the other hand on the dorsomedial aspect of the foot. Instruct the patient to invert the foot and dorsiflex it with the toes and the extensors of the great toe relaxed. It is crucial that the toe extensors be relaxed because they can supplement the tibialis anterior in dorsiflexion. The foot should be in inversion as opposed to a neutral position or eversion to eliminate the action of the extensors and peroneus tertius. A weak tibialis anterior is often accompanied by a talipes equinus deformity. The tibialis anterior can also be tested by having the patient walk on his or her heels with the feet inverted (Fig. 7.**8**).

Tibialis posterior. The patient is in a lateral position lying on the affected side so that the lateral margin of the foot is in contact with the examining table. In the presence of severe weakness, the foot should dangle over the end of the examining table. Immobilize the distal calf with one hand while applying pressure to the medial side of the forefoot to move the foot into

Fig. 7.**9** Tibialis posterior test with muscle weakness. To test the tibialis posterior, have the patient supinate the foot from a lateral position.

Fig. 7.**11** Extensor digitorum longus test. To test the extensor digitorum longus, immobilize the tarsus and apply dorsolateral pressure to the distal small toes.

Fig. 7.**13** Peroneus brevis longus test. To test the peroneus brevis, immobilize the calf slightly proximal to the ankle with one hand while pressing the lateral margin of the foot into adduction and inversion with the other hand.

eversion and abduction and to move the ankle into dorsiflexion. Make sure the toes are in a neutral position and are not actively flexed to eliminate the action of the flexor hallucis longus (Fig. 7.**9**).

Extensor hallucis longus. The patient is seated or supine on the examining table. A lateral position may be used for muscle weakness. Immobilize the tarsus with one hand so that the foot is in the neutral-0 position. Press the great toe on the distal phalanx into plantar flexion with the other hand. Now have the patient dorsiflex the great toe. It is difficult to separate the action of the extensor hallucis brevis from that of the extensor hallucis longus. In paralysis of the extensor hallucis longus, the extensor hallucis brevis will only be able to dorsiflex the proximal phalanx of the great toe. Aside from this, the great toe will be moved slightly toward the second toe (Fig. 7.**10**).

Fig. 7.**10** Extensor hallucis longus test. To test the extensor hallucis longus, immobilize the tarsus and apply dorsal pressure to the distal phalanx of the great toe.

Fig. 7.**12** Extensor digitorum brevis longus test. To test the extensor digitorum brevis, immobilize the tarsus and apply dorsolateral pressure to the proximal phalanges of the small toes.

Extensor digitorum longus. The patient is seated or supine. Immobilize the forefoot in the neutral-0 position with one hand and apply pressure to the dorsum of the four lateral toes with the fingers of the other hand to move the toes into plantar flexion. Then have the patient extend the toes. If isolated muscle weakness is present, each toe can be tested individually (Fig. 7.**11**).

Extensor digitorum brevis and extensor hallucis brevis. The patient is seated or supine. Again, hold the metatarsus in a neutral position with one hand. Apply pressure to the proximal phalanges with the fingers of the other hand, moving them into plantar flexion against the patient's resistance. Instruct the patient to extend the toes (Fig. 7.**12**).

Peroneus brevis. The patient is in a semi-lateral position on the contralateral side with the ankle in the neutral-0 position. Immobilize the distal calf with one hand proximal to the ankle while pressing the lateral margin of the foot into inversion with the other hand. Instruct the patient to evert the foot and the talocalcaneonavicular joint in a neutral position. Make sure that the long extensors are relaxed and the toes are held in slight flexion (Fig. 7.**13**).

Fig. 7.**14** Peroneus longus test. To test the peroneus longus, immobilize the calf slightly proximal to the ankle with one hand, and press the head of the first metatarsal into inversion and the ankle into dorsiflexion with the thumb and index finger.

Fig. 7.**15** Gastrocnemius test II with normal muscle strength. To test the gastrocnemius, have the patient lift the heel off the floor into a tiptoe stance.

Fig. 7.**16** Gastrocnemius test I with muscle weakness. Test the gastrocnemius with the patient supine and the knee extended. Have the patient move the ankle into plantar flexion.

Peroneus longus. The patient is in a semi-lateral position on the contralateral side. The ankle is in plantar flexion. Immobilize the distal calf proximal to the ankle with one hand. At the same time, press with the other hand against the head of the first metatarsal to elevate it, invert the foot, and move the ankle into dorsiflexion. Instruct the patient to evert the foot and bring the head of the first metatarsal into plantar flexion. Make sure that the toe extensors are relaxed for this maneuver (Fig. 7.**14**).

Triceps surae. This test is performed with the patient standing on one leg. Instruct the patient to stand on tiptoe without flexing the knee. The rest results are considered normal when the patient can successfully complete this maneuver ten times. Five successful maneuvers are considered good, one is satisfactory, and inability to achieve full plantar flexion is poor (Fig. 7.**15**).

With normal and poor results, repeat the test without weight bearing. Have the patient lie prone with the knee and ankle in the neutral-0 position. Immobilize the calf with one hand while pressing the posterior portion of the heel into dorsiflexion with the other. Now instruct the patient to move the foot into plantar flexion (Fig. 7.**16**). If the foot is not in the neutral-0 position but inverted, the tibialis posterior can contribute to the movement when the peroneal group is elongated. The same maneuver can be performed with the knee flexed 90° to test the soleus

Fig. 7.**17** Soleus test. To test the soleus, place the knee in flexion to eliminate the action of the gastrocnemius and have the patient move the ankle into plantar flexion.

since the gastrocnemius components are relaxed in this position (Fig. 7.**17**).

The Silverskjöld test has proven effective in distinguishing the gastrocnemius and the soleus in talipes equinus deformities. The patient is supine. Grasp the heel to avoid any deviations in the valgus or varus alignment. If possible, bring the foot into 10°–20° dorsiflexion with the hip and knee flexed. This position eliminates the action of the gastrocnemius so extending the knee will produce an uncorrectable talipes equinus position. This is referred to as a positive gastrocnemius sign.

Fig. 7.**18**   Flexor hallucis longus test. To test the flexor hallucis longus, apply pressure to the distal phalanx of the great toe.

Fig. 7.**19**   Flexor hallucis brevis test. To test the flexor hallucis brevis, apply pressure to the proximal phalanx of the great toe.

Fig. 7.**20**   Flexor digitorum longus test. To test the flexor digitorum longus, apply pressure to the distal phalanges of the small toes.

Fig. 7.**21**   Flexor digitorum brevis test. To test the flexor digitorum brevis, apply pressure to the proximal phalanges of the small toes.

Flexor hallucis longus. The patient is seated or supine. Stabilize the metatarsophalangeal joint with one hand. Hold the proximal phalanx of the great toe in a neutral position with the ankle in 30°–40° plantar flexion. Apply pressure to the distal interphalangeal joint with the other hand, moving it into dorsiflexion. Instruct the patient to flex the distal interphalangeal joint of the great toe. Make sure that the ankle is not completely dorsiflexed because the interphalangeal joint of the great toe flexes passively in dorsiflexion. On the other hand, complete plantar flexion weakens the muscle by moving its origin and insertion closer together (Fig. 7.**18**).

Flexor hallucis brevis. The patient is seated or supine. One hand stabilizes the head of the first metatarsal with the ankle held in plantar flexion to eliminate the action of the flexor hallucis longus. With the other hand, press against the plantar surface of the proximal phalanx of the great toe to dorsiflex it while instructing the patient to flex the toe (Fig. 7.**19**).

Flexor digitorum longus. The patient is seated or supine. One hand immobilizes the proximal and mid-

dle phalanges in a neutral position with the ankle in a neutral position. With the other hand, press against the plantar surface of the distal phalanges of the small toes to dorsiflex them while instructing the patient to flex the distal phalanges.

Because the two heads of the quadratus plantae insert into the lateral, dorsal, and plantar margin of the flexor digitorum tendon, it can contribute, to a certain extent, to flexion in the distal interphalangeal joint (Fig. 7.**20**).

Flexor digitorum brevis. The patient is supine. One hand immobilizes the proximal phalanges with the ankle flexed about 40°. With the other hand, press against the plantar aspect of the middle phalanges to move them into dorsiflexion while instructing the patient to flex the toes (Fig. 7.**21**).

Abductor hallucis. The patient is supine. Holding the foot in a neutral position with one hand, press the great toe toward the small toes with the other while instructing the patient to abduct the great toe.

Abductor digiti quinti. The patient is supine. Hold

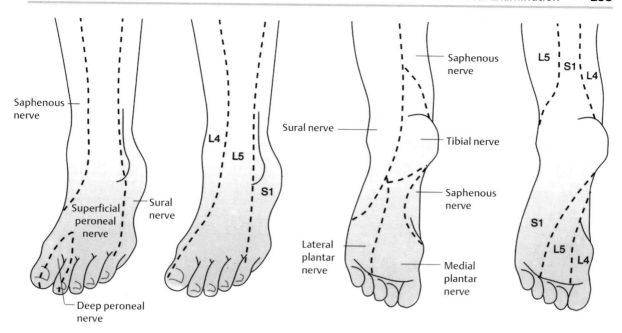

Fig. 7.**22** Sensation in the foot.

the forefoot in the neutral-0 position with one hand. Instruct the patient to abduct the small toe against your resistance as you press with the other hand against the lateral aspect of the small toe to move it into adduction. The dorsal interossei abduct the third and fourth toes. However, the average patient is unable to abduct the small toe.

Adductor hallucis and digitorum. The patient is seated or supine. Abduct the toes and press the great toe medially. Now have the patient move the great toe toward the small toes.

To evaluate the function of the plantar interossei, hold the metatarsals of the third, fourth, and fifth toes in abduction. Instruct the patient to adduct against this resistance.

Lumbrical muscles. The anatomy of these muscles is highly variable in contrast to the lumbricals of the hand, and the muscles may even be missing. For this reason, they are not usually tested.

Neurologic Examination

Preliminary neurologic examination of the foot includes evaluation of the Achilles tendon, tibialis posterior, and patellar tendon reflexes, testing the Babinski reflex, and testing for atrophy in the intrinsic musculature of the foot (see p. 228). Sensation is tested on the lateral and medial margin of the foot and in the first and second web to evaluate the sensory supply of the deep peroneal nerve (Fig. 7.22).

If muscle weakness is present, it is evaluated and documented according to the degree of neurologic strength. Peripheral neuropathies such as are seen in

diabetes, Charcot–Marie–Tooth disease, Friedreich's ataxia, disorders of the spinal cord, tabes dorsalis, and other neurologic disorders are often initially identified in an examination of the foot.

Mild, undiagnosed cerebral palsy occasionally causes spastic flatfoot syndrome in one or both feet. In this case, the spasm can be associated with a positive Babinski reflex.

Specific Examination of Individual Regions of the Foot

Heel and Achilles Tendon

Examine the heel for varus or valgus deviation with the patient standing. Normally the heel will have a strong, uniformly rounded heel pad that may be atrophied in older patients, causing plantar heel pain.

Pain and sensitivity in the anterior portion of the medial tubercle of the calcaneus is a classic finding in heel spur syndrome. Pressure in this anatomic region can elicit pain (Fig. 7.**23**).

Less frequently, these symptoms may be located further posterior in the middle of the plantar aspect of the heel, particularly in association with heel pad atrophy.

Sensitivity in the plantar heel can occur in rheumatoid arthritis. Painful swelling of the heel pad may occur. Laboratory studies and other clinical signs of rheumatoid arthritis will confirm the diagnosis.

As has been mentioned, tenderness 2 cm distal to the medial calcaneal tubercle can be a sign of tenosynovitis of the flexor hallucis longus tendon. With the hallux in extreme passive dorsiflexion, the course of the tendon will be more readily palpable under the

Fig. 7.**23**   Palpation of a heel spur.

Fig. 7.**24**   Palpation of the flexor hallucis longus tendon.

Fig. 7.**25**   Palpation of the plantar fascia.

Fig. 7.**26**   Palpation of the Achilles tendon bursa.

plantar fascia. The pain will be more superficial than in a heel spur syndrome and can be localized distally along the longitudinal arch (Fig. 7.**24**). In distance runners, one should consider plantar fascitis as the more probable caused of the discomfort (Fig. 7.**25**).

Examine the Achilles tendon for shortening or elongation. A torn Achilles tendon, whether spontaneous or chronic, usually results in elongation. Significant pain will not necessarily be present, although the patient will usually be unable to stand on tiptoe. Soft swelling in the region of the Achilles tendon will confirm the diagnosis. In contrast, soft-tissue swelling in the bursa of the Achilles tendon usually suggests bursitis. This should be distinguished from synovial thickening of the posterior ankle (Fig. 7.**26**).

Subtalar Joint

Diagnosis and treatment of disorders of the subtalar joint are difficult and time-consuming. With injuries and diseases of the subtalar joint, the patient will frequently have a history of pain anterior and distal to the lateral malleolus. The range of motion of the talocalcaneonavicular joint should be evaluated in inver-

Fig. 7.**27** Palpation of the tarsal sinus.

sion and eversion according to the axis of motion. Grasp the heel with one hand and the forefoot with the other to evaluate range of motion. This grip technique is also used to evaluate the range of motion in the talocalcaneal joint and in the Chopart joint.

Normally, motion in the subtalar joint is uniform and painless.

Painless limitations of motion are usually encountered in older patients. Limited motion associated with pain may be a sign of a subtalar disorder. Often these limitations of motion are associated with tenderness to palpation over the tarsal sinus, inferior and anterior to the lateral malleolus (Fig. 7.27).

Subtalar symptoms can be cause by tarsal coalitions, rheumatoid arthritis, cerebral palsy, posttraumatic arthritis following fractures of the talus or calcaneus, Sudeck atrophy following ankle injuries, arthrofibrosis, prolonged immobilization in a plaster cast or traction through the calcaneus, and degenerative disorders in severe chronic pes planovalgus. However, the cause of these disorders often remains unclear. Abnormal subtalar findings are frequently overlooked.

Longitudinal Arch

Often the longitudinal arch is flat in children but can reach normal height by puberty. The small cushion of fat above the longitudinal arch combined with the natural flexibility of the foot in children, which tends to flatten when bearing weight, will make the longitudinal arch appear flatter than it actually is.

Pes planus with normal subtalar mobility is a normal finding and does not require special shoes or inserts. On the other hand, pes planus can influence the normal subtalar mobility and biomechanics, and

can be the presenting feature in a congenital vertical talus. Usually, further examination of pes planus in children is only necessary when range of motion is limited or other conditions such as poliomyelitis or cerebral palsy are present.

The lack test describes the rise in the longitudinal arch when the great toe is dorsiflexed in the presence of flexible pes planus.

Tarsals

One of the most common diseases of the tarsus is osteoarthritis, which is observed most frequently in older obese people. Involvement of one or more tarsal joints manifests itself as typical localized joint pain, tenderness to palpation, and possibly palpable osteophytes.

Charcot–Marie–Tooth disease of the foot usually begins in the tarsal region with palpable bone thickening. Pain is relatively slight in comparison to the palpable findings. Solid, rounded, and hard ganglia will occasionally be palpable in the tarsals and may be mistaken for bony exostoses. These ganglia typically increase or decrease in size and can be drained by aspiration. The aspirate will be the typical gelatinous fluid of a ganglion.

Metatarsals and Transverse Arch of the Foot

Metatarsalgia is a frequent foot symptom in women. Pain in the region of the metatarsal heads is usually described as burning. Generally there will be local pain directly under the heads of the metatarsals, usually at the second metatarsal.

Normally the anterior transverse arch describes a convex dorsal arc that flattens out with weight bearing. This occurs due to dorsoplantar play in the shafts of the first, fourth, and especially the fifth metatarsals. The second and third metatarsals are rigid in comparison. Plantar keratosis under the second, third, and fourth metatarsal heads is usually pathologic.

In many cases, the anterior transverse arch describes a rigid dorsal concave arc, especially in splayfoot syndrome. This causes calluses under the second, third, and sometimes fourth metatarsal heads.

Any shortening of the metatarsal shaft, particularly of the first metatarsal, or dorsal displacement of the distal portion of the metatarsal increases the stress on the other metatarsal heads. Plantar flexed toes normally reduce the weight load on the metatarsal heads, whereas hammer toes increase the load. Pain under a metatarsal head adjacent to a healed metatarsal fracture or osteotomy is referred to as a transfer lesion.

Any cavus deformity, talipes equinus, or superior displacement of the heel increases the load on the metatarsal heads. Hallux valgus can produce increased callusing under the second metatarsal head due to the metatarsus varus.

Fig. 7.**28**   Characteristic pain is elicited by compressing the interdigital space with the thumb and index finger in the presence of a Morton neuroma.

Fig. 7.**29**   Palpation of the bunion at the medial metatarsophalangeal joint in hallux valgus.

Fixed dorsal deviation of one or more of the metatarsal heads is usually seen in rheumatoid arthritis and is exacerbated by the associated hammer toe deformities and the atrophy of the plantar fat cushion. Occasionally there will be a slight depression proximal to the metatarsal heads. Normal elasticity of the plantar fat cushion can usually be verified by applying moderate pressure with the fingertips. In some disorders only a slight depression will appear despite a well-developed fat cushion, whereas finger pressure against a thin fat cushion will produce increased elasticity or even form a depression.

Plantar hyperkeratoses frequently develop in the region of the metatarsal heads as a sequela to scarring, superficial retention of foreign bodies, or plantar warts. They are often found in the vicinity of the metatarsal heads as opposed to directly beneath them. Sometimes plantar warts can simulate skin calluses but they can also rapid development of projecting calluses. Removing the hyperkeratosis exposes the plantar wart beneath it, which can be multilocular. One identifying characteristic of plantar warts is that direct pressure will only cause slight pain, while indirect compression can cause acute pain.

Painful rubbery edema on the dorsal aspect of a metatarsal is frequently a sign of a stress fracture.

Another clinical syndrome encountered in the forefoot is Morton neuroma, usually seen between the third and fourth interdigital space. Pain will typically occur when the metatarsal heads are subjected to transverse compression and during simultaneous dorsal and plantar palpation of the interdigital spaces with the thumb and index finger. Patients will feel tingling pain (Fig. 7.**28**). Injection of local anesthetic through the intermetatarsal ligament can confirm the diagnosis by anesthetizing this neuroma.

Great Toe

Disorders that involve the great toe include ingrown toenails, hallux valgus, hallux rigidus, and bursitis.

In hallux rigidus, evaluate the severity of the deformity and the degree to which it is passively correctable. As mentioned in the preceding section, first determine whether proximal pathology such as pes planus is responsible for the hallux valgus deformity. Determine if the disorder is metatarsus varus, or is in the metacarpophalangeal or interphalangeal joint.

Also document any pronation deformities of the great toe (Fig. 7.**29**).

Lesser Toes

The most frequent deformity of the lesser toes is hammer toe. A combination of hallux valgus, bursitis, and several hammer toes is a sign of rheumatoid arthritis. Findings of uncommonly rigid lesser toes, or associated rheumatoid involvement of the subtalar joint, support this tentative diagnosis; radiographic and laboratory studies can confirm this. Other peripheral joints will not necessarily be affected in rheumatoid arthritis. However, concurrent involvement is most frequently encountered in the wrists.

Describe the type of hammer toe deformity. An isolated hammer toe, frequently the second toe, will usually be congenital and will appear flexible, semiflexible, or rigid. The metatarsophalangeal joint can be in extension while the proximal or distal interphalangeal joint can be in flexion. Attempting to reduce the deformity to a neutral position will reveal whether the severity of the contracture involves only the flexor and extensor tendon, or to what extent associated capsular contractures may be present that produce rigidity in the soft tissue including the collateral ligaments and lumbricals. Palpable subluxation or dislocation can be present in severe cases. Usually, the metatarsophalangeal joints are involved.

Precise diagnosis of the individual deformity is crucial to effective conservative therapy; it is important to evaluate the patient's specific hammer toe deformity.

Tenderness in the region of the toe extensors, including the extensor hallucis longus, is exacerbated when the foot is in plantar flexion and alleviated when the ankle is dorsiflexed. The contracted extensors are most easily palpated over the dorsal aspects of the metatarsophalangeal joints with the toes slightly flexed. However, flexing the toes completely flattens out the tendons over the bone so that they are no longer palpable. Tightening a tourniquet over the ankle can be helpful in evaluating the deformity because the resulting ischemia can produce involuntary extension spasm in the toe extensors, which will recede when the tourniquet is loosened.

Evaluate the interdigital spaces of the toes for fungus and chronic eczema, which can coexist. The fifth toe can exhibit callusing on its laterodorsal aspect. This will often be found with splayfoot deformities. The lateral calluses are due to pressure from the shoe. The fifth toe presses against the base of the fourth toe and can produce a corn in the interdigital space.

Any ulceration, infection, or swelling beneath, or in the region of a soft corn is a sign of disturbed vascular supply or drainage and is frequently associated with diabetes mellitus.

Congenital hammer toes should be distinguished from acquired deformities because they are treated completely differently. A congenital hammer fifth toe will flatten out in comparison to the fourth toe and does not normally produce significant symptoms. In contrast, an acquired hammer toe usually causes symptoms that require treatment.

Exostosis of the lateral aspect of the fifth metatarsal head is frequently associated with a broad forefoot and with splayfoot syndrome.

Other rare toe deformities include polydactyly and syndactyly.

Sole

Any excessive pressure or friction in the skin of the sole will cause ulceration or increased callusing, consisting mainly of hypertrophy of the stratum corneum. Proper evaluation of stresses in the sole requires examination of the foot while it is bearing weight. Clinical inspection, palpation, and functional examination of the foot are supplemented by methods such as barographs, gait analyses, and electromyographic studies.

Foreign-body granulomas are frequently found in the sole, although the patient may not remember any injury. Deep wood splinters in the sole can migrate slowly dorsally, and frequently cannot be reliably demonstrated in radiographic studies.

7.3 Radiology

Indications, Diagnostic Value, and Clinical Relevance

The anterior to posterior (dorsal to plantar) view does not adequately image all areas of the foot due to the varying thickness of the forefoot and hindfoot in the dorsoplantar projection. When radiographs of the foot are requested, the exposure technique is normally chosen according to the thickness of the tarsals so that the toes are overexposed. Routine lateral radiographs of the foot are generally not very helpful because overlapping shadows in the metatarsals, toes, talocalcaneonavicular joint, and tarsals limit the amount of useful information.

The forefoot is distorted in lateral radiographs of the ankle. However, the lateral and medial articular surfaces of the talus in the ankle do not appear parallel to each other in normal lateral radiographs. Special views are required for specific lines of inquiry, such as the tangential sesamoid view in hallux valgus.

Frequently, radiographic examination alone is insufficient to identify a cause for the presenting symptoms. However, radiographic studies are especially important for preoperative planning. Routine foot radiographs occasionally reveal unexpected, previously asymptomatic pathology such as a calcaneocuboid coalition.

In studies of the hindfoot, the calcaneus is best imaged in the lateral and tangential calcaneus projection. This projection reveals sagittal fractures of the calcaneus and talocalcaneal coalitions. The subtalar joint is best imaged in the direct lateral view. However, if the articular surface is rotated, as can occur in a severe valgus deformity or spastic flatfoot, the articulating members will overlap in the projection and the central ray will not enter the joint parallel to the articular surfaces. Visualization of the joint can be improved by changing the position of the foot or the axis of projection. The anterior, middle, and posterior joint facet of the subtalar joint is best demonstrated in special oblique and axial views. However, these views are not part of the routine examination. Many views have also been described for the various tarsal bones. With the advent of CT, many of the older special views of the hindfoot have fallen out of use.

The routine medial oblique view of the foot is best for revealing calcaneonavicular coalitions, fractures of the superior portion of the anterior process of the calcaneus, a secondary calcaneus, or a fracture of the lateral talus. One of the most important views of the hindfoot is the dorsoplantar projection. It can demonstrate structures in the region of the calcaneus, cuboid, and talus.

The weight-bearing and non-weight-bearing dorsoplantar view is recommended for diagnosing the severity of a splayfoot. Splayfoot and metatarsus varus are usually more pronounced in a weight-bearing stance.

Oblique views of the forefoot can demonstrate the toes and metatarsals more clearly than the lateral view. The medial oblique view is preferable to the lateral oblique view because the first metatarsal tends to appear in the middle of the image where it can obscure possible abnormal findings.

Radiographs of the toes should be precisely planned.

Dorsoplantar views demonstrate the metatarsophalangeal joints well, but not the phalangeal joints of hammer toes. Subluxations and dislocations of the metatarsophalangeal joints can be visualized in the dorsoplantar projection. Lateral views are unsatisfactory for imaging toe deformities because the toes overlap. One possible technique for obtaining a useful radiograph is to place a small dental film between the toes. Alternatively, oblique radiographs should be obtained.

A tangential sesamoid view should be obtained to evaluate joint congruity and degenerative processes in hallux valgus. The patient may be positioned sitting or supine and can extend the toes while holding the foot in 20°–30° plantar flexion with a bandage or strap.

A radiopaque marker can be placed on the center of a corn prior to the examination to aid in detecting bony projections or foreign bodies under corns or calluses in the forefoot or toes. This technique makes it possible to precisely determine the bony landmarks for the subsequent surgical procedure.

Radiographs obtained with the patient standing are helpful for demonstrating static deformities. Standard views yield results that are more easily comparable.

Standard Views

Radiographs of the foot and ankle are no substitute for careful clinical examination; radiographic studies should be obtained only after thorough clinical examination. Routine foot radiographs include the following views:

— AP view
— Lateral view
— Dorsoplantar view
— Oblique view

Standardized views are necessary to evaluate the foot in a neutral position. The skeletal configuration of the foot may be described using a number of different measuring angles. However, many authors prefer to use the contours of individual bones of the foot as the basis of analysis.

AP View of the Ankle

The exposure technique is described on page 229, Chapter 6.

The articular surfaces of the malleoli are nearly vertical. In the AP projection there is almost no overlapping of bony structures in the ankle, with the exception of the lateral portion of the tibial pilon and the distal fibular metaphysis. The tangents lateral and medial to the foot form a truncated pyramid. If the standard AP view includes the sole, the bed of the sesamoid beneath the first metatarsal can also be visualized.

Lateral View of the Foot

The foot is in a neutral position with the fibula in contact with the film cassette. The central ray is directly perpendicular and aimed at the tarsus. This view documents the talus and calcaneus. However, there is some overlapping in the tarsus, metatarsals, and phalanges.

In the weight-bearing lateral view, the patient stands with the lateral aspect of the foot against the cassette, with the foot and calf in a neutral-0 position. The contralateral foot must be placed in front of or behind the affected foot to avoid overlapping. The central ray enters at a right angle to the medial aspect of the tarsus and the cassette.

The posterior fibular cortex is immediately anterior to the posterior margin of the tibia.

Dorsoplantar View of the Foot

The patient is supine with the knee flexed and the sole fixed against the cassette. The central ray is vertical and directed at the base of the first metatarsal.

For the weight-bearing view, the patient stands on the film cassette. The central ray is at a right angle to the metatarsals and aimed between both feet by tilting the tube anteriorly 15°. This tilt is necessary to avoid overlap.

This projection demonstrates portions of the tarsus and the forefoot in particular. It provides an overview of the foot, showing bone relationships, contours, and structures, and articulating members. Tangents to the medial and lateral aspects of the tarsus and the metatarsals should be continuous from posterior to anterior, diverging anteriorly. Seventy-five percent of the talar head normally articulates with the navicular. Lisfranc's joint between the tarsals and metatarsals is visualized, as is Chopart's joint between the talus and navicular, and calcaneus and cuboid.

Tangents through the cortex of the first and fifth metatarsals diverge toward the toes. Lines through the middle axis of the talus and calcaneus diverge at an angle of about 30°. The entire head of the talus is covered by the navicular.

Oblique View of the Foot

The plantar aspect of the foot is against the cassette with the lateral aspect raised. The angle for the oblique view is usually 45° to the plantar surface of the foot. To achieve better standardization, a 45° wedge of radiolucent material can be placed beneath the lateral side of the foot.

The central ray is aimed directly at the sinus tarsi. This view is particularly suitable for demonstrating the anterior portion of the subtalar joint, calcaneus, and cuboid; the talonavicular, naviculocuneiform, and calcaneonavicular joints; and the lateral cuneiforms and lateral metatarsals.

This view is particularly helpful in demonstrating avulsion fractures of bifurcate ligaments occurring in the dorsomedial aspect of the anterior process of the calcaneus.

Special Views

Dorsoplantar View of the Toes

The patient is seated on the examining table with the hip and knee flexed so that the sole of the forefoot lies flat on the cassette; the cassette is raised 15° on the toe side. The central ray is aimed perpendicular to the proximal phalanx of the third toe. This projection should allow unobscured visualization of all joints, including the metatarsophalangeal joints.

Lateral View of the Toes

The patient is in a lateral position so that the medial margin of the foot or the great toe is in contact with the cassette in a true lateral projection. The fourth and fifth toes are plantar flexed with a strap. The central ray is aimed perpendicular to the proximal phalanx of the third toe, passing through the foot lateromedially. The great toe, including the metatarsophalangeal joint, should be visualized in a true lateral projection.

Tangential View of the Sesamoid

The patient is seated on the examining table with the hip and knee flexed and the ankle in slight plantar flexion. The patient holds the great toe in maximum dorsiflexion with a strap so that the central ray can enter the metatarsosesamoid joint space. This view is useful for evaluating joint congruity, degenerative changes, and fragmentation.

Spot Views of the Subtalar Joint

Oblique views in internal rotation are obtained to supplement standard views and to aid in evaluating processes in the talocalcaneonavicular joint and calcaneus. The patient is supine with the knees extended, the ankle in a neutral position, and the calf internally rotated 45°. The central ray is angled 15° craniocaudally and enters directly distal to the lateral malleolus.

In this position, the talocalcaneonavicular joint and calcaneus are well visualized with minimal overlapping.

The view in 45° internal rotation is also referred to as the Broden projection.

Alternatively, the view of the talocalcaneonavicular joint can be obtained as an oblique supine view in external rotation.

The patient and X-ray tube are positioned as described, except that the calf is externally rotated 45° and the central ray is aimed at a point distal to the tip of the medial malleolus. This view visualizes the talocalcaneonavicular joint including the calcaneal sulcus.

In the Isherwood view, the patient sits on the examining table with the foot and calf internally rotated and the medial side of the foot angled 30° from horizontal. The foot is inverted in plantar flexion, and the central ray is aimed 2.5 cm distal and anterior to the lateral malleolus and angled 10° cranially. The sustentaculum talus and the middle facet of the subtalar joint are clearly visualized in this view, as is the sinus tarsi.

Anterior Tangential View

The patient stands on the film cassette, as for the dorsoplantar view, with the foot at a right angle to the calf. The X-ray tube is tilted 45° to horizontal in front of the patient and aimed at the level of the distal malleoli. This view clearly visualizes the talonavicular joint. The position of the sustentaculum talus is also visible; it appears as an oval, radiopaque area on the medial side of the calcaneus. In a normal foot, the sustentaculum will extend to the medial cortex of the talus.

In a clubfoot deformity, the sustentaculum of the talus is rotated under the medial talar cortex and talar neck.

In a flatfoot deformity, the head and neck of the talus will be visible medially next to the sustentaculum of the talus.

Posterior Tangential View

The patient stands with the sole of the foot on the cassette. The X-ray tube is behind the patient, angled 45° to horizontal, with the central ray aimed at the ends of the malleoli. This technique provides good exposure of the posterior portion of the calcaneus and the posterior and middle facets of the subtalar joint. However, the 45° setting represents an empirical value. To determine the precise angle to horizontal, the inclination of the posterior facet is measured on the standard lateral radiograph. This angle is then used as the tilt angle of the X-ray tube. This view is also helpful for detecting talocalcaneal coalitions. Angling the X-ray tube 45° provides a good reproduc-

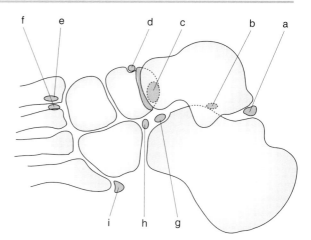

Fig. 7.**31**   Schematic diagram of the most frequent accessory bones in the foot as seen in a lateral view. For key, see Figure 7.**30**.

Fig. 7.**30**   Schematic diagram of the most frequent accessory bones in the foot as seen in a dorsoplantar view. **a** Os trigonum, **b** os subtibiale, **c** os tibiale externum, **d** os supranaviculare, **e** os intermetatarseum, **f** pars peronea metatarsalia, **g** calcareus secundarium, **h** processus uncinatus, **i** os peroneum

ible overview for describing contours and deformities. Exposure of the middle and posterior joint facets can be improved by increasing and decreasing the imaging angle. This is helpful in evaluating deformities in the subtalar joint.

Stress Views

The primary purpose of stress views is to evaluate ankle injuries. See the relevant section in the ankle chapter for a discussion of this topic.

Sesamoid and Accessory Bones

There two types of bones in a normal foot that are separate from the main structure of the foot. These are the sesamoid and the accessory bones.

Sesamoid

Sesamoid bones are found in tendons, over bony prominences, or in locations at which tendons change direction. They are embedded in the substance of the tendon, and one surface forms a kind of joint with the respective adjacent bone. The sesamoids glide with the tendons. In the foot, they are located immediately beneath the plantar surface. Usually there are two sesamoid bones beneath the head of the first metatarsal.

Less frequently, individual sesamoid bones are found beneath the heads of the second, third, and

fourth metatarsals. Very rarely, two sesamoid bones will be seen beneath the head of the fifth metatarsal and on the plantar aspect of the interphalangeal joints. It is also rare to find sesamoid bones beneath the head of every metatarsal.

Sometimes a sesamoid bone will be found in the peroneus longus tendon. This bone will then appear at the transition to the cuboid where the tendon enters the sole of the foot. Another frequent location is in the tibialis posterior tendon at the navicular tuberosity. This must not be confused with an accessory navicular.

Sesamoid bones are also subject to degenerative changes and often cause pain. Like the patella, they can have bipartite and multipartite morphologic anomalies. These are usually found near the head of the first metatarsal and must not be confused with fractures.

Usually bipartite sesamoids are larger than their "twin" on the contralateral side.

Accessory Bones

Accessory bones are located in the tarsus and are evaluated separately from normal bones. Tendons or ligaments can insert into accessory bones, but, unlike sesamoids, accessory bones will not glide with movement of the tendon. The consensus is that accessory bones form as secondary ossification centers of normal bones. As a rule they are asymptomatic; they should not be confused with fractures.

There are many accessory bones, the most frequently encountered ones being (Figs. 7.**30** and 7.**31**):

— **Os trigonum.** This bone varies in size and is located at the posterior process of the talus. The tendon of the flexor hallucis longus courses through a groove in the os trigonum. The tibiotalar and posterior talofibular ligaments and the posterior portion of the capsule of the ankle and talocalcaneonavicular joint insert at this process. This bone can persist throughout the life of the individual and is found in 10% of the population.

— **Os sustentaculi.** This is a small pyramidal bone on the posterior and medial aspect of the sustentaculum talus.

— **Os tibiale externum or accessory navicular.** This ossicle is located at the medial navicular tuberosity and is not connected to the rest of the navicular. Even when the tibialis posterior tendon inserts there, it is not considered a sesamoid bone.

However, a sesamoid bone within the substance of this tendon is described separately. Frequently the os tibiale externum is bilateral (Fig. 7.**32**).

— **Os supranaviculare.** This small triangular ossicle is found at the dorsal navicular joint and must be distinguished from possible fractures of osteoarthritic projections.

— **Pars peronaea metatarsalis primi.** This ossicle is a separated peroneal tubercle on the proximal end of the first metatarsal where the peroneus longus tendon inserts.

— **Os intermetatarseum.** This isolated ossicle is occasionally found between the proximal ends of the bases of the first and second metatarsals.

— **Secondary calcaneus.** This ossicle appears as a prominence at the dorsal distal end of the calcaneus. It articulates with the cuboid and the navicular.

— **Secondary cuboid.** This ossicle may be somewhat larger. It is located on the plantar tibial aspect of the cuboid and articulates with the navicular and possibly with the anterior process of the calcaneus.

— **Os vesalianum.** This ossicle is a part of the tubercle on the base of the fifth metatarsal. The peroneus brevis tendon inserts at this location.

Radiologic Foot Analysis

Radiologic evaluation of the foot provides the physician with insight into structural abnormalities and changes caused by local or systemic disorders. Non-weight-bearing radiographs should be used to evaluate congenital abnormalities, neoplasms, infections, metabolic diseases, or injuries. Weight-bearing films demonstrate functional abnormalities.

A number of angles and lines have been mentioned in the literature for describing various deformities in standard radiographs. Measuring the foot according to these radiographic parameters is intended to permit a more accurate description of the deformity. The reproducibility of these measured values depends on standardization of radiographic posi-

Fig. 7.**32** Dorsoplantar view of an accessory navicular with a medial bipartite sesamoid.

tioning. Since absolute standardization is not possible, these measured values must be regarded in conjunction with clinical findings. Despite these shortcomings, descriptions of foot morphology using angles and lines are a valuable aid in the diagnosis and treatment of foot disorders.

Analysis in the AP Projection

● **Linear measurements**
Length of the distal and proximal phalanges of the hallux. The length of the phalanges of the hallux is important for detecting deformities of the forefoot. The distance between the proximal and distal end of the bone is measured in millimeters. The length of the distal phalanx ranges between 19 and 28 mm in an adult foot, the proximal phalanx between 21 and 35 mm. This measurement provides information about mechanical and cosmetic aspects.

Relative length of the toes. The relationship between the distal limit of the hallux and the small toes allows classification of the structural configuration of the forefoot. The comparison of the length of the small

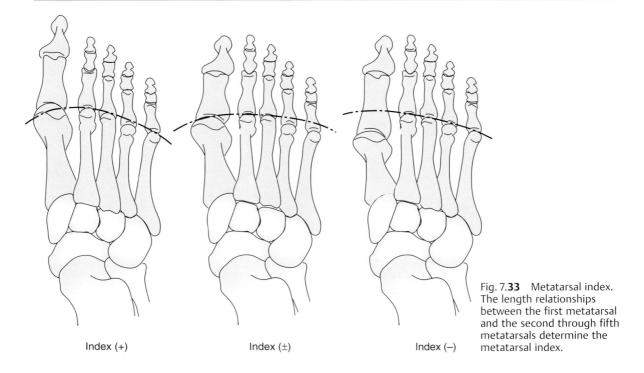

Index (+)   Index (±)   Index (−)

Fig. 7.**33** Metatarsal index. The length relationships between the first metatarsal and the second through fifth metatarsals determine the metatarsal index.

toes with the length of the hallux falls into one of three basic groups. The most frequent configuration is the so-called Egyptian form in which the hallux is the longest toe. The small toes become progressively shorter moving from medial to lateral.

In what is known as the Greek foot, the great toe is shorter than the second toe. In the square foot, the great toe is the same length as the second toe. These various foot configurations are associated in the literature with various forefoot deformities. The foot configuration is important when planning surgical correction of forefoot deformities.

Absolute and relative length of the metatarsals. The absolute length of each metatarsal can be quantified by measuring the longitudinal axis of each bone from its proximal to distal endpoints. Of greater clinical significance than the absolute length is the relationship between the distal ends of the metatarsals. To determine the relative metatarsal length, draw a uniform arc across the ends of the second through fifth metatarsals. If the head of the first metatarsal is distal to this arc, the configuration is referred to as a plus index. If the distal limit of the first metatarsal head touches the arc, the configuration is referred to as a plus-minus index. If the first metatarsal head is significantly proximal to the arc, one refers to a minus index.

This evaluation is significant in that a minus index combined with an Egyptian forefoot tends to result in a hallux valgus and metatarsalgia due to increased stress on the second and third metatarsal heads (Fig. 7.**33**).

In the United States, four other methods of describing the relative length of the first and second metatarsals are used (Figs. 7.**34 a–d**).

Morton method. In the Morton method, lines are drawn perpendicular to the longitudinal axis of the second metatarsal at the distal margin of the first and second metatarsals, and the difference is defined as the distance between the lines. However, these results can be distorted by a valgus or varus deformity of the first digit.

Harris and Beath method. This method uses the posterior end of the calcaneus as the center of a circle around which an arc is drawn through the distal margin of the first metatarsal. The respective distal limits of the second through fifth metatarsals are compared with this arc. This method can only be used on radiographs that also visualize the posterior portion of the calcaneus.

Stokes method. This method compares the absolute lengths of the first two metatarsals. The weaknesses of this method are that the proximal limit of the first metatarsal varies and is not that important for weight bearing in the region of the metatarsal heads.

Hardy and Clapham method. This method is widely used. The center of an arc is placed in the center of the talus, similar to the Harris and Beath method, and an arc is drawn through the distal portions of the first and second metatarsal heads. The distance between

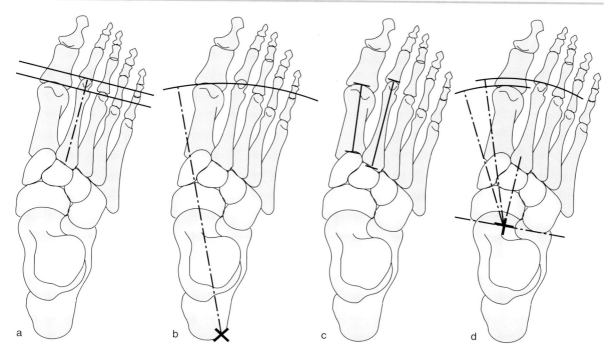

Figs. 7.**34a–d** Alternative methods of determining metatarsal relationships. (**a**) Morton method. (**b**) Harris and Beath method. (**c**) Stokes method. (**d**) Hardy and Clapham method.

these two arcs is the measurement of the distance between the two bones.

Measuring forefoot width. This parameter describes the distance between the medial aspect of the head of the first metatarsal and the lateral aspect of the head of the fifth metatarsal. A normal width is between 71 and 90 mm.

Another method consists of drawing two lines parallel to the anatomic axis of the foot. One line is tangent to the most medial part of the head of the first metatarsal, while the other line is tangent to the most lateral part of the head of the fifth metatarsal. The distance between both straight lines is a measure of the width of the forefoot and, accordingly, of a splayfoot deformity as well.

Steel's measurement of hindfoot width. Hindfoot width is measured similarly to forefoot width with two straight lines drawn parallel to the longitudinal axis of the foot through the most medial part of the talus and the most lateral part of the calcaneus. The values of this measurement range from 40–50 mm. This parameter has proven valuable in evaluating calcaneus fractures.

Measurement of the position of the first metatarsophalangeal joint. Subluxation and deviations in the first metatarsophalangeal joint are seen especially in hallux valgus. The extent of the hallux valgus deformity is determined by deviations in this joint in particular. Subluxation is measured by drawing two lines parallel to the longitudinal axis of the second metatarsal through the lateral articular portion of the proximal phalanx and the head of the metatarsal. The distance between both lines is measured in millimeters. First-degree subluxation is described as a distance of 2 mm or less, and second-degree subluxation as more than 2 mm.

Measurement of the excursion of the first medial exostosis. In hallux valgus the prominence of the medial exostosis is determined by measuring the distance between two parallels. The first is drawn tangential to the medial diaphyseal cortex, and the second is drawn through the point representing the farthest medial distance to the exostosis. The distance is specified in millimeters (Fig. 7.**35**).

Harris and Beath's measurement of the overlap of the talus and calcaneus. Harris and Beath described this parameter for quantifying pes planus deformities. They cite the loss of talocalcaneal overlap as an index for the weak support of the talar head by the calcaneus in the dorsoplantar view. The first step in quantifying the overlap is to measure the distance between two parallel lines. The first line is drawn through the lateral margin of the talus, and the second through the medial margin of the calcaneus. The second step involves establishing the relationship between the overlap and the diameter of the talar head.

Fig. 7.**35**   Metatarsophalangeal joint subluxation. (**A**) measurement of subluxation in the metatarsophalangeal joint. (**B**) measurement of the projection of the medial metatarsal eminence.

Measurement of the calcaneonavicular ligament. Approximate estimation of the length of the calcaneonavicular ligament should be possible by measuring the distance between two perpendiculars to the longitudinal axis, one drawn through the anterior margin of the sustentaculum tali and the other through the proximal articular margin of the navicular. The authors describing this method maintain that this distance is comparable to the length of the calcaneonavicular ligament.

Measurement of the distance between the sustentaculum talus and the anterior aspect of the calcaneus. This also involves measuring the distance between two perpendiculars to the longitudinal axis of the talus in millimeters. The first line is drawn anterior to the sustentaculum talus and the second line at the most anterior margin of the anterior process of the calcaneus. This measurement is used in evaluating pes planus deformities.

Measurement of the projection of the talar head and the anterior aspect of the calcaneus. The first line is drawn at the most anterior portion of the calcaneus as described above, and a second line is drawn at the most anterior portion of the talus. The distance between these lines is intended to represent the hyperpronation of the fund.

Measurement of the sesamoid position. To quantify the proximal displacement of the sesamoids, two

Fig. 7.**36**   Measurement of sesamoid subluxation in the dorsoplantar view. **1** Distance between the lateral sesamoid and the lateral cortex of the head of the first metatarsal. **2** Relationship of the medial sesamoid to the longitudinal axis of the first metatarsal.

lines are drawn parallel to the longitudinal axis of the first metatarsal. The first line divides the sesamoid into two equal parts, the second line is tangent to the convexity of the head of the first metatarsal. The distance is specified in millimeters.

The lateral displacement of the sesamoids, especially in a hallux valgus deformity, is viewed in relation to the middle longitudinal axis of the first metatarsal. The position of the medial sesamoid relative to this axis is specified in four degrees of dislocation (Fig. 7.**36**).

Dimension of the talonavicular joint. This dimension can be measured with the foot in pronation. Determine the midpoint of the articular surface of the talar head and the proximal articular surface of the navicular. The distance between these two points is measured in millimeters. Normal values are specified as 6–7 mm. Higher values are a sign of hyperpronation.

● **Axes of the foot**
Anatomical axis of the foot (Fig. 7.**37**). This is defined as a line through the center of the head of the second metatarsal and the midpoint of the posterior tubercle of the calcaneus. This line can be used as a landmark for other parameters. It has proven neutral in describing morphology of the forefoot and hindfoot.

A transverse line is drawn from the medial aspect of the talonavicular joint to the lateral aspect of the calcaneocuboid joint. Normally, the anatomic axis divides this line into two equal segments. A decrease in one or the other is a sign of increased supination or pronation of the forefoot.

Fig. 7.**37** Axes of the foot in the dorsoplantar view.
AB: anatomical axis.

EF: transverse naviculocuboid line to describe the position of the forefoot and hindfoot.

BCD: triangular weight-bearing area of the foot obtained by connecting the centers of the heads of the first and fifth metatarsals and the tubercle of the calcaneus.

GH: transmalleolar line. Together with line **CD**, this can be used to determine deviations in the horizontal plane.

Fig. 7.**38** Mechanical axes of the foot in the dorsoplantar view. The midline of the foot (**A**) forms a 15° angle with the longitudinal axis of the talus and is parallel to the lateral margin of the foot (**C**). The midline divides the sinusoidal articular line of Chopart's joint into two approximately equal segments and forms a right angle with the transverse axis of the navicular (**E**).

Mechanical axis of the foot. According to the literature, the mechanical axis should run through the middle of the first metatarsal.

The weight-bearing platform of the foot is defined as a triangle. The mechanical axis forms the first side, the axis through the center of the head of the fifth metatarsal and the center of the tubercle of the calcaneus forms the second side, and the line connecting the heads of the first and fifth metatarsal forms the third side. These bony landmarks are helpful in describing structural abnormalities in the foot.

The connecting line between the heads of the first and second metatarsals should normally be parallel to a line connecting the lateral and medial malleoli. Increased lateral convergence suggests increased abduction of the fund; increased medial convergence suggests increased adduction.

The midline of the foot. This extends from the center of the calcaneus to the medial aspect of the head of the third metatarsal (Fig. 7.38). The line forms an angle of 15° to the longitudinal axis of the talus or the first metatarsal and is parallel to the margin of the foot. The midline intersects the articular margin of

the talonavicular joint, appearing as a sinusoidal curve, and passes through the calcaneocuboid joint. This line is also perpendicular to the transverse axis of the navicular.

● **Measuring angles in the foot.**

Interphalangeal angle (Figs. 7.**39**). This angle is used to evaluate interphalangeal hallux valgus. The longitudinal axes of the proximal and distal phalanx form an angle that should normally be less than 5°.

Metatarsophalangeal angle (Fig. 7.**40**). Also referred to as the hallux valgus angle, this angle quantifies a significant aspect of this deformity. The angle is formed by the longitudinal axes of the first metatarsal and the proximal phalanx of the first digit. An angle of 15° is regarded as normal; angles exceeding 15° indicate a hallux valgus deformity.

Angle of incongruity in the metatarsophalangeal joint. To determine incongruity in the metatarsophalangeal joint, the tangent is drawn at the base of the proximal phalanx of the first digit, and a line is drawn through the medial and lateral osteochondral margin

Fig. 7.**39**   The interphalangeal angle is determined by the longitudinal axes of the proximal and distal phalanx.

Fig. 7.**40**   Hallux valgus angle. The metatarsophalangeal angle is formed by the longitudinal axes of the proximal phalanx and the first metatarsal.

Fig. 7.**41**   The angle of incongruity in the metatarsophalangeal joint is formed by the line through the osteochondral margins of the head of the metatarsal and the tangent to the base of the proximal phalanx.

Fig. 7.**42**   The proximal metatarsophalangeal joint angle (proximal articular set angle = PASA) is used to determine valgus deviation of the proximal articular surface. It is formed from the line through the osteochondral margins of the head of the metatarsal and the longitudinal axis of the metatarsal.

of the head of the metatarsal. This angle can vary from 4° to 24° (Fig. 7.**41**). Since radiographic findings often differ from intraoperative findings, this angle is of limited value in preoperative planning.

Proximal metatarsophalangeal joint angle (proximal articular set angle = PASA) (Fig. 7.**42**). This parameter is described for measuring the deviation of the articular surface of the head of the metatarsal. The angle is formed from the longitudinal axis of the first metatarsal and the perpendicular to the line connecting the medial and lateral osteochondral margins of

the head of the metatarsal. Normal feet show a variation between 0° and 15°. However, this angle is of limited value because the actual margins of the articular surface are often not clearly discernible in radiographs.

Angle of the proximal articular surface of the first metatarsal. This angle is formed by the longitudinal axis of the first metatarsal and the tangent to the articular surface of the proximal base of the first metatarsal. It is rarely used.

Fig. 7.**43** Angle between the first and second metatarsals for determining metatarsus varus.

Fig. 7.**44** Angle between the first and fifth metatarsals for determining the width of the forefoot.

angle is formed by the longitudinal axes of the first and second metatarsals. It is required to determine the possibilities for correcting hallux valgus.

Intermetatarsal angle between the first and fifth metatarsals (Fig. 7.**44**). This angle is formed by the longitudinal axes of the first and fifth metatarsals. It may range between 14° and 35° in a normal foot. Larger values correlate closely with splayfoot deformities.

Angle between the fourth and fifth metatarsals. This angle is formed by the longitudinal axes of the fourth and fifth metatarsals and may be as high as 5° in normal feet. It is used for evaluating metatarsus valgus of the fifth digit. It can also be significant in describing splayfoot deformities, where it can assume values of approximately 10°.

Metatarsophalangeal angle of the fifth toe. This angle is determined as in the great toe and is required for correction of varus deformities. In a normal foot, this angle will range from 1° to 21°.

Metatarsal depth angle (Fig. 7.**45**). This angle is defined by the tangent to the distal portion of the heads of the first and second metatarsals and the tangent to the distal portion of the heads of the second and fifth metatarsals. This obtuse angle, whose sides are important for further measurements, normally has a value of 140°. Values below 135° are a sign of relative shortening of the metatarsal.

Fig. 7.**45** The metatarsal depth angle is formed by the tangent of the articular surfaces of the heads of the first and second metatarsals and the tangent of the heads of the second and fifth metatarsals. It is used to describe hallux valgus and splayfoot deformities.

Angle between the first and second metatarsal (Fig. 7.**43**). This angle is important in evaluating forefoot deformities because it describes the extent of metatarsus varus, associated with hallux valgus. The

Fig. 7.**46**   The angle between the longitudinal axis of the talus and the second metatarsal describes the position of the hindfoot relative to the forefoot.

Fig. 7.**47**   The Giannestra dorsoplantar talonavicular angle is formed by the longitudinal axis of the talus and the axis of the cuneonavicular joint.

Fig. 7.**48**   The tarsometatarsal angles are formed by the tarsometatarsal axis and the longitudinal axes of the metatarsals. This angle is approximately 40° in the first metatarsal and increases laterally to approximately 65° in the fifth metatarsal.

Angle between the longitudinal axis of the talus and the second metatarsal (Fig. 7.**46**). The longitudinal axes of the talus and metatarsal form an angle that normally lies between 5° and 10° in a normal foot, and describes a normal relationship between hindfoot and forefoot.

The Giannestra dorsoplantar talonavicular angle (Fig. 7.**47**). This angle can be used to describe a pes planus deformity. The angle is formed by the longitudinal axis of the talus and the tangent drawn through the naviculocuneiform joint. It varies between 60° and 80° in a normal foot. A decreased angle is frequently associated with a pes planus deformity.

Tarsometatarsal angles (Fig. 7.**48**). The relationship between the forefoot and the metatarsus is described using a series of angles obtained by drawing a straight line from the medial metatarsocuneiform joint to the matatarsocuboid joint. This line intersects with the longitudinal axes of the individual metatarsals. The angles created by these intersecting lines increase from 41° in the first metatarsal to 66° in the fifth metatarsal.

Talocalcaneal angle (Fig. 7.**49**). This angle is frequently used to quantify congenital and acquired foot deformities. The longitudinal axis of the talus forms an angle with the longitudinal axis of the calcaneus. This angle can normally vary between 15° and 50°. In children up to the age of five, it will measure between

Fig. 7.**49** Talocalcaneal angle. This angle in the dorsoplantar view is important in quantifying pes planus and pes cavus deformities.

Fig. 7.**50** Feiss' line is formed by the distal aspect of the head of the first metatarsal, the center of the navicular, and the dorsal aspect of the talus.

Foot height. The height of the foot is quantified at a number of different points by drawing lines perpendicular to the plane of the plantar surface. The tip of the talar dome is the highest point of the foot and represents the total height. This value ranges from 73–95 mm in a normal foot, with a difference of up to 2 mm between left and right feet. Other parameters describe the height of the calcaneus, cuboid, and navicular. The height of the bases of the first and fifth metatarsals are also measured.

Length of the calcaneus. The length of the calcaneus is measured parallel to the horizontal line extending between its anterior and posterior aspects. A long calcaneus is thought to provide less support for the talar head, which can be seen in a pes planus deformity. This reveals the problem with studies of foot deformities. For example, a clubfoot is frequently imaged in a true lateral view so that the forefoot or tarsus are imaged laterally. However, in this view the calcaneus will be visualized obliquely due to the adduction of the forefoot and will appear foreshortened.

Height of the talar head. This value is thought to best describe the height of the longitudinal arch. The distance from the inferior margin of the talar head to the sole of the foot is measured. An increased value is seen in pes cavus and a decreased value in pes planus.

Height of the fat cushion. The height of the fat cushion in the heel and at the heads of the metatarsals is measured from the most inferior portion of the calcaneus or the heads of the metatarsals to the horizontal plane of the foot. The thickness of the heel cushion ranges from 4–17 mm. The fat cushion beneath the head of the first metatarsal varies between 7 and 25 mm, and between 1 and 16 mm beneath the head of the fifth metatarsal.

- **Axes of the foot in the lateral plane**

Feiss' line (Fig. 7.**50**). This line extends from the center of the navicular and the trochlea of the talus to the inferior
margin of the head of the first metatarsal. The presence of this line defines a normally shaped foot because normally all of the points described will lie in a straight line.

30° and 50°; in children above the age of five and adolescents, this angle will measure only 30°.

In a normal foot, the longitudinal axis of the talus points toward the head of the first metatarsal, and the longitudinal axis of the calcaneus toward the head of the fourth metatarsal. In a clubfoot deformity, the talocalcaneal angle is small; occasionally, longitudinal axes will even be parallel. In congenital vertical talus, the talocalcaneal angle will be increased, with medial deviation in relation to the first metatarsal. A pes planus deformity will also show a larger talocalcaneal angle.

Analysis in the Lateral Plane

- **Linear measurements**

Total length of the foot. Total length is measured from the most posterior aspect of the heel to the hip of the distal phalanx of the longest toe. Foot length in adults normally ranges between 23 and 28 cm. The left and right feet may differ in length by up to 3 cm.

The literature mentions length measurements for the various sections of the foot. The posterior aspect of the calcaneus is used as a reference. Length is measured to the distal portion of the first metatarsal, the distal margin of the fifth metatarsal, the proximal margin of the first metatarsal, the proximal margin of the fifth metatarsal, the distal margin of the talar head, the proximal margin of the cuboid, and the apex of the talar dome.

Fig. 7.51   Schade's line is formed by the center of the head of the first metatarsal, the medial cuneiform, the navicular, and the talus.

Fig. 7.52   Giannestra's tarsal relationships are represented by the position of the articular axes of the talonavicular joint and the first tarsometatarsal joint relative to the Meary-Tomeno axis.

Fig. 7.53   The Meary-Tomeno axis is the line that bisects the angle with its apex in the center of the head of the first metatarsal and its sides tangential to the inferior and superior cortex of the talus.

Schade's line (Fig. 7.51). Another line describes the structural configuration of the foot. Here, the reference points are in the center of the head of the first metatarsal, the cuneiform, the navicular, and at the posterior aspect of the trochlea of the talus. Here too, the points should lie in a straight line.

Diagonal axis of the talus. This line is drawn as a tangent to the superior cortex of the talar neck. It describes the relationship between the talus and calcaneus. Normally this line will be horizontal.

The line of Chopart's joints. This line describes the shape of the talonavicular and calculating calcaneocuboid joint. It should be a smooth, uniform curve. An interruption of the uniform line is a sign of joint incongruity and structural abnormality.

Description of the tarsometatarsal relationship. To describe the tarsometatarsal relationship, tangents are drawn along the superior and inferior margins of the cortex of the talar head, the navicular, and the cuboid. These two lines should normally be parallel and perpendicular to the joint lines of the metatarsocuneiform joint.

Giannestra's description of metatarsal relationships (Fig. 7.52). In this method, a longitudinal axis is drawn through the first metatarsal and the talar head, and the joint planes of the talonavicular and first tarsometatarsal joints are drawn in. These two should be parallel and perpendicular to the longitudinal axis of the first metatarsal and the talar neck.

The Meary–Tomeno axis (Fig. 7.53). This axis may be used to describe structural abnormalities. It is formed by the line bisecting the angle whose sides extend as tangents to the inferior and superior cortex of the talus.

Description of hindfoot relationships. Certain bony structures in the hindfoot can be described in the lateral view. The sustentaculum talus, the lateral tubercle of the calcaneus, and the peroneal sulcus at the cuboid should be identifiable. Varus and valgus deviations of the hindfoot alter these structures. Complete visualization of the sinus tarsi as a radiolucent oval area is an indication of normal hindfoot anatomy.

- **Measuring angles of the foot in the lateral plane**

Reference angle at the base of the talus. This angle is created by the longitudinal axis of the talus and a line parallel to the plane of the plantar surface of the foot. It ranges between 14° and 30° in a normal foot and describes the inclination of the talus. A larger angle is measured in plantar and medial displacement of the talus.

Anterior and posterior angles of the longitudinal arch (Fig. 7.54). The angle of the anterior longitudinal arch is formed by a tangent along the inferior cortex of the talar neck, navicular, cuneiform, first metatarsal, medial sesamoid of the great toe, and the plane of the plantar surface of the foot. When combined with the angle of the posterior longitudinal arch, formed by the longitudinal axis of the calcaneus and the plane of the plantar surface of the foot, the two superior sides meet a point referred to as the apex of the longitudinal arch.

Reference angle at the base of the calcaneus. This angle is created by the intersection of the longitudinal axis of the calcaneus and the plane of the plantar surface of the foot. It ranges between 15° and 39°. Generally this angle is congruent to the posterior angle of the longitudinal arch.

Tarsal joint angle. This angle can be used to measure the orientation of the articular surfaces of the tarsus.

Fig. 7.**54** Construction of the angle of the longitudinal arch from the anterior and posterior inflation angles of the calcaneus and forefoot.

Fig. 7.**55** The tarsal joint angle is formed by a line parallel to the plantar surface and the tangents of the talonavicular and naviculocuneiform joints and the proximal tangent of the base of the first metatarsal.

Böhler angle

Fig. 7.**56** Flattened Böhler angle in a comminuted fracture of the calcaneus.

Fig. 7.**57** The Philip-Fowler angle describes the size of the posterior surface of the tubercle of the calcaneus.

The angles are created by a line parallel to the plantar surface and the lateral joint planes of the talonavicular, naviculocuneiform, and metatarsocuneiform joints (Fig. 7.**55**). The talonavicular angle ranges from 54°–74°, the naviculocuneiform angle ranges from 51°–78°, and the metatarsocuneiform angle from 55°–72°. Deviations from these values suggest a pes planus or pes cavus deformity.

The anterosuperior and posterosuperior angles of the surface of the calcaneus. The anterosuperior angle of the surface of the calcaneus is created by a tangent to the anterosuperior surface of the calcaneus and the plantar surface. It ranges between 2° and 30°. A similar angle describes the inclination of the posterior calcaneus. A tangent to the posterosuperior surface of the calcaneus forms an angle ranging from 10°–35° in a normal foot.

The Böhler angle. This angle is an important parameter for determining deformities after a calcaneus fracture. It is formed by tangents to the posterosuperior and anterosuperior aspects of the calcaneus. Usually this angle lies between 28° and 40°. Fractures in the anterior process of the calcaneus can result in significant flattening or even a negative Böhler angle. For this reason, this angle can occasionally be used as a criterion for open reduction of fractures of the calcaneus (Fig. 7.**56**).

Inclination of the calcaneus. The inclination of the calcaneus is determined by the angle of the tangent to the interior calcaneal cortex to horizontal. A normal angle lies between 20° and 30°.

The Philip-Fowler angle (Fig. 7.**57**). This angle is formed by the inferior calcaneus tangent and the tangent to the posterosuperior aspect of the tubercle of the calcaneus. Normal values for this angle range between 44° and 69°. An angle exceeding 75° is a sign of prominence of the tubercle of the calcaneus. Such a configuration is frequently associated with Achilles tendinitis or bursitis beneath the Achilles tendon caused by mechanical impingement of soft-tissue structures between the prominence of the calcaneus, the tendon, and the shoe.

Lateral talometatarsal angle. This angle is significant in defining pes planus or pes cavus. It is formed by the longitudinal axis of the first metatarsal and the longitudinal axis of the talus. In a normal arch, the angle will range between 4° and –4° (except for the talocalcaneal joint). Values exceeding 4° are a sign of a pes cavus deformity; values below 4° indicate a pes planus deformity. This angle is also significant with respect to the flexibility of the foot because it can vary significantly at rest and during weight-bearing stance. A difference of more than 8° in these comparative radiographs suggests a hyperflexible foot (Fig. 7.**58**).

Lateral talocalcaneal angle. This angle is formed by the intersection of the longitudinal axes of the talus

Pes planus

Pes planus

Normal

Normal

Pes cavus

Pes cavus

Fig. 7.**58** Significance of the talometatarsal angle in the lateral view for diagnosing pes planus and pes cavus.

Fig. 7.**59** Significance of the talocalcaneal angle in the lateral view for diagnosing pes planus and pes cavus.

and calcaneus. Normally this angle ranges from 25°–50°.

Since the talar head in pes planus is tilted medially and plantarly, the talocalcaneal angle will be increased. An increased angle is also observed in metatarsus varus. This is in contrast to a varus deformity of the hindfoot or pes cavus, in which the talocalcaneal angle will frequently be reduced (Fig. 7.**59**).

Inclination of the metatarsals. The longitudinal axes of the metatarsals form a cone whose apex lies dorsal and superior. The angle of inclination is 20° for the first metatarsal, 15° for the second, 10° for the third, 8° for the fourth, and 5° for the fifth.

Radiologic Findings with Specific Foot Deformities

Hallux Valgus and Hallux Rigidus

Comprehensive radiologic evaluation of hallux valgus deformities requires several measurements.

The actual deformity itself is described by the metatarsophalangeal angle in the dorsoplantar view. An angle exceeding 15° is a sign of a hallux valgus deformity.

The interphalangeal angle is determined to distinguish true hallux valgus from hallux interphalangeus. This angle should not exceed 5°.

Measuring the interphalangeal angle between the first and second digits determines whether metatarsus varus of the first digit is present. Depending on

Fig. 7.**60** Dorsoplantar radiograph of the phalangeal and metatarsal region in the presence of a severe hallux valgus deformity with an enlarged metatarsophalangeal angle, sesamoid displacement, metatarsophalangeal subluxation, and secondary lateral displacement of the small toes.

Fig. 7.**61** Hallux rigidus with complete loss of the joint space, increased sclerosis, and marginal osteophytes at the metatarsophalangeal joint.

the author, an angle exceeding 15° or 20° represents metatarsus varus of the first digit.

Evaluation of the orientation of the metatarsophalangeal joint requires measurement of the articular set angle. A value exceeding 20° is a sign of subluxation of the metatarsophalangeal joint. As has been mentioned, the articular set angle in the first metatarsal joint is of limited value in evaluating subluxation in the metatarsophalangeal joint.

The relative length of the metatarsals is important for preoperative planning. A shortening correction should be performed if a minus index is present (Fig. 7.**60**).

Determining the extent of the medial exostosis has already been discussed in the section Analysis in the AP Projection, page 263.

The lateral displacement of the sesamoids should be defined in relation to the mean longitudinal axis of the first metatarsal. The position of the medial sesamoid relative to this axis is defined according to one of four degrees of dislocation.

When evaluating hallux valgus deformities, radiographic signs of arthritic changes should also be identified, such as increased subchondral sclerosis, wear, and osteophytes. Arthritic change in the meta-

tarsophalangeal joint of the great toe is referred to as hallux rigidus because of the painfully limited motion (Fig. 7.**61**).

Motion limited by a structure such as a dorsal osteophyte while articular structures are otherwise intact is referred to as hallux limitus (Fig. 7.**62**).

Pes Planus

Radiographs of a pes planus deformity are two-dimensional images of a three-dimensional geometric deformity. The transition to standard radiographs has improved reproducibility of the radiographs and measurements. However, clinical examination is still the primary means of describing the deformity. To describe congenital pes planus, useful radiographs cannot be obtained until the age of six at the earliest. However, even these can only be approximately evaluated because the ossified centers of the bones do not accurately represent the actual bone contours (Fig. 7.**63**).

The measurements below are useful for preoperative documentation and postoperative radiographic follow-up examination.

The Giannestra talonavicular angle is reduced to less than 60° in pes planus. The talocalcaneal angle is

Fig. 7.**62**   Lateral view of hallux limitus. The image shows congruent articular surfaces with dorsal osteophytes that limit dorsiflexion.

Fig. 7.**63**   Dorsoplantar radiograph of both feet showing pes planus with talonavicular subluxation in the left foot.

especially significant; in adult flatfoot deformities it exceeds 30°.

The talometatarsal angle is equally as important as the talocalcaneal angle. In a pes planus deformity, the talometatarsal angle will have negative values of less than 4° (Fig. 7.**64**).

Pes planus deformities can be documented in lateral views by the increased reference angle at the base of the talus (exceeding 30°), and a reduction in the anterior angle of the longitudinal arch and the reference angle at the base of the calcaneus. The tarsal joint angle can also be used to describe the pes planus deformity.

The angle of the longitudinal arch resulting from the reference angle at the bases of the calcaneus and talus provides an excellent description of the deformity. In this case it achieves values exceeding 160°.

Pes Cavus

Radiographic examination can only approximately describe pes cavus as a three-dimensional deformity; the same limitations apply as in descriptions of pes planus or talipes equinovarus. Again, standard radiographs should be obtained for better reproducibility.

In lateral views, pes cavus is demonstrated by a reduced reference angle at the base of the talus (less

Fig. 7.**64**   Lateral radiograph of the left foot shown in Figure 7.**63**. The image shows a negative talometatarsal angle.

Fig. 7.**65** Lateral view of a pes cavus deformity with a normal talocalcaneal angle and a significantly increased talometatarsal angle. Note the hammer toe deformity resulting from increased activity of the extensors.

than 14°), and an increased anterior angle of the longitudinal arch and reference angle at the base of the calcaneus. The tarsal joint angle can also be used to describe the pes cavus deformity. Feiss' and Schade's lines are particularly useful since they help to identify the deformity in the metatarsus. A pes cavus deformity in the tarsus is characterized by an increased talometatarsal angle while the talocalcaneal angle is normal (Fig. 7.**65**).

The angle of the longitudinal arch resulting from the references angle at the bases of the calcaneus and talus provides an excellent description of the deformity. In this case its values are less than 150°.

In the method described by Giannestra for evaluating metatarsal configuration, the axes of the talonavicular joint and the tarsometatarsal joint are no longer parallel but diverge dorsally. Both axes are no longer perpendicular to the axis through the first metatarsal and talar neck.

Clubfoot

Radiologic description of clubfoot concentrates on the talocalcaneal complex. Kite describes the talocalcaneal angle in the dorsoplantar view as less than 20° in a clubfoot deformity. Occasionally the two axes are parallel.

The talocalcaneal angle is less than 30° in the lateral view. Again, the two axes can be parallel. The tibiocalcaneal angle is reduced to less than 25° because of the superior displacement of the heel.

The talometatarsal angle is increased, indicating increased adduction of the forefoot.

In addition to performing radiologic measurements, be alert to talonavicular and calcaneocuboid subluxation and dislocation. These findings can be readily quantified using the methods described above. On the whole, these measurements are of secondary importance in clinical practice because they can only provide approximate results in infants.

In adult clubfoot deformities, the degree of talocalcaneal coverage should also be determined.

Xeroradiography

Xeroradiography uses a selenium-coated charged plate for radiographic imaging. During X-ray exposure, the surface of the plate with the selenium coating changes its charge proportional to the radiation that is passing through. The plate is then covered with a negatively charged powder that accumulates in the positively charged areas. This image is then fixed on plastic-coated paper.

A characteristic feature of xeroradiography is the enhanced resolution that accentuates the borders between areas of different radiodensity. This characteristic provides a highly detailed image of areas of significantly different radiodensity. This technique has proven effective in diagnosing subtle initial changes in metabolic diseases or arthritic processes.

Xeroradiography can also be helpful in detecting hairline fractures. Despite these advantages, this diagnostic imaging modality has not come into widespread use.

The disadvantages of the modality compared to conventional radiography include contrast suppression where there are larger areas of similar radiodensity and increased radiation exposure for the patient. However, the hands and feet can be imaged using radiation doses comparable to conventional radiography.

Conventional Tomography

Conventional tomography is used in locations where overlapping structures prevent plain radiography from providing clear images. In this type of tomography, layer images are produced by simultaneously moving the X-ray tube and film. Only the layer in which the plane of focus lies is sharply visualized on the radiograph. The greater the range of adjustment of the X-ray tube, the thinner will be the slices that can be obtained. However, this requires sacrificing contrast.

A disadvantage of this method is the imaging time required, particularly when images must be obtained in several planes. The time can be reduced by using cassette cartridges that permit simultaneous imaging of multiple planes. A further disadvantage is the increased radiation exposure for the patient compared with plain radiography.

With the advent of CT, the use of conventional tomography has declined. However, it can still be superior to CT in diagnostic imaging of the foot. Fractures in the plane of Lisfranc's joint are poorly visualized in axial CT images but clearly visualized in conventional tomography. Visualization of osteochondral fractures is also often superior in conventional tomography than in CT images.

Radiographic Magnification Techniques

Radiographic magnification techniques were developed to improve the quality and diagnostic value of radiographs. Optical magnification should be distinguished from direct radiographic magnification. Both techniques can be used to look for subtle initial changes in arthritis, metabolic diseases, and infections of the foot and hand. A purely optical magnification requires high-quality X-ray film. The magnification is achieved photographically using a projector. This technique requires X-ray film with higher resolution, higher contrast, and decreased granularity than in standard radiography. However, in contrast to the microfocus technique, there is no improvement in spatial resolution.

The greatest disadvantage is the increased radiation exposure for the patient.

The direct radiographic magnification technique, or microfocus technique, requires a special microfocus X-ray tube that achieves higher spatial resolution by decreasing the focal spot. This imaging technique provides a magnified radiographic image that is significantly superior in quality to optical magnification. The smaller focal spot means that there is less loss of definition than in conventional radiography and higher spatial resolution. Although the radiation exposure is greater than in conventional radiography, it is significantly less than the radiation dose required for optical magnification. A disadvantage of this technique is that it can only visualize small areas.

Microfocus technique is used in skeletal radiography in oncologic settings for typing bone and soft-tissue tumors using the Lodwick classification. It is used in rheumatology for early detection of rheumatic diseases by visualizing changes in border layers, destruction, and erosion in the extremities.

7.4 Pedobarography

Pedobarography can be used to measure the distribution of pressure exerted by the sole of the foot while the patient stands or walks. Using carbon paper to measure the static distribution of foot pressure has been common since the 1930s. The disadvantage of this method is that it can only document weight distributions with the patient standing.

Computerized capacitive measuring methods can be used to determine pressure distribution while the patient walks. The load in the stress zones can then be displayed as a three-dimensional pressure graph. This method can record up to 20 images per second. The measured parameters include the area used, total force, maximum pressure, the area curve, the curve of the center of gravity, and the curve of peak total force.

Piezoelectric measuring systems can document dynamic processes and high stresses with respect to the resulting force vector, the point at which force is applied, the frontal component, the sagittal component, the vertical component, and the torque.

With the advent of instrumented inserts for shoes, measurements of pressure distribution can be obtained without influencing the individual gait. Piezoelectric ceramic sensors allow up to 1000 measurements per second.

Neither capacitive nor piezoelectric methods have yet become common in everyday clinical practice. However, more widespread use of these systems would be advantageous for preoperative diagnostic studies and in the development of orthopedic inserts.

7.5 Ultrasound

Ultrasonography is used in the foot primarily to evaluate the Achilles tendon. Tears and changes in the Achilles tendon can be imaged with a high degree of precision in B-mode ultrasound studies. This modality is also used to detect intra-articular and periarticular fluid accumulations or vascular cysts.

Ultrasound is a valuable adjunctive diagnostic procedure for detecting soft-tissue changes in the plantar fascia in the presence of inflammation or tumor.

Except for the Achilles tendon, there has been little clinical experience with ultrasound diagnostic studies of the foot.

The future will reveal whether the benefits of ultrasound examination of the foot justify its costs.

7.6 Nuclear Medicine Studies

See chapter 1 (Shoulder, p. 54) for a general discussion on the utility of nuclear medicine studies.

7.7 Computed Tomography

Indications, Diagnostic Value, and Clinical Relevance

A sequence of cross-sectional images provides a three-dimensional perspective that significantly expands the understanding of normal and abnormal anatomy of the foot. Parts of the anatomy are often obscured in plain radiographs by overlapping bones. For example, the subtalar joint is obscured by the tarsal joints. Soft-tissue structures can be visualized with far greater clarity in CT and MR images than is possible in conventional radiographs. CT images tissue according to its radiodensity and specific radiation absorption. This offers significant advantages in evaluating articular and cortical surfaces in various different bones.

Technique, Instrumentation, and Examination Procedure

When working with cross-sectional images, it is particularly important to maintain a clear idea of the perspectives and the cross-sectional plane of the foot. Usually, perpendicular slices in the coronal, transverse, and sagittal planes are used. These terms refer to the anatomy of the foot in the standing position.

The coronal plane is perpendicular to the plantar surface and to the longitudinal axis of the foot. The perspective is chosen so that the structures of the foot are imaged sequentially, usually beginning at the tip of the toes and proceeding proximally to the dorsal aspect of the heel.

The transverse plane, often referred to as the axial plane, lies parallel to the plantar surface of the foot. The perspective is comparable to an AP radiograph of the foot.

The sagittal plane permits a perspective similar to that of a plain lateral radiograph.

Metal implants significantly reduce the imaging quality of CT because of the image artifacts generated. If the metal is not too close to the area of examination, though, imaging quality may be sufficient to justify such an examination.

However, if the metal is immediately adjacent to the area of examination, well prepared radiographic diagnostic studies can provide more information than CT.

- **Requesting CT studies from the radiologist**

When requesting CT studies, remember that the imaging plane should always be perpendicular to the articular surface or fracture plane. When making the request, inform the radiologist of the anatomical region of the suspected pathology so that the appropriate area can be better imaged in thinner slices or magnified images.

It is a good idea to give the radiologist copies or originals of existing radiographs. The rule of thumb is that the more precisely the requirements for a CT examination are described, the greater the efficacy of the study and radiologic interpretation will be.

Normal Findings

The hindfoot includes the talus and calcaneus, and the talocalcaneal, talonavicular, and calcaneocuboid joints. The hindfoot is the region of the foot that is most frequently examined in CT studies. The subtalar joint is an important joint but is poorly visualized in AP and lateral plane radiographs because of the overlapping shadows of the talus and calcaneus. One of the most frequent indications for CT examination of the hindfoot is limited subtalar motion and exclusion of a tarsal coalition.

The talocalcaneal joint is divided into three radiographic and anatomic sections: the posterior, middle, and anterior facets.

In the coronal plane, the posterior facet extends across the entire width of the talocalcaneal overlap and lies parallel to the tibiotalar articular surface.

The middle talocalcaneal facet is short and lies on the medial aspect of the talocalcaneal joint. The articular surfaces of the middle facet are parallel to the posterior talocalcaneal facet. The anterior talocalcaneal facet is not well defined. In a normal foot, in contrast to a flatfoot, the lateral aspect of the talus will slightly but visibly overlap the medial aspect of the calcaneus.

In the coronal plane, the sinus tarsi will appear at the level between the middle and anterior facet. The contour of the sinus tarsi varies in depth according to the arch of the foot.

The longitudinal axis of the talus closely approximates the transverse plane. A small groove for the flexor hallucis longus tendon will be seen at the posterior process of the talus, and the os trigonum (also known as the Stieda process) can be visualized.

There will be variations in the coronal plane between the talus and calcaneus, depending on whether the foot is more in a pes cavus or pes planus position.

In a severe pes planus deformity, the joint imaging plane of the posterior talocalcaneal facet will be valgus to the tibiotalar joint imaging plane of the ankle.

The calcaneonavicular space can be visualized in the transverse plane. This area can also be visualized in plain radiographs in an oblique projection. CT studies do not offer any significant advantages over plain radiography in the examination of this area.

Several intrinsic muscle groups and tendons of the dorsum of the foot can be visualized using soft-tissue techniques. Tenography facilitates visualization of the peroneal tendons in CT examination.

Fig. 7.**66**   The lateral radiograph of the talocalcaneonavicular joint shows three oval radiolucencies with indistinct perifocal marginal sclerosis in the talus on the posterior joint facet.

Fig. 7.**67**   CT image in the coronal plane of the posterior facet of the patient in Figure 7.**66** shows three lobulated cysts that communicate with the talocalcaneonavicular joint.

CT Procedure and Findings in the Presence of Specific Pathologic Changes

Pes Planus and Pes Cavus

In contrast to a normal foot, the posterior talocalcaneal facet is parallel to the superior tibiotalar facet in pes cavus. However, the foot with a pes planus deformity will have a narrow articular surface at the level of the middle talocalcaneal facet and a deep sinus tarsi. In pes cavus, the middle talocalcaneal facet is relatively wide and the sinus tarsi narrow.

There is no bony overlap at the levels of the anterior talocalcaneal facet in pes planus. In pes cavus, however, the anterior portion of the calcaneus provides a well-developed bony support for the anterior portion of the talus.

In pes planus, the navicular tuberosity has a plantar alignment in the coronal plane at the level of the navicular. In pes cavus, the bony plane of the navicular is aligned horizontally.

Fractures of the Talus

CT images in the transverse plane are useful in distinguishing os trigonum from a fracture of the Stieda process (the posterior process of the talus). Comparison with the asymptomatic side is often helpful in evaluating the posterior portion of the talus. Asymmetric irregularities between a dorsal portion of a bone and the posterior portion of the body of the talus suggests trauma.

Fractures of the body of the talus are best visualized in the sagittal or coronal plane. If the fracture plane is aligned in a sagittal line, coronal slices are indicated for evaluation. Fractures in the coronal plane can be more precisely visualized with transverse imaging planes.

Regardless of the fracture plane, a coronal imaging plane should be favoured when the subtalar joint is involved.

Severe fractures in the hindfoot and tarsal region can occur in diabetes patients with a neuropathic foot. Occasionally, tiny compression fractures of the talus can be visualized. CT studies can reproduce the fracture lines of these fractures significantly more faithfully than plain radiography because overlapping of the distal tibia, distal fibula, and calcaneus can be avoided.

Fractures of the talar neck are normally visualized in the coronal plane, more so in the transverse plane if evaluation of medial or lateral displacement is required. In some cases, the severe swelling of a lateral dislocation can obscure the valgus deformity of the foot.

Abnormal Findings in the Subtalar Joint

Examinations of patients with rheumatoid arthritis can document soft-tissue swelling, joint-space narrowing, bone erosion, and the pes planus valgus deformity. A clear image of the hindfoot and talocalcaneonavicular joint in the coronal plane is helpful in deciding whether arthrodesis should be performed.

CT studies can provide important information about bone structure and density of subtalar or multiarticular arthrodeses in the hindfoot. Coronal slices permit good evaluation of the talocalcaneal joint (Figs. 7.**66** and 7.**67**); a transverse imaging plane facilitates evaluation of possible pseudarthrosis in the talonavicular joint.

Fig. 7.**68**   Lateral view of a comminuted calcaneus fracture showing a negative Böhler angle.

Occasionally, lateral displacement of the dorsal portion of the calcaneus, with contact to the distal lateral malleolus, can be diagnosed in patients suffering from pain after a calcaneal fracture involving the subtalar joint that was subsequently treated by arthrodesis.

In other cases, subtalar pseudoarthrosis may be the reason for persistent pain.

Rotation subluxation of the subtalar joint is diagnosed in over two-thirds of examinations of a residual clubfoot deformity. The posterior portion of the calcaneus at the level of the posterior talocalcaneal facet is often subluxed lateral to a tangent of the cortex of the distal tibia.

In over one-third of patients, CT studies will reveal lateral talocalcaneal subluxation despite normal findings in plain radiographs.

Fractures of the Calcaneus

CT has come into widespread use in diagnosing fractures of the calcaneus (Fig. 7.**68**). CT studies are performed with acute and chronic fractures and malunited fractures. In the coronal plane, they provide information about the interruption of the subtalar joint and the lateral dislocation of the lateral surface of the calcaneus and its impingement in the calcaneofibular space.

Depression of the calcaneal tubercle can also be measured in the coronal plane. This examination can influence the treatment of both acute and malunited fractures.

The posterior articular facet is involved in an injury to the subtalar joint, which can occur when the patient falls on the calcaneus (for example, falling off a ladder). The middle facet can be involved in higher-energy fractures, occurring for example in automobile accidents. The fracture line can continue through the middle facet or cause dislocation so that the congru-

Fig. 7.**69**   Comminuted calcaneus fracture in CT in the transverse plane. Medial dislocation of the calcaneal tubercle.

ity between middle facet of the calcaneus and the corresponding talar facet is disturbed.

Occasionally a fracture can also involve the anterior calcaneocuboid aspect. Depending on the severity of the injury to the calcaneocuboid joint, plain radiographs may not be sufficient. In this case, CT studies in the transverse plane are a recommended adjunctive diagnostic procedure (Fig. 7.**69**).

Coronal CT slices of the hindfoot clearly define the lateral extent of the calcaneus fracture. Normally, the lateral margin of the talus converges with that of the calcaneus to form a line. In any calcaneus fractures, this line will be interrupted and the lateral cortex of the calcaneus will be displaced into the soft tissue between the calcaneus and fibula.

Even when the peroneal tendons are not displaced, this lateral wall fracture can show clinical symptoms. However, the peroneal tendons are often dislocated, coming to rest at the lateral side of the lateral malleolus. In one series of 24 patients, damage to the peroneal tendon was found in 92% of calcaneus fractures. This injury involved lateral displacement in 58% of the cases, impingement by bone fragments in 33%, and subluxation or dislocation in 25% of all cases. CT examination allows a more precise understanding of the morphology of the calcaneus fracture and aids in planning the surgical procedure.

Three-dimensional reconstruction of calcaneus fractures has been available for several years. This method provides improved spatial understanding of the fracture, which aids in preoperative planning.

Abnormal Findings in the Tarsals

The talonavicular and calcaneocuboid joints can also be involved in acute injuries or in systemic or degenerative disorders. These joints lie in the coronal plane and are best imaged in the transverse plane.

The navicular can be injured by overuse or acute trauma. Stress fractures of the navicular are often difficult to diagnose because they are poorly visualized in plain radiographs. Usually the fracture lies in the sagittal plane and is visible in the coronal CT plane. The cause of persistent pain in the tarsal region and increased uptake in the navicular in nuclear medicine studies can be identified in a CT examination in the coronal plane. Navicular injuries are usually the result of severe acute trauma involving the body of the navicular. Findings can include dorsal dislocation, comminuted lateral or plantar fragments, and a loss of congruity in the talonavicular joint. Both the coronal and transverse imaging planes permit better visualization of such injuries than is possible in plain radiographs. CT of navicular injuries should include examination of the hindfoot.

Many navicular fractures are associated with fractures of the calcaneus. When evaluating avulsion fractures of the dorsal and medial aspects of the navicular, pay close attention to the calcaneocuboid joint in the transverse CT plane because a compression fracture may be present here.

The ability to identify injuries and arthritis of the tarsometatarsal joints (Lisfranc's joint) is increased by CT studies. Plain radiographs of the metatarsal region are plagued by significant overlapping of the bones. In contrast, CT studies permit better evaluation of the degree of joint involvement in arthritis or in dislocations secondary to fractures, which explains the increasing popularity of this imaging modality.

Abnormal Findings in the Metatarsals

The articular surfaces of the metatarsal region lie in the coronal and sagittal planes so that they are best visualized in the transverse plane. The transverse slices of the tarsometatarsal section of the foot should be thinner to allow more precise evaluation of the narrow articular sections.

A complete CT examination of the injury of tarsometatarsal joints includes obtaining slices in both the transverse and coronal planes. The transverse imaging plane clearly visualizes the tarsometatarsal articular surfaces. However, a vertical dislocation may be present that can be more precisely visualized in the coronal imaging plane. An injury at the base of the metatarsals without significant dislocation can also be precisely reproduced in the coronal plane.

A fracture at the bases of the metatarsals often puts the physician in the difficult position of deciding whether open or closed reduction is indicated. A CT examination in the coronal plane is also helpful in this diagnostic setting.

CT studies in the transverse imaging plane are helpful in diagnosing patients who may require metatarsocuneiform arthrodesis for treatment of arthritis. The transverse CT examination shows the extent of joint involvement with this indication.

Coronal imaging planes are useful in evaluating fractures and determining the positioning of the heads of the metatarsals. Measure the distance of the plantar margin of the heads of the metatarsals to the underlying plantar surface in the coronal plane. Several authors recommend obtaining thin coronal and transverse CT slices where there is pain at the sesamoids of the head of the first metatarsal.

Coronal slices faithfully reproduce the relationship between the two sesamoids and the undersurface of the head of the metatarsal. The transverse plane is used for imaging fractures and fragmentation. Three-dimensional reconstructions of the metatarsals will visualize the congruity of the sesamoids with the metatarsal articular surface if thin slice-thicknesses are used. However, the high cost of this examination relative to plain radiography prohibits its use in clinical practice (Fig. 7.**70**).

Coalitions

One of the most common indications for CT studies of the hindfoot is to demonstrate or exclude a tarsal coalition. Tarsal coalitions primarily occur in the talocalcaneal and calcaneonavicular joints. A calcaneonavicular coalition can be readily visualized in plain radiographs. However, talocalcaneal coalitions are often difficult to discern. Their morphology can be more clearly visualized in CT studies in the coronal plane (Figs. 7.**71** and 7.**72**).

Characteristics of a talocalcaneal coalition in the coronal plane include the partial or complete formation of a bony bridge, the AP direction of the coalition, and the alignment of the aberrant articular facet.

Fig. 7.**70**   The three-dimensional reconstruction of the distal metatarsals and toes shows congruent alignment of the sesamoids to the distal head of the metatarsal.

Fig. 7.**72**   CT image in the coronal plane of the patient in Figure 7.**71** showing a talocalcaneal coalition.

Fig. 7.**71**   The posterior oblique view of the talocalcaneonavicular joint shows a talocalcaneal coalition at the sustentaculum of the talus.

Information about these characteristics is helpful for preoperative planning in the treatment of a symptomatic coalition.

Be careful not to overread CT studies of a talocalcaneal coalition. If the imaging plane is parallel to the plane of the facet, the facet may not be properly visualized and may simulate a coalition (pseudocoalition).

A genuine talocalcaneal coalition can be identified in a CT image by the significant irregularity of the articular surfaces of the talocalcaneonavicular joint and by the loss of parallelism between the posterior and middle facets in the coronal plane. Despite this, the talocalcaneal coalition may be so subtle that it can only be identified by the absence of the tarsal canal.

Not every patient with limited motion in the hindfoot will have a verifiable coalition. However, the CT examination can exclude a coalition, particularly when images are obtained in both planes (coronal and transverse).

Tumors

CT examinations can demonstrate tumors in the tarsal region that may escape detection in plain radiographs because of overlapping shadows. CT has significant advantages over plain radiography; CT studies can precisely demonstrate the dorsoplantar and dorsoanterior dimensions of the tumor and the extent of bone destruction (Fig. 7.**73**).

CT has been largely supplanted by MRI in the diagnosis of soft-tissue tumors. However, the use of various contrast media can prove the diagnostic value of CT studies of soft-tissue processes.

Fig. 7.**73**   Transverse CT image of a benign bone cyst in the calcaneus without erosion of the cortex.

Infections and Foreign Bodies

CT studies have proven effective in detecting foreign bodies in the foot that cannot be visualized in plain radiographs. Several authors emphasize the importance of CT in evaluating plantar compartment infections in the foot in diabetes patients, noting that these studies provide information on the extent of the processes for preoperative planning. Thin slices in two planes should be obtained. Axial slices are preferable in the hindfoot, and coronal slices in the metatarsals.

7.8 Magnetic Resonance Imaging

Indications

MRI is indicated for suspected radiographically occult fractures, especially stress fractures, avascular osteonecroses, nerve compress (Morton neuroma), arthritis, soft-tissue infections, osteomyelitis, and tumors.

Examination Procedure (Figs. 7.**74a–c**)

Patient positioning, coils, and sequences are the same as for examinations of the ankle. For small lesions, superficial coils can be used to improve the resolution.

Pathologic Findings

Fractures (Fig. 7.**75**)

Forced abduction can tear the tarsometatarsal ligaments with resultant lateral dislocation of the metatarsals. This is frequently accompanied by a fracture of the second metatarsal base. The dislocation can be detected on axis-oriented coronal images. The osseous lesion is recognized as signal intensity that is increased on the STIR (short-time inversion recovery) image and decreased on the T1-weighted image. The fracture line is best seen on the gradient-echo (GRE) image.

Stress fractures of the metatarsals, also referred to as march fracture, frequently do not show a fracture line. The STIR image exhibits an ill-defined increase in signal intensity within the bone marrow of the affected metatarsal surrounded by a bright periosteal bulge.

Microfractures close to the distal epiphysis can cause avascular necrosis of the metatarsal head. Second and third metatarsals are most often affected. The necrotic zone is well demarcated as a dark signal on the T1-weighted image and a bright signal on the STIR image.

Neuromas

Morton neuromas consist of painful thickening of the perineurium of the interdigital nerves, mostly found between the fourth and fifth metatarsal heads. The thickening exhibits an increased signal on the STIR image. In contrast to a neurinoma, the nerve itself only shows a weak increase in signal intensity.

Osteoarthritis (Fig. 7.**76**)

The first metatarsophalangeal articulation is most frequently involved. The STIR image and the T2-weighted image show an effusion with high signal intensity. After intravenous administration of contrast medium, the T1-weighted GRE image with phase contrast reveals the inflammatory synovial changes

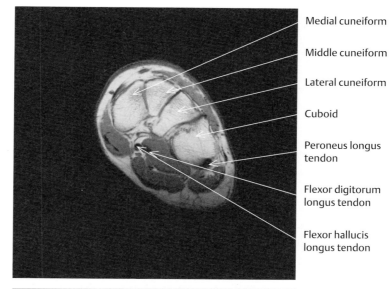

Medial cuneiform

Middle cuneiform

Lateral cuneiform

Cuboid

Peroneus longus tendon

Flexor digitorum longus tendon

Flexor hallucis longus tendon

Fig. 7.**74a**   Transverse image (SE 500/20) showing normal metatarsus.

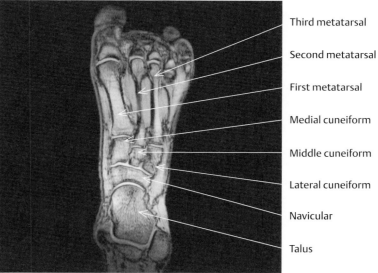

Third metatarsal

Second metatarsal

First metatarsal

Medial cuneiform

Middle cuneiform

Lateral cuneiform

Navicular

Talus

Fig. 7.**74b**   Coronal image (GRE 600/11 out of phase) showing normal metatarsus and forefoot.

Talus

Navicular

Medial cuneiform

First metatarsal

Flexor hallucis brevis

Proximal phalanx of the hallux

Flexor hallucis longus tendon

Distal phalanx of the hallux

Fig. 7.**74c**   Sagittal image (GRE 600/11 out of phase) showing normal metatarsus and forefoot.

Periostitis with
contrast medium
enhancement

Intramedullary
edema

Fig. 7.**75** Sagittal image
(GRE 500/11 out of phase
after administration of intravenous gadolinium contrast
medium) showing a march
fracture of the third metatarsal. The cortical defect is
barely discernible.

Inflamed hyper-
trophic joint
capsule

Fig. 7.**76** Coronal image
(GRE 500/11 out of phase
after administration of intravenous gadolinium contrast
medium) showing arthritis of
the first and second metatarsophalangeal joints. There is
significant contrast medium
enhancement of the joint
capsule.

as marked enhancement. The articulating surfaces are irregularly outlined and bear marginal osteophytes. The periarticular erosions are seen on all sequences.

Soft-Tissue Infections and Osteomyelitis
(Fig. 7.**77**)

Because of the serious clinical implications, MRI should be used early whenever a soft-tissue infection of the sole of the foot is suspected. The infected area is seen as increased signal intensity on the STIR image. The infection spreads along the muscular fasciae and within the plantar muscles.

Osteomyelitis develops after injuries and occurs as a frequent complication of diabetes mellitus. The bone-marrow space exhibits an increased signal intensity on the STIR image. If an abscess develops, the abscess cavity is surrounded by an enhancing rim

on the phase contrast image, while its content remains only moderately signal intense.

Tumors (Fig. 7.**78**)

Tumors of the midfoot and forefoot are rare. Angiomatous tumors are recognized by their spongiose structure, sometimes also by stellar, converging, linear structures. Furthermore, lipomas are recognized by their signal pattern, appearing bright on T1-weighted and T2-weighted images. The tissue diagnosis of other tumors is rarely possible. Most tumors have a heterogeneous pattern of increased signal intensities on STIR and T2-weightened images and show intense enhancement as evidence of an impaired blood-tissue barrier.

Fig. 7.**77** Transverse image (GRE 600/11 out of phase after administration of intravenous gadolinium contrast medium) showing a suppurative inflammation of the soft tissue of the ball of the foot. Contrast medium enhancement is seen in the infected tissue.

Contrast medium enhancement in infected tissue of the ball of the foot

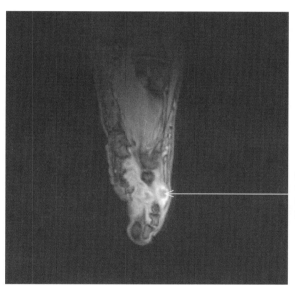

Fig. 7.**78** Sagittal image (GRE 500/11 out of phase after administration of intravenous gadolinium contrast medium) showing a tumor arising from the metaphysis of the fourth metatarsal. Histologic examination revealed a chondrosarcoma.

Cauliflower tumor with halo of contrast medium enhancement

References

Bernau A. *Orthopädische Röntgendiagnostik – Einstelltechnik.* Munich–Vienna–Baltimore: Urban & Schwarzenberg; 1990

Camasta CA, Sinnott Vickers N, Ruch JA. *Reconstructive Surgery of the Foot and Leg.* The Podiatry Institute, Inc; 1993

Endler F, Fochem K, Weil UH. *Orthopädische Röntgendiagnostik.* Stuttgart–New York: Thieme; 1984

Burgener F, Kormano M. *Differential Diagnosis in Conventional Radiology.* Stuttgart–New York: Thieme; 1985

Gould JS. *Operative Surgery.* Philadelphia: Saunders; 1994

Greenspan A. *Skelettradiologie.* Weinheim: VCH Verlagsges. edition medizin; 1993

Jahss MH. *Disorders of the Foot and Ankle.* Philadelphia: Saunders; 1991

Kaphandji IA. *Funktionelle Anatomie der Gelenke.* Vol 3. Stuttgart: Enke; 1992

Köhler/Zimmer, Schmidt H, Freyschmidt J, eds. *Grenzen des Normalen und Anfänge des Pathologischen im Röntgenbild des Skeletts.* Stuttgart–New York: Thieme; 1989

Mann RA, Coughlin MJ. *Surgery of the Foot and Ankle.* St Louis: Mosby; 1987

McGlamry ED, Banks AS, Downey MS. *Comprehensive Textbook of Foot Surgery.* Williams & Wilkins: Baltimore; 1992

Neale D, Adams IM. *Common Foot Disorders.* New York: Churchill Livingstone; 1989

Rabel CRH, Nyga W. *Orthopädie des Fußes.* Stuttgart: Enke; 1982

Ruland WO. *Dopplersonographische Diagnostik.* Cologne: Deutscher Ärzte-Verlag; 1993

Shereff MJ. *Atlas of Foot and Ankle Surgery.* Philadelphia: Saunders; 1993

Tachdjian MO. *The Child's Foot.* Philadelphia: Saunders; 1985

Wirth C-J, Ferdini R, Wülker N, ed. *Vorfußdeformitäten.* Berlin–Heidelberg–New York: Springer; 1993

8 Spine

8.1 Introduction

The spinal column forms the keel of the human body and is exposed to a variety of metabolic, mechanical, and circulatory stresses. Many of these stresses can lead to acute or chronic syndromes. Back pain is a symptom. In some cases, the symptom can be matched to a specific diagnosis, but in many cases this is not possible. Back pain is common in the industrialized world. Very rarely does an individual never suffer from back pain in his or her lifetime. Various studies have demonstrated that up to 80% of the population will suffer from back pain. Approximately 30% of the population has back pain at any moment. The cost of treating back pain is high; the cost of disability payments to workers with back pain may be two or three times the cost of treatment. With increased concern over medical spending, it is clear that diagnosis and treatment of back problems are of crucial importance for the individual and for society. This is not always an easy task, as is illustrated by the example of a prolapsed disk. In light of the fact that myelography (Hitselberger and Witten 1968), CT (Wiesel et al. 1984), and MRI (Boden et al. 1990, Jensen et al. 1994) can demonstrate prolapsed disks in a relatively high percentage of asymptomatic patients, the physician may not automatically presume that the presence of a prolapsed disk on imaging is the cause of symptoms in a patient suffering from pain in the back and legs. The enormous number of operations performed to treat prolapsed disks suggests that this sort of reasoning is widespread in day-to-day practice. The presumption that an imaging abnormality is the cause of the patient's pain is not always correct. Surgical treatment based on erroneous diagnostic decisions can have long-lasting consequences for the patient. Symptoms may persist because the surgically treated disk was not the cause of the symptoms, but a purely incidental finding. The persisting symptoms might then be categorized as a "post-discectomy syndrome," and not infrequently fusion of the affected segment of the spine is performed. The authors emphasize the importance of precise diagnosis prior to surgery on the lumbar spine (Castro et al. 1995) because the sequelae of an operation based on a faulty diagnosis can be more detrimental to the patient's health than the original disorder. The history and clinical examination are of extreme importance for a precise diagnosis. The changes documented in diagnostic imaging studies must always be evaluated in light of the patient's history and the findings of the clinical examination. The diagnostic significance of provocative tests such as discography or diagnostic infiltration such as selective nerve root blocks in the evaluation of back symptoms will be discussed in detail in the following sections.

References

Boden SD, Davis DO, Dina TS et al. Abnormal magnetic resonance scans of the lumbar spine in asymptomatic subjects; a prospective investigation. *J Bone Joint Surg.* 1990; 72–A: 403

Castro WHM, Bongartz G, Schulitz KP. Stellenwert der CT-Diskographie in der differenzierten Therapie des Bandscheibenvorfalles. *Deutsches Ärzteblatt.* 1995; 92: 352

Hitselberger WE, Witten RM. Abnormal myelograms in asymptomatic patients. *J Neurosurg.* 1968; 28: 204

Jensen MC, Brant-Zawadzki MN, Obuchowski N, et al. Magnetic resonance imaging of the lumbar spine in people without back pain. *N Engl J Med.* 1994; 331: 69

Wiesel SW, Tsourmas N, Feffer, et al. A study of computer-assisted tomography. The incidence of positive CAT scans in an asymptomatic group of patients. *Spine.* 1984; 9: 549

8.2 Clinical Standard Examination

The standard examination for the spine is similar to the procedure for the examination of the rest of the musculoskeletal system. However, physical examination techniques and neurologic examination play a more important role (Table 8.1). Performing the respective individual steps of the examination with the patient standing, sitting, and supine is a proven approach during inspection, palpation, and range-of-motion testing.

Table 8.1 Standard examination procedure

- History
- Inspection
- Palpation
- Range-of-motion testing and manual medicine examination
- Neurovascular examination
- Diagnostic imaging studies

Table 8.**2**   Overview of the clinical value of individual diagnostic imaging procedures according to the clinical syndrome

	Radiography	Myelography	Nuclear medicine studies	CT	MRI	Discography
Bone structure	++	–	–	+++	++	–
Facet arthritis	+++	–	++	+++	++	–
Prolapsed disk	–	++	–	+++	+++	++
Symptomatic disk (without prolapse	–	–	–	–	(+)	+++
Trauma	+++	+	++	+++	+++	–
Spondylitis	++	–	+++	++	+++	–
Deformities	+++	–	–	–	–	–
Tumor	+++	+	+++	+++	+++	–
Central spinal stenosis	+	+++	–	+++	+++	–
Lateral stenosis	(+)	–	–	+++	+++	–

–   No information content
(+)   Low information content
+   Moderate information content
++   High information content
+++   Very high information content

The examination begins when the patient's name is announced in the waiting area. Observe how the patient arises from the chair. Are arm rests used? Is he or she standing erect? Observe the patient's gait. Note any pain-related behaviour such as groaning or grimacing. Are ambulatory aids used? This period of observation and assessment is invaluable because it provides an opportunity to note how the patient functions outside of the examination room. Document your observations. Upon occasion, the formal examination may be different from these informal observations.

The formal examination begins by obtaining the history. Usually this will provide the basis for a working diagnosis. Next, inspect the patient's torso and cervical spine from behind. The patient should be undressed for this examination. Note any deviations from vertical, shoulder or pelvic obliquity, defective posture, scoliosis, and muscle contour. When inspecting the patient from the front, document any asymmetry in the face, neck, and rib cage, and note the muscle contour and skin folds.

The next phase of the examination is palpation of the posterior aspect of the spine to identify painful points at the spinous processes, vertebral articulations, transverse processes, capsular ligaments, and musculature of the back. Palpation can verify paravertebral spasms. It is important to exclude peripheral causes of pain in radiating pain syndromes by examining adjacent joints. These include primarily the sacroiliac joints, hips, and shoulders. After palpation, preliminary range-of-motion tests are performed for

the various segments of the spine in all three planes of motion. Again, adjacent joints should be examined to exclude referred pain. Once you have an initial overview and have assessed the range of motion of the spine, specific physical examination techniques help to more precisely localize and quantify dysfunction. Finally, neurologic examination is performed to exclude sensory deficits and paralysis of the upper and lower extremities. This includes testing intrinsic muscular reflexes and testing for nerve stretch signs. The standard examination procedure may be supplemented by special tests detailed in the following section depending on the tentative diagnosis.

The tentative diagnosis arrived at during clinical examination can be verified by diagnostic imaging studies. The choice of modalities supplementing plain radiography will depend on the working diagnosis. For example, CT with its higher contrast between bone and soft tissue is more suitable for visualizing changes in bone than MRI, whose advantage lies in its high-resolution visualization of soft tissue. Table 8.**2** provides an overview of the respective value of the individual diagnostic imaging modalities.

Patient History

As in all other areas of medicine, diagnosis of acute and chronic spinal disorders initially relies on obtaining a history. Chronic symptoms of underlying degenerative changes usually occur in the third or fourth decade of life and are either due to repetitive overuse

Table 8.3   Differential diagnosis of low-back pain

Spinal causes	Extraspinal causes
Discogenic Arthrogenous Spondylolisthesis Muscle or ligament insufficiency Osteoporosis Osteopathy Fracture Spondylitis, vertebral osteomyelitis Tumor, metastasis Ankylosing spondylitis Psoriatic arthritis Reactive spondylarthritis Baastrup disease Coccygodynia	**Urologic causes** (urolithiasis, cystitis, prostatitis, prostate tumor) **Gynecologic causes** (pregnancy, prolapsed uterus and vagina, retroflexion of the uterus, myomatosis, ovarian tumors, endometriosis) **Neurologic causes** (Borrelia or zoster infection, polyradiculoneuritis, angioma, intradural and extramedullary tumors) **Intra-abdominal causes** (gastric ulcer, duodenal ulcer, pancreatitis, cholecystitis, hepatitis, pyelonephritis, diverticulitis, visceral tumor) Aneurysm of the abdominal aorta **Psychological causes**

or misuse or occur as a response to the natural aging process. These symptoms have often been present in a milder form for years or even decades, and they may be intermittent or totally asymptomatic for long periods. Radiating pain often has its origin in the spinal column. Conversely, extravertebral disorders may initially manifest as pain in the spine.

Table 8.3 provides an overview of the various vertebral and extravertebral causes of pain in the low back.

Krämer (1994) differentiates between **discogenic pain** and **joint or ligamentous pain** in discussing the cause of pain in the low back. The former is characterized by a sudden onset that is dependent on position and stress. Hip and knee flexion usually alleviate the symptoms. Joint and ligamentous pain in the low back begins gradually and is characterized by a chronic, recurrent course. Pain is often more intense in the evening than in the morning.

Obtaining a detailed history often permits a differentiation to be made between disk pain, as in a prolapsed disk, and joint pain, as can occur in facet syndrome (Tables **8.4** and **8.5**).

Ask the patient to describe the symptoms as precisely as possible. The following questions are helpful:

Where?
How?
When?
How long?

Table 8.4   Typical symptoms reported by the patient in lumbar disk syndrome

- Sudden onset
- Erratic development
- Position dependent
- Pain increased by coughing, sneezing, and pressing

It is important to **localize** the pain as precisely as possible. Is it solely low-back pain, as in ankylosing spondylitis, or low-back and leg pain as in a prolapsed disk? Is pain concentrated at one point or does it radiate? The former suggests a muscular cause; radiating pain requires further distinguishing between radicular and nonradicular pain. Classic **radicular** pain, such as occurs with a prolapsed disk, is characterized by pain limited to one dermatome, occasionally in combination with sensory dysfunction and loss of strength in the muscle supplied by the nerve root. **Nonradicular** radiating pain, such as occurs with facet syndrome, is often diffuse, not limited to any particular dermatome, and rarely extends beyond the knee or elbow.

It is important to inquire about **sensory** or **motor deficits.** Ask the patient to describe these in detail. Inquire specifically about bowel and bladder dysfunction and, in addition, about alteration in sexual sensation or sexual function. The history can provide important information for differentiating radicular from nonradicular pain, and can permit an inference of the level of the affected segment. Bladder or rectal paralysis can occur with lesions in the cauda equina or conus medullaris. Weakness in dorsiflexors of the foot is attributable to a lesion of L5; weakness in the plantar flexors is attributable to a lesion of S1.

Table 8.5   Typical findings reported by the patient with facet syndrome (Hoppenfeld)

- Dull or stabbing pain in the low back
- Pseudoradicular pain radiating into both legs
- Pain rarely extends beyond the knee
- Radiating pain is difficult to localize
- Pain cannot be reliably localized in a specific dermatome
- Pain increases during the day
- Lying down eases pain

Table 8.**6** Typical symptoms of various spinal disorders

Prolapsed disk	Pain increased by coughing, sneezing, and pressing Segmental radiation Neurologic deficits
Facet syndrome	Pain in the small of the back with pseudoradicular radiation
Spinal stenosis	Intermittent spinal claudication Improves when the spine is moved out of lordosis
Ankylosing spondylitis	Deep-seated nighttime pain in the small of the back Morning stiffness Extravertebral findings

Table 8.**7** Relative age-dependence of certain clinical syndromes

Age	Clinical syndrome
First decade of life	Torticollis, Klippel–Feil syndrome
Second decade	Scoliosis, Scheuermann disease
Second to fourth decades	Ankylosing spondylitis
Third to fifth decades	Discogenic disorders
Fifth to eighth decades	Spinal stenosis

The type of pain and its **progression over time** can often be used to identify clinical syndromes. For example, **rheumatic spondylarthritis** and **ankylosing spondylitis** frequently present as deep-seated pain in the low back that increases late at night and improves during the course of the day. Morning stiffness is typical. Accompanying symptoms can include extravertebral findings such as monarthritis, polyarthritis, tendinitis at muscular insertions, chest pain with limited respiratory excursion, iridocyclitis, conjunctivitis, and urethritis.

Where the pain is chronic and progressive, a **spinal tumor** must be excluded. Inquire in detail about conditions that provoke the pain. For example, increased intra-abdominal pressure such as coughing, sneezing, or pressing increases intrathecal pressure and can produce pain in discogenic disorders. **Spinal stenosis** characteristically causes symptoms when the patient stands or walks, referred to as **neurogenic claudication.** Increased lumbar lordosis with these postures will narrow the spinal canal. The patient will finding walking uphill easier than walking downhill. Forward flexion typically alleviates pain. Vascular claudication must be excluded. Typically, vascular claudication is worse with exercise and improves with sitting. With vascular claudication there may be findings of decreased peripheral pulses or diminished vascular indices. Consultation with a vascular surgeon may be appropriate.

Several typical syndromes are summarized in Table 8.**6.**

The patient's age should always be considered. As Table 8.**7** shows, certain syndromes become clinically relevant in specific age-groups.

Not all spinal disorders involve pain. An example of this is scoliosis that is rarely painful in juveniles. However, other aspects of the history are important in this clinical syndrome. First, it is important to determine the extent to which other family members are affected by the disorder. Inquire about the extent of their respective deformities. It is helpful to query the patient about complications during pregnancy and birth, motor development, neuromuscular dysfunction, and other diseases such as connective-tissue disorders (Marfan syndrome or Ehlers-Danlos syndrome) or other syndrome disorders such as von Recklinghausen disease that are frequently associated with scoliosis (Table 8.**8**). The amount of curvature and the patient's physical maturity are factors used to predict curve progression (Table 8.**9**).

After an **accident,** inquire about the precise mechanism of injury, the use of seat belts, headrests, and air bags, cuts, bruises, impacts inside a vehicle, emergency medical treatment, and the degree of

Table 8.**8** Overview of the various causes of scoliosis

Idiopathic neuromuscular
  Infantile cerebral palsy
  Poliomyelitis
  Spinal muscle atrophy
  Cerebrospinal ataxia
  Muscular dystrophy
  Other disorders

Congenital
  Developmental disorders
  Failure of segmentation

Neurofibromatosis
Collagen development disorders
  Marfan syndrome
  Ehlers-Danlos syndrome

Chondrodystrophy
Osteogenesis imperfecta

Table 8.**9** Important history data for scoliosis patients

- Family history
- Complications during pregnancy or birth
- Motor development during childhood
- Associated disorders
- Neurologic deficits
- Time of menarche
- Signs of cardiopulmonary insufficiency
- Time of initial diagnosis
- Increase in the deformity

Table 8.**10** Important history questions for diagnosing injury to the cervical spine following an acceleration mechanism (adapted from Ludolph)

- Was the patient surprised by the accident, or could it be anticipated by looking in the rear-view mirror?
- From which side did the collision occur?
- Did the patient's head hit the windshield or other parts of the passenger compartment, or did it move freely?
- Was the patient wearing a seat belt?
- Did the car have air bags?
- Was the patient's head stopped by a headrest?
- What was the exact sitting position of the patient when the collision occured?

Table 8.**11** Clinical classification of whiplash-associated injuries

Grade	Clinical presentation
0	No complaints about the neck, no physical signs
I	Neck complaints of pain, stiffness, or tenderness only No physical signs
II	Neck complaints *and* musculoskeletal sign(s)*
III	Neck complaints *and* neurologic sign(s)+
IV	Neck complaints *and* fracture/dislocation

* Musculoskeletal sign(s) include decreased range of motion and point tenderness
+ Neurologic sign(s) include decreased or absent deep-tendon reflexes, weakness, and sensory deficits
Symptoms and disorders manifest in all grades include deafness, dizziness, tinnitus, headache, memory loss, dysphagia, and temporomandibular joint pain

Table 8.**12** Examples of sports involving minimal stress to the spine or detrimental to the spine (Castro and Schilgen, 1995)

Minimal-stress sports	Higher-rate sports
Swimming (especially backstroke)	Tennis
	Downhill skiing
Jogging (on soft ground)	Volleyball
Cross-country skiing	Basketball
Cycling (with high handlebars)	Football
	Soccer

damage to the vehicle. The forces acting on the body can provide important information about the structures that may be injured. An example is injury to the cervical spine after an acceleration or deceleration mechanism (whiplash). Without a history of an accident this is very difficult to diagnose because most patients in whiplash associated disorders (WAD) report symptoms that cannot be correlated with corresponding traumatic physical examination findings, and imaging studies are usually normal. Elements needed to define WAD often include an unexpected or surprise impact, an unsupported head and neck, and an immobilized torso. This indicates that no direct trauma has occurred to the cervical spine. Blunt trauma to the head resulting from collision with the windshield excludes the diagnosis of WAD from a rear-end collision (Ludolph 1995) (Table 8.**10**).

The report of the Quebec Task Force on Whiplash-Associated Disorders is important in clinical spine science. In the exhaustive synthesis of the literature, the task force identified five grades of whiplash-associated disorder (Table 8.**11**). These grades are not diagnoses but serve as adequate descriptions of the presentations, given that spine science has not yet identified with certainty what the injuries are. An increasingly important question is whether a technical analysis of the collision has been prepared; a change in velocity due to a collision provides information about the amount of force and resulting biomechanical stress (Weber 1995, Castro et al. 1997).

The history should include **occupational** and **leisure activities.** Repetitive overuse and misuse can be the cause of back pain.

Epidemiologic studies have demonstrated a relationship between low-back pain and the effects of vibration, for example in helicopter pilots or truck and tractor drivers. Behavior when sitting and posture appear to be more significant than the vibration itself with respect to the incidence of low-back pain.

Discogenic disorders of the cervical spine are less frequent than those of the lumbar spine. Repetitive

torsional stresses, high axial forces, and asymmetric loads on the cervical spine over an extended period of time are particularly detrimental. Military pilots and meat packers are occupational groups with these stresses.

The history should also include the patient's **athletic activities.** Sports that involve axial loads on the spinal column or strong torsional motions of the spinal column are particularly detrimental to the back. Sports that place minimal stresses on the spine include those whose motions relieve stress on the spine or those involving gentle, harmonic motions (Castro and Schilgen 1995) (Table 8.**12**).

Remember to ask about private circumstances that may coincide with the occurrence of symptoms. Often, factors such as personal or occupational problems coincide with the onset of symptoms. A history of the patient's **psychosocial situation** is particularly important for patients with chronic back pain. We know that the longer the duration of occupational disability the lower the chance of rejoining the workforce. The degree to which the patient is satisfied with his or her job is highly significant in this context.

Carefully inquire about the patient's psychosocial situation with respect to any planned surgical treatment. An unfavorable psychosocial profile can doom even the most carefully performed operation to failure. Patients in a worker's compensation setting show significantly poorer response to treatment than do patients who are not.

It is important to inquire about **smoking** since there is a known correlation between smoking and discogenic back pain.

To complete the patient's history, ask about **previous therapy.** Compile a list of operations, physical therapy, medication, and injections that is as comprehensive as possible and documents the respective success of these treatments. You will often find that patients with chronic back pain have previously consulted other physicians and that comprehensive diagnostic examinations have been performed.

Physical Examination

Physical examination begins with **inspection.** This provides the experienced examiner with a rough overview of function, alignment, and muscle development. Any abnormal findings can be investigated in greater detail during the further course of the examination.

Inspection begins the moment the patient arises from the chair in the waiting room and ambulates to the examining room. Evaluate the patient's gait, swing of the arms, and overall coordination. Watching the patient undress can provide important infor-

Fig. 8.**1**   Fifteen-year-old patient with severe spondylolisthesis at L5–S1 and pathologic lordosis.

Table 8.**13**   Diagnoses that can be made by inspection

- Torticollis
- Scoliosis
- Contour irregularities (such as thoracic hyperkyphosis)
- Spondylolisthesis and spondyloptosis

Table 8.**14**   Overview of selected findings at inspection

Inspection from posterior	Lateral inspection
Deviation from vertical in the coronal plane	Deviation from vertical in the sagittal plane
Shoulder obliquity	Sagittal profile
Pelvic obliquity	– Kyphosis of the thoracic spine
Triangles at the waist	– Lordosis of the lumbar spine
Michaelis rhomboid (visible rhomboid-shaped depression over the sacral area)	– Lumbosacral junction
Body hair	Active and passive posture
Muscle contour	

mation about impaired motion. Table 8.**13** summarizes a few diagnoses that can be made by observation.

Examination with the Patient Standing

Have the patient undress down to his or her underwear for further inspection. The patient should stand as erect as possible with both legs fully extended. Observe the patient from behind, from the side, and from the front. The patient's arms should hang down relaxed at the sides. Table 8.**14** lists important points for inspection. Palpation and range-of-motion tests can be integrated into the inspection phase of the examination. First, obtain a general impression of the patient's posture, musculature, and axial symmetry. Note the position of the hips, knees, and ankles. In extreme spondylolisthesis or spondyloptosis, extreme lordosis will be present; slender patients will show a step sign in the spinous processes (known as a "ski-jump" phenomenon; Fig. 8.**1**). **Skin changes** such as café-au-lait spots or neurofibromas can be clinical signs of generalized neurofibromatosis (von Recklinghausen disease), a systemic disorder frequently asso-

b

a

Figs. 8.**2a, b** Patient with generalized neurofibromatosis. Findings include multiple fibromas and several café-au-lait spots (**a**); café-au-lait spot in the same patient (**b**).

ciated with scoliosis (Figs. 8.**2a, b**). Localized hypertrichosis in the region of the spinous processes suggests failure of fusion of the vertebral arches (Fig. 8.**3**).

Inspection from behind may proceed from superior to inferior or in the opposite direction. The important point is to inspect systematically to minimize the risk of overlooking pathologic changes. Beginning from superior, note the **posture of the head** that is characteristically altered in torticollis. The course of the **spinous processes** provides further information; palpation permits more precise evaluation. Follow the spinous processes from the cervical spine into the thoracic spine. Significant deviation of the row of spinous processes from the midline of the coronal plane is usually due to severe scoliosis since the rotational component is only sufficient to shift the row of spinous processes away from the coronal midline in severe cases. The level of the shoulders and scapulae (Figs. 8.**4** and 8.**5**) provides important information about scoliotic deformities. Shoulders should be level and the scapulae should blend smoothly and symmetrically into the posterior musculature. Peripheral neuropathy should be excluded as a possi-

ble cause of asymmetry in this region. **Muscle contour** should be symmetric on both sides; document any muscular atrophy or hypertrophy. The **triangles at the waist,** bounded by the arms hanging loosely at the patient's sides, should be symmetric. Asymmetric triangles at the waist are seen primarily in scoliosis and are an important clinical sign of an underlying deformity (Fig. 8.**4**). A vertical plumb line suspended from the spinous process of C7 should intersect the gluteal cleft in a balanced spine. Scoliosis should be excluded whenever the spine is seen to deviate from vertical (Fig. 8.**6**). Inspect the **Michaelis rhomboid** for symmetry. This figure is formed by the two iliac spines, the spinous process of L5, and the most proximal point of the gluteal cleft (Fig. 8.**7**).

Bending test. Instruct the patient to bend forward. Document the projection of the ribs and the lumbar bulge, both of which are important signs of scoliotic deformity of the spine. Rib projection is due to rotation of the ribs in an angular deformity frequently associated with scoliosis (Figs. 8.**8**–8.**10**). The lumbar bulge is caused by projection of the paravertebral musculature on one side as a result of the rotational deformity. A scoliometer can be used to clinically quantify the severity of the rotational deformity (Fig. 8.**11**).

Table 8.**15** summarizes the range-of-motion tests described in the following section.

The results of this test should be compared to the degree of hip flexion achieved during manual motor testing of hip flexors. A discrepancy between formal and informal tests of lumbar spine motion suggests a nonanatomic cause for decreased motion.

Distance between fingers and floor. To test the range of motion of the spine, first instruct the patient

Table 8.**15** Overview of range-of-motion tests of the spine

- Distance between fingers and floor
- Ott test
- Schober test
- Neutral-zero method

Fig. 8.**3**   Lumbosacral hypertrichosis

Fig. 8.**4**   Fourteen-year-old patient with idiopathic right convex thoracic scoliosis. Note the asymmetric level of the scapulae and the reduced triangle at the waist on the right side.

Fig. 8.**5**   Twenty-two-year-old patient with right convex thoracic scoliosis and a high thoracic left convex countercurvature that lowers the level of the right shoulder.

to bend over as far as possible with the knees fully extended. Measure the distance between the patient's fingers and the floor (Fig. 8.**12**). Normally this should be 0–10 cm, but it may be greater without underlying pathology. The bending test can also be evaluated as a nerve-stretch test (Lasègue test with the patient standing); findings can be compared with the results of the Lasègue test with the patient sitting and supine.

Ott and Schober signs. Next, check for the Ott and Schober signs. Locate the most prominent spinous process (C7). Measure 30 cm caudal to this landmark and mark the site. Note any changes in the length of this line that occur as the patient bends forward and backward. Ott cites lengthening of 2–4 cm and shortening of 1 cm as normal.

To perform the Schober test, use S1 as the starting point for measuring a line extending 10 cm craniad. Document changes in the length of this line as the patient bends forward and backward as far as possible. Normal values for this test are 4–7 cm of lengthening and 3 cm of shortening (Figs. 8.**13a–c**). The thoracolumbar spine can be further evaluated by defining a 10 cm line with its midpoint at L1 and measuring the changes in length as the patient bends forward and backward.

Neutral-zero method. The neutral-zero method permits a more precise measurement of the range of motion of the spine in all three planes. Measurements are performed with the patient standing or sitting (see Table 8.**19** for normal values).

Fig. 8.**6**   Fifteen-year-old patient with idiopathic right convex thoracic scoliosis in a long arc, deviating from vertical to the right.

Fig. 8.**7**   Symmetric Michaelis rhomboid.

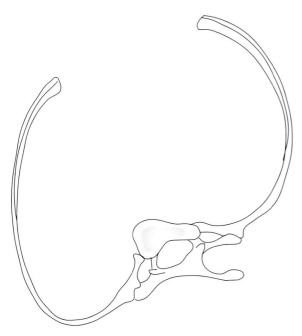

Fig. 8.**8**   Diagram of a rib with an angular deformity. The rotation of the vertebra in thoracic scoliosis raises the rib and causes it to project when the patient bends over.

To evaluate **pelvic version in the coronal plane** palpate the highest point of each iliac crest, ensuring the best possible contact with the bone to minimize measurement errors. Locate and compare first the anterior iliac spines, then the posterior iliac spines. Palpate them from distal to proximal according to their anatomic orientation. This permits precise evaluation of pelvic version in the coronal plane. Isolated **pelvic obliquity** may be recognized by the difference in height of both the iliac spines and iliac crests. Asymmetric iliac crests without a difference in leg length can be excluded by evaluating the AP pelvis radiograph.

Isolated pelvic obliquity without a rotational component is a reliable sign of a **leg-length difference** (Lewit 1977) (Fig. 8.**14**). To obtain a more accurate measurement of the leg-length difference, place standardized measuring plates under the shorter leg until the pelvis is level. Precise evaluation of the leg length and axis deviation requires radiographic measurements.

Pelvic obliquity can occur without a difference in leg length. In these cases, it is usually accompanied by a **rotational deformity of the pelvis.** This is recognized by the asymmetric position of the iliac spines.

Fig. 8.**9**   Anterior view of forward-bending test in a 15-year-old patient with right convex thoracic scoliosis and severe projection of the ribs on the right side.

Fig. 8.**10**   Posterior view of the same patient as in Fig. 8.**9**.

Fig. 8.**11**   Projection of the ribs is measured in degrees using a scoliometer placed at the level of maximum projection.

Fig. 8.**12**   The distance between the patient's fingers and the floor is measured to evaluate the range of motion of the spine.

Scoliosis is a frequent cause of pelvic rotation of this type (Fig. 8.**15**). Table 8.**16** lists important landmarks for palpation of the spine and pelvis.

Table 8.**16**   Important landmarks for palpation of the spine and pelvis

- Spinous process
- Iliac crest
- Anterior inferior iliac spine
- Anterior superior iliac spine
- Sacroiliac joint
- Greater trochanter

Figs. 8.**13a–c**   Overview of the Ott and Schober signs in evaluating the range of motion of the spine (FFD = Finger-floor distance).

- **Pathologic anterior movement of the posterior iliac spines**

Next locate the posterior iliac spines and instruct the patient to forward flex again. Observe whether the iliac spines move anteriorly. This is a sign of limited motion in the sacroiliac joints. If motion in the sacroiliac joints is limited, the posterior superior iliac spine on the affected side will move superiorly (Figs. 8.**16a, b**). Pathologic anterior movement of the posterior iliac spine can be tested with the patient supine (Figs. 8.**17a, b**) if there is a difference in leg length.

Spine test. This is a further test for examining the sacroiliac joints. Locate the posterior superior iliac spine on one side with your thumb. Mark the position of the median sacral crest at the same level with your other thumb. Then instruct the patient to lift the leg on the palpated side. Normally the iliac spine will dip as a result of the motion of the sacroiliac joint. If the sacroiliac joint is impaired, compensatory tilting of the pelvis will cause the iliac spine to move superiorly (Figs. 8.**18a, b**).

Trendelenburg sign. Instruct the patient to stand on one leg to evaluate the pelvic and trochanteric musculature (gluteus medias and minimus). Pelvic version in the coronal plane can be evaluated at the same time. If muscular weakness results in poor stabilization of the pelvis, a positive Trendelenburg sign will be present: the pelvis will dip toward the side of the flexed leg (Figs. 8.**19a, b**).

Next, inspect the standing patient from the side. This will reveal posture and structural changes such as thoracic hyperkyphosis (Figs. 8.**20** and 8.**21**) or gibbus. Thoracic hyperkyphosis can occur in combination with lumbar hyperlordosis. However, this is more difficult to detect by inspection because of the thicker mantle of soft tissue covering the lumbar spine. Spondylolisthesis appears as a step sign; the severe forms produce what is known as a "ski-jump" phenomenon (see Fig. 8.**1**). Normally, the spine forms a slightly curved double S profile with kyphotic curves in the

Fig. 8.**14**   Genuine leg-length difference in a scoliosis patient that manifests itself in pelvic obliquity with a left tilt. The measurement is made with a pelvic scale.

Fig. 8.**15**   Severe pelvic obliquity in a patient with neuromuscular left convex lumbar scoliosis; the cause is pelvic version resulting from an underlying spinal deformity.

spine and sacrum and lordotic curves in the cervical and lumbar spine.

Postures are categorized as lumbar hyperlordosis, thoracic hyperkyphosis, thoracic hyperkyphosis and lumbar hyperlordosis in combination, and flat back (Figs. 8.**22a–f**).

Inspection from anterior completes this phase of clinical examination. This reveals facial asymmetry as can occur in muscular torticollis, deformities of the rib cage, or deformities such as the transverse folds in the abdominal wall that are often present in thoracic hyperkyphosis (Table 8.**17**). Inspection of the anterior musculature is important in conjunction with pelvic obliquity and lumbar hyperlordosis. The axis of vision is clinically relevant in ankylosing spondylitis (Bechterew disease) in particular. Kyphotic stiffening of the

Table 8.**17**   Findings during anterior inspection

- Axis of vision
- Facial asymmetry
- Rib cage deformities
- Transverse abdominal folds

entire spine, including the cervical spine, means that the patient can no longer see straight; a horizontal visual axis can no longer be achieved.

After inspection is completed, test the **range of motion of the cervical spine** and measure the distance between the chin and sternum. This should measure 0 cm with the cervical spine in flexion, and approximately 20 cm with the cervical spine in maximum extension. The range of motion may be reassessed with the patient sitting.

In ankylosing spondylitis measure also the distance between the external occipital protuberance and the wall, with the patient's heels touching the wall. This distance should normally be 0 cm and is typically higher in ankylosing spondylitis (Fig. 8.**23**). This measurement should allow for possible hip contractures that often accompany the disorder, possibly also contributing to the deviation of the torso. Finally, measure the **excursion of the rib cage during respiration** at the level of the nipples. Normally, this is 5–10 cm in young adults. In ankylosing spondylitis, it can be reduced at an early age (Table 8.**18**).

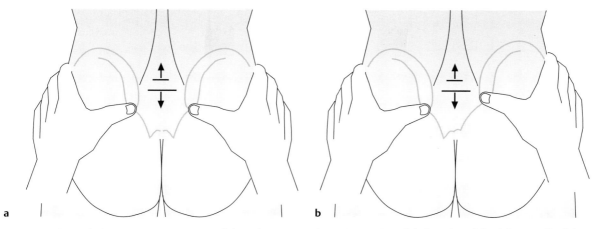

Figs. 8.**16a, b**   Pathologic anterior movement of the right posterior iliac spine is a sign of dysfunction of the right sacroiliac joint.

Figs. 8.**17a, b**   Changing length of the right leg is observed with dysfunction of the right sacroiliac joint. As the patient sits up with the legs extended (**b**), asymmetric superior motion of the right medial malleolus is observed relative to findings with the patient supine (**a**). This is a sign of impaired motion in the right sacroiliac joint.

Figs. 8.**18a, b**   In a normal spine test, the motion of the sacroiliac joint as the ipsilateral hip is flexed causes the iliac spine to dip.

a   **b**

Figs. 8.**19a, b**   Schematic diagram of a positive Trendelenburg sign.

Table 8.**18**   Important clinical findings in ankylosing spondylitis

- Axis of vision
- Distance between external occipital protuberance and wall
- Chest excursion during respiration
- Hip contractures
- Spinal curvature

Examination with the Patient Sitting

The rest of the examination is performed with the patient sitting. Normal values of the cervical spine are approximately 45°–50° for lateral bending, and 80° for rotation from a neutral position. The **cervical spine** is the most mobile segment of the spinal column. Only its lateral bending is limited to any great extent, primarily by the uncinate processes.

Where extension of the cervical spine is reduced, instruct the patient to repeat the test with the mouth open to relax the anterior musculature of the neck. If the patient then achieves greater extension, shortening of the musculature is responsible for the limited motion.

The **thoracic spine** is the least mobile segment of the spinal column. This is due to its articulations with the rib cage. Only the lower thoracic spine is somewhat more mobile because of the floating lower ribs. Extension is greatly limited due to the shingle-like arrangement of the articular processes.

▲
Fig. 8.**21**   The same patient as in Fig. 8.**20**. The kyphotic deformity is even more apparent when the patient bends over.

◄ Fig. 8.**20**   Eighteen-year-old patient with thoracic hyperkyphosis in Scheuermann disease. The severity of the kyphosis can be measured in degrees during clinical examination using a kyphometer.

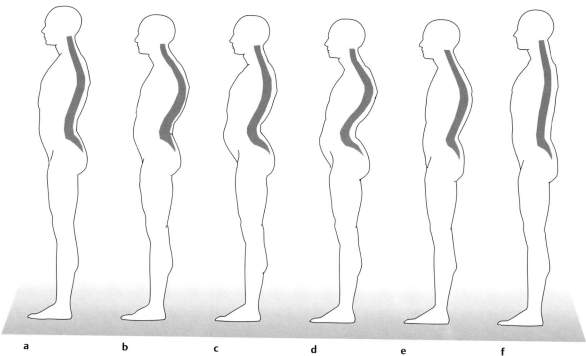

Figs. 8.22a–f Overview of various types of posture: (**a**) physiologic, (**b**) thoracic hyperkyphosis, (**c**) lumbar hyperlordosis, (**d**) thoracic hyperkyphosis and lumbar hyperlordosis in combination, (**e**) total kyphosis, (**f**) flat back.

Fig. 8.23 Measurement of the distance between the occipital bone and the wall with the patient standing erect.

The **lumbar spine** has a relatively large range of motion in the sagittal and coronal planes but limited rotation due to the sagittal orientation of the facet joints. Rotation in the cervical and thoracic spines is about 30° in both directions. Next measure the range of lateral bending toward both sides. Normal values are 20°–40° (Table 8.**19**).

Examination with the Patient Lying Down

• Examination with the patient prone

The patient is prone for the next part of the examination. First palpate the spinous processes, beginning proximally. The first palpable spinous process is usually the second cervical vertebra. C7 can readily be localized because of its prominence and the fact that the spinous process of C6 disappears next to C7 as the patient extends the cervical spine. The iliac crests are other important landmarks that are usually at the same level as the spinous process of the fourth lum-

Table 8.**19**   Normal values in degrees for the range of motion of the spine according to the neutral-zero method

Cervical spine		Thoracic and lumbar spine	
Flexion/extension	50/0/70	Flexion/extension	120–130/0/20–30
Lateral bending	45/0/45	Lateral bending	20–40/0/20–40
Rotation (in neutral position)	80/0/80	Rotation	30/0/30
Rotation (flexion)	45/0/45		
Rotation (extension)	60/0/60		

Fig. 8.**24**   Kibler fold in the region of the thoracic spine.

Fig. 8.**25**   Springing test in segmental examination of the thoracic spine.

bar vertebra. Palpation of the row of spinous processes helps to detect common sites of pain, axial deviations, failure of fusion of the vertebral arches, and step signs in spondylolisthesis. The interspinous ligaments should also be examined for painful sites. Comparative palpation of the paravertebral musculature on both sides can reveal differences in tone indicative of segmental dysfunction.

Palpate the iliolumbar ligaments at the point where the spine joint the pelvis. These ligaments originate on the transverse processes of the fifth lumbar vertebra and extend to the medial aspect of the iliac crest. Continue by palpating the sacrum and sacroiliac joints. The sacrospinal and sacrotuberal ligaments and the clinically significant piriformis will be palpable in the deep plane in slender patients. The relaxed gluteal musculature permits palpation of the ischial tuberosities and the hamstrings that originate there. The adductor magnus is also palpable. **Rectal palpation of the coccyx** may be necessary to evaluate coccygodynia injury following a fall on the buttocks (see Fig. 9.**12**, p. 428).

Kibler fold. Examine the paravertebral musculature for spasm. Placing the cervical spine in extension relaxes the muscle fascia and facilitates palpation. To localize muscle tension, grasp a fold of skin adjacent to the spine with the thumb and index finger and displace it superiorly (Fig. 8.**24**). An experienced examiner can determine differences in muscle tone by locally reduced suppleness that may be painful.

Springing test. This test may be used to examine joint play and tenderness in the individual segments. Place your index and middle fingers on the vertebral arch or the inferior articular processes and test the segment by applying slight pressure to the fingers with the ulnar edge of the other hand (Fig. 8.**25**).

Reversed Lasègue sign. You can test for the reversed Lasègue sign with the patient prone (Fig. 8.**26**). Passively hyperextend the leg at the hip while flexing the knee to apply an additional stretching stimulus. Radiating pain on the anterior thigh can suggest a nerve root irritation syndrome at L3–L4 (stretching pain in the femoral nerve) or shortening of the rectus femoris or iliopsoas. With nerve-root irritation syndromes, it is essential to compare both sides.

Mennel's first sign. This sign is elicited by a stress test of the sacroiliac joint performed with the patient prone. Immobilize the pelvis on one side by applying pressure to the sacrum and placing the ipsilateral hip in hyperextension. The sign is positive if the patient feels pain in the sacroiliac joint (Fig. 8.**27**). The test for Mennel's second sign is performed with the patient supine (Fig. 8.**28**).

Three-step test. This test is performed to differentiate symptoms in the lumbar spine, sacroiliac joint, and hip. In contrast to the test for Mennell's first sign, begin by immobilizing the superior lumbar spine while placing the ipsilateral hip in hyperextension. This places stress on the inferior facet joints of the lumbar (first step). The second step is the same as in testing for Mennell's first sign, although your immobilizing hand now only stabilizes the sacrum to place stress on the sacroiliac joint. In the third step, evaluate irritation in the ipsilateral hip by moving your

Fig. 8.**26** Reversed Lasègue sign. The hip is in hyperextension. Flexing the knee creates an additional stretching stimulus.

Fig. 8.**27** Mennell's first sign. Immobilize the sacrum with one hand while placing the ipsilateral hip in hyperextension with the other.

Fig. 8.**28** Mennell's second sign. This test places stress on the left sacroiliac joint.

Fig. 8.**29** Shaking test of the right sacroiliac joint.

Fig. 8.**30** Kneeling test for evaluating the flexibility of kyphotic deformities.

Fig. 8.**32** Bragard sign

Fig. 8.**31** Lasègue sign

hand further inferior to immobilize the pelvis in the acetabular region while placing stress on the hip by hyperextending the leg.

Shaking test. Palpate the sacroiliac joint inferomedial to the posterior superior iliac spine. With your other hand, grasp the wing of the contralateral ilium at the level of the anterior superior iliac spine. Now apply slight posterior shaking motions (Fig. 8.**29**). Where there is normal joint play in the sacroiliac joints, you will be able to feel fine movements with your palpating hand. Lack of, or limited motion in comparison to the contralateral side suggests hypomobility.

Valleix points. Deep palpation can subject the sciatic nerve to direct pressure between the ischial tuberosity and greater trochanter. Additional Valleix points are located along the course of the sciatic nerve on the posterior thigh. An irritated nerve will react with increased tenderness to palpation.

Kneeling test. This final test may be used to evaluate the flexibility of kyphotic deformities. Instruct the patient to assume a kneeling position and to attempt

to stretch out on the examining table or floor with the arms extended as far as possible (Fig. 8.**30**).

● **Examination with the patient supine**
The patient is supine for the next part of the examination. It can be difficult to distinguish pseudoradicular pain from radicular pain. For example, irritation of the lumbar roots of the sciatic nerve from a prolapsed disk can elicit the nerve stretching sign.

Lasègue sign. With the Lasègue sign, passively lifting the extended leg 60° or less elicits pain extension from the low back into the calf or foot (Fig. 8.**31**).

It is important to distinguish this from a **false Lasègue sign** that involves pain radiating only as far as the knee due to stretching of the hamstrings. As a result of the one-sided pelvic version, pain with a Lasègue sign can also be a function of sacroiliac joint disease. In this case, differential diagnosis is made by repeating the test with both hips flexed and the legs extended; this eliminates the twisting of the pelvis so that the test will be negative if isolated dysfunction of the sacroiliac joint is present.

Bragard sign. The Lasègue sign can be intensified by passive dorsiflexion of the foot Fig. 8.**32**). Document the degree of hip flexion that causes pain.

Sit-up with legs extended. A final version of the test for the Lasègue sign should be performed by instructing the patient to sit up with the legs extended. This test and previous findings with the patient standing should be considered when evaluating the Lasègue

a b

Figs. 8.**33a, b** In the reclining test, nerve root irritation when expanding the leg will cause the patient to move backward in compensation (**b**).

sign to eliminate the possibility that the patient may be simulating symptoms.

Kernig sign. A different version of the Lasègue sign is the Kernig sign. This produces the same pain when the knee is passively extended with the hip flexed 90°. The same test can be performed with the patient sitting by having the patient extend the knee. This so-called **reclining test** is positive if the patient's torso moves backward (Figs. 8.**33a, b**). The various nerve-stretch signs are listed in Table 8.**20**.

An important differential diagnosis with back and leg pain is piriformis syndrome. In this syndrome, the piriformis is tender to palpation with noticeable pain in internal rotation (stretching) or painful external rotation and abduction against resistance (contraction) in the affected hip.

Patrick four-part sign. The Patrick test may be performed to further evaluate sacroiliac joint dysfunc-

Table 8.**20**   Stress tests for nerve root irritation

- Lasègue sign
- Bragard sign
- Sit-up with legs extended
- Reclining test
- Kernig sign
- Reversed Lasègue sign

tion that can simulate S1 nerve root irritation symptoms. The patient's leg is extended and the pelvis is immobilized on the examining table by applying pressure to the anterior superior iliac spine to eliminate pelvic motion. Flex the patient's other knee and abduct the other hip, keeping the foot of the leg supported by the contralateral knee (Fig. 8.**34**). Normally the knee of the abducted sign will reach the examining table. However, comparison of both sides is more important. Difference in mobility between the two sides with painfully restricted hyperabduction suggest dysfunction in the ipsilateral sacroiliac joints if hip disorders can be excluded and if the adductors are normal. Hip disorders can be eliminated by evaluating the range of motion of the hip (particularly rotation) and palpating the capsule of the hip in the deep plane of the groin. Other signs of a hip disorder include tenderness of the trochanter to palpation and pain upon axial compression.

Mennell's second sign. Mennel signs are also regarded as tests that place stress on the sacroiliac joint. Compared to Mennel's first sign with the patient prone, the pelvis can be more effectively immobilized with the patient supine and the contralateral knee and hip in maximum flexion (Thomas grip). At the same time, the affected hip is hyperextended past the edge of the examining table, which places stress on the sacroiliac joint. Mennell's second sign is positive if pain is elicited in the region of the sacroiliac joint (Fig. 8.**28**).

Fig. 8.**34**   In the test for the Patrick four-part sign, stress is placed on the ipsilateral sacroiliac joint by abducting and externally rotating the hip.

Fig. 8.**35**   Elasticity test of the left sacroiliac joint.

Elasticity test of the sacroiliac joint (including femur). To directly test the play in the sacroiliac joint, flex the contralateral knee and hip with the patient supine. Adduct the leg toward you until the pelvis begins to follow (the other leg remains extended). Next, grasp the knee of the adducted side and briefly apply elastic axial pressure to the knee while palpating the sacroiliac joint with the other hand. Normally this will produce elastic motion in the sacroiliac joint that will be palpable as relative motion between the posterior iliac spine and sacrum (Fig. 8.**35**). Lack of joint play in this test is typical of joint dysfunction (Eder and Tilscher 1995). This elasticity test is based on the principle that the range of motion of any intact joint can be increased, even when the joint is at the end of its range of motion, by applying elastic pressure. In principle, this type of test can be used to manually diagnose dysfunction in any joint. However, it is important to place stress on the joint before performing the test (Lewit 1977).

Changing leg length (Figs. 8.**17 a, b**, p. 301). The variant of the test for pathologic anterior movement of the posterior iliac spines can be performed with the patient supine. The length of both legs is evaluated using the medial malleoli as reference points as the patient sits up from a supine position. Loss or limitation of movement in the sacroiliac joint will produce a relative increase in leg length on the affected side. Table 8.**21** summarizes the individual stress tests of the sacroiliac joint.

- **Examination with the patient in a lateral position**

Segmental range-of-motion testing in the lumbar spine is performed with the patient in a lateral position with both hips and knees flexed. Stand facing the patient, grasping both calves with one hand. The patient's legs may rest on your thighs to give you more information about the respective motion. With your free hand, palpate two adjacent spinous pro-

Fig. 8.**36** Segmental range-of-motion testing of the lumbar spine (lateral bending) with the patient in a lateral position.

cesses and the respective interspinal space. Successively test each segment in flexion, extension, and in a neutral position by passively moving the lower extremities. The same examining technique can be used to detect a limited range of motion in lateral bending. Evaluate lateral bending by lifting and lowering the patient's calves (Fig. 8.**36**). Locally limited or increased mobility, indicative of segmental dysfunction, is regarded as pathologic.

Neurologic Examination

Neurologic examination of the spine includes the upper and lower extremities and the torso. Initially this entails testing muscles, sensation, reflexes, and coordination, including relevant autonomous functions.

Motor deficiencies involving paralysis are categorized as flaccid or spastic paralysis. The former occurs when the lower motor neuron is damaged or in spinal shock; the latter occurs as a result of a lesion of the upper motor neuron. This can be demonstrated by

Table 8.**21**   Stress tests for the sacroiliac joints

- Mennell's first sign
- Mennell's second sign
- Elasticity test including femur
- Shaking test
- Test for pathologic anterior movement of the posterior iliac spines with patient standing
- Changing leg length
- Spine test
- Patrick four-part sign
- Three-step test

what is known as the jackknife phenomenon in which increased muscle tone is suddenly overcome after maximum muscle extension. Other clinical signs include the so-called pyramidal tract signs that are discussed in the individual sections.

Neurologic Examination of the Upper Extremities

Neurologic examination of the upper extremities may begin by having the patient clasp the hands behind the head and behind the back (Figs. 8.**37** and 8.**38**). This will give you a rough overview of the patient's capacity for abduction, external or internal rotation in the shoulder, and flexion in the elbow. Joint diseases should be distinguished from neurologic deficits.

Detailed examination of **muscle strength** involves testing the strength of individual muscle groups with the patient sitting. Elbow flexion against your resistance can be used to test segments C5 and C6. Segment C7 and C8 are tested by evaluating elbow extension. Muscle strength is graded on a scale of 0 (no palpable contractility) to 5 (normal muscle strength) as shown in Table 8.**22**. Latent paralysis of the upper examination can be tested by instructing the patient to extend both arms in supination with the eyes closed (**arm-extension test).** Pronation and subsequent lowering of one arm suggest a latent central hemiparesis. An arm that drops before the hand moves into pronation while the patient's eyes are closed may be attributable to psychogenic influence (Figs. 8.**39a, b**).

Sensory supply to the upper extremities is divided into band-shaped dermatomes (Figs. 8.**40a, b**).

The important **intrinsic muscle reflexes** of the upper extremity include the biceps and brachioradialis reflexes (C5 and C6), the triceps reflex (C7), and Trömner reflex (C8) that involves tapping the

Fig. 8.**37**   Clasping the hands behind the head.

Fig. 8.**38**   Clasping the hands behind the back.

a

b

Figs. 8.**39a, b**   Arm extension test for evaluating latent central hemiparesis characterized by pronation and subsequent lowering of the affected arm.

Table 8.**22**   Muscle grading chart

Muscle gradation	Muscle reaction
0	No palpable contractility
1	Evidence of slight contractility, but insufficient to move the extremity with gravity eliminated
2	The muscle is able to move the extremity with gravity eliminated
3	The muscle is able to move the extremity against gravity
4	The muscle moves the extremity against some resistance
5	Normal muscle strength against resistance

Table 8.**23**   Examination of the neurologic levels of the cervical spine

Nerve root	Intrinsic muscle reflex	Muscles involved
C5	Biceps reflex	Deltoid, biceps
C6	Brachioradialis reflex	Biceps, brachioradialis
C7	Triceps reflex	Triceps, thenar eminence
C8	Trömner reflex	Flexors of the fingers, hypothenar eminence

patient's fingertips to elicit reflexive flexion of the distal phalanges including the thumb (Figs. 8.**41**–8.**44**). The Trömner and snap reflexes are both intrinsic reflexes of the flexors of the fingers. If they can be elicited on both sides, they only indicate a greater sensitivity to reflex stimuli; unilateral response is regarded as a pyramidal tract sign. Table 8.**23** summarizes the individual intrinsic muscle reflexes and the respective muscles involved.

According to Krämer (1994) most monoradicular cervicobrachial syndromes involve the intervertebral disk C5–C6, affecting nerve root C6 (C6 syndrome). This is followed by intervertebral disk spaces C6–C7 and C7–T1 with the associated C7 and C8 syndromes. Table 8.**24** shows the incidence of nerve-root involvement in monoradicular cervicobrachial syndrome.

For a preliminary test of coordination, instruct the patient to close his or her eyes and to touch the nose with the index finger in a long sweeping motion. Another coordination test is the **diadochokinesis test**

Table 8.**24**   Incidence of monoradicular cervicobrachial syndromes (Krämer)

Affected nerve root	Incidence
C5	4.1%
C6	36.1%
C7	34.6%
C8	25.2%

Figs. 8.**40a, b**   Overview of the sensory dermatomes of the upper extremities (**a**) and lower extremities (**b**).

Fig. 8.**41**   Biceps reflex

Fig. 8.**42**   Brachioradialis reflex

Fig. 8.**43**   Triceps reflex

Fig. 8.**44**   Trömner reflex

Fig. 8.**46**   Heel position with weakness of the extensors of the left great toe in a prolapsed disk at L4–L5.

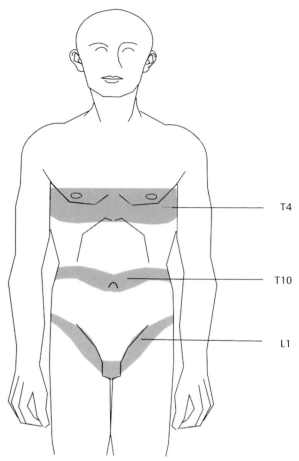

Fig. 8.**45**   Anatomical landmarks on the surface of the torso for determining the level of transverse paralysis.

in which the patient alternately performs supination and pronation motions, as if screwing in a lightbulb.

Neurologic Examination of the Surface of the Torso

Neurologic examination of the surface of the torso is useful primarily in determining the level of transverse lesions. Note that the cord usually ends at the level of L1 or L2 where it joins the cauda equina. From about T1 on, the segments are shifted superiorly because of the early cessation of growth of the spinal cord so that segment T12 lies at about the level of the ninth thoracic vertebra. The sacral segments begin at about the 11th or 12th thoracic vertebra.

Only the spinal groups between C8 and L2 have sympathetic fibers so that sympathetic deficiencies such as disturbed sweat secretion should not be expected in injuries below the 10th thoracic vertebra. The nipples (T4–T5), umbilicus (T10), and the groin (L1) are helpful anatomic landmarks on the torso (Fig. 8.**45**). Transverse lesions superior to the fourth cervical vertebra results in loss of function in the phrenic nerve that produces bilateral paralysis of the diaphragm and respiratory insufficiency.

The **superficial abdominal reflexes** are physiologic reflexes that may be used to evaluate segments T6 through T12. These reflexes are tested by rapidly moving a needle across the skin from lateral to medial at the level of the inferior costal arch and umbilicus, and superior to the inguinal ligament. A polysynaptic reflex arc produces contraction of the abdominal musculature.

Neurologic Examination of the Lower Extremities

Neurologic examination of the lower extremities in patients capable of standing and walking begins by observing their gait. Instruct the patient to stand and walk on tiptoe and on the heels (Fig. 8.**46**). This is usually performed to exclude major motor deficiencies. With the patient supine, evaluate the strength of the quadriceps in knee extension (L3–L4), the extensor digitorum and hallucis longus in dorsiflexion of the toes (L5), and the triceps surae in plantar flexion of the foot (S1). The patient should perform these motions against your resistance. Where there are negative findings, exclude latent central hemiparesis

Fig. 8.**47** Leg-holding test to detect latent hemiparesis of the lower extremities.

Fig. 8.**48** "Saddle anesthesia" with loss of sensation in dermatomes S3–S5.

in the **leg holding test.** Instruct the patient to close his or her eyes and flex both hips and knees at right angles. Lowering of the calf is a sign of latent central hemiparesis (Fig. 8.**47**).

Sensory supply to the torso and lower extremities is divided into band-shaped dermatomes (Figs. 8.**40a, b**). The most important areas of sensory supply are in order of their clinical significance in nerve-root irritation syndromes: 1 segment S1 that extends in a posterolateral strip from the buttock to the lateral margin of the foot; 2 the region supplied by segment L5 extending from lateral and passing slightly inferior to the patella and across the lateral malleolus into the great toe; 3 segment L4 with its dermatome extending from the thigh across the knee to the medial malleolus. A prolapsed disk between L5 and S1 can affect nerve roots L5 and S1. In a mediolaterally prolapsed disk, the inferior root is affected (in this case S1); a laterally prolapsed disk affects the superior root (in this case L5). Combined compression of both nerve roots can also occur.

The **perianal region** receives its sensory supply from segments S3–S5 and is important in cauda equina syndrome. In these cases, what is known as "saddle anesthesia" typically occurs due to loss of sensory supply from segments S3–S5, with disturbed micturition, defecation, and sexual function (Fig. 8.**48**). The tone of the anal sphincter in such cases is reduced and clinically significant. It can be evaluated by instructing the patient to close it around your palpating finger during rectal examination. Other clinical signs of cauda equina syndrome include lack of anal and bulbocavernosus reflexes that present as extrinsic differences of segments S3–S5 (Masuhr and Neumann 1992; Table 8.**27**). With a medially prolapsed disk, partial flaccid paralysis will often be present with radicular loss of sensation.

The next phase of the examination involves testing reflexes. Table 8.**25** lists the respective muscles tested with their segments. The two most important intrinsic muscle reflexes in the lower extremities are the patellar reflex (L3–L4) and the Achilles tendon reflex (S1–S2). Other intrinsic muscle reflexes include the tibialis posterior reflex (L5), elicited by tapping the tibialis posterior tendon superior of inferior to the medial malleolus, and the adductor reflex (L3–L4), which can be elicited by tapping the medial femoral condyle (Figs. 8.**49**–8.**52**). The adductor reflex is difficult to elicit. Since the patellar reflex tests the same segment, it can be used instead. If reflex response is weak, the **Jendrassik maneuver** (Figs. 8.**53a, b**) can be used to emphasize the patellar reflex and facilitate evaluation.

Table 8.**25** Examination of the neurologic levels of the lumbar spine

Nerve root	Intrinsic muscle reflex	Muscles involved
L3	Adductor reflex, patellar reflex	Hip adductors, quadriceps femoris
L4	Patellar reflex	Quadriceps femoris, tibialis anterior
L5	Tibialis posterior reflex	Extensor hallucis, tibialis anterior
S1	Achilles tendon reflex	Triceps surae, gluteus maximus

Fig. 8.**49**   Patellar reflex

Fig. 8.**50**   Achilles tendon reflex.

Fig. 8.**51**   Tibialis posterior reflex.

Fig. 8.**52**   Adductor reflex

If a lumbar nerve root is irritated or injured, **monoradicular lumbar syndrome** will result. 98% of the time the L5-S1 or L4-L5 segments are affected (Krämer 1994). The rest is distributed among the proximal lumbar segments (Table 8.**26**).

However, a purely monoradicular syndrome is present in only about half of all cases. Often several nerve roots are affected simultaneously. For example, a prolapsed disk in the most distal segment of a five-

Table 8.**26**   Incidence of monoradicular lumbar syndromes (Krämer)

Affected nerve root	Incidence
L2	0.5%
L3	0.5%
L4	1.0%
L5	43.8%
S1	54.2%

segment lumbar spine can compress both the nerve roots L5 and, laterally, S1 (Fig. 8.**54**). A far lateral disk prolapse at this level can also produce only an L5 syndrome. However, a mediolateral prolapse with predominantly S1 symptoms is frequent.

Numerous **variations of the lumbar spine** can make neurologic diagnosis difficult. For example, in a four-segment lumbar spine, the nerve root L5 courses through the first sacral foramen. In a six-segment lumbar spine, the nerve root S2 courses through this foramen (Figs. 8.**55a–c**).

The **physiologic superficial reflexes** are polysynaptic and exhaustible proprioceptive reflexes, in contrast to the monosynaptic intrinsic muscle reflexes. These include the cremasteric reflex in which contraction of the cremaster may be elicited by stroking the medial side of the upper thigh (L1–L2), the bulbocavernosus reflex in which contraction of the bulbocavernosus is elicited by stroking the dorsum of the penis, and the anal reflex in which stroking of the perianal region causes contraction of the anal sphincter (S3–S5) (Table 8.**27**).

Figs. 8.**53a, b** Jendrassik maneuver (**a**) applied when eliciting the patellar reflex (**b**).

The physiologic superficial reflexes require central stimulation and are weakened or absent when the upper motor neuron is damaged. Subsequently, flaccid paralysis will develop into spastic paralysis with increased intrinsic muscle reflexes due to the lack of inhibition from central efferents. The severity of the spastic paralysis will increase, the higher the neurologic level of injury. Where the lower motor neuron is damaged, both intrinsic muscle reflexes and superficial reflexes will be absent.

After this examination, test for pathologic reflexes (**pyramidal tract signs**). These signs are positive if injury to the upper motor neuron, the pyramidal tract, is present. They can be elicited by stroking

Table 8.**27** Neurologic level of the various physiologic superficial reflexes

Physiologic reflex	Neurologic level
Cremasteric reflex	L1–L2
Bulbocavernosus reflex	S3–S4
Anal reflex	S3–S5

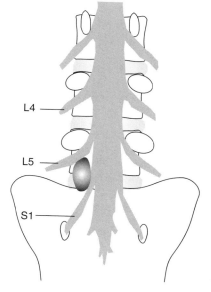

Fig. 8.**54** A sufficiently severe laterally prolapsed disk at L5–S1 can compress nerve root L5 inside the foramen and nerve root S1 laterally.

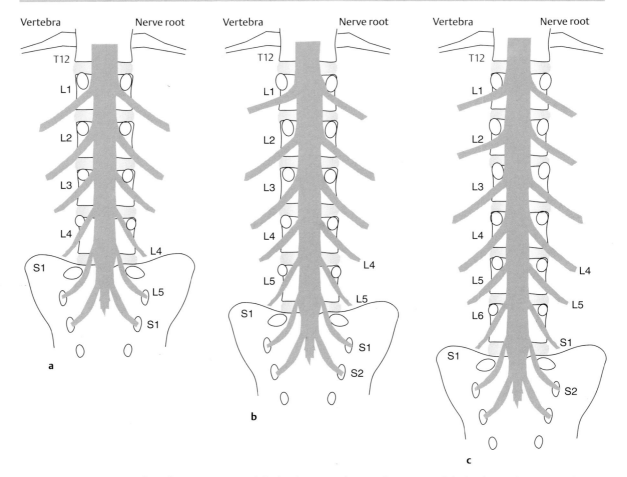

Figs. 8.**55a–c** Overview of numbering variations of the lumbar spine showing the courses of the lumbar and upper sacral nerve roots ([a] four non-rib-bearing lumbar-type vertebrae; [c] six non-rib-bearing lumbar-type vertebrae).

the lateral sole of the foot (Babinski) or by pressing on the muscles of the calf (Gordon). Tonic dorsiflexion of the great toe with abduction of the other toes is characteristic.

A brief coordination test concludes examination. Instruct the patient to touch the patella with the contralateral heel with his or her eyes closed.

References

Castro WHM, Schilgen M. *Kreuzschmerzen. Ursachen, Behandlung, Vorbeugung.* Berlin–Heidelberg–New York: Springer; 1995

Castro WHM, Schilgen M, Meyer S, Weber M, Peuker C, Wörtle K. Do "whiplash injuries" occur in low speed rear impacts. Eur Spine J. 1997; 6: 366–375.

Eder M, Tilscher H. *Chirotherapie.* Stuttgart: Hippokrates; 1995

Hoppenfeld S. *Klinische Untersuchung der Wirbelsäule und der Extremitäten.* Stuttgart–New York: Fischer; 1992

Krämer J. Kreuzschmerzen aus orthopädischer Sicht. *Deutsches Ärzteblatt.* 1994; 5: 227

Lewit K. *Manuelle Medizin.* 2nd ed. Munich–Vienna–Baltimore: Urban & Schwarzenberg; 1977

Ludolph E. Das Halswirbeltrauma nach geringer Belastung. In: Weber M, ed. Die Aufklärung des Kfz-Versicherungs-betruges – Grundlagen der Kompatibilitätsanalyse und Plausibilitätsprüfung. *Schriftenreihe Unfallrekonstruktion.* MS; 1995

Masuhr KF, Neumann M. *Neurologie.* Stuttgart: Hippokrates; 1992

Weber M, ed. Die Aufklärung des Kfz-Versicherungsbetruges – Grundlagen der Kompatibilitätsanalyse und Plausibilitätsprüfung. *Schriftenreihe Unfallrekonstruktion.* MS; 1995

8.3 Radiology

Indications, Diagnostic Value, and Clinical Relevance

As in all other imaging of the musculoskeletal system, films taken in two planes at right angles to each other provide the basic studies for radiologic diagnosis of the spinal column. The AP and lateral projections of the spinal column can be taken with the patient supine or standing. In an AP radiograph with the patient supine, flexing the patient's hips during the exposure will compensate for physiologic curves of the spine. This will expose the intervertebral spaces although the radiograph will only show the bony details. If there are anomalies in the sagittal and coronal planes, a standing radiograph should be prepared.

Table 8.**28** Clinical value of plain-film radiographs of the spine

Bone structure	++
Facet arthritis	+++
Disk prolapse	−
Symptomatic disk without prolapse	−
Trauma	+++
Spondylitis	++
Deformities	+++
Tumor	+++
Spinal stenosis (central)	+
Lateral stenosis	(+)

−	No information content
(+)	Low information content
+	Moderate information content
++	High information content
+++	Very high information content

Full-length spine radiographs should always be prepared to allow sufficient evaluation of all secondary curves, the position of the pelvis, and deviations from vertical that may be present.

Certain situations will require additional **special views** such as the open-mouth odontoid view for diagnosing a dens fracture. Right and left oblique views are obtained to image the facet joints and the foramina for diagnosing spondylolysis. **Flexion and extension views** of the spine are used to diagnose instability or loss of motion in patients with back pain. Side bending views are used to assess curve flexibility.

Plain-film radiographs are of limited value in diagnosing soft-tissue conditions (Table 8.**28**). However, these conditions must be evaluated in patients with back pain or in the presence of injuries to the spinal cord. CT and MRI are valuable in such cases. Invasive studies such as myelography, and in rare cases discography, can provide important information.

Cervical Spine

Standard Views

AP view (Figs. 8.**56** and 8.**57**). The AP radiograph may be taken with the patient standing or supine. The central ray is aimed at the fourth cervical vertebra (at the level of the Adam's apple) and angled cranially

Fig. 8.**56** In the AP radiograph of the cervical spine, the central ray is angled cranially, approximately 15°–20° from horizontal.

15°-20°

Fig. 8.**57** Plain PA radiograph of the cervical spine. Normal findings in a 30-year-old female patient.

a

b

Figs. 8.**58a, b** The lateral radiograph may be taken with the patient supine or standing. The central ray is aimed at the middle of the fourth cervical vertebra.

Fig. 8.**59** Plain lateral radiograph of the cervical spine. The image shows normal findings.

approximately 15°–20°. This projection provides good exposure of the cervical vertebrae C3–C7 (and in young patients often the atlas and axis as well), the uncovertebral joints (Luschka joints) with the uncinate process, and the disk spaces. The spinous processes are imaged almost head on and cast oval tear-shaped shadows.

The atlas and axis are visualized by having the patient quickly open and close his or her mouth to obscure the mandible. This provides a good image of the first two cervical vertebrae.

Lateral views (Figs. 8.**58a, b** and 8.**59**). The lateral radiograph may be taken with the patient supine, standing, or sitting. This view of the cervical spine is valuable because the important traumatic changes to the cervical spine are discernible. Visualized structures include the anterior and posterior arch of the atlas, the dens in profile, and the distance between atlas and dens. The vertebral bodies and the spinous processes are visible from C2–C7, and the disk spaces and prevertebral soft tissue can be evaluated. The central ray is aimed at the middle of the fourth cervi-

cal vertebra in this projection. The entire seventh cervical vertebra and the top plate of the first thoracic vertebra should be visualized on a lateral radiograph. Failure to do so could lead to missing a fracture (Figs. 8.**82a, b**, see p. 327).

The lateral radiograph of the cervical spine, including the base of the skull, is important to evaluate subsidence involving the atlantoaxial joint and migration of the dens to the foramen magnum. The extent of cranial displacement of the dens can be reliably determined using Chamberlain's line from the posterior margin of the foramen magnum, McGregor's line from the lowest point of the base of the occiput to the posterior margin of the hard palate, or McRae's line to the anterior margin of the foramen magnum (Figs. 8.**60**–8.**62**). Normally, the dens should not be more than 3 mm above Chamberlain's line, and no more than its tip should intersect McRae's line. The dens should not project more than 4.5 mm beyond McGregor's line. Since the hard palate is often difficult to define on the conventional lateral radiograph, Ranawat et al. (Greenspan, 1993) developed another method for measuring the superior protru-

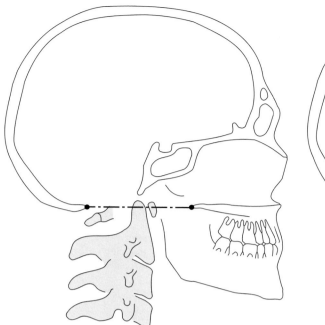

Fig. 8.**60** Chamberlain's line extends from the posterior margin of the hard palate to the anterior margin of the occiput. The tip of the dens axis should normally not project to more than 3 mm above this line.

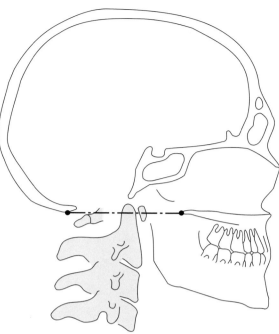

Fig. 8.**61** McGregor's line extends from the posterior margin of the hard palate to the inferior margin of the occiput. The tip of the dens axis should normally not project to more than 4.5 mm above this line.

Fig. 8.**62** McRae's line extends from the anterior margin of the foramen magnum to the anterior margin of the occiput. The tip of the dens axis should normally not project above this line.

sion of the dens. First, the coronal axis of the atlas is marked with a line. Next, the center of the anterior sclerosed ring of the axis is located and a line is drawn cranially, parallel to the axis of the dens. The distance to the point of intersection with the atlas line should average 17 mm in men and 15 mm in women (Fig. 8.**63**).

Special Views

Open-mouth odontoid view (Figs. 8.**64** and 8.**65**). To measure the dens axis, an AP radiograph is prepared with the patient's mouth open and the central ray aimed at the middle of the open mouth. The patient should say "ah" to avoid shadows from the tongue. This view provides good exposure of the cervical articular pillars (lateral masses) of the atlas, the entire axis with the dens, and the atlantoaxial joints with the lateral spaces. The Fuchs odontoid process position can be useful for better visualizing the tip of the dens in particular. In this position the cervical spine is overextended and the central ray is aimed slightly below the tip of the chin.

Oblique views (Figs. 8.**66a, b** and 8.**67**). These views are used for visualizing the intervertebral foramina. The actual oblique radiographs of the cervical spine are taken in an AP or PA projection with the patient sitting upright. The patient is turned 45° to one side of the room and the respective contralateral foramina are imaged in an AP projection. The central ray is

Fig. 8.**63** Ranawat's method for measuring the protrusion of the dens axis. The coronal axis of the atlas is marked with a line; another line, parallel to the axis of the dens, is drawn cranially from the center of the anterior sclerosed ring of the axis. The distance to the point of intersection with the atlas line is then measured.

Fig. 8.**64**   The open-mouth odontoid view is an AP protection with the mouth open. The X-ray beam is aimed at the middle of the open mouth.

Fig. 8.**65**   Plain radiograph of an open-mouth odontoid view. The image shows normal findings.

Figs. 8.**66a, b**   To image the facet joints and the intervertebral foramina of the cervical spine, the patient stands at an angle of approximately 45° to the X-ray beam. The beam is angled cranially, at approximately 15°–20°.

Fig. 8.**67**   Plain radiograph of the cervical spine in an oblique projection. The image shows narrowing of the foramen at the C6–C7 level.

Figs. 8.**68a, b**   The AP axial oblique position allows evaluation of the lateral masses. The patient is supine with the cervical spine overextended and the X-ray beam angled 30°–35° caudally toward the thyroid from vertical. It can also be prepared as an oblique projection by turning the patient's head 45°, aiming the central ray at a point 3 cm below the earlobe, and angling the tube 35°–40° caudally from vertical.

Fig. 8.**69**   The swimmer's view is used to image the cervicothoracic region. The arm on the side of the film cassette is placed alongside the body. The arm on the side of the X-ray beam is abducted 180° and the beam is aimed at the axilla.

aimed at the fourth cervical vertebra and is angled cranially 15°–20°.

AP axial oblique position (Figs. 8.**68a, b**). This position permits visualization of the lateral masses of the cervical vertebrae (Greenspan 1993). The radiograph

can be prepared with the patient supine and the neck overextended and the central ray aimed at the thyroid cartilage and angled 30°–35° caudally. It can also be prepared as an oblique projection of the lateral masses by turning the patient's head 45°, aiming the central ray at a point 3 cm below the earlobe, and angling the tube 35°–40° caudally.

Swimmer's position (Figs. 8.**69** and 8.**70**). This position is used for visualizing vertebrae C7, T1, and T2, which are often obscured by the clavicle and shoulder in conventional views. This view is prepared with the patient supine. The arm on the side of the film cassette is placed alongside the body. The contralateral arm is abducted 180°, and the X-ray beam is aimed at the axilla.

Fig. 8.**70**   Plain radiograph of the swimmer's view with the patient prone. Postoperative image after treatment of a teardrop fracture at C6/C7.

Figs. 8.**71a, b**   The flexion and extension views of the cervical spine can be obtained with the patient sitting. It is important to demonstrate the seventh cervical vertebra. It may be necessary to give the patient weights to hold to prevent the shoulders from obscuring the C7–T1 level. The X-ray beam is aimed at the center of the cervical spine as in the lateral projection.

Dynamic Views

These views should only be obtained after bony instability has been excluded. They are helpful in evaluation of the function of the cervical spine. Various methods are used to measure mobility.

Flexion and extension views are taken in a lateral projection. These are done with a fully conscious, cooperative patient without neurologic deficits. The patient is encouraged to obtain maximum voluntary flexion and extension. The study may be done with fluoroscopic visualization or plain films in maximum flexion and extension (Figs. 8.**71a, b** and 8.**72 a, b**).

Dynamic views represent an important method for diagnosing **atlantoaxial instability** resulting from lesions of the transverse ligament of the atlas or the alar ligaments. They can be traumatic, inflammatory, or congenital in origin (os odontoideum). In the flexion radiograph, less than 3 mm between the anterior margin of the dens and the posterior margin of the anterior arch of the atlas is regarded as physiologic (Greenspan 1993). Values between 3 mm and 5 mm indicate a lesion of the transverse ligament of the atlas, and values between 5–8 mm suggest the presence of an additional lesion of the alar ligaments.

The **lateral flexion radiographs** are taken in an AP projection. The lateral borders of the dens and lateral masses are the bony landmarks. Atlantoaxial instability manifest itself in the lack of physiologic

a

b

Figs. 8.**72a, b**   Plain radiographs of the cervical spine in flexion and extension. Note the AP translation at C2–C3; (**a**) flexion, (**b**) extension.

forced rotation of the dens in the direction of inflammation and in the failure of the atlas to shift in the same direction (Drerup 1985). Increasing lateral flexion will also cause the other cervical vertebrae to rotate; the degree of rotation decreases from cranial to caudal.

The motion components of the axis (rotation, tilting, and transverse shift) are tightly integrated. The tilting and transverse shift increase as rotation increases. A disturbance in this motion pattern is apparent in the so-called dissociation phenomenon in which the extent of rotation of the axis and the combined tilting and transverse shift appear dissociated (Dihlmann 1987).

Traumatic Changes in the Cervical Spine

Injuries to the cervical spine almost always result from indirect forces acting on the head and skull. The site and nature of damage are determined by the position of the head and cervical spine at the time of the accident. According to Daffner (1986), a force acting on the cervical spine always produces a similar pattern of injury, regardless of the site. A differentiation is made between flexion, extension, compression, shear, rotation, and distraction injuries. The stability of such an injury can be evaluated by examining

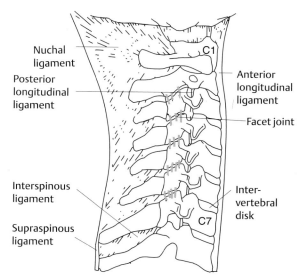

Fig. 8.**73**   Important ligamentous structures in the cervical spine.

the spinal ligaments (Fig. 8.**73**). Holdsworth has defined the so-called *posterior ligamentous complex,* consisting of the supraspinous ligament, interspinous ligament, and flaval ligaments, and the capsules of the small vertebral joints. If these structures are intact,

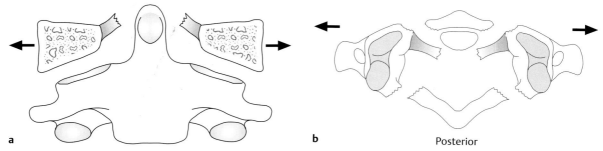

Figs. 8.**74a, b** Schematic diagram of a Jefferson fracture. When both transverse ligaments of the atlas are torn, the lateral masses of the atlas are shifted laterally.

Figs. 8.**75a–c** Schematic diagram of classification of dens fractures according to Anderson and D'Alonzo.
Type I: oblique fracture in the upper dens axis area.
Type II: transverse fracture at the base of the dens axis.
Type III: fracture at the base of the dens axis extending into the body of the axis.

the fracture can be regarded as stable. Radiologic signs of instability include vertebral displacement an increase in the distance between spinous processes or laminae, gaping facet joints, a widened or elongated spinal canal, or an interruption in the posterior longitudinal line (Daffner 1986). If only one of these criteria is present, then the injury to the cervical spine must be regarded as unstable. However, precise evaluation of the bony architecture of the spinal canal will require CT studies. Soft tissue is best visualized using MRI.

● **Frequently encountered injuries to the cervical spine**

Jefferson fracture. Axial forces acting through the occiput on the atlas and axis can shatter the atlas, causing symmetric fractures of the anterior and posterior arches and tearing the transverse ligament. In a plain radiograph this compression injury is best imaged in the open-mouth odontoid view (Figs. 8.**74a, b**).

Dens fracture. Hyperflexion of the cervical spine can shift the dens anteriorly. It can also sublux anteriorly between the atlas and axis. In rare cases, hyperexten-

Fig. 8.**76** Plain lateral radiograph of the upper cervical spine. Dens fracture in a child.

Fig. 8.**77** Plain radiograph of the dens (tomography) in the coronal plane. Pseudarthrosis of the dens.

Fig. 8.**78** Plain radiograph (lateral tomography) of the upper cervical spine. The image shows typical radiologic changes suggestive of os odontoideum.

sion can result in injury to the dens with posterior subluxation. Dens fracture are also classified according to Anderson and D'Alonzo (Figs. 8.**75a–c**). Type I generally involves a diagonal fracture line superior to the base of the dens. Type II describes a fracture through the base of the dens. In type III, the fracture spreads into the body of the axis. These injuries are best diagnosed in a plain radiograph obtained using the conventional open-mouth odontoid view or the Fuchs odontoid process position (Fig. 8.**76**). Type II fractures according to Anderson and D'Alonzo are accompanied by a higher rate of pseudarthrosis (Fig. 8.**77**). The differential diagnosis of dens fractures should always exclude an os odontoideum (Fig. 8.**78**).

Hangman fracture. In 1912 Wood-Jones studied the pathologic mechanism of execution by hanging. He found that simultaneous hyperextension and distraction causes bilateral fractures of the base of the arch of the axis with anterior subluxation and subsequent severing of the spinal cord. This form of fracture is also observed in injuries to the cervical spine involving extension. The lateral projection is best for imaging the fracture in these patients (Figs. 8.**79a, b**).

Compression fracture. Hyperflexion of the cervical spine results in compression of the anterior aspect of the vertebral body without injury to the posterior ligamentous complex. This is a stable form of fracture and can be demonstrated in a conventional lateral radiograph.

Burst fracture. Axial force acting on the lower cervical vertebrae (C3–C7) can cause a fracture of the endplate of the vertebra that may extend to the anterior and posterior margin of the body of the vertebra, rupturing the anulus fibrosus and compressing the nucleus pulposus into the neighboring vertebra. The retropulsion of the posterior fragments can result in narrowing of the spinal canal. If the posterior ligamentous complex is also ruptured, then it should be assumed that the fracture is unstable. The commi-

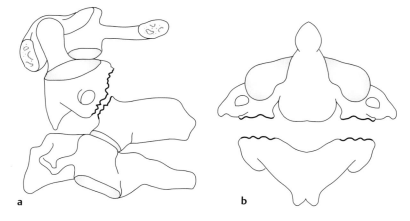

Figs. 8.**79a, b**   Schematic diagram of a hangman fracture. Bilateral fractures of the base of the arch of the axis with anterior subluxation and subsequent severing of the spinal cord.

Figs. 8.**80a, b**   Plain radiograph of the cervical spine in two planes showing a burst fracture of C5.

nuted fracture and the posterior margin of the affected vertebral body can be seen on the lateral radiograph (Figs. 8.**80a, b**).

Teardrop fracture. This flexion injury is regarded as the most unstable form of all injuries to the cervical spine. Subluxation or dislocation of the affected vertebra, accompanied by a tear in the posterior capsular ligamentous structures (Fig. 8.**81**), is the cause of this frequently observed syndrome with immediate quadriplegia and loss of sensitivity to pain and temperature. The teardrop fragment is created by avulsion of the anterior longitudinal ligament which generally

remains attached to a fragment of bone. This fracture can be reliably diagnosed in the lateral radiograph (Figs. 8.**82a, b**). It is important to distinguish the classic teardrop fracture from the stable avulsion teardrop fracture, in which an anterior bony projection may be seen but the capsular ligaments remain intact and subluxation is not present (Greenspan 1993). These two fractures can be differentiated using CT with a sagittal reconstruction (Fig. 8.**198**, see p. 388).

Clay-shoveler fracture. Forceful flexion or, in rare cases, direct trauma, can cause an oblique fracture of the spinous process in the sixth or seventh cervical vertebra. This is a stable fracture that can generally be readily diagnosed in the lateral radiograph. If the seventh cervical vertebra is obscured, the swimmer's position should be used. In the AP radiograph, the displacement of the fragment will appear as a double-contour spinous process.

Perched facets. A flexion rotation injury causes a rupture of one or both facet joint capsules and the posterior ligamentous complex (Fig. 8.**83**). This is an unsta-

Fig. 8.**81** Schematic diagram of a teardrop fracture. In this unstable fracture, a teardrop-shaped bone fragment is avulsed from the anterior margin of the body of the vertebra (**1**). The posterior capsular ligaments are also torn (**2**).

Fig. 8.**83** Schematic diagram of a perched facet. The capsule of the facet joints and the posterior ligaments are ruptured. The facet joint has dislocated and the superior joint facet has become wedged in front of the inferior joint facet.

Figs. 8.**82a, b** Plain radiographs in two planes (**a**) and lateral spot view (**b**) of the cervicothoracic region (as shown in Fig. 8.**198**, p. 388). (**a**) A fracture is not discernible in the standard radiographs in two planes. However, only six vertebrae are visible in the lateral image. (**b**) The fracture dislocation is only revealed in the spot view.

Fig. 8.**84** Plain lateral radiograph of the cervical spine. The image shows changes in the cervical spine with degenerative joint disease and degenerative disk disease.

Fig. 8.**85** Plain lateral radiograph of the cervical spine. The image shows pseudospondylolisthesis at C5–C6.

Fig. 8.**86** Plain AP radiograph of the cervical spine. Uncovertebral arthritis in a 25-year-old female patient.

ble injury that is recognizable in the lateral radiography by the subluxation or dislocation of the facet joints in which the articular pillars appear to be shaped like a bat's wing.

Degenerative Changes in the Cervical Spine

As in the other synovial joints of the human body, degeneration of the cervical spine occurs in the form of arthritic changes (see section Degenerative Changes in the Lumbar Spine). The classic signs of arthritis such as narrowing of the joint space, subchondral sclerosis, and formation of osteophytes are observed here as well (Figs. 8.**84** and 8.**85**). Since the thickness of the intervertebral disks decreases with age, uncovertebral arthritis will often develop (Fig. 8.**86**), which is readily discernible in the AP radiograph. The foramina and the small vertebral joints are easier to evaluate in the oblique views (Fig. 8.**87**). Extensive spondylarthritis can cause irritation of the nerve roots with pain radiating into the back of the neck, shoulders, and arms. For this reason, oblique views of the cervical spine can provide valuable information in diagnosing a shoulder-arm syndrome. In addition, dynamic views provide important

Fig. 8.**87** Plain radiograph of the cervical spine, oblique view. The image shows narrowing of the C3–C4 foramen.

Fig. 8.**89** Plain AP radiograph of the thoracic spine. Thirty-four-year-old patient with symptomatic thoracic spine. Radiologic findings are normal for this age (see also Fig. 8.**92**).

Fig. 8.**88** To obtain the AP radiograph of the thoracic spine with the patient supine, the patient's hips and knees are slightly flexed. The X-ray beam is aimed at the midline approximately 3 cm superior to the xiphoid process.

indications of disturbed motion with segmental hypomobility or hypermobility. White et al. (1975) have an instability grading system of the cervical spine. One component of this system includes more than 3.5 mm of AP translation between flexion and extension.

Thoracic Spine

Standard Views

AP view (Figs. 8.**88** and 8.**89**). The thoracic spine can be imaged with the patient standing or lying down. When a radiograph is obtained in the supine position, the patient's hips and knees should be flexed slightly to compensate for physiologic kyphosis. This provides exposure of the intervertebral spaces. The central ray is aimed at the midline approximately 3 cm superior to the xiphoid process.

The end-plates of the vertebrae are readily discernible in the supine radiograph, as are the intervertebral spaces. The pedicles appear as oval radiolucencies that form the lateral margin of each vertebra. This position also permits evaluation of the costotransverse joints. The spinous processes appear as drop-shaped projections in the midline.

Lateral view (Figs. 8.**90**–8.**92**). A technique similar to tomography is used to image the thoracic spine. The patient breathes shallowly to obscure the surrounding soft tissue and to enhance the section of the spine being imaged. The radiograph can then be obtained with the patient standing with his or her arms raised or lying down. The central ray is aimed at the sixth thoracic vertebra.

The vertebral bodies and intervertebral disk spaces can be readily evaluated in the lateral view. The pedicles and the intervertebral foramina are also imaged. The kyphotic angle in the normal thoracic spine is +20°–+40° according to Cobb (Bernard and Bridwell 1989; Bradford et al. 1974; Moe et al. 1994; Propst-Prockor and Bleck 1983; Roaf 1960). The meas-

Fig. 8.**90** For the lateral view of the thoracic spine, the patient stands with arms raised. The X-ray beam is aimed at the middle thoracic spine at the level of the sixth thoracic vertebra.

a

b

Figs. 8.**91a, b** Lateral view of the thoracic spine with the patient lying down. The X-ray beam is aimed at the middle thoracic spine at the level of the sixth thoracic vertebra.

urement is taken from the superior end-plate of the fourth vertebral body and the inferior end-plate of the 12th vertebral body. Stagnara et al. (1982) examined 100 test subjects and found an average kyphotic angle of +37° within a range extending from +7°–+63°. The thoracolumbar junction from T10–L2 marks the transition from kyphosis to lordosis and should normally have a neutral orientation. Bernard and Bridwell (1989) observed an average kyphotic value for the superior thoracolumbar spine (T10–T12) of +5.5° within a range from –3°–+20°. The inferior thoracolumbar spine (T12–L2) showed an average lordosis value of –3° within a range extending from –23°–+13°.

Special Views

Special views such as oblique views or dynamic studies are less common in imaging the thoracic spine. Oblique projections can provide information about bony structures constricting the intervertebral foramina in intracostal neuralgia. Flexion and extension views or lateral bending views can provide important evidence of disturbed motion with segmental hypermobility or hypomobility.

Fig. 8.**92** Plain lateral radiograph of the thoracic spine. The image shows the sagittal view of the spine shown in Fig. 8.**89**. This projection shows normal radiologic morphology for this age.

Scoliosis views (full-spine radiographs in two planes, AP and lateral) are special views to evaluate the entire spine in three dimensions. These views are obtained with the patient standing. Possible differences in leg length are equalized by placing standardized spacers under the shorter leg. A 30 × 90 cm film cassette allows imaging of the entire spine, including the pelvis and femoral heads.

Traumatic Changes in the Thoracic Spine

Changes to the thoracic spine due to trauma are similar to those in the lumbar spine. The thoracolumbar junction is the region of the spine most frequently affected by spinal injuries. For a detailed classification of individual fractures, see the section on the lumbar spine.

Degenerative Changes in the Thoracic Spine

As in the cervical and lumbar spine, degenerative changes in the thoracic spine are characterized by narrowing of the joint spaces with subchondral sclerosis and especially with development of osteophytes. Spondylosis deformans (Figs. 8.**93a, b**) is charac-

terized by the development of anterior and lateral osteophytes. The intervertebral disks may be intact or may exhibit symptoms of degenerative disk disease. In the lateral view, spondylosis must be distinguished from ankylosing spondylitis (Bechterew disease) with fine syndesmophytes and from Forestier disease, diffuse idiopathic skeletal hyperostosis (DISH). An anterior prolapsed intervertebral disk can appear as a small triangular bony projection, the limbus vertebrae, which should not be confused with a fracture (Greenspan 1993).

Lumbar Spine

Standard Views

AP view (Figs. 8.**94** and 8.**95**). The lumbar spine can be imaged with the patient standing or lying down. When a radiograph is obtained in the supine position, the patient's hips and knees should be flexed slightly to compensate for the physiologic lordosis. This provides exposure of the intervertebral spaces. The central ray is aimed at the midline at the level of the iliac crests. The image with the patient standing is also suitable for documenting functional changes. You can

Figs. 8.**93a, b** Plain radiographs of the thoracic spine in two planes. Degenerative changes of the thoracic spine.

a

b

Fig. 8.**94** AP radiograph of the lumbar spine with the patient supine. The patient's hips and knees are slightly flexed. The X-ray beam is aimed at the midline at the level of the iliac crests.

Fig. 8.**96** Lateral view of the lumbar spine with the patient lying down. The X-ray beam is aimed at the middle lumbar spine at the level of the third lumbar vertebra.

Fig. 8.**95** Plain AP radiograph of the lumbar spine. The image shows normal findings in the lumbar and lumbosacral spine (see also Fig. 8.**97**).

evaluate whether the axis of the pelvis and sacrum is vertical. Evaluating the sacral axis is particularly important since the iliac crests will often be asymmetric.

The end-plates of the vertebrae with the adjacent intervertebral disk spaces, pedicles, the drop-shaped projection of the spinous processes, and the transverse processes are readily discernible. The inferior end-plates of the lumbar spine have the characteristic form of Cupid's bow.

Special views may be used to evaluate the lumbosacral junction. Accurate identification of the number of lumbar vertebrae is necessary. This may require obtaining a full-length spine radiograph; the vertebrae are counted starting at C1. It is possible for S1 to be included in the lumbar spine, i.e., six lumbar vertebrae, and conversely for L5 to be included in the sacrum, i.e., four lumbar vertebrae (Heine 1980) (Figs. 8.**55a–c**, p. 316).

Lateral view (Figs. 8.**96** and 8.**97**). The lateral radiograph of the lumbar spine may be obtained with the

patient standing or lying down. The central ray is aimed at the middle of the third lumbar vertebra.

The lateral view allows evaluation of the vertebral bodies as well as of the height of the intervertebral spaces, pedicles, intervertebral foramina, and spinous processes. The lordosis of the lumbar spine measured from L1–L5 ranges from –14°– –69° with a mean value of –44°according to Cobb. Other authors (DeSmet 1985; Propst–Proctor, Bleck 1983) have determined similar ranges for lumbar lordosis extending from –20°– –60°.

Special Views and Dynamic Studies

Oblique views. The patient is placed in a 45° lateral oblique position (Fig. 8.**98**). The PA projection images the side to which the patient is turned. This imaging technique allows evaluation of the facet joints with the superior and inferior articular processes (Fig. 8.**99**), the intervertebral foramen, the bases of the vertebral arch, and the pars interarticularis. The oblique view shows the characteristic arrangement of

Fig. 8.**97**   Plain radiograph, lateral projection, of the lumbar spine. The image shows the sagittal view of the spine shown in Fig. 8.**95** with normal findings.

Fig. 8.**98**   The oblique view of the lumbar spine for evaluating the facet joints and the intervertebral foramina can be obtained with the patient placed in a 45° lateral oblique position. The X-ray beam is aimed at the middle lumbar spine at the level of the third lumbar vertebra and images the ipsilateral facet joints.

a "Scottie dog" (Fig. 8.**114**) and is an important projection for diagnosing spondylolysis and degenerative changes of the lesser vertebral joints.

Dynamic views. These include the lateral **flexion-extension view** and the AP **bending views.** The latter are especially important for evaluating scoliosis and segmental hypermobility in the coronal plane. They are obtained with the patient positioned supine and at the maximum lateral bend (see section Scoliosis, Radiographic Studies). The lateral dynamic views are used to detect disturbed motion with segmental hypermobility or hypomobility in patients with back pain (see section Degenerative Changes in the Lumbar Spine, Figs. 8.**100a, b** and 8.**101a, b**).

Conventional tomography. Before the era of CT, this was regarded as a valuable means of imaging. In current use, it has fallen from favor due to its relatively high radiation doses and limited utility. CT has replaced plain tomography except in the evaluation of spondylolysis (Brant-Zawadzki et al. 1981).

Fig. 8.**99**   Plain radiograph of the lumbar spine in an oblique position. This is a normal study. The individual facet joints are readily discernible in this view.

Figs. 8.**100a, b** The lateral dynamic views of the lumbar spine are obtained with the patient standing. The X-ray beam is aimed at the middle of the lumbar spine at the level of the third lumbar vertebra.

a   b

Figs. 8.**101a, b** Plain radiograph of the lumbar spine showing lateral dynamic views. Aside from slight anterior osteophytes at the superior end-plate of the fourth vertebra, the image shows a lumbar spine with normal mobility. There is no evidence of hypermobility of individual segments of the spine. (**a**) Flexion, (**b**) extension.

Traumatic Changes in the Lumbar and Thoracic Spine

Since the middle of the century there have been efforts to classify spinal injuries (Böhler 1951). Nicoll was the first to separate fractures into the two large groups of stable and unstable fractures. Holdsworth contributed decisively to the understanding of spinal injuries by developing his **two-column concept** (Fig. 8.**102**). He distinguished between the anterior

column and the so-called posterior ligamentous complex which he viewed as crucial to stability. Denis minimized the importance of the posterior column and proposed the **three-column concept** of the spinal column (Fig. 8.**103**). Here, the anterior column included the anterior longitudinal ligament, the anterior margin of the vertebral body with the superior and inferior end-plates, and the intervertebral disk with the anterior aspects of the anulus fibrosus and

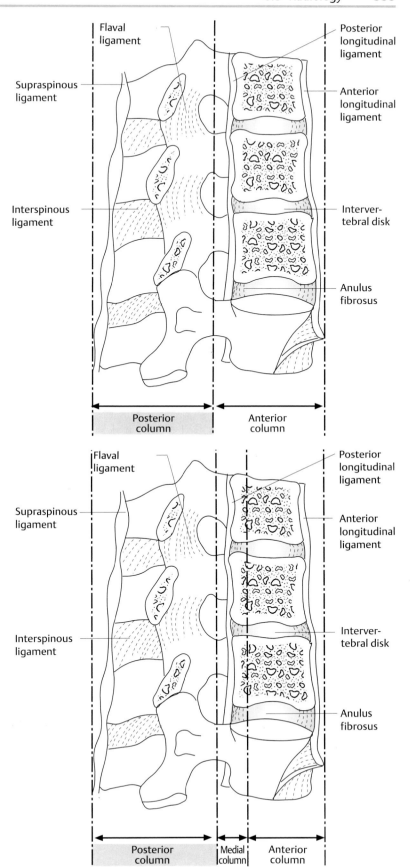

Fig. 8.**102** Schematic diagram of the most important ligamentous structures in the lumbar spine as seen in a lateral projection. Holdsworth in his two-column concept distinguishes between the posterior ligamentous column composed of the so-called posterior ligamentous complex and the anterior bony column.

Fig. 8.**103** Schematic diagram of Denis' three-column concept as seen in a lateral projection.

the nucleus pulposus. The posterior column is formed by the bases of the vertebral arch, the facet joints with their capsular attachment, and the spinal ligaments (the flaval ligaments, the interspinous ligament, and the supraspinous ligament), corresponding to Holdsworth's posterior ligamentous complex. The posterior aspects of the anulus fibrosus, the posterior margin of the vertebral body, and the posterior longitudinal ligament represent the medial column that is crucial for stability of the injury. If the middle column is compromised there is a risk of damage to the spinal cord due to fracture fragments projecting into the spinal canal.

The **Denis classification** differentiates between compression, burst, seat-belt, and dislocation injuries. **Compression fractures** represent a collapse of the superior or inferior end-plate without involvement of the posterior margin of the vertebral body and are classified as types A–D (Figs. 8.**104a–d** and 8.**105**).

Burst fractures are compression factors involving the posterior margin of the vertebra and are

Figs. 8.**104a–d**   Schematic classification of compression fractures according to Denis.

Fig. 8.**105**   Plain lateral radiograph of the thoracic spine showing an old compression fracture of the ninth thoracic vertebra with osteoporosis.

Figs. 8.**106a–e**   Schematic diagram of the burst fractures according to Denis.

a

b

Figs. 8.**107a, b**   Plain radiographs of the lumbar spine in two planes. The image shows a burst fracture of the first lumbar vertebra and a compression fracture of the twelfth thoracic vertebra.

divided into five types (Figs. 8.**106a–e**, 8.**107a, b** and 8.**108**). **Seat-belt injuries** represent a group of flexion-distraction injuries and are classified according to the bony structures involved (Figs. 8.**109a–d**). The final category, **dislocation injuries,** consists of all injuries involving all three columns and includes flexion-rotation, shear, and flexion-distraction injuries (Figs. 8.**110a–d**, 8.**111**, and 8.**112**). According to Denis, the stability of an injury to the spinal column is determined by the number of affected columns. Single-column injuries are generally stable, three-column injuries are always unstable, and two-column injuries may be stable or unstable depending on the severity. The transition from stable to unstable can be gradual. Denis introduced the concepts of mechanical and neurologic instability. According to this system, severe compression fractures and flexion-distraction

Fig. 8.**108**   Plain lateral radiograph of the lumbar showing a ▶ severe burst fracture of the first lumbar vertebra.

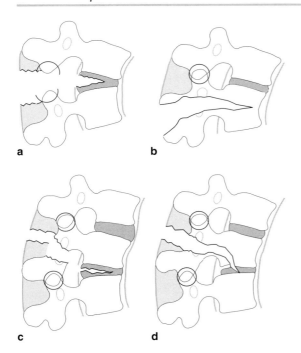

Figs. 8.**109a–d** Schematic diagram of the flexion-distraction injuries (known as seatbelt injuries) according to Denis. The upper right diagram (**b**) shows the so-called chance fracture.

Figs. 8.**110a–d** Schematic diagram of dislocation fractures according to Denis.

Fig. 8.**111**   Plain radiograph of the thoracolumbar spine in two planes showing a fracture dislocation at T9–T10.

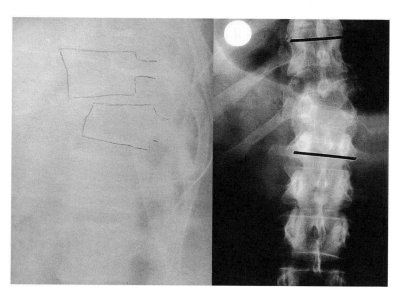

Fig. 8.**112**   Plain radiograph of the thoracolumbar spine in two planes showing a fracture dislocation at T9–T10 (from Castro W. M., Schilgen, M., Kreuzschmerzen, Springer Verlag 1995).

injuries should be regarded as mechanically unstable because they involves a risk of subsequent deformity. Burst fractures without primary loss of neurologic function belong to the class of neurologically unstable fractures. They can lead to progressive deformation with resulting secondary neurologic deficits. Burst fractures with primary neurologic symptoms and fracture dislocations are among the fractures that are both mechanically and neurologically unstable.

McAfee et al. (1983), Magerl et al. (1994), and Harms (1987) have developed further classifications of spinal column injuries based on Denis' three-column principle according to pathogenesis. McAfee described three different forces that can act on the medial column in a spinal injury. These include axial compression, axial distraction, and translation in the transverse plane. Where there is simultaneous translation and compression or distraction, the transverse force is the decisive factor in evaluating the instability of the injury.

Based on the form of injury to the medial column, injuries are classified as follows: **wedge compression fractures** (exclusively involving compression of the anterior column); **stable burst fractures** (with the posterior column intact) and **unstable burst fractures** (with compression, rotation, or translation of the posterior column); **chance fractures** (flexion injury with its axis anterior to the anterior longitudinal ligament that results in a distraction injury to all three columns); **flexion-distraction injuries** (flexion injury with its axis posterior to the anterior longitudinal ligament as results in a compression injury to the anterior column and a distraction injury of the middle and posterior columns); **translational injury** in the form of a shear dislocation injury as described by Denis.

Fig. 8.**113**   Tension/compression mechanism of the spinal column compared to a tension/compression mechanism of a crane. The relationship between tension and compression is the basis for Whitesides' two-column model.

The most current classification system was developed by Magerl et al. This system is again based on a two-column model, this time the one described by Whitesides (Fig. 8.**113**). According to this system, the anterior column formed by the vertebral bodies is the section of the spinal column that is subjected to compressive loads, whereas the posterior column consisting of the posterior bony structures and the ligaments is primarily subjected to tensile loads. This classification system is based on the respective pathomorphologic characteristic of the injury. It uses a rigid three-tier scheme, each with three sublevels, corresponding to the AO/ASIF classification system. Fractures are first divided into three large groups according to the mechanism of injury.

Type A injuries involve compression of the vertebral body, **type B injuries** involve distraction of the anterior and/or posterior column, and **type C injuries** involve a rotation injury to the anterior and posterior columns.

Each group is divided into three subgroups according to the respective severity of the injury. These subgroups are themselves divided into further subgroups that specify the injury in greater detail.

Type A injuries. These injuries are caused by axial compression of the vertebral body with or without flexion. **A1 injuries** include the less severe forms in which there is no risk to the spinal canal. **A2 injuries** involve fragmentation of the vertebral body in the sagittal or coronal plane due to axial compression ("split fractures"). The posterior margin of the vertebral body remains intact so that loss of nerve function is rare. **A3 injuries** include the forms of the classic burst fracture. Depending on the severity, the vertebral body will burst to a certain extent with a fracture of the posterior margin of the vertebral body and loss of neural function corresponding to the degree to which the spinal canal is narrowed. The vertebral arch or spinous process may be vertically fractured, but this will have a negligible effect on stability. **A3 injuries** are always regarded as unstable, especially

flexion-compression injuries. The overall incidence of neurologic complications is cited at 14%.

Type B injuries. These injuries are caused by distraction in a flexion or extension injury. **B1 and B2 injuries** are flexion injuries involving either primarily ligamentous structures (B1) or bony structures (B2). **B1 injuries** involve a tear in the posterior ligamentous structure; often the classic joints will be subluxed, dislocated, or fractured. This may be associated with a type A injury to the vertebral body. **B2 injuries** are characterized by transverse fractures of the laminae or pedicles. The greater the transverse tear, the greater the instability of the injury. Neural involvement is generally higher than in type A injuries. These injuries are generally unstable in flexion; more extensive forms are also unstable in the transverse plane (in the direction of shear) and axially if accompanied by a type A injury. **B3 injuries** are hyperextension injuries with distraction of the anterior column that can extend posteriorly. This form of injury is relatively rare and involves a high rate of neurologic complications. The overall incidence of neurologic complications in type B injuries is cited at 32%.

Type C injuries. This form of injury describes a rotational injury of the spinal column that involves the anterior and posterior columns and must be regarded as the most unstable form of spinal injury. **C1 injuries** are type A injuries with a rotational component; accordingly, **C2 injuries** are type B injuries with a rotational component. **C3 injuries** are rotational shear injuries and are regarded as the most unstable of all spinal injuries. The overall incidence of neurologic complications in type C injuries is cited at 55%.

Spondylolysis and Spondylolisthesis

Spondylolysis is characterized by a congenital or acquired defect in the pars interarticularis. In 90% of all cases, the L4 or L5 vertebrae are affected. The defect is clearly discernible in the oblique radiograph as a "collar" on the "Scottie dog" figure (Figs. 8.**114**,

Fig. 8.**114** Schematic diagram of the "Scottie dog" figure visible in each segment of the lumbar spine on oblique radiographs.

Superior articular process

Transverse process

Contralteral superior articular process

Pars interarticularis (isthmus)

Lamina and spinous process

Inferior articular process

Contralateral inferior articular process

Fig. 8.**115** Schematic diagram of an oblique radiograph of the lumbar spine showing the "Scottie dog" figure. Its "collar," the defect in the pars interarticularis, is a sign of spondylolysis.

Fig. 8.**116** Plain radiograph of the thoracolumbar spine in an oblique projection. The arrows indicate the "Scottie dog's collar," a sign of spondylolysis.

8.**115**, and 8.**116**). As a result of the defect, the superior vertebra can slide over the inferior one, resulting in spondylolisthesis.

Wiltse (1976) classifies spondylolisthesis into five different types:

— Dysplastic form with a congenital defect of the pars interarticularis.
— Isthmic form with a lesion in the pars interarticularis due to a fatigue fracture or from elongation without lysis.
— Degenerative form as a result of chronic segmental instability.
— Traumatic form with a fracture of the pars interarticularis.
— Pathologic form with local or generalized bone disease.

Genuine spondylolisthesis, with lysis of the pars interarticularis, should be distinguished from **pseudo-**

spondylolisthesis, which is characterized by an intact pars interarticularis and results from subluxation of the small vertebral joints due to degenerative processes. In the conventional lateral view of the lumbar spine, spondylolisthesis can be diagnosed from the slippage of the superior vertebra over the inferior one. A step will be visible in the row of spinous processes. In genuine spondylolisthesis this step will be superior to the level of slippage; in pseudo-spondylolisthesis it will be inferior to it in the form of a spinous process sign (Figs. 8.**117a, b**). The severity of spondylolisthesis is diagnosed on a scale of 1–4 using the Meyerding system according to the extent of anterior slippage (Figs. 8.**118a–d**). This is done using the lateral radiograph (Figs. 8.**119a, b** and 8.**120a, b**).

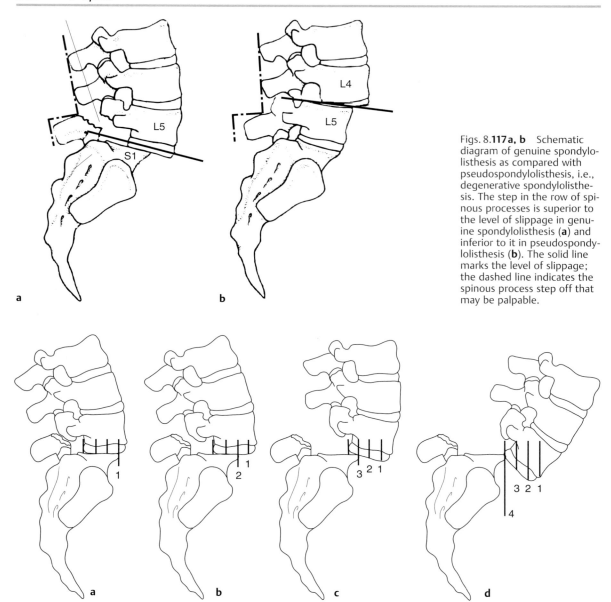

Figs. 8.**117a, b** Schematic diagram of genuine spondylolisthesis as compared with pseudospondylolisthesis, i.e., degenerative spondylolisthesis. The step in the row of spinous processes is superior to the level of slippage in genuine spondylolisthesis (**a**) and inferior to it in pseudospondylolisthesis (**b**). The solid line marks the level of slippage; the dashed line indicates the spinous process step off that may be palpable.

Figs. 8.**118a–d** Schematic diagram of Meyerding's system for classifying the severity of lumbar spondylolisthesis: (**a**) grade I, (**b**) grade II, (**c**) grade III, (**d**) grade IV.

In spondyloptosis, the most severe form, the superior vertebra will be seen to completely slip off the inferior one (Fig. 8.**121**). Severe spondylolisthesis of L5 or S1, with an anteroinferior shift of L5 in relation to S1, will appear on the AP radiograph as a figure resembling an upside-down Napoleon's hat (Fig. 8.**122**). Generally, spondyloptosis will occur as the result of a tilting and rolling motion. However, cases have been described in which the fifth lumbar vertebra slips anteriorly on to S1 and drops down without tilting (Imhäuser 1988). Even the less severe forms of spondylolisthesis will produce lumbosacral kyphosis in addition to the translational deformity. This kyphosis

can significantly influence the overall stability of the spinal column. The kyphotic angle is calculated from the tangent of the posterior margin of the sacrum and the inferior end-plate of slipping vertebra (Fig. 8.**123**).

Degenerative Changes in the Lumbar Spine

Degenerative changes in the lumbar spine affect the intervertebral disks, joints, vertebral bodies, and spinal ligaments. These changes appear as osteochondrosis, spondylosis, and spondylarthritis and are frequent observed together. **Degenerative disk disease** is characterized by a reduction in the height of the

a

b

Figs. 8.**119a, b**   Plain lateral radiographs of the lumbar spine in the sagittal plane. These dynamic views demonstrate abnormal motion in the second to the last segment of the lumbar spine in the presence of first-degree to second-degree spondylolytic spondylolisthesis (Meyerding).

a

Figs. 8.**120a, b**   Lateral (**a**) and oblique (**b**) plain radiographs of the lumbar spine showing dysplastic spondylolisthesis of the lumbar spine (Meyerding grade II).

b

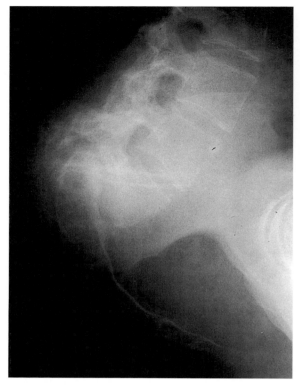

Fig. 8.**121**   Plain lateral radiograph of the lumbar spine show-ing spondyloptosis with a typical round sacrum plateau.

Fig. 8.**122**   Plain AP radiograph of the lumbosacral spine showing spondyloptosis with the figure of Napoleon's hat upside down.

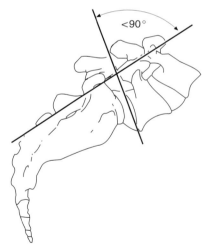

Fig. 8.**123**   Schematic diagram for calculating the angle of lumbosacral kyphosis.

Fig. 8.**124**   Plain lateral radiograph of the lumbar spine. In addition to Schmorl nodules on the second and third lumbar vertebrae, the image shows narrowing of the intervertebral space in the two lower segments accompanied by subchond-ral sclerosis. A posterior spondylophyte can be seen on the inferior end-plate of the fourth lumbar vertebra.

intervertebral space with an increase in the radiodensity of the end-plate of the vertebrae due to subchondral sclerosis (Fig. 8.**124**). According to Krämer, degeneration of the intervertebral disk and the resulting loss of height cause segmental loosening with secondary overloading of the vertebral joints. Aside from the reduction in height, disk degeneration is occasionally discernible in the plain radiograph from the "vacuum phenomena" resulting from gas inclusions within the disks (Fig. 8.**125**). Degeneration of the intervertebral disk with advancing age can be readily evaluated with discography and MRI. The role of discography in degenerative disk disease is controversial.

Spondylosis (Figs. 8.**126a, b**) refers to the development of osteophytes on the end-plates of the vertebrae, frequently associated with degenerative disk disease (known as marginal spondylophytes). Submarginal spondylophytes occur more frequently in intervertebral spaces of normal height and result in a reaction to increase tensile loading of the anterior longitudinal ligaments with segmental hypermobility. MacNab studied this phenomena in 1971 and referred to this form of spondylophytes as "traction spur" (Fig. 8.**127**).

Spondylarthritis refers to degeneration of the facet joints, also known as degenerative joint disease of the spine. This disorder is best detected in oblique radiographs that will reveal the classic signs of arthritis of the small vertebral joints, including narrowing of the joint space, subchondral sclerosis, and formation of osteophytes (spondylophytes; Figs. 8.**128** and

Fig. 8.**125** Plain lateral radiograph of the lumbar spine. In addition to spondylolisthesis at L3–L4, the image demonstrates a "vacuum phenomenon," in the two inferior segments associated with degeneration of the intervertebral disk (see also Fig. 8.**130**).

Figs. 8.**126a, b** Plain radiograph of the lumbar spine in two planes. The image shows degenerative changes, particularly in the two inferior lumbar spine segments where narrowing of the intervertebral disk and spondylosis is present. A vacuum phenomenon can be seen at L4–L5 (from Castro W. M., Schilgen, M., Kreuzschmerzen, Springer Verlag 1995).

a   b

Fig. 8.**127**   Plain lateral radiograph of the lumbar spine. The image shows a submarginal spondylophyte, the "traction spur" at the level of the body of the fourth lumbar vertebra.

Fig. 8.**128**   Plain radiograph of the lumbar spine in an oblique ▶ projection. The facet joint L3–L4 shows a vacuum phenomenon in addition to degenerative changes. The other facet joints, particularly L4–L5 and L5–S1 (only partially visible) show degenerative changes but without a vacuum phenomenon.

Fig. 8.**129**   Plain radiograph of the lumbar spine in an oblique projection showing arthritis of the lumbosacral facet joints.

Fig. 8.**130**   Plain radiograph of the lumbar spine showing lateral dynamic views. The images demonstrate degenerative spondylolisthesis at L3–L4 (see also Fig. 8.**125**).

a

b

Figs. 8.**131a, b**   Plain radiograph of the lumbar spine. The AP image (**a**) shows the "clothespin sign" (particularly at L2–L3), and the lateral image (**b**) shows short pedicles indicative of central spinal stenosis.

8.129). When the sacrum is included in the AP radiograph, the sacroiliac joints are readily visible. If arthritic changes are present in this region, the possibility should be considered of ankylosing spondylitis in its early stages that will often manifest itself as sacroiliitis.

Degenerative segmental instability, or degenerative spondylolisthesis from subluxation of the small vertebral joints, spinal stenosis resulting from development of osteophytes on the articular processes, and hypertrophy of the flaval ligament are regarded as results of degenerative spinal disease. **Degenerative segmental instability** can be diagnosed in plain radiographs using lateral flexion and extension views. Normal values and pathologic values cited by various studies overlap. According to Boden and Wiesel (1990), dynamic AP translation (after allowing for the translation inherent in the extension and flexion view) that exceeds 3 mm, or 8% of the width of the vertebral body, is indicative of segmental hypermobility (Boden and Wiesel 1990) (Fig. 8.**130**). The normal values of segmental sagittal translation and seg-

mental sagittal angular rotation are shown in Tables 8.**29** and 8.**30**.

Plain radiographs are inferior to myelography, CT, and MRI for detecting **spinal stenosis**. The "clothespin sign" in the AP image and short pedicles in the lateral radiograph may be signs of central spinal stenosis (Figs. 8.**131a, b**).

"Kissing spine," where the spinous processes are seen to impinge on the lateral radiograph, can be

Table 8.**29**   Overview of the normal values for sagittal translation in the lumbar spine (according to Boden and Wiesel)

Dynamic sagittal translation in mm	
L1–L2	1.4 mm
L2–L3	1.3 mm
L3–L4	1.2 mm
L4–L5	1.2 mm
L1–S1	1.0 mm

Table 8.**30** Overview of the normal values for rotation in the sagittal plane (flexion/extension) in the lumbar spine

Level	White and Panjabi	Hayes et al.	Pearcy et al.	Dvo-rak et al.	Boden and Wiesel
L1–L2	12°	7°	13°	11.9°	8.2°
L2–L3	14°	9°	14°	14.5°	7.7°
L3–L4	15°	10°	13°	15.3°	7.7°
L4–L5	16°	13°	16°	18.2°	9.4°
L1–S1	17°	14°	14°	17°	9.4°

Table 8.**31** Overview of the various forms of vertebral osteophytes

	Spondy-lophytes	Hyper-ostoses	Syndes-mophy-tes	Parasyn-desmo-phytes
Cause	Degener-ative	Forestier disease (DISH)	Ankylos-ing spon-dylitis	Reiter syn-drome, psoriatic arthritis
Localiza-tion	Marginal, submar-ginal	Anterior aspect of vertebral body	End-plates	Lateral, occasion-ally iso-lated
Form	Hook-shaped	Conical	Comma-shaped, fine	Horn-shaped, hairpin-shaped
Direction of growth	Horizon-tal	Vertical	Vertical	Vertical

either an incidental finding or a painful idiopathic disorder (Figs. 8.**132a, b**).

Inflammatory Changes in the Spine

Vertebral osteomyelitis is almost always the result of hematogenous dissemination of pyogenic pathogens that often begin in the subchondral region of the vertebral body. If the focus of the infection breaks through the end-plate of the vertebra and spreads to the intervertebral disk, **diskitis** will result. This will appear on the plain radiograph as a narrowing of the intervertebral space with destruction of the adjacent end-plates and a soft-tissue abscess visible in the form of a paraspinal mass. In the AP radiograph, a soft-tissue abscess will generally appear as a paravertebral widened area in the shape of an hourglass. Primary hematogenous diskitis only occurs in children because at this age the intervertebral disk still has its own blood supply. In adults, disk infection occurs as a result of direct inoculation of pathogens during surgery or discography.

In an appropriate clinical setting, isolated narrowing of an intervertebral disk seen on a standard radiograph (Figs. 8.**133a, b** and 8.**134a–c**) should be regarded as vertebral osteomyelitis and diskitis until proven otherwise. Appropriate diagnostic studies include nuclear medicine scans and MRI. Disk space aspiration and vertebral body biopsy will be required to identify the organism.

Spinal tuberculosis (Pott disease) is most frequently observed in the inferior thoracic and superior lumbar spine. The radiologic features of this disorder resemble a pyogenic infection and frequently include paraspinal masses; occasionally a psoas abscess can burst forth from beneath the inguinal ligament. MRI is the imaging study of choice following plain films.

Rheumatoid arthritis is the primary nonbacterial inflammatory disorder of the cervical spine. Erosion of the dens and destruction of the ligamentous structure posterior to the dens can result in severe atlantoaxial instability, including subluxation. Subluxation can be documented by an increase in the anterior atlantodental distance to more than 3 mm when inclined. For further diagnostic information, an axial imaging process such as CT or MRI is helpful for evaluating the spinal canal and the inflammatory soft-tissue changes (Krämer 1994).

With progression of the disease, subsidence of the lateral masses and the vertebral body of C2 can cause the skull to sink relative to the dens so that it becomes invaginated in the foramen ovale. This is known as pseudobasilar impression (Krämer).

Rheumatoid arthritis can also affect the intervertebral disks, vertebral joints, spinous processes, and the ligamentous structures (Figs. 8.**135a, b**). The resulting segmental loosening can appear in the radiograph as a characteristic step sign (Krämer).

Facet ankylosis is also observed with rheumatoid disorders. Ankylosis occurs in association with primary chronic polyarthritis, although it occurs more frequently with ankylosing spondylitis. Fine syndesmophytes and ankylosis of the facet joints are typical signs of this disorder (Greenspan 1993).

Forestier disease or diffuse idiopathic skeletal hyperostosis (DISH) is typified by continuous ossification of the anterior aspects of the vertebral bodies, extending past the intervertebral disk spaces that are generally well preserved (Figs. 8.**136a, b**). Differential diagnosis should also include **psoriatic arthritis**, which can be associated with solitary paraspinal ossifications (parasyndesmophytes). In contrast to the syndesmophytes in ankylosing spondylitis, these rarely bridge the intervertebral space and are almost always limited to one vertebra or occur without bony connections in paravertebral connective tissue (Table 8.**31**).

Figs. 8.**132a, b**   (**a**) Schematic diagram of "kissing spine" disease of the lumbar spine (Baastrup disease) as seen in a lateral projection. Impingement of the spinous processes occurs. (**b**) Plain radiograph of the lower lumbar spine in the coronal plane. The image shows "kissing spine" disease of the inferior lumbar spine.

Figs. 8.**133a, b**   Plain radiograph of the lower lumbar spine in two planes. The image shows vertebral osteomyelitis at the L3–L4 level in a 55-year-old patient.

a

b

11/94

1/95

c

Figs. 8.**134a–c**   Plain radiographs of the thoracic spine in two planes. The images show vertebral osteomyelitis at the T9–T10 level (**a, b**) which led to complete resorption within 3 months (**c**).

Tumors of the Spine

When radiologic examination reveals pathologic findings in the spine, tumor should always be excluded. Malignant changes are generally observed in the vertebral body; benign tumors will more frequently involve the posterior vertebral structures (Greenspan 1993). On the whole, however, it is extremely difficult to distinguish between benign and malignant tumors in the spine (Wolf and Gnann 1984). Benign lesions tend to be regular and sharply demarcated by a sclerotic halo. In contrast, malignant tumors tend to appear as ill-defined lesions without a sclerotic halo. The most common malignant processes in the spinal column is metastases (Gradinger et al. 1989, Wuisman et al. 1989). Metastases are often localized in the inferior segments of the spinal column, particularly between the second and fourth lumbar vertebrae (Thümler et al. 1987). Table 8.**32** provides an overview of the various types of malignant spinal tumors.

Primary malignant bone tumors include **Ewing sarcomas, chondrosarcomas,** and **osteosarcomas,** although these rarely affect the spinal column. Osteosarcoma of the spinal column generally occurs after

Table 8.**32**   Malignant spinal tumors

• Metastases	• Osteosarcoma
• Multiple myeloma	• Ewing sarcoma
• Chordoma	• Chondrosarcoma

a   b

Figs. 8.**135a, b**   Plain radiographs of the cervical spine showing lateral dynamic views. In this patient with rheumatoid arthritis, the dynamic views document increased translation at C2–C3, C3–C4, and C4–C5, in addition to degenerative changes in the inferior cervical spine; (**a**) flexion, (**b**) extension.

Figs. 8.**136a, b**   Plain radiographs of the thoracic spine in two planes. The images show typical changes associated with Forestier disease (DISH).

a   b

Table 8.**33**   Primary tumors that most frequently develop spinal metastases

• Breast	• Thyroid
• Lung	• Kidney
• Prostate	• Melanoma

exposure to radiation or in association with underlying Paget disease. Chondrosarcomas generally grow more slowly than osteosarcomas and Ewing sarcomas (Salzer-Kuntschik 1984) (Figs. 8.**137a, b**).

A **chordoma** is a malignant tumor derived from persistent portions of the notochord; it occurs exclusively in the midline of the skeleton (Salzer-Kuntschik 1984) and is generally localized in the sacrum.

The primary malignant bone tumor most frequently encountered is **multiple myeloma** (Greenspan 1993). On plain radiographs it will appear as diffuse osteoporosis with subsidence of the vertebral body and multiple-level compression fractures with osteolysis at multiple sites, some accompanied by reactive sclerosis. The bases of the vertebral arch are rarely affected in the early stages of the disorder due to their relatively low content of red bone marrow.

Metastatic disease is the most frequent form of spinal tumor. It will often cause destruction of the bases of the vertebral arch (Jacobson sign; Fig. 8.**138**).

In the AP radiograph, the destruction of the pedicle is readily discernible as a lack of an oval window or a lytic reaction. The profuse vascularization of bone permits hematogenous dissemination of carcinomas such as breast, prostate, and bronchial cancers (Table 8.**33**). Due to the paired or segmental vascular supply, most metastases will begin in the vertebral body (Gradinger et al. 1989). In a plain radiograph, bone metastases will appear as circumscribed areas of osteolysis with or without a sclerotic halo or as radiodense foci. In other cases, subsidence of a vertebra is the first sign of metastatic disease. Among the primarily osteolytic metastases are metastases of kidney and thyroid cancers. Breast carcinoma can occur in a mixed form (Figs. 8.**139a, b**); metastases of prostate carcinomas are generally osteoblastic (Figs. 8.**140a, b**).

Benign bone tumors that involve the spinal column relatively frequently (Table 8.**34**) include **aneurysmal bone cysts,** frequently visible as multicystic, eccentrically expanding lesions with a narrow clamshell-shaped periosteal reaction. Since these lesions frequently recur after resection, they are regarded as aggressive benign tumors. A **hemangioma** is a tumor originating in the blood vessels with characteristic coarse vertical stripes on the vertebral body resembling corduroy or a honeycomb pattern (Figs. 8.**141a–c**). Another benign lesion that can affect the spinal column is the **osteoid osteoma,** a bony tis-

a   b

Figs. 8.**137a, b**   Plain radiographs of the thoracic spine in two planes. The images show a large tumor at the lumbosacral junction. Diagnosis: chondrosarcoma.

Table 8.**34**   Benign spinal tumors

- Osteoid osteoma
- Osteoblastoma
- Eosinophilic granuloma
- Isolated bone cyst
- Hemangioma
- Aneurysmal bone cyst
- Giant cell tumor

Fig. 8.**138**   This Ap tomogram shows massive lytic reaction ▶ (Jacobson sign) due to metastasis from melanoma.

Figs. 8.**139a, b**   Plain radiographs of the lumbar spine in the coronal plane (**a**) and thoracic spine in the sagittal plane (**b**). The image shows diffuse skeletal metastases of a breast carcinoma of mixed osteolytic and osteoblastic type. Fig. 9.**25** (p. 432) demonstrates the pelvis and hips of the same patient.

▼

a

b

a   b

Figs. 8.**140a, b** Plain radiograph of a lumbar spine in two planes. The image shows changes in the bone structure of vertebral body L3, typical of osteoblastic metastasis, in a 75-year-old patient with known prostate cancer.

sue change with a typical central nidus. A relatively frequent location of this lesion is the posterior bony column of the spinal column. The nidus, which consists of osteoid or mineralized immature bone, can either be radiolucent or sclerotic. If the nidus is calcified, it will be almost impossible to distinguish it from an osteoblastoma, a related lesion (Wolf and Gnann 1984).

The **osteoblastoma** is a benign bone tumor involving the spinal column in 30-40% of all cases (Huvos 1979, Marsh et al. 1975). Generally the posterior vertebral elements will be affected, with possible spreading to the vertebral body; the tumor is rarely limited to the vertebral body (Nemoto et al. 1990). In the plane radiograph, it will generally appear as a lobular, well-defined contour (Figs. 8.**142a, b**).

Eosinophilic granulomas belong to the group of reticuloendothelial proliferations. When they involve the spinal column, almost complete subsidence of the vertebral body can be observed with the intervertebral spaces unaffected. This appears as vertebra plana on the lateral radiograph (Figs. 8.**143a, b**).

Giant cell tumors involve the spinal column relatively frequently. Wuisman et al. (1989) cite the incidence of involvement of the spinal column as approximately 7%. Because of its high incidence of recurrence and aggressive local growth, the giant cell tumor is regarded as aggressive but benign. However,

metastases of giant cell tumors have also been described.

Isolated bone cysts are among the lesions that resemble tumors. They are benign and only rarely involve the spinal column (Dahmen and Bernbeck 1987).

Spinal Deformity

Scoliosis

Spinal deformity is understood to mean deviations from normal in the coronal and sagittal planes. Scoliosis is defined as a structural lateral curve in the spinal column with a rotational component and resulting deformity in the sagittal plane. Curves of less than 10° do not represent scoliosis. Depending on location, a differentiation is made between thoracic, thoracolumbar, lumbar, and double curve scoliosis (Fig. 8.**144a–d**). Ponseti and Friedman (1950) first defined a systematic classification of scoliotic curves that was slightly modified by Moe et al. (1994).

According to this scheme, **lumbar scoliosis** is defined as having its apex at L2 with predominantly left convex curves. If the apex of the curve is at T12 or L1, the disorder is a **thoracolumbar scoliosis** that is predominantly right convex. **Thoracic scoliosis** is predominantly right convex with the apex of its curve between T7 and T11.

Figs. 8.**141 a–c**   Plain radiographs and spot views of the lumbar spine in two planes (**a, b**) and lateral tomography (**c**). The image shows vertical stripes on the vertebral body typical of hemangioma.

a   b

Figs. 8.**142a, b**   Plain AP radiograph of the lumbar spine (**a**) and tomography in the coronal plane (**b**). The images show a sclerotic tumor in the first lumbar vertebra, diagnosed as an osteoblastoma.

a   b

Figs. 8.**143a, b**   Plain radiographs of the thoracolumbar spine in two planes. The images demonstrate subsidence of vertebral body T11, diagnosed as eosinophilic granuloma.

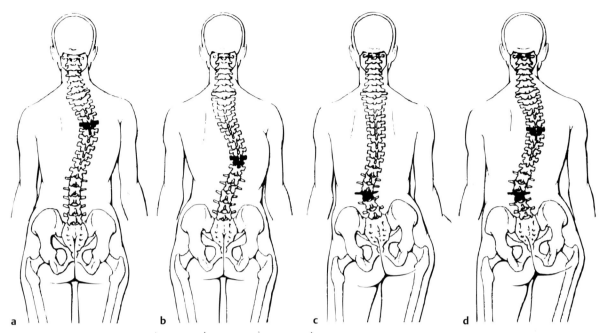

Figs. 8.**144a–d**   Schematic diagram of various scoliotic curves. The change in the contour of the trunk will vary according to the height of the apical vertebra: (**a**) thoracic, (**b**) thoracolumbar, (**c**) lumbar, (**d**) thoracic and lumbar (double curve).

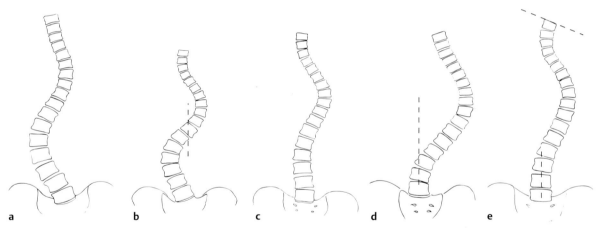

Figs. 8.**145a–e**   Schematic diagram of five types of scoliotic curves (I–V) according to King. (**a**) type I, (**b**) type II, (**c**) type III, (**d**) type IV, (**e**) type V.

Idiopathic right convex thoracic scoliosis, which comprises by far the largest share of idiopathic scoliotic disorders, is further subdivided according to King's classification (King et al. 1983) (Table 8.**35**, Figs. 8.**145a–e** and 8.**146**–8.**157**).

A new classification by Lenke (Lenke et al. 1999) subdivides adolescent idiopathic scoliosis into 6 types (primary thoracic, double thoracic, double major, triple major, primary thoracolumbar and primary thoracolumbar with structural secondary thoracic curve). Depending on the shift of the lumbar curve, these types are classified as lumbar modifier type A, B or C. Aim of this classification is to clearly define the fusion

length in anterior and posterior correction and fusion in scoliosis surgery.

Scoliosis frequently occurs with von Recklinghausen disease and collagen disorders such as Marfan syndrome. Dystrophic changes in the vertebral body are typical in von Recklinghausen disease (Fig. 8.**158**).

Congenital scoliosis involves failure of formation and of segmentation, or a mixed form. Formation of wedge-shaped vertebra, hemivertebrae, or vertebral bars leads to congenital scoliosis or kyphosis that tends to be progressive (Figs. 8.**159a–d** and 8.**160**). This includes **Klippel–Feil syndrome** that involves congenital failure of segmentation of the cervical

Fig. 8.**146** Plain radiographs of the entire spine in two planes, obtained with the patient standing. The images show a 15-year-old female patient with idiopathic adolescent right convex thoracic scoliosis, type I according to King. At 82° according to Cobb, the left convex lumbar lateral curve is more pronounced than the right convex thoracic lateral curve. Pronounced leftward deviation from vertical of approximately 3.5 cm is visible.

Fig. 8.**147** Plain radiographs of the spine in two planes, obtained with the patient standing. The images show a 14-year-old female patient with idiopathic adolescent right convex thoracic scoliosis, type II according to King. At 48°, according to Cobb, the right convex curve is more pronounced than the left convex lumbar curve of 28°. The lateral radiograph shows the typical flattened thoracic spine of thoracic lordoscoliosis with lordosis between T4 and T12, measuring −20° according to Cobb, accompanied by flattening of the lumbar lordosis.

Fig. 8.**148** Plain radiographs of the spine in two planes, obtained with the patient standing. The images show a 15-year-old female patient with idiopathic adolescent right convex thoracic scoliosis, type III according to King, with pronounced lordosis of the entire thoracic and lumbar spine.

Table 8.**35** Classification of the right convex thoracic curves according to King

King type	Criteria	Incidence
Type I	Double curve scoliosis, in which the thoracic and lumbar curves both cross the midline. The lumbar curve is larger and more rigid than the thoracic curve. "Genuine" double curve scoliosis	13%
Type II	Double curve scoliosis, in which the thoracic and lumbar curves both cross the midline. The thoracic curve is larger and more rigid than the lumbar curve. "False" double curve scoliosis	33%
Type III	Thoracic scoliosis in which the secondary lumbar does not cross the midline	33%
Type IV	Thoracic scoliosis with a long curve. The second last lumbar vertebra is tilted	9%
Type V	Double structural thoracic scoliosis with the first thoracic vertebra tilted along the convex superior curve (positive T1 tilt)	12%

Fig. 8.**149** Plain radiograph of the spine in the coronal plane, obtained with the patient standing. The image shows right convex thoracic scoliosis of type IV according to King, measuring 62° according to Cobb. The second to last lumbar vertebrae is tilted along the main right convex thoracic curve.

Fig. 8.**150** Plain radiographs of the spine in two planes, obtained with the patient standing. The images show a 15-year-old female patient with idiopathic adolescent double-arc thoracic scoliosis, type V according to King, with positive T1 tilt. The lateral radiograph shows a largely physiologic profile.

Fig. 8.**151** Plain radiographs of the spine in two planes, obtained with the patient standing. The images show double-curve scoliosis in a 14-year-old male patient with a left convex thoracic lateral curve measuring 58° according to Cobb and a right convex lumbar lateral curve measuring 48° according to Cobb. The lateral view shows a physiologic profile.

58°

48°

THORACIC SPINE +42°

TLJ +13°

LWS −61°

68°
(36°)

Fig. 8.**152** Plain radiographs of the spine in two planes, obtained with the patient standing. The images show a 16-year-old female patient with idiopathic adolescent left convex low thoracic scoliosis measuring 68° according to Cobb. The lateral radiograph shows abnormal low thoracic kyphosis with kyphosis of the thoracolumbar junction measuring +13° according to Cobb.

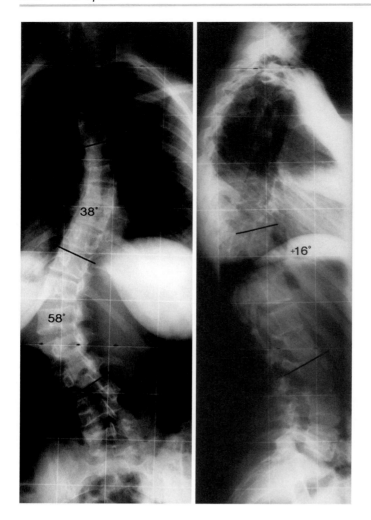

Fig. 8.153 Plain radiographs of the spine in two planes, obtained with the patient standing. The images show a 21-year-old female patient with idiopathic left convex thoracolumbar scoliosis measuring 58° according to Cobb and thoracic right convex curvature measuring 38° according to Cobb. There is a pronounced leftward deviation from vertical in the coronal plane (5 cm). The lateral radiograph shows abnormal thoracolumbar kyphosis measuring +16° according to Cobb.

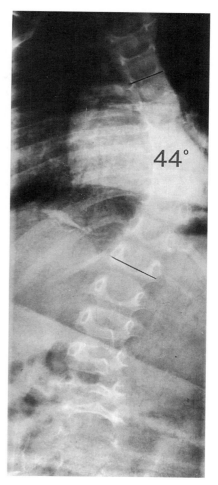

Fig. 8.**155**   Plain radiograph of the spine in the coronal plane, obtained with the patient supine. The images show infantile right convex thoracic scoliosis measuring 44° according to Cobb in a 2-year-old boy.

Fig. 8.**154**   Plain radiographs of the spine in two planes, obtained with the patient standing. The images show a 16-year-old female patient with left convex lumbar scoliosis, measuring 77° according to Cobb, and thoracic curve of 48°. The lateral radiograph shows abnormal thoraco-lumbar kyphosis measuring +16° according to Cobb.

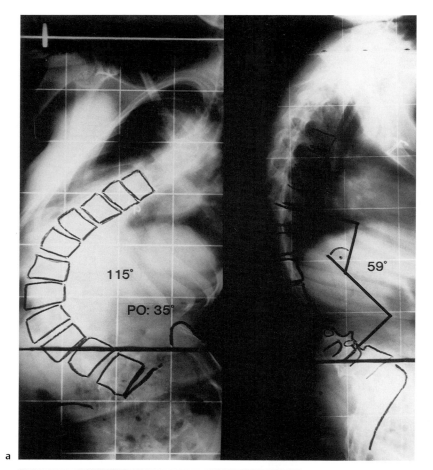

115°

PO: 35°

59°

a

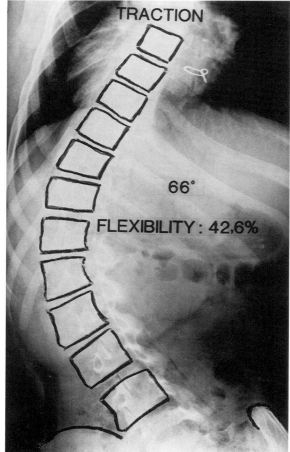

TRACTION

66°

FLEXIBILITY: 42,6%

b

Figs. 8.**156a, b** Plain radiographs of the spine in two planes, obtained with the patient sitting, and a traction view to evaluate flexibility. The images show a 15-year-old male patient with spastic tetraparesis. Long-arc C-shaped neuromuscular left convex scoliosis of 115° according to Cobb and pelvic obliquity of 35° are present. The lateral radiograph shows pronounced rotational kyphosis measuring +59° according to Cobb. The traction view shows reduction of the lateral curve to 66° according to Cobb, corresponding to 42.6% flexibility.

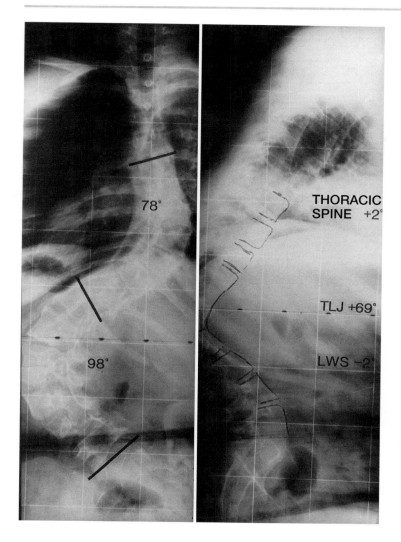

Fig. 8.**157** Plain radiographs of the spine in two planes, obtained with the patient sitting. The images show a 14-year-old female patient with a history of poliomyelitis. Pronounced neuromuscular double-arc scoliosis is present with a left convex lumbar lateral curve measuring 98° according to Cobb and a right convex thoracic curve measuring 70° according to Cobb. There is pronounced rotational kyphosis in the thoracolumbar junction measuring +69° according to Cobb.

Fig. 8.**158**   Plain radiograph of the thoracolumbar spine in the sagittal plane. The image shows a 31-year-old female patient known to have von Recklinghausen disease after spinal fusion with Harrington rods. The dystrophic changes in the vertebral body typical of von Recklinghausen disease (scallop sign) can be seen.

Fig. 8.**160**   Plain radiograph of the lumbar spine in the coronal plane. The image shows a segmented hemivertebra on the right side and a nonsegmented hemivertebra on the left side (corresponding to Figs. 8.**217a, b**, p. 396).

spine, possible shortening of the neck, and also if limited to one side, cervical scoliosis (Figs. 8.**161a, b**). Spina bifida and **Sprengel's deformity,** congenital elevation of the scapula, often accompany this deformity.

According to the age at which the deformity occurs, scoliosis is referred to as infantile (up to age 3 years) (Fig. 8.**155**), juvenile (age 4–10 years), or adolescent (age 11 years until completion of growth).

a   b   c   d

Figs. 8.**159a–d**   Examples of segmentation failure in the spinal column. (**a**) Unilateral unsegmented bar. Progressive scoliosis will result. (**b**) Anterior segmentation failure. Progressive kyphosis will result (Fig. 8.**171**, see p. 371). (**c**) Segmented hemivertebra with scoliosis. (**d**) Nonsegmented hemivertebra with scoliosis.

a   b

Figs. 8.**161a, b**   Plain radiograph of the cervical spine in two planes. The images show a 9-year-old female patient with Klippel–Feil syndrome. The failure of segmentation and of formation typical of Klippel–Feil syndrome, with an anterior vertebral bar in the mid-cervical spine, are readily discernible.

There are three major categories of adult scoliosis:

— Young adults with previous scoliosis no degenerative changes.
— Older adults with previous scoliosis now with superimposed degenerative changes.
— Older adults with degenerative scoliosis where there is no evidence of scoliosis before the age of 40 (de-novo scoliosis).

• Radiographic studies

The AP radiograph should be obtained as a radiograph of the entire spinal column, including the entire cervical spine and pelvis, with the patient standing. In this projection, scoliosis is discernible from the **lateral curve** that is measured using the Cobb angle. To do this it is necessary to locate the respective neutral vertebrae that mark the transition from convexity to concavity and to determine the angle between the superior end-plate of the superior neutral vertebra and the inferior end-plate of the inferior neutral vertebra (Fig. 8.**162**).

Rotation, according to the method described by Nash and Moe (1969), is the deviation of the convex pedicle from the concavity. The percentage of shift within the width of the vertebral body corresponds to the rotation in degrees (Fig. 8.**163**). An alternative method to measure vertebral rotation is the method according to Perdriolle (Perdriolle 1981). A deviation from vertical, which is frequently observed, can be measured in centimeters by drawing a vertical line from C7 and measuring the deviation of the spinous process of S1. Aside from this, pelvic or sacral obliquity must be excluded because this is closely related to scoliosis.

Bending views are useful in the treatment of scoliosis. These are obtained by positioning the patient supine and instructing him or her bend to each side. They differentiate between structural and flexible components of the curve (Figs. 8.**164a, b**).

Every scoliosis patient should have a **full-length lateral radiograph** to permit evaluation of the extent of sagittal profile abnormalities, which are frequently present. Thoracic scoliosis will frequently be associated with thoracic hypokyphosis (known as lordoscoliosis), and thoraculumbar scoliosis will frequently be associated with pathologic kyphosis of the thoracolumbar junction. In the full-length radiograph, the vertical line may be drawn from the opening of the external acoustic meatus. Normally, the axis will run through the anterior column (Lewit 1977).

Whenever a spinal deformity is present in children, **skeletal age** should be determined to evaluate remaining growth and the risk of curve progression.

Fig. 8.**162** Schematic diagram for measuring scoliosis according to Cobb.

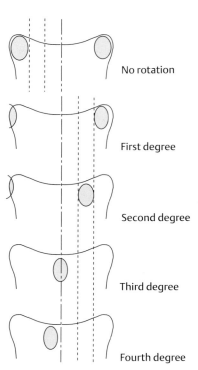

No rotation

First degree

Second degree

Third degree

Fourth degree

Fig. 8.**163** Schematic diagram for determining rotation of a vertebral body according to Nash and Moe.

a

b

Figs. 8.**164a, b** Plain radiograph of the thoracolumbar spine in the coronal plane. Bending views obtained with the patient supine show a left convex thoracolumbar scoliosis. At maximum left bending, the thoracolumbar curve is seen to straighten to 8° according to Cobb (**a**). The secondary right convex thoracic curve is also seen to straighten to 8° according to Cobb when the patient bends maximally to the right (**b**).

Fig. 8.**165** Schematic diagram of the Risser sign for determining skeletal age. At Risser I, the radiograph shows the onset of ossification of the apophysis of the iliac crest. At Risser V, ossification is complete (Table 9.**7**, see p. 439).

Recommended methods include evaluation of the apophyses of the iliac crests according to Risser (see chapter 9, p. 438) which is often possible using the full-spine AP radiograph (Fig. 8.**165** and Table 9.**7**) or Greulich and Pyle's method of determining skeletal age using a radiograph of the left hand (Table 8.**36**).

Kyphosis

Isolated changes occur particularly as hyperkyphosis of the thoracic spine with Cobb angles exceeding 40°.

Fig. 8.**166**   Plain lateral radiograph of the thoracic spine. The image shows a 16-year-old boy with radiographic changes typical of Scheuermann disease including several wedge-shaped vertebrae with narrowing of the intervertebral spaces.

Fig. 8.**167**   Plain lateral radiograph of the spine. The image shows Scheuermann disease with thoracic kyphosis measuring 76°.

Fig. 8.**166**

Fig. 8.**167**

Adolescent kyphosis, or **Scheuermann disease,** is a clinically significant idiopathic form (Figs. 8.**20,** 8.**21,** p. 302). The cause of this disorder is controversial, but it primarily involves the thoracic spine. Typical radiologic changes with Scheuermann disease include:

Table 8.**36**   Overview of the individual views and measuring methods for evaluating scoliosis

View	Radiographic measuring parameters
Full-spine AP radiograph	Cobb angle Rotation Deviation from vertical in coronal plane Shoulder position Pelvis position Risser sign
Full-spine lateral radiograph	Thoracic kyphosis Thoracolumbar spine Lumbar lordosis Deviation from vertical in sagittal plane
Bending views	Cobb angle
Left hand AP radiograph	Skeletal age

— Schmorl nodes
— Irregular vertebral end-plates
— Pronounced narrowing of the intervertebral sections
— Three or more adjacent vertebrae with 5° or more of anterior wedging
— Thoracic hyperkyphosis of more than 45° (Figs. 8.**166** and 8.**167**).

There is also a lumbar form of the disease.

Ankylosing spondylitis is a rheumatic disorder that primarily affects the synovial joints of the spinal column, neighboring soft tissues, and the sacroiliac joints. Ossification that shortens the anterior longitudinal ligament, accompanied by formation of syndesmophytes, leads to kyphotic deformities involving the entire spine. Different types of kyphosis can result, depending on the pattern of involvement (Figs. 8.**168a–e**). The disease often emanates from the sacroiliac joints, which in the plain radiograph simultaneously show signs of erosion, sclerosis, and ankylosis (Krämer et al. 1993). Involvement of the spinal column progresses superiorly during the course of the disease. The disorder is characterized by **rectangular vertebrae,** resulting from erosion of the normally biconcave vertebral end-plates and the typical syndesmophytes. The syndesmophytes tend to be aligned more vertically than degenerative spondylo-

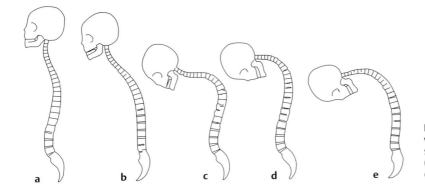

Figs. 8.**168a–e**   Schematic diagram of various forms of kyphosis. (**a**) Normal spinal column. (**b**) Lumbar kyphosis. (**c**) Thoracic kyphosis. (**d**) Cervicothoracic kyphosis. (**e**) Full-spine kyphosis.

Fig. 8.**169**   Fig. 8.**170**

Fig. 8.**169**   Plain AP radiograph of the lumbar spine. The image shows the "railroad sign" of ankylosing spondylitis. Only the facet joints are affected.

Fig. 8.**170**   Plain lateral radiograph of ankylosing spondylitis.

phytes and have a finer appearance. Increasing ossification of the facet joints as the disease progresses leads to a typical **"railroad sign"** in the AP radiograph, which can appear to have three tracks as the ossification of the interspinal ligaments progresses (Fig. 8.**169**). In the final stage of the disease, complete ossification of the apophyseal joints will give the spinal column an appearance referred to as **"bamboo spine."** The pathologic ossification can be classified according to surgically relevant criteria (Fig. 8.**170**) (Hehne and Zielke 1990).

A secondary kyphosis is generally characterized by a short arc, i.e., a gibbus. It can occur as the result of trauma, infection, or tumor, but may also be a result of congenital deficiencies (Fig. 8.**171**).

Vertebral Arch Defects

Failure of fusion of the vertebral arches represents the most frequent congenital deformity of the spinal column. These range from harmless spina bifida occulta, a variation of the normal spine, to meningomyelocele or myelocele, which involve symptoms typical of a transverse lesion. Common sites include the lumbar spine and the lumbosacral spine, although the atlas can be affected in rare cases. Spina bifida occulta is the result of incomplete bony fusion of the vertebral arches in a closed cartilaginous spinal canal in which the neural structures are usually intact. Spina bifida cystica involves prolapse of the arachnoid with either a normal spinal cord (meningocele) or involvement of the spinal cord (meningomyelocele; Figs. 8.**172a–d**).

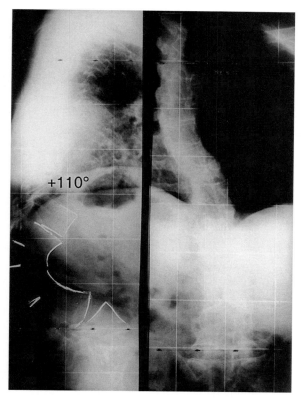

Fig. 8.**171** Plain radiograph of the spine in two planes. The image shows congenital kyphosis with anterior failure of segmentation (see Fig. 8.**159**, page 366).

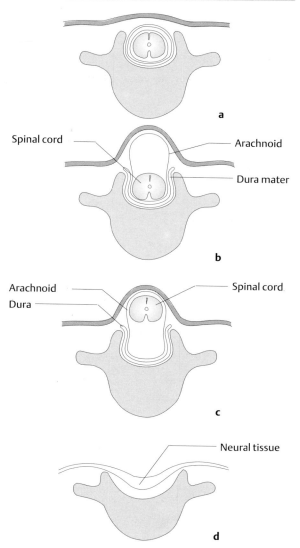

Figs. 8.**172a–d** Schematic diagram of various types of failure of fusion of the vertebral arches.
(**a**) Spina bifida occulta: incomplete bony fusion of the vertebral arches without displacement of the spinal cord or the meninges.
(**b**) Meningocele: displacement of the meninges without displacement of the spinal cord and with a bony defect of the vertebral arch.
(**c**) Meningomyelocele: displacement of the spinal cord and the meninges through the bony defect of the vertebral arch. The neural structures are either covered by skin or exposed.
(**d**) Spina bifida aperta (rachischisis): embryologic failure of fusion of the neural tube with exposure of neural tissue at the surface.

Both forms are usually associated with sensorimotor transverse paralysis at the level of the bony defect. Spina bifida aperta is the most serious form of fusion failure of the vertebral arches since the spinal cord is exposed without a layer of covering skin. Failure of fusion of the vertebral arches is recognizable in the plain AP radiographs by the respective defect (Figs. 8.**173a, b** and 8.**174**). CT or MR studies may be performed to further determine the extent of the disorder.

Osteoporotic Changes in the Spine

Osteoporosis is characterized by a quantitative decrease in the bone matrix, i.e., a decrease in both the organic and mineral content of the bone tissue. In the plain radiograph, this is seen as an increase in radiolucency, although this phenomenon will only be discernible once the decrease in bone matrix has exceeded 30% (MacNab 1971). The cancellous trabeculae are rarefied and the cortex narrowed. In the spine these changes will be most apparent in the cancellous vertebral bodies. Since the cancellous parts of the vertebra are affected first, it will appear on the radiograph as a **hollow vertebra** due to the relative increase in density of the cortex. During the further course of the disease, the thinned end-plates of the vertebrae can collapse under the intervertebral disk tissue, producing biconcave **vertebral deformities** known as fish vertebrae. Further subsidence of the anterior and posterior margins of the vertebral body lead to flattening of the vertebrae. In its advanced stages, osteoporosis is characterized by multilevel **compression fractures** that result in wedge-shaped vertebrae (Figs. 8.**175a, b**).

a

b

Figs. 8.173a, b   Plain radiograph of the lumbosacral spine in two planes showing sacral spina bifida.

Fig. 8.174   Plain Ap radiograph of the cervical spine. The image shows spina bifida occulta of the sixth cervical vertebra.

Table 8.37   Overview of the processes used to measure bone density

- Single and dual photon absorptiometry
- Single and dual X-ray absorptiometry
- Quantitative CT

Various processes are available for diagnosing osteoporosis (Table 8.37).

Single photon absorptiometry was the first process that permitted routine measuring of bone density (Gugliemi et al. 1995). Single and dual photon absorptiometry are nuclear medicine studies that measure the photon absorption in bone and thus provide and indication of bone density. Single and dual X-ray absorptiometry measures the absorption of X-rays. This value can also be used to calculate bone density (see also pp. 387 and 395).

References

Anderson LD, D'Alonzo RT. Fractures of the odontoid process of the axis. *J Bone Joint Surg.* 1974; 56-A; 1663

Bernard M, Bridwell KH. Segmental analysis of the sagittal plane alignment of the normal thoracic and lumbar spines and thoracolumbar junction. *Spine.* 1989; 7: 717

Boden S, Wiesel S. Lumbosacral segmental motion in normal individuals. *Spine.* 1990; 15: 571

a   b

Figs. 8.**175a, b**   Plain radiographs of the thoracic spine in two planes showing multilevel osteoporotic compression fractures.

Böhler L. *Die Technik der Knochenbruchbehandlung.* Vienna: Maudrich; 1951: 318

Bradford D, et al. Scheuerman's kyphosis and roundback deformity; Results of Milwaukee brace treatment. *J Bone Joint Surg.* 1974; 46-A: 740

Brant-Zawadzki M, Miller E, Federle M. CT in the evaluation of spine trauma. *AJR.* 1981; 136: 369

Cobb JR. Outline for the study of scoliosis. In: *American Academy of Orthopedic Surgeons; Instructional course letters.* Ann Arbor, Edward Brothers Inc. 1948; 5: 261

Daffner RH. Fingerprints of vertebral trauma — a unifying concept based on mechanism. *Skeletal Radiol.* 1986; 15: 518

Dahmen G, Bernbeck R. *Entzündungen und Tumoren der Wirbelsäule.* Stuttgart–New York: Thieme; 1987

Denis F. The three column spine and its significance in the classification of acute thoracolumbar spine injuries. *Spine.* 1983; 8: 817

Denis F. Spinal instability as defined by the three-column spine concept in acute spinal trauma. *Clin Orthop.* 1984; 189: 65.

DeSmet A, ed. Radiographic evaluation. Chap. 2. *Radiology of Spinal curvature.* St. Louis:Mosby; 1985.

Dihlmann W. *Gelenke-Wirbelverbindungen; klinische Radiologie einschließlich Computertomographie-Diagnose, Differentialdiagnose.* Stuttgart–New York: Thieme; 1987.

Dvorak J. Funktionelle Röntgendiagnostik der oberen Halswirbelsäule. *Orthopäde.* 1991; 20: 121

Dvorak J, et al. Functional radiographic diagnosis of the lumbar spine — flexion-extension and lateral bending. *Spine.* 1991; 16: 562

Gradinger R, et al. Operative Therapie von primären und sekundären malignen Tumoren der BWS und LWS. *Z Orthop.* 1989; 127: 410

Greenspan A. *Skelettradiologie.* 2nd ed. Weinheim–London: Chapman & Hall; 1993

Guglielmi G, et al. Current methods and advances in bone densitometrie. *Eur J Radiol.* 1995; 5: 129

Harms J. Klassifikation der BWS- und LWS-Frakturen. *Fortschr Med.* 1987; 105: 545

Hayes M, et al. Roentgenographic evaluation of lumbar spine flexion-extension in asymptomatic individuals. *Spine.* 1989; 14: 327

Hehne HJ, Zielke K. *Die kyphotische Deformität bei Spondylitis ankylosans. Klinik, Radiologie, Therapie* (Die Wirbelsäule in Forschung und Praxis, vol 112). Stuttgart; Hippokrates; 1990

Heine J. *Die Lumbalskoliosis.* Stuttgart: Enke; 1980

Holdsworth FW. Fractures, dislocations, and fracture dislocations of the spine. *J Bone Joint Surg.* 1963; 45-B: 6

Holdsworth F, Chir M. Fractures, dislocations, and fracture dislocations of the spine. *J Bone Joint Surg.* 1970; 52-A: 1534

Huvos AG. *Bone Tumors: Diagnosis, treatment and prognosis,* Philadelphia: WB Saunders; 1979

Imhäuser G. Knöcherne Abstützung bei Spondylolisthesis. Ein kausuistischer Beitrag. *Z Orthop.* 1988; 6: 647

King H, et al. The selection of fusion levels in thoracic idiopathic scoliosis. *J Bone Joint Surg.* 1983; 65-A: 1302

Krämer KL, Stock M, Winter M. *Klinikleitfaden Orthopädie; Untersuchung, Diagnostik, Therapie, Notfall.* Stuttgart: Jungjohann; 1993

Lenke L. A new surgical classification of idiopathic scoliosis: predicting and assessing treatment. Paper read at the 6th International Meeting on Advanced Spine Techniques (IMAST) in Vancouver, Canada. July 1999

Lewit K. *Manuelle Medizin.* 2nd ed. Munich–Vienna–Baltimore: Urban & Schwarzenberg; 1977

Link T, et al. Conventional CT versus spiral CT in the diagnosis of vertebral fractures. *Radiology.* 1996; 198: 515–519

MacNab I. The traction spur. *J Bone Joint Surg.* 1971; 53-A: 663

Magerl F. *Klassifizierung von Wirbelsäulenverletzungen.* (Hefte zur Unfallheilkunde, Heft 189). Berlin–Heidelberg: Springer, 1987: 597

Magerl F, et al. A comprehensive classification of thoracic and lumbar injuries. *Europ. Spine J.* 1994; 3: 184

Marsh B, et al. Benign osteoblastoma: Range of manifestations. *J Bone Joint Surg.* 1975; 57-A: 1

McAfee P, Youan H, Fredrickson B, Lubicky J, et al. The value of computed tomography in thoracolumbar fractures. *J Bone Joint Surg.* 1983; 65-A: 461

Moe J, Winter R, Bradford D, Lonstein J. *Scoliosis and other spinal deformities.* Philadelphia: WB Saunders; 1994

Nash CL, Moe JH. A study of vertebral rotation. *J Bone Joint Surg.* 1969; 51-A: 223

Nemoto O, Moser R, Van Dam B, Aoki J, Gilkey F. Osteoblastoma of the spine. *Spine.* 1990; 15: 1272

Nicoll EA. Fractures of the dorso-lumbar spine. *J Bone Joint Surg.* 1949; 31-B: 376

Pearcy M, Portek I, Shepherd J. Three-dimensional X-ray analysis of normal movement in the lumbar spine. *Spine.* 1984; 9: 294

Perdriolle R, Vidal J. Etude de la courbure scoliotique: importance et l'extension et de la rotation vertebral. *Rev. Chir. Orthop.* 1981; 67: 25

Ponseti I, Freidman B. Prognosis in idiopathic scoliosis. *J Bone Joint Surg.* 1950; 32-A: 381

Propst-Proctor S, Bleck E. Radiographic determinations of lordosis and kyphosis in normal and scoliotic children. *J Pediatr Orthop.* 1983; 3: 344

Roaf R. Vertebral growth and its mechanical control. *J Bone Joint Surg.* 1960; 42-B: 40

Salzer-Kuntschik M. *Tumoren der Wirbelsäule.* Stuttgart: Hippokrates; 1984

Stagnara P, DeMauroy JC, Dran G. Reciprocal angulation of vertebral bodies in a sagittal plane. Approach to references for the evaluation of kyphosis and lordosis. *Spine* 1982; 7: 335

Thümler P, Püttmann H, Metz-Stavenhagen P. Möglichkeiten und Grenzen der operativen Behandlung und orthetischen Versorgung von Wirbelsäulentumoren. *Orthopädie-Technik.* 1987; 10: 578

White AA, Johnson RM, Panjabi MM, Southwick WO. Biomechanical analysis of clinical stability in the cervical spine. *Clin. Orthop.* 1975; 109: 85

White AA, Southwick WO, Panjabi MM. Clinical instability in the cervical spine. *Spine* 1976; 1: 15

White AA, Panjabi MM. *Clinical biomechanics of the spine.* Philadelphia: JP Lippincott; 1990

Whitesides T. Traumatic kyphosis of the thoracolumbar spine. *Clin Orthop.* 1977; 128: 78

Wiltse L, Newman P, MacNab J. Classification of spondylolisthesis. *Clin Orthop.* 1976; 117: 23

Wolf KJ, Gnann H. Röntgendiagnostik der Wirbelsäulentumoren. In: Schmitt E, ed. *Tumoren der Wirbelsäule.* Stuttgart: Hippokrates; 1984

Wuisman P, Härle A, Nommensen B, Reiser M, Erlemann R, Roessner A. Der Riesenzelltumor des Knochens. *Z Orthop.* 1989; 127: 89

Wuisman P, Polster J, Härle A, Matthias HH, Brinckmann P. Das Wirbelkörperimplantat als Behandlungsprinzip bei Tumoren und Metastasen der thorakalen und lumbalen Wirbelsäule. *Z. Orthop.* 1989; 127: 25

8.4 Ultrasound

Indications, Diagnostic Value, and Clinical Relevance

The goal of diagnostic imaging of the spine is to reproduce spinal structures in a precise and reliable manner. Ultrasound is a second-line imaging modality. Its primary use is in evaluating postoperative changes such as hematomas and seromas, or for imaging pseudomeningoceles after disk operations. With current technology, ultrasound is not suitable as a diagnostic aid in evaluating a prolapsed lumbar disk (Jerosch et al. 1992). Although prolapsed disks can be successfully imaged under certain conditions, ultrasound alone is not sufficient for diagnostic purposes (Jerosch and Marquardt 1993). CT and MRI are significantly superior imaging modalities for disks.

Due to the cartilaginous structure of the spinal column in fetuses and infants, posterior ultrasound can provide relatively high quality images up to the age of 6 months (Graf and Schuler 1995).

Instrumentation, Transducers, and Examination Technique

The intraoperative examination is performed by filling the posterior wound with Ringer solution and imaging the operative site through a small laminotomy (Eismont and Barth 1984).

The posterior approach is used primarily when imaging the spinal column in children to evaluate the neural tube.

Normal Findings

The PA projection is used in newborns to image and evaluate the disks, the spinal cord with the spinal nerve roots and central canal, and the dural sac its epidural fatty tissue. The intervertebral disk itself will appear hypoechoic; only the posterior margin of the disk will appear as a strong echo. The dura will appear hyperechoic, while the epidural fatty tissue in between will be moderately echogenic. The nerve roots and the cauda equina produce fine echo structures.

The fetal spinal column can be imaged from the 15th week of pregnancy (Filly and Golbus 1982). Three bony cores are already discernible at this time, one each at the vertebral arches and another in the vertebral body (Graf and Schuler 1995).

Pathologic Findings

Ultrasound can image cleavages and deformities with or without involvement of parts of the spinal cord. A meningocele will appear as a hypoechoic hollow space; fine echo structures within the hernia sac are signs of spinal cord involvement and are indicative of a meningomyelocele (Graf and Schuler 1995).

Intraoperative ultrasound studies can detect involvement of the nerve roots, dural changes such as hematoma or edema, and extradural stenoses of the spinal canal in spinal injuries. Intraoperative ultrasound can demonstrate that extensive decompression is indicated, and it can be used to verify the results of decompression (Eismont and Barth 1984).

References

Eismont F, et al. The role of intraoperative ultrasonography in the treatment of thoracic and lumbar spine fractures. *Spine.* 1984; 9: 782

Filly R, Golbus M. Ultrasonography of the normal and pathologic fetal skeleton. *Radiol Clin North Am.* 1982; 20: 311

Graf R, Schuler P. *Sonographie am Stütz- und Bewegungsapparat bei Erwachsenen und Kindern.* Weinheim–London: Chapman & Hall; 1995

Jerosch J, Marquardt M. *Sonographie des Bewegungsapparates.* Ch 7, Sonographie der Wirbelsäule. Zülpich: Bierman; 1993

Jerosch J, Strauss J, Castro W, Schlicker U. Sonographische Diagnostik des lumbalen Bandscheibenvorfalles — eine klinisch relevante Methode? *Ultraschall Med.* 1992; 13: 187

8.5 Myelography

Indications, Diagnostic Value, and Clinical Relevance

Before the era of CT and MRI, myelography was regarded as one of the most important diagnostic methods for demonstrating changes in the subarachnoid space or the effects on these structures of extradural tumors in the spinal canal. As an invasive procedure, this method involves certain risks (infection, fistula of cerebrospinal fluid, bleeding, post-procedure headache, and anaphylactic shock). The introduction of CT and, later, MRI as noninvasive modalities relegated myelography to a supportive role. Compared with discography, myelography has the disadvantage of not being able to image the anatomy of the intervertebral disks and not permitting pain propagation testing. Myelography used in combination with CT (CT myelography) remains one of the most important modalities for evaluating spinal stenosis (Table 8.**38**).

Technique, Instrumentation, and Examination Procedure

First, the AP radiograph should be examined to exclude degenerative stenoses and ossification, espe-

Table 8.38 Clinical value of myelography

Bone structure	–
Facet arthritis	–
Disk prolapse	++
Symptomatic disk without prolapse	–
Trauma	+
Spondylitis	
Deformities	–
Tumor	+
Spinal stenosis (central)	+++
Lateral stenosis	–

– No information content
(+) Low information content
+ Moderate information content
++ High information content
+++ Very high information content

cially in the flaval ligaments, which could interfere with injection. The patient is placed in a lateral position with the hips and knees flexed and at maximum kyphosis or is positioned sitting and bent far forward. The iliac crests can be used as landmarks to locate the spinous processes of L3 and L4. Next the skin is disinfected and the area surrounding the injection site sterilely draped. Injection is performed under sterile conditions (i.e., sterile gloves, mask, cap, and perforated draping) with a 22-G spinal needle between the spinous processes L3 and L4 or L2 and L3. The dura mater can be recognized by the resistance of the tough tissue. This resistance must be overcome to advance the needle into the subarachnoid space. The cerebrospinal fluid that begins to drip after the stylet is removed indicates that the needle is in the proper position (Fig. 8.**176**). If you suspect that the passage of cerebrospinal fluid is locked, apply the Queckenstedt-Stookey test and compress the jugular veins, which should increase the drip speed. Failure of the fluid to drip faster after pressure is applied suggests a block in the subarachnoid channels. A few drops of CSF should

Fig. 8.176 Schematic diagram of lumbar myelography. The needle is advanced into the subarachnoid space at the L3–L4 level.

Fig. 8.**178**   Lumbar CT myelography in the transverse plane, showing normal findings. Note how the two nerve roots are clearly demonstrated by the contrast medium.

Fig. 8.**177**   Lumbar myelography in the sagittal plane, showing normal findings. Notice the slight impressions in the dural sac at the level of the intervertebral disks (from Castro W. M., Schilgen, M., Kreuzschmerzen, Springer Verlag 1995).

routinely be saved for laboratory analysis. A lateral radiograph should be obtained to verify and document correct needle positioning.

After injection of contrast medium into the subarachnoid space, the contrast medium will mix with the CSF. Since the contrast medium has a higher specific gravity than the cerebrospinal fluid, gravity and patient positioning can be used to influence its spread through the spinal canal. Proper evaluation requires obtaining images of the respective structures in each of four planes (AP, lateral, left oblique, and right oblique; Fig. 8.**177**); lateral dynamic views obtained under fluoroscopy are also important. CT studies can follow the myelogram (CT myelography) to provide further diagnostic images (Fig. 8.**178**).

Normal Findings

In myelography, the dural sac and the nerve roots with their sheath are discernible as gaps in the contrast medium. The union between the medullary cone and the cauda equina is visualized as a transition from the solid gap in the contrast medium produced by the medullary cone to the striped pattern of individual nerve roots in the cauda equina. In the lateral view, slight impressions in the dural sac at the level of the intervertebral spaces in the deep lumbar spine are visible. This pattern is caused by the disks that are larger than the vertebral bodies and bulge outward (Rauschning 1990) (Fig. 8.**177**).

In the AP projection you should verify that the sheaths of the nerve roots exit the spinal column symmetrically.

◀ Fig. 8.**179**   Lumbar myelography in the coronal plane. The image shows a prolapsed disk with a central contrast medium defect (Jerosch and Castro 1994).

Fig. 8.**180** Lumbar myelography in the sagittal plane, showing subtotal contrast-medium blockage at two levels due to stenosis of the spinal canal.

Fig. 8.**181** Lumbar myelography in the sagittal plane. The dural sac is compressed at the L4–L5 level as a result of a prolapsed disk. Note the cut-off of the L5 nerve root.

Abnormal Findings with Degenerative Changes

Bear in mind that in the deep lumbar spine the lower intervertebral disks have larger sagittal diameters than the vertebral end-plates. This means that a slight bulge in the disks in this part of the spine is regarded as physiologic (Rauschning 1990) (Fig. 8.**177**).

Central stenoses of the spinal canal will be reliably visualized. Heithoff cites a true positive rate of 100% in this regard. The stenoses may be the result of posterior osteophytes, hypertrophy of the flaval ligaments, medial disk prolapse (rare) (Fig. 8.**179**), or other masses (neoplasms). In the lateral projection, myelography depicts spinal stenosis as a reduction in the sagittal diameter of the column of contrast medium (which may include a complete contrast-medium block if there is medial prolapse of a mass) and as posterior impressions resulting from the hypertrophic articular processes (Verbiest 1990) (Fig. 8.**180**).

Mediolateral prolapsed disks are also easily detected in the oblique and AP views as displacement of the column of contrast medium, which may include a complete contrast-medium block (Figs. 8.**181** and 8.**182a, b**). The accuracy of myelography in

diagnosing disk prolapse is cited at 60–100% (Haag et al. 1985; Jackson and Jacobs 1990; Simon 1981; Zsernaviczky and Juppe 1989). In the same connection, the incidence of false positive results cited ranges from 6–30%; false negative results range from 4–30% (Haughton et al. 1982; Heithoff 1990; Jackson and Jacobs 1990; Zsernaviczky and Juppe 1989). Studies by Jackson and Jacobs (1990) in which CT is performed immediately after myelography (CT myelography) have improved accuracy by 7% (Fig. 8.**183**).

Lateral stenoses, and even **lateral prolapsed disks,** often elude detection in myelography because the compression of the nerve root occurs outside its sheath. Heithoff (1990) cites a 100% incidence of false negative findings in the myelogram for surgically confirmed lateral stenosis.

Whereas radiographic diagnosis of spinal stenosis once relied entirely on myelography, the modality today serves primarily to locate the segment of the spine which is to undergo subsequent CT evaluation (Verbiest 1990). CT myelography is regarded as one of the most important modalities for diagnosing spinal stenosis (see section Spinal Stenosis).

As in other spinal imaging modalities, findings must always be correlated with the clinical examina-

a

b

Figs. 8.**182a, b** Cervical myelography in the sagittal and oblique planes, showing a mediolateral disk prolapse at C5–C6.

tion and history of the respective patient. Hitselberger and Witten (1968) detected pathologic changes in the lumbar myelogram ranging from nerve-root compression to complete contrast-medium block in 37% of asymptomatic patients.

Abnormal Findings with Traumatic Changes

Pathologic findings include asymmetry or compression of the nerve sheaths and leakage of contrast due to avulsion of nerve roots in traumatic plexus lesions that may even include complete contrast-medium block (Figs. 8.**184a, b** and 8.**185**). Burst or dislocation fractures can also lead to stenosis of the dural sac including complete compression with contrast-medium block in the myelogram. In the surgical treatment of spinal injuries, intraoperative myelography can provide important information about the success of the fracture reduction. In operative procedures through a posterior approach, a dislocated fragment of the posterior margin of a burst fracture may be reduced by distracting the spine (ligamentotaxis).

Fig. 8.**183** Axial lumbar CT, post myelogram, showing compromise of the left S1 nerve root due to a mediolateral disk prolapse.

Since ligamentotaxis may not be feasible or sufficient in the presence of a ruptured posterior longitudinal ligament or rotated or impinged fragments, intraoperative myelography is crucial. The subarachnoid space is aspirated intraoperatively and filled with

Figs. 8.**184a, b** Lumbar myelography in two planes, showing traumatic avulsion of the left L5 nerve root in a fracture dislocation at L5–S1. (corresponding to Fig. 8.**185**).

a   b

Fig. 8.**185** Axial lumbar CT, post myelogram (corresponding to Figs. 8.**184a, b**).

Fig. 8.**186** Lateral intraoperative thoracolumbar myelogram following reduction and stabilization of a burst fracture of the first lumbar vertebra and showing good contrast-medium flow.

contrast medium following open reduction of the fracture. If there are still fragments in the spinal canal, an anterior procedure should be considered (Fig. 8.**186**).

References

Haag M, Beck A, Wimmer B. Korrelation von Radiologischem und intraoperativem Befund bei lumbalen Bandscheibenvorfällen. *Orthopädische Praxis*. 1985; 4: 287

Haughton V, et al. A prospective comparison of computed tomography and myelography in the diagnosis of herniated lumbar disks. *Radiology*. 1982; 142: 103

Heithoff K. Computed Tomography and Plain Film Diagnosis of the lumbar spine. In: Weinstein J, Wiesel S, eds. *The Lumbar Spine*. Philadelphia: WB Saunders; 1990

Hitselberger W, Witten R. Abnormal myelograms in asymptomatic patients. *J Neurosurg*. 1968; 28: 204

Jackson R, Jacobs R. Computed Tomography — Discography. In: Weinstein J, Wiesel S, eds. *The Lumbar Spine*. Philadelphia: WB Saunders; 1990

Jerosch J, Castro WHM. *Das Facettensyndrom: Ursachen, Diagnostik, Therapie,* Prophylaxe. (Bücherei des Orthopäden, vol. 62). Stuttgart: Enke; 1994

Rauschning W. Imaging Anatomy of the Lumbar Spine. In: Weinstein J, Wiesel S, eds. *The Lumbar Spine.* Philadelphia: WB Saunders; 1990

Simon W. Stimmen Röntgendiagnose und OP-Befund bei der lumbalen Myelographie überein? *Radiologe.* 1981; 21: 347

Verbiest H. Lumbar spinal stenosis. Morphology, classification, and long-term results. In: Weinstein J, Wiesel S, eds. *The Lumbar Spine.* Philadelphia: WB Saunders; 1990

Zsernaviczky J, Juppe M. A Comparison of myelography and computer tomography in lumbar disk herniation. *Int. Orthop.* 1989; 13: 51

8.6 Nuclear Medicine Studies

Indications, Diagnostic Value, and Clinical Relevance

Nuclear medicine studies for diseases of the spine and pelvis may be indicated by a tentative clinical diagnosis (Tables 8.**39** and 8.**40**). Radiographic and nuclear medicine imaging studies used in combination, i.e., as stages in a well-ordered diagnostic scheme, will complement each other so as to increase the yield of diagnostic information in most cases.

Basic advantages of all nuclear medicine studies include their high sensitivity and the fact that they image the entire body, which is particularly advantageous in disorders with possible systemic manifestations. However in changes that proceed from the marrow, bone metabolism may be affected only relatively late. Bone marrow scintigraphy or positron emission tomography (PET) scans are often more sensitive.

Bone scans and bone marrow scintigraphy are less specific studies because the activation of bone metabolism or the destruction of the hemopoietic

Table 8.**39** Indications for nuclear medicine studies of the spinal column and pelvis

Tumors	Primary tumors (malignant and benign) Metastases
Inflammation	Bacterial Rheumatic
Trauma	Fractures (including stress fractures) Multiple trauma Child abuse Pseudarthrosis
Postoperative	After spinal fusion After implantation of autologous or allograft bone Implant loosening Infection
Degenerative	Arthritis Osteochondrosis
Other	Bone pain or restricted movement with unclear canse

Table 8.**40** Clinical value of nuclear medicine studies of the spinal column and pelvis

Bone structure	–
Facet arthritis/arthritis of the sacroiliac joints	++
Disk prolapse	–
Symptomatic disk without prolapse	–
Trauma	++
Spondylitis/osteomyelitis/sacroiliac arthritides	+++
Deformities	–
Tumor	+++
Spinal stenosis (central)	–
Lateral stenosis	–

–	No information content
(+)	Low information content
+	Moderate information content
++	High information content
+++	Very high information content

marrow can represent an unvarying reaction to a variety of stimuli. However, the specificity can be significantly increased by documenting the arrangement, shape, size, localization, number, and intensity of the changes while taking clinical information into account. There are also other nuclear medicine studies that utilize certain mechanisms of increased focal uptake to permit tissue-specific visualization of tumors or infections.

Technique, Instrumentation, and Examination Procedure

The most frequently used scintigraphic method for disorders of the spine and pelvis is the **bone scan** with **technetium-99m phosphonate complexes**. Please refer to section 1.6 for a discussion of the underlying pathophysiology, examination procedure, and acquisition techniques.

Unobscured tomographic visualization using **SPECT** (single-photon emission computed tomography) often provides valuable additional information, particularly in spinal and pelvic disorders. Generous criteria should be used in determining if this method is indicated. Obtaining the additional tomographic images does not involve any further exposure to radiation, and these images can supplement the results of planar diagnostic studies.

In addition to conventional bone scans, other scintigraphic examination methods are used for specific disorders of the spine and pelvis. These include bone marrow scintigraphy, labeled leukocyte studies, and special sensitive or specific tumor-detecting methods. PET warrants special mention in this regard as this method has now become an important modality in diagnosing tumors and infections of the axial skeleton.

Primary Bone Tumors

Even in the age of modern cross-sectional imaging processes, primary bone tumors are best classified using conventional radiographic studies. CT and MRI supplement this classification with precise information on tumor localization, orientation, extent, and organ involvement (Reiser and Semmler 1992).

Bone scans supplement these imaging modalities. The three-phase technique in particular is able to confirm or disprove the tentative classification. Increased metabolism in all three phases (high blood-flow rate, increase in soft-tissue concentration, and intensive bone metabolism) is frequently suggestive of a malignant bone tumor and is often observed with osteosarcomas and Ewing sarcomas (Fig. 8.**187**). If we only observe the metabolic behavior of such a lesion, it cannot be differentiated from a florid inflammatory process in its form. Such a pattern can also be detected in benign skeletal tumors, such as an osteoid osteoma or lesions similar to tumors, such as Paget disease. Morphologic parameters such as the size and orientation of the lesion, its pattern of dissemination, and whether it respects anatomic borders, skip lesions, detection of a nidus, inhomogeneity, or multifocal growth, aid in scintigraphic differential diagnosis.

Conversely, normal blood flow and only slight activation of bone metabolism will sometimes be observed in primary bone tumors as well, especially in Ewing sarcomas or in primarily osteolytic osteosarcomas. Otherwise a normal or only slightly activated metabolism in a bony lesion is suggestive of a benign cause.

Bone scans represent an ideal **screening method** in the presence of pain syndromes of unidentified origin or limited motion. On occasion, skeletal tumors causing such syndromes are detected before there are any pathologic radiographic findings (Fig. 8.**188**).

Metastases

Depending on the prevalence of the disorder, **bone scans** continue to represent a simple, fast, and inexpensive screening method for detecting suspected metastases (Munz 1994).

This modality offers the advantages of whole-body imaging and a sensitivity of over 90%. Metastases can be detected on average 3–6 months earlier than in conventional radiographic studies (Rieden 1987). The low specificity, in the order of 60–70%, usually requires further radiographic or other diagnostic imaging studies in the presence of a pathologic scan.

In addition to the typical appearance of lesions showing increased bone metabolism, metastases can appear less often as circumscribed osteopenic defects without an osteoblastic halo, or as a homogeneous diffuse, increased concentration in the axial skeleton.

Bone scans fail to detect osteolytic metastases more often than osteoblastic ones since osteopenic foci are harder to detect. Several studies have described the superiority of MRI in the early diagnosis of metastases in the spine in particular (Algra et al. 1991, Link et al. 1995). However, MRI is too complicated to use as a screening method and the field of view is limited.

In the postoperative care of breast cancer, the most frequent primary tumor with skeletal metastases, the indications for bone scans are controversial. A routine bone scan in the early stages is not indicated due to the low prevalence of metastatic disease and the minimal amount of additional diagnostic information (Schünemann and Jourdain 1989).

Fig. 8.**187** Osteosarcoma of the left iliac wing. Three-phase bone scan in the posterior projection. Increased metabolism is discernible in all three phases: vascular phase (6 seconds), blood pool phase (2 minutes), and bone phase (3 hours). The size of the tumor itself is overestimated due to the reactive activation of osteoblasts.

Fig. 8.**188**   Twelve-year-old female patient with unidentified pain in the thoracolumbar spine. Conventional radiographic studies were normal. The bone scan reveals an intense, unifocal increase in concentration in the 12th vertebral body, diagnosed histologically as an osteoid osteoma.

Fig. 8.**189**   Multiple metastases showing activation of bone metabolism. The intensity of the lesions is typical of carcinoma of the prostate.

If the indication criteria is limited to high-risk and symptomatic patients, the value of bone scans as a screening method is undisputed. Bones scans are a standard diagnostic method for monitoring the clinical course of metastases under treatment. There is good correlation between the scintigraphic behavior of the metastases and the duration of clinical remission and patients' survival time.

Usually it is not possible to draw conclusions regarding the primary tumor, except for the highly intensive accumulation with metastases of prostate carcinoma (Fig. 8.**189**). The detection of early metastases in the axial skeleton can be proved by use of **bone marrow scintigraphy** (Reske et al. 1990).

The bone marrow scintigram will often detect foci of destruction in cases where a bone scan fails to reveal pathologic findings. This is particularly true with primary myelogenic metastasizing or infiltrative tumors such as lymphomas, plasmocytomas, or breast cancer.

However, the concentration defects in bone marrow scintigraphy are not specifically characteristic of metastases but are as similarly unspecific as the "hot" foci in bone scans (Fig. 8.**190**).

Inflammation

Nuclear medicine studies for diagnosing inflammation include three-phase bone scans and labeled-white-cell studies. Labeled-white-cell studies utilize a wide variety of radiopharmaceuticals, each with various advantages and disadvantages. In the following section we will refer exclusively to technetium-99m-labeled monoclonal antigranulocyte antibodies. This is an antibody with the surface antigen NCA 95 of mature granulocytes, as well as with myelopoietic cells. This means that this substance can be used for two indications, for detecting foci of infections and for imaging the hemopoietic marrow.

Peripheral foci of osteomyelitis, i.e., foci in parts of the skeleton containing yellow bone marrow, lead to an increased concentration of the antibody that is both sensitive and specific and clearly marks the actual area of infection. In contrast, infections in parts of the skeleton containing hemopoietic marrow (these infections can include spondylitis or osteomyelitis of the pelvis) destroy the hemopoietic medulla, producing a storage tissue defect (Fig. 8.**191**). These

Fig. 8.**190** Metastasis of an unknown primary tumor in the body of the 12th thoracic vertebra. The left bone scan is normal whereas the bone marrow scan in the right image shows a storage tissue defect.

Fig. 8.**191** Leukocyte scintigraphy with technetium-99m-labeled monoclonal antigranulocyte antibodies, showing a storage tissue defect in the body of the fifth lumbar vertebra in chronic vertebral osteomyelitis.

storage-tissue defects are unspecific manifestations of displacement or destruction of bone marrow. They cannot necessarily be linked to a specific cause since other disorders such as metastases, trauma, postoperative sequelae, or severe degenerative processes can also produce similar defects. Even after spondylitis has healed, bone marrow depression may persist for a long time. Increased concentration of monoclonal antigranulocyte antibodies in bone marrow will only predominate over lesser concentration in the presence of an acute florid infection, producing a positive contrast. This means that leukocyte scintigraphy in the axial skeleton does not have nearly the diagnostic value it has in the peripheral skeleton, where it is a highly accurate method (Bartenstein et al. 1989; Schauwecker 1989; Sciuk et al. 1992; Whalen et al. 1991). Usually it only provides specific additional information in acute infections and in evaluating the involvement of soft tissue surrounding bony structures.

In a **bone scan,** the location of a focus of infection does not significantly impair its visualization. An increase in activity will typically be seen in all three phases in osteomyelitis or spondylitis (Fig. 8.**192**). The pathologic findings in the first two phases will decrease the more chronic the infection becomes. In chronic osteomyelitis, the late phase almost always shows an increased level of bone metabolism; "normal" bone metabolism almost certainly excludes a chronic bone infection. However, false negative findings can occasionally occur in acute spondylitis. Metal implants do not reduce the accuracy of nuclear medicine studies. Alternatively, scans with gallium-67 citrate or human immunoglobulin can provide additional information in patients with axial skeletal infections since the physiologic concentration in the hemopoietic marrow is not significant in these cases.

Other Abnormal Findings

Nuclear medicine studies may also be indicated in trauma, pediatric orthopedics, and rheumatology, for postoperative syndromes, uncertain clinical symptoms such as pain or limited motion, degenerative processes, and metabolic systemic disorders, and in other specific lines of inquiry (Fig. 8.**193**).

The opportunities offered by scintigraphy are rarely utilized in **trauma treatment**. Radiographic studies are the method of choice, particularly in the cervical spine and pelvis. However, the physician should consider additional nuclear medicine indications such as the clarification of discrepancies between clinical and radiographic findings, the verification of suspected stress fractures, the exclusion of fractures, child abuse, multiple trauma cases, and in follow-up (Spitz and Tittel 1990).

Remember that fractures of the vertebral body often appear in the scintigram as a metabolic reaction only after a latency period of several days, whereas injuries to the hands or feet are usually detectable on the first day. Follow-up examinations permit conclusions regarding the **age of the fracture,** which can be highly significant in cases of child abuse or in patients who have suffered multiple trauma. Bone scans are well suited for detecting **stress fractures** and for evaluating **disturbed healing of fractures,** such as pseudarthrosis. Here, we differentiate between hypertrophic pseudarthrosis, which is characterized by a strong concentration of activity, and the atrophic form with a band of diminished activity concentration (Winkel 1990). In spondylolysis, scintigraphy can be helpful in distinguishing an older or congenital lesion from a fresh fatigue fracture. The same applies to postoperative follow-up examinations, such as after spinal fusion, after implantation of autologous or allograft bone, and especially in evaluating implant loosening or periprosthetic infections.

Fig. 8.**192**   Acute vertebral osteomyelitis with diskitis at L2–L3, showing increased activity in all three phases of the scan.

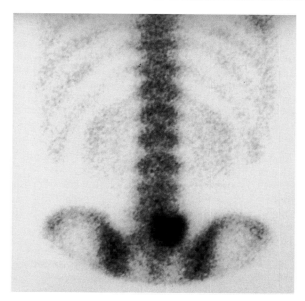

Fig. 8.**193** Sixteen-year-old male patient with intense concentration in the lumbosacral spine, histologically diagnosed as a chordoma.

Fig. 8.**195** Spondylarthritis. SPECT reconstruction in the coronal plane. The foci that could not be definitely localized in the planar views are projected on the small vertebral joints in the SPECT image.

In **rheumatic disorders,** nuclear medicine techniques detect inflammatory changes in joints early. Here, early diagnosis of sacroiliitis in Bechterew disease is particularly significant because it can be standardized by a semiquantitative evaluation of bone metabolism in the sacroiliac joints (Fig. 8.**194**). Further indications include primary chronic polyarthritis and psoriatic arthritis involving the spine.

Whereas **degenerative changes** are the most common pathologic changes in the bone scan, they are generally incidental to other findings. Reactive metaplastic processes in bone produce positive findings more often seen than in radiographs and often do not correlate with the extent of visible morphologic changes. Arthritis of the intervertebral joints of the cervical spine generally shows a typical pattern with paravertebral and posterior concentrations so that a specific diagnosis can be made in these cases (Büll and Hör 1990). Evaluation of the configuration and location of the foci and follow-up studies aid in differential diagnosis. SPECT in particular is very important in the axial skeleton and should be used generously (Fig. 8.**195**). When in doubt, further radiographic studies are indicated.

Fig. 8.**194** Sacroiliitis on the left side. The image shows a pathologic relation between the activity of the sacroiliac joints and sacrum on the left side and a normal relation on the right.

Sacroiliac joint / Sacrum

(Reference: 1.35)

Right: 1.1

Left: 1.5

References

Algra PR, Bloem JL, Tissing H, et al. Detection of vertebral metastases: comparison between MR imaging and bone scintigraphy. *Radiographics.* 1991; 11: 219

Bartenstein P, Sciuk J, Erlemann R, et al. Leukozytenszintigraphie und Kernspintomographie in der Diagnostik muskuloskelettaler Infektionen. *Nuklearmediziner.* 1989; 5 (12): 327–336

Büll U, Hör G. *Klinische Nuklearmedizin.* Weinheim–London: Chapman & Hall; 1990

Link M, Sciuk J, Fründt H, et al. Wirbelsäulenmetastasen-Wertigkeit diagnostischer Verfahren bei der Erstdiagnostik und im Verlauf. *Radiologe.* 1995; 35: 21

Munz DL. Ist die Skelett-Szintigrafie als Metastasenscreening erforderlich? *Nuklearmedizin.* 1994; 33: 5

Reiser M, Semmler W. *Magnetresonanztomographie.* Berlin–Heidelberg–New York: Springer; 1992

Reske SN, Karstens HJ, Glöckner, et al. Nachweis des Knochenmarkbefalls beim Mammakarzinom und bei malignen Lymphomen durch Immunszintigraphie des hämatopoetischen Knochenmarks. *Fortschr. Geb Röntgenstr Nuklearmed Ergänzungsband.* 1990; 152: 60

Rieden K. *Knochenmetastasen. Radiologische Diagnostik, Therapie und Nachsorge.* Berlin–Heidelberg–New York: Springer; 1987

Schauwecker DS. Osteomyelitis: Diagnosis with In-111-labeled leukocytes. *Radiology.* 1989; 171: 141

Schünemann H, Jourdain M. Stellenwert der Skelettszintigraphie in der Nachsorge des Mammakarzinoms. *Dtsch Med Wochenschr.* 1989; 114: 3

Sciuk J, et al. Bildgebende Diagnostik der Osteomyelitis. *Deutsches Ärztebl.* 1992; 89: 2462

Spitz J, Tittel K. Indikationen und Ergebnisse der Skelettszintigraphie in der Traumatologie. In: Brussatis F, Hahn K, eds. *Nuklearmedizin in der Orthopädie.* Berlin–Heidelberg–New York: Springer; 1990: 280

Whalen J, et al. Limitations of Indium leukocyte imaging for the diagnosis of spine infections. *Spine.* 1991; 16: 193

Winkel K. *Nuklearmedizin.* Berlin–Heidelberg–New York: Springer; 1990

sue, it can reliably determine the extent of the injury and precisely visualize fracture lines. The posterior margin of the vertebra plays an important role in the classification of the fracture. This part of the vertebra is often poorly visualized in plain radiographs. Reconstruction views should be requested in spinal injuries. These images permit good two-dimensional visualization of the fracture, evaluation of the spinal canal and retropulsed fragments. However, reliable evaluation of intramedullary changes is not always possible (Schubiger 1984). In these cases, MRI is the diagnostic imaging modality of choice.

CT is also important in evaluating osteoporosis. Bone densitometry permits precise evaluation and allows judgement of risk factors and the response to treatment (Table 8.**41**).

Table 8.**41**   Clinical value of CT of the spine (without three-dimensional CT)

Bone structure	+++
Facet arthritis	+++
Disk prolapse	+++
Symptomatic disk without prolapse	–
Trauma	+++
Spondylitis	++
Deformities	–
Tumor	+++
Spinal stenosis (central)	+++
Lateral stenosis	+++

–   No information content
(+) Low information content
+   Moderate information content
++ High information content
+++ Very high information content

8.7 Computed Tomography

Indications, Diagnostic Value, and Clinical Relevance

CT provides precise visualization of the vertebrae with their joints and ligaments, the intervertebral disks, and the spinal canal including the neuroforamen. CT complements plain radiography in the evaluation of degenerative spinal processes. It is regarded as a standard adjunctive imaging modality after plain radiography for diagnosing back and leg pain in patients who have not had previous surgery (Heithoff 1990). Patients who have undergone previous surgery may have fibrotic tissue of the same radiodensity as nerve or disk tissue. This can make the CT image difficult to interpret. MRI with its higher soft-tissue resolution permits more precise differentiation of these structures.

CT is a valuable imaging modality in spine injuries. With its high contrast between bone and soft tis-

Technique, Instrumentation, and Examination Procedure

CT is a process in which X-rays are used to visualize slices of the body. A narrowly focused bundle of X-rays scans the desired slice to produce a **cross-sectional image.** The thickness of the slices can vary from 1–12 mm. A computer calculates appropriate shades of gray from the X-ray absorption values and forms an image from these gray-scale levels. A density scale specifies the respective density value in Hounsfield units. Water has a density of zero, air –1000, and cortical bone +1000.

Two-dimensional or three-dimensional reconstructions can be requested (Figs. 8.**198,** 8.**205b,** and 8.**217a, b**). Two-dimensional sagittal reconstructions are important in the diagnosis of spinal injuries. Three-dimensional reconstructions are used primarily with complex injuries of the skull or pelvis.

Fig. 8.**196** Axial CT image of the cervical spine showing a normal cervical vertebra.

Fig. 8.**197** Axial CT image of the lumbar spine showing a normal lumbar vertebra/disk.

Quantitative CT is used in bone densitometry to provide precise information. Density values of the lumbar vertebrae (usually the second or third lumbar vertebra) are calculated, averaged, and compared with a reference body of hydroxylapatite or potassium dihydrogen phosphate placed next to the patient. This procedure is used in the early diagnosis of osteoporosis (plain-film radiography is only positive if the reduction in calcium salt exceeds 30%) and as a follow-up diagnostic procedure during treatment (Niethard 1992) (see also pp. 371 and 395).

Normal Findings

The **atlas** does not have a vertebral body as such and appears as a biconvex ring-shaped structure with an anterior and posterior arch. The dens projects posterior to the thin anterior arch of the atlas. The two lateral masses articulate with the occiput. The atlas and axis are connected to one another via the atlantoaxial joints, the two lateral vertebral joints, and the atlantodental joint. The transverse ligament holds the dens in the joint of the anterior arch of the atlas. The other **cervical vertebrae** appear in axial CT images as oval structures with their greatest diameter in the coronal plane. The intervertebral joints lie in an anteriorly tilted coronal plane. The transverse processes of each cervical vertebra contain the transverse foramen. The vertebral artery courses through this foramen from the first to the sixth cervical vertebrae on both sides. The spinous processes of the second through sixth cervical vertebrae are bifurcated; the spinous process of the seventh cervical vertebra is not bifurcated and is significantly longer than the rest (Fig. 8.**196**).

Like the cervical vertebrae, the twelve **thoracic vertebrae** are oval. Their greatest diameter is in the sagittal plane. In contrast to the cervical spine, their articular surfaces are in an oblique plane between the coronal and sagittal planes.

In the **lumbar spine** from cranial to caudal, the intervertebral joints progressively rotate, increasingly coming into the sagittal plane. The lateral recess is bounded anteriorly by the vertebral body, superiorly by the pedicle, and posteriorly by the superior articular process (Fig. 8.**197**).

The intervertebral disks are imaged as homogeneous structures in CT scans. It is not possible to distinguish between the anulus fibrosus and the nucleus pulposus. The spinal ligaments are only rarely visualized if they are embedded in soft tissue, primarily fat (Schubiger 1984). In contrast to the flaval ligament, which is well visualized, the longitudinal ligaments close to the bone are poorly visualized (Fig. 8.**197**).

The **spinal canal** is bounded anteriorly by the posterior aspect of the body of the vertebra or the disk, and posteriorly by the ligamentum flavum and the vertebral arches or facet joints. The spinal cord and the two respective nerve roots are surrounded by epidural fatty tissue.

Abnormal Findings in the Cervical Spine

Traumatic Changes

As early as 1977, Kerschner et al. cited the superior performance of CT in the diagnosis of **Jefferson fractures of the atlas** (see p. 324). Since fracture lines of the arches are perpendicular to the axial plane, they can be reliably diagnosed even with larger slice thicknesses (Heithoff 1990). The higher contrast between soft tissue and bone in CT readily visualizes the position of a dislocated dens against surrounding tis-

Fig. 8.**198**   CT image of the cervical spine. Lateral reconstruction of the cervicothoracic spine in a 25-year-old female patient after a swimming accident. This teardrop fracture was accompanied by neurologic findings of sensory loss in the left hand (corresponding to Figs. 8.**82a, b**).

a   b

Figs. 8.**199a, b**   Axial CT of the cervical spine showing a burst fracture of the fifth cervical vertebra in a 14-year-old male patient.

Fig. 8.**200**   Axial CT of the cervical spine showing a burst fracture of a vertebral body with fragments in the spinal canal and compression of the spinal cord.

sue, especially the spinal cord. An isolated horizontal dens fracture can be overlooked in CT scans if slice thicknesses are too thick. However, sagittal and coronal reconstruction provides an image that permits reliable evaluation of the fragments. For this reason, CT evaluation of spinal injuries should include appropriate reconstruction images (Fig. 8.**198**).

Another fracture of the cervical spine is the stable compression fracture in which the posterior margin of the vertebral body remains intact. This must be distinguished from a **burst fracture.** In this fracture, the fracture line courses through the posterior margin of the vertebral body, making it an unstable fracture with possible nerve involvement (Figs. 8.**199a, b** and 8.**200**). Another unstable fracture of the cervical spine is the **teardrop fracture.** This is caused by hyperflexion and involves a tear of the posterior ligaments (described by Holdsworth) (see p. 323) and avulsion of the anterior margin of the vertebral body. The vertebral joints can dislocate in these injuries, producing

Fig. 8.**201**   Axial CT of the cervical spine showing a mediolateral prolapsed disk at the level of segment C6–C7.

Fig. 8.**202**   Axial CT of the cervical spine showing marginal osteophytes constricting the nerve root canal.

severe neurologic injury including quadriplegia. CT is essential in these cases because a fracture dislocation is difficult to distinguish from the far less ominous hyperextension teardrop fracture in plain radiographs (Fig. 8.**198**).

Injuries in the **cervicothoracic spine** cannot always be reliably evaluated in CT scans because of the artifacts frequently seen in this region. In these cases, MR studies are indicated as an adjunctive diagnostic imaging procedure.

Helical CT is a quick and effective method for diagnosing spinal trauma that offers certain advantages over conventional CT. Continuous data acquisition as the X-ray tube describes a helical path around the patient can reduce examination time to less than 1 minute. This minimizes motion artifacts and improves the quality of the reconstructions. The short duration of the examination is a decisive advantage particularly for severely injured patients. However, helical CTs lower resolution entails a sacrifice in image quality, particularly where larger volumes are involved. An experimental study of artificial fractures in cadaver spines demonstrated that conventional CT is more precise than helical CT in diagnosing spinal fractures (Link et al. 1996). Technological progress will further improve the quality of this imaging technique so that helical CT can be expected to play a greater role in the diagnosis of spinal fractures in the future.

Degenerative Changes

Prolapsed cervical disks most frequently involve the C5–C6 and C6–C7 disks (Schubiger 1984) (Fig. 8.**201**). Diagnosing disk changes in CT images of the cervical spine can be difficult for two reasons. First, the shoulders can often produce strip-shaped artifacts in the cervicothoracic spine. Second, the epidural space is poorly visualized. This is due to the fact that the cervical dural sac is directly adjacent to the bone. In contrast to the lumbar spine, it is not possible to diagnose a suspected prolapsed disk on the basis of the obliterated epidural space (Schubiger 1984). For this reason, myelography followed by CT (CT myelography) or MRI is the imaging method of choice for radicular or pseudoradicular symptoms.

CT can reliably distinguish discogenic and bone causes of nerve root compression syndromes. Marginal osteophytes that compress the intervertebral foramen or constrict the spinal canal are easily diagnosed, even in the presence of strip-shaped artifacts in the lower cervical spine (Schubiger 1984) (Fig. 8.**202**).

Abnormal Findings in the Thoracic Spine

Traumatic Changes

Spinal injuries most often occur in the cervical spine and thoracolumbar junction. Because the thoracic spine is integrated into the relatively rigid rib cage, it is less frequently the site of fractures. The same types of fractures that occur in the cervical and lumbar spine are seen in the thoracic spine (Figs. 8.**203a, b**).

Degenerative Changes

Symptomatic degenerative changes are rare in the thoracic spine. Although bony structures are visualized in CT scans, MRI is more commonly used in addition to plain-film radiography in this part of the spine.

Abnormal Findings in the Lumbar Spine

Traumatic Changes

Injuries to the lumbar spine can be categorized according to the classification described by Magerl

a

b

Figs. 8.**203a, b** Axial CT image of the thoracic spine in a 28-year-old male patient after a motorcycle accident. Neurologic examination was normal. The image shows a fracture dislocation with fracture of both pedicles.

Fig. 8.**204** Axial CT image of the lumbar spine. The image shows a burst fracture with fragments almost completely blocking the spinal canal and compression of the spinal cord. The vertebral arch is fractured.

et al. (1994) (see p. 340). In **type A injuries,** it is often not possible to evaluate the stability of the posterior aspect of the vertebral body, which is crucial to the stability of the fracture. CT can clearly distinguish A1 and A2 injuries from A3 injuries in such cases. Sagittal reconstruction is particularly helpful for this purpose (Figs. 8.**205a, b**). Retropulsion of fragments (Fig. 8.**204**) in burst fractures can be identified as one of the four fracture types described by Atlas et al. (1986) in the conventional axial image. The singular type, in which a solid fragment is displaced into the spinal canal, occurs most frequently. The second most common injury is the sagittal or asymmetric cleft form. The unilateral cleft type involving bursting of one side of the vertebral body is less common. Eighty-five percent of all fractures involve the posterior column, usually in the form of a unilateral arch fracture. There is a notable lack of correlation between the degree of spinal stenosis and the extent of neurologic deficits.

CT can be used to image **type B injuries** involving bony structures, although MRI can provide more information in injuries involving only soft tissue. The same basically applies to **type C injuries** (Figs. 8.**203a, b**). The bony component of the injury can be better visualized in the sagittal reconstruction while the MR image better visualizes soft tissue. Intramedullary changes can be visualized in MR images with significantly higher sensitivity.

Degenerative Changes

• Prolapsed disk

CT scans are regarded as an accurate method of diagnosing a prolapsed disk in patients who have not undergone surgery. However, Heithoff (1985) emphasizes several criteria that must be fulfilled for diagnosing a prolapsed disk in a CT image. The prolapse must be focal and asymmetric (frequently posterolateral), and compression or displacement of the nerve root must be demonstrated (Figs. 8.**206a, b**). The final criterion is the presence of postimpingement swelling distal to the compressed nerve root; this appears as an ill-defined area in the image, occasionally accompanied by inflammatory changes or venous stasis. These criteria may be used to distinguish a prolapsed disk from diffuse posterior bulging of the disk without clinical significance. Note that in the distal lumbar spine the intervertebral disks project slightly

a   b

Figs. 8.**205a, b** Axial CT image of the lumbar spine (**a**) and lateral reconstruction (**b**) of a 32-year-old male patient who fell downstairs. The images show a burst fracture with retropulsion of a fragment into the spinal canal. Neurologic examination was normal.

a   b

Figs. 8.**206a, b** (**a**) Axial CT image of the lumbar spine showing lateral disk prolapse into the foramen with nerve root compression (Jerosch and Castro, 1994). (**b**) Axial CT image of the lumbar spine showing mediolateral disk prolapse with compression of nerve root S1.

posterior to the posterior aspect of the vertebral body, a physiologic phenomenon that must not be confused with a prolapsed disk. An exception in which a symmetric and diffuse projection of an intervertebral disk can lead to compression of a nerve root is spinal stenosis in a cloverleaf-shaped spinal canal. Since this type of spinal canal is already narrowed, a constellation of such findings can be symptomatic.

Unlike MRI, CT cannot distinguish between the nucleus pulposus and the anulus fibrosus (Heithoff 1990). As a result, it is not usually possible to differentiate between **protrusion** with an intact anulus fibrosis (contained disk) and **extrusion** with rupture of the anulus fibrosis (noncontained disk; see pp. 402 and 414). In CT it may be difficult to differentiate between

a **subligamentous prolapsed disk** and an **extraligamentous prolapsed disk** with rupture of the posterior longitudinal ligament (Schubiger 1984). Where precise differentiation between protrusion and extrusion is of clinical significance, such as in determining whether percutaneous or open disk surgery is indicated, MRI or discography followed by CT (**CT discography**) should be performed (Figs. 8.**207**–8.**210**).

The accuracy of CT in diagnosing a prolapsed disk as cited in the literature ranges from 48–100%, with the incidence of false negative findings between 2% and 29%, and false positive findings between 2% and 24% (Heithoff 1985, Jackson and Jacobs 1990). Other studies (Milette et al. 1990) of patients with chronic back pain without neurologic deficits and suspected

Fig. 8.**207** Axial CT following lumbar discography. The contrast medium lies in the nucleus pulposus and does not extend into the periphery of the disk. These are normal findings in a CT discogram.

Fig. 8.**208** Axial CT following lumbar discography. The contrast medium shows broad-based protrusion into the disk. The disk is seen to protrude posteriorly with compression of the nerve structures, i.e., broad-based protrusion.

Fig. 8.**209** Axial CT following discography showing narrow-based protrusion of the disk. The contrast medium diffuses into the disk and protruding area in an hourglass-shaped pattern after injection. Nerve structures are compressed.

Fig. 8.**210** Axial CT following discography showing a contrast-medium depot posterior to the vertebral body. This suggests a sequestered disk or fragment.

discogenic pain who underwent CT and comparative discography resulted in incidences of false negative results ranging from 0–64% and false positive findings from 0–19% for CT. The ranges of error are attributed to the inability of CT to identify penetration of nucleus pulposus tissue into the degenerated anulus fibrosis without projecting past the posterior aspect of the vertebral body (Williams et al. 1982). For this reason, discography is recommended for these patients, in applicable cases followed by CT (Milette et al. 1990). Jackson and Jacobs (1990) demonstrated improved accuracy of up to 87% in studies on the

diagnosis of prolapsed disks using a combination of discography and CT (CT discography) where CT alone had an accuracy of 74%. The rate of false negative findings was 8% and false positive findings 19%.

As with MR studies, abnormal CT findings should only be interpreted as significant where they correlate with the history and clinical findings in the patient. Wiesel et al. (1984) found pathologic changes such as prolapsed disks, spondylarthritis, or spinal stenosis in over 35% of 52 patients without back symptoms. A prolapsed disk was diagnosed by independent neuroradiologists in over 19% of the patients below the age of 40. Every second patient over the age of 40 showed degenerative changes, primarily in the form of severe spondylarthritis or spinal stenosis.

CT in conjunction with discography (CT discography) or myelography (CT myelography) clearly demonstrates the intervertebral disk, spinal canal, and recess (Jackson and Jacobs 1990). Some authors favor high-resolution CT over myelography, and even MRI in the diagnosis of lateral prolapsed disks (Broom 1993, Jackson and Jacobs 1990).

CT discography (see p. 391) is regarded as the best method for diagnosing painful disk degeneration. This modality can visualize changes within the disk, while discography can be used to perform a pain provocation test (Tervonen et al. 1991). CT discography allows precise differentiation of disk prolapse into broad-based protrusion, narrow-based protrusion (hourglass form), and extrusion with or without sequestration (Castro et al. 1995) (Figs. 8.**208**–8.**210**). This differentiation is significant as regards the choice of therapy because a sequestrated disk prolapse cannot be treated by automated percutaneous lumbar discectomy, chemonucleolysis, or laser treatment. Studies by Jackson and Jacobs on the diagnosis of prolapsed disks have demonstrated that CT discography produces an 8% incidence of ambiguous findings, whereas the incidence from myelography is 16%, from CT myelography 18%, from plain CT 23%, and from discography 71%.

Gas inclusions similar to the vacuum phenomenon in the small vertebral joints (Fig. 8.**128**, p. 346) are frequently observed in abnormal intervertebral disks (Schubiger 1984). **Calcifications of the flaval ligament** can be signs of pathologic changes in the intervertebral disks or spinal stenosis. Avrahami et al. (1990) demonstrated a correlation between calcification of the flaval ligament and corresponding degenerative changes. The level of calcification did not always correspond to the level of disk pathology or stenosis.

Facet ganglia represent a rare cause of nerve root compression. Cysts developing in the capsule of the joints can cause symptoms similar to a prolapsed disk (Fig. 8.**214**).

● **Spinal stenosis**

According to the proposal of the nomenclature committee of the North American Spine Society in 1988, spinal stenosis can be categorized as central, lateral recess, or extraforaminal according to the location of nerve compression.

Aside from decreased height resulting from disk degeneration, spondylosis and spondylarthritis, with degenerative increase in size of the facet joints, play an important role in the cause of spinal stenosis (Kirkaldy-Willis 1978). The resulting nerve compression can occur in the center of the canal (**central stenosis;** Fig. 8.**211**) or further distal in the nerve root canal (**lateral recess stenosis;** Fig. 8.**212**). For example, the L5 nerve root can be compressed either mediolaterally at the level of segment L4–L5 or further distal in the nerve root canal between L5 and S1. Lateral recess stenosis is encountered more frequently than extraforaminal stenosis. However, the two forms should not be considered in isolation because they often occur in combination with the same cause (Heithoff 1990). Lateral recess stenosis is cited by many authors as the most frequent cause of "failed back surgery syndrome."

CT, CT myelography, or MRI can precisely visualize central and lateral recess stenosis. Sagittal reconstruction images are helpful in addition to the conventional axial views. These reconstructions also help in preoperative planning by precisely visualizing

Fig. 8.**211**   Axial CT image of the lumbar spine. Spinal stenosis with bony narrowing of the spinal canal: central stenosis.

Fig. 8.**212**   Axial CT image of the lumbar spine. Bilateral lateral stenosis with bony narrowing of both lateral recesses.

Fig. 8.**213** Axial CT image of the lumbar spine. Central spinal stenosis due to degenerative facet hypertrophy, especially on the left side.

Fig. 8.**214** Axial CT image of the lumbar spine. Facet joint ganglion at the L4–L5 level with compression of nerve root L5.

topographic relationships. The accuracy of CT in diagnosing central and lateral recess stenosis is cited at 100% (Heithoff 1990). The severity of facet joint hypertrophy and marginal osteophytes in the vicinity of the nerve root can be readily evaluated in **axial views** (Fig. 8.**213**). One disadvantage of CT compared to MRI is its inability to distinguish soft-tissue structures in the nerve root canal; disk tissue, ganglia, veins, the flaval ligament, and fibrous structures are all equally radiodense. **Sagittal reconstruction views** permit further differentiation of lateral recess stenosis. Craniocaudal, anteroposterior, and combined forms may be differentiated. The latter was first described by Ray (Heithoff 1990). Compression can occur on four sides (cranially from the pedicle, caudally from the intervertebral disk, anteriorly from the body, and posteriorly from the superior articular process). **Craniocaudal** stenosis is attributable to compression of the nerve root between the pedicle and intervertebral disk, due either to decrease in height with reactive osteophyte formation or to the prominence of the intervertebral disk. Craniocaudal stenosis, or "up-down" stenosis, is regarded as the most frequent form of lateral recess stenosis. In over 90% of all cases, it occurs in the lumbosacral junction (Lifson et al. 1982). The **anteroposterior form** results from hypertrophy of the superior articular process or anterior subluxation of the process in ligamentous instability with compression of the nerve root against the vertebral body or, more frequently, due to formation of bony spurs on the posterior aspect of the vertebral body.

Extraforaminal stenosis is a special form of spinal stenosis characterized by compression of the fifth nerve root between the pedicle of vertebra L5, the intervertebral disk at L5–S1, and the wing of the sacrum. Failure to diagnose extraforaminal stenosis is frequently the cause of unsuccessful surgical intervention for a proximally located lesion imaged with CT. Heithoff (1985) describes five such cases in 100

patients who underwent surgery for lateral recess stenosis. For this reason, it is always important to visualize the entire length of the nerve root canal in CT or MR images. Sagittal reconstruction views in sufficiently lateral imaging-planes should always be obtained to supplement these studies (Heithoff 1990).

Degenerative spondylolisthesis is closely associated with central and subarticular spinal stenosis (Heithoff 1990). In CT studies, it is characterized by degenerative hypertrophy of the facet joints, thickening of the flaval ligament, and erosion of medial portions of the articular process with subsequent anterior subluxation of the cranially adjacent vertebra and nerve root compression. Segment L4–L5 is the most frequently affected.

Other Abnormal Findings

Because of its high resolution, CT is regarded as a valuable supplement to plain-film radiography in the diagnosis of **spinal tumors.** The most frequent malignant tumors in the spine are bone metastases (see p. 350). A tentative diagnosis can be established on the basis of plain-film radiographs or nuclear studies. However, CT is helpful in evaluating the proliferation of the tumor and the degree of structural and neurologic instability it causes. CT does not permit pathologic diagnosis although it can differentiate between osteolytic and osteoblastic processes.

Hemangiomas and aneurysmal bone cysts are benign spinal tumors that occur relatively frequently. Spinal hemangiomas can be identified by their characteristic appearance; the inner structure of the vertebral body will appear spotty (Sartor 1984). Aneurysmal bone cysts frequently appear as polycystic eccentric expanding lesions (Fig. 8.**215**).

Chondrosarcomas are frequently characterized by destructive deforming changes and extensive calcifications that may also be visible in the surrounding soft tissue. In contrast, osteosarcomas, Ewing sarcomas, and malignant hemangiopericytomas do not show specific identifying characteristics (Sartor 1984).

Other applications of CT in orthopedics include postoperative follow-up studies for evaluating pedicle screws. CT permits precise evaluation of the position of the pedicle screw, which can be particularly helpful where new neurologic symptoms occur postoperatively (Figs. 8.**216a, b**). Titanium implants or special protocols are necessary to eliminate artifacts that can degrade images.

Three-dimensional reconstructions are possible in addition to two-dimensional reconstructions if sufficiently thin slice thicknesses are used. These three-dimensional reconstructions provide detailed images that are of diagnostic value in preoperative planning for correction of **complex vertebral deformities** (Figs. 8.**217a, b**).

Fig. 8.**215**   Axial CT image of the lumbar spine in a 34-year-old female patient with a large cystic tumor at the fifth lumbar vertebra. Pathologic diagnosis was an aneurysmal bone cyst.

a

b

Figs. 8.**216a, b**   **(a)** CT image obtained as a follow-up study to evaluate the position of a pedicle screw after spinal fusion for scoliosis. The image demonstrates the correct position of the screw that extends through the pedicle, without injuring the pedicle cortex, at the level of the eleventh thoracic vertebra. **(b)** The image demonstrates that the screw at the level of the fifth thoracic vertebra is now correctly positioned and passes through the pedicle after revision surgery to correct its position. The previous screw channel is clearly visible, and plastic deformation of the cortex is present. The cortex is almost in direct contact with the wall of the aorta to the right of the previous location of the tip of the screw.

Bone Densitometry

Quantitative CT can be used to obtain precise measurements in bone density in diagnosing osteoporosis. This is done by obtaining slices in the lumbar spine (usually between L1 and L3) and comparing them with a calibration phantom. The bone density values obtained in this manner are expressed in grams of hydroxylapatite per cubic centimeter. The mean value is then calculated and evaluated compared with the respective age and sex-specific stan-

Figs. 8.**217a, b**   Three-dimensional CT reconstruction of the lumbar spine showing a fully segmented hemivertebra in congenital scoliosis (corresponding to Fig. 8.**160**, p. 366).

dard values. Quantitative CT is particularly valuable in the spine because of its high sensitivity, its ability to differentiate between cancellous and cortical bone, and its ability to provide precise three-dimensional images (see also pp. 371 and 387).

References

Atlas S, Regenbogen V, Rogers L, et al. The characterization of burst fractures of the spine. *AJR*. 1986; 147: 575

Avrahami E, Wigler I, Stern D, et al. Computed tomographic demonstration of the ligamenta flava of the lumbosacral spine associated with protrusion of the intervertebral disk. *Spine* 1990; 15: 21

Broom M. Foraminal and extraforaminal lumbar disk herniations. *Clin Orthop*. 1993; 289: 118

Castro WHM, Bongartz G, Schulitz KP. Stellenwert der CT-Diskographie in der differenzierten Therapie des Bandscheibenvorfalles. *Deutsches Ärzteblatt*. 1995; 92: 352

Heithoff K. *Cooperative sudy of the efficacy of metrizamide myelography and CT in the study of lumbar disk disease and spinal stenosis*. 71st Scientific Assembly, Radiological Society of North America. Chicago, November 1985

Heithoff K. Computed Tomography and Plain Film Diagnosis of the Lumbar Spine. In: Weinstein J, Wiesel S, eds. *The Lumbar Spine*. Philadelphia: WB Saunders; 1990

Heuchemer Th, Waidelich H, Häberle H, et al. Diagnostik des Wirbelsäulentraumas: Indikation zur CT und Myelo-CT am Unfalltag. *Fortsch Geb Rontgenstr Nuklearmed*. 1992; 156: 156

Jackson R, Jacobs R. Computed Tomography — Discography. In: Weinstein J, Wiesel S, eds. *The Lumbar Spine*. Philadelphia: WB Saunders; 1990

Kerschner M, Goodman G, Perlmutter G. Computed tomography in the diagnosis of an atlas fracture. *AJR*. 1977; 128: 688

Kirkaldy-Willis W, Wedge J, Yong-Hing K, Reilly J. Pathology and pathogenesis of lumbar spondylolysis and stenosis. *Spine*. 1978; 3: 319

Lifson A, Heithoff K, Burton C, Ray C. High resolution computed tomographic scanning of the lumbosacral spine. *Modern Neurosurgery*. 1982; 1: 31

Magerl F, Aebi M, Gertzbein SD, et al. A comprehensive classification of thoracic and lumbar injuries. *Europ Spine J*. 1994; 3: 184

Milette P, Raymond J, Fontaine S. Comparison of high-resolution computed tomography with discography in the evaluation of lumbar disk herniations. *Spine*. 1990; 15: 525

Niethard F, Pfeil J. *Orthopädie*. Stuttgart: Hippokrates; 1992

Sartor K. Computertomographie bei Tumoren der Wirbelsäule. In: Schmitt E, ed. *Tumoren der Wirbelsäule*. Stuttgart: Hippokrates; 1984

Schubiger O. *Die Computertomographie der Wirbelsäule*. Stuttgart: Hippokrates; 1984

Tervonen O, Lähde S, Vahnaranta H. Ultrasound diagnosis of lumbar disk degeneration. *Spine*. 1991; 16: 951

Wiesel S, Tsourmas N, Feffer H, et al. A study of computer-assisted tomography. I. The incidence of positive CAT scans in an asymptomatic group of patients. *Spine*. 1984; 9: 549

Williams A, Haughton V, Meyer G, Ho K. Computed tomographic appearance of bulging anulus. *Radiology*. 1982; 142: 403

8.8 Magnetic Resonance Imaging

Indications, Diagnostic Value, and Clinical Relevance

MRI has supplanted CT as the gold standard in diagnostic imaging of the spine. MRI is an instrument of morphologic analysis and tissue identification. The advantages of MRI over CT include freely selectable imaging planes and image windows, and excellent soft-tissue resolution. The patient is not exposed to radiation, and acquisition times are now comparable with CT. Disadvantages include contraindications such as artificial heart valves with metallic components or foreign bodies in the vitreous humor, and higher costs.

MRI is indicated in the diagnosis of **traumatic injuries** when intraspinal sequelae of injuries such as hematoma or edema with compression of the spinal cord must be excluded (Table 8.**42**). CT, otherwise preferred for the diagnosis of spinal fractures, is subject to increased artifacts from the shoulders in the cervicothoracic junction (vertebrae C5–T1) and plays

Table 8.**42**   Clinical value of MRI of the spine

Bone structure	++
Facet arthritis	++
Disk prolapse	+++
Symptomatic disk without prolapse	(+)
Trauma	+++
Spondylitis	+++
Deformities	–
Tumor	+++
Spinal stenosis (central)	+++
Lateral stenosis	+++

–   No information content
(+)   Low information content
+   Moderate information content
++   High information content
+++   Very high information content

a secondary role in this region. MRI has advantages over CT in diagnosing injuries in this region. MRI is also indicated in the diagnosis of spinal injuries in children, where ossification of the spinal column is still incomplete. MRI examination of a child requires sedation, which itself holds risks, therefore strict criteria should be used to determine which method is to be used. MRI can demonstrate occult fractures in post-trauma cases with persistent symptoms of uncertain cause, where plain films and CT scans are negative (see p. 444).

In the diagnosis of **degenerative disorders** of the cervical spine, MRI can be used to evaluate conditions where pain radiates into the arms. CT in the cervico-thoracic junction is subject to the artifacts described above, and MRI is preferred for visualizing this region. Myelography combined with CT (CT myelography) is equally as reliable as MRI in imaging in the clinical setting of radicular and pseudoradicular pain, although this method entails several disadvantages. Myelography is an invasive procedure, and CT scans of several segments are required to minimize the risk of overlooking pathology. Discography may be performed to reproduce pain where purely discogenic symptoms are suspected, although this is an invasive procedure and involves certain risks.

MRI is preferred to CT in the rare case of degenerative pathology in the thoracic spine, as it will be better able to locate the process. MRI is indicated in the lumbar spine where radicular pain is present. Again, CT myelography will provide equally reliable results but involves the disadvantages discussed above. Isolated back pain may require MRI if a discogenic cause is suspected. In the diagnosis of disk degeneration, discography offers the advantage of reproducing pain with a provocative test. Subsequent CT scans (CT discography) help to determine whether minimally invasive treatment such as percutaneous discectomy or chemonucleolysis may be used to manage a prolapsed disk.

MRI is the diagnostic imaging modality of choice in all regions of the spine where there are secondary degenerative changes such as focal edema, venous stasis, or nerve root edema, and where pathology inside or outside the foramen is suspected. This applies to end-plate reaction, an inflammatory change in the subcortical region of the vertebral endplates, thought to be a sequela of disk degeneration with resulting instability.

Further indications for MRI include **spinal tumors, dysraphism,** and **"tethered-cord syndrome."** MRI can visualize early changes in **spondylitis** or spondylolisthesis. It can usually visualize postoperative infection within 6 days of surgery. While MRI is regarded as superior to nuclear medicine studies in the early diagnosis of metastatic disease (Algra et al. 1991, Link et al. 1995), it is relatively expensive as a screening method and the examination requires a long time.

Technique, Instrumentation, and Examination Procedure

Usually the patient is positioned supine. Take whatever steps are necessary to ensure the patient is comfortable to minimize motion artifacts. The patient should be supplied with ear protection because of the high noise level of the examination. MRI examinations in children may only be performed with the patient under sedation.

Surface coils are used for better resolution. Since several tissue parameters (chemical shift, flow effects, susceptibility characteristics, proton density, T1 and T2 relaxation, and T2* relaxation) contribute to the imaging process, different **excitation sequences** must be selected depending on the clinical setting. The imaging plane is freely selectable (Table 8.**43**). Minimum slice thickness is 1 mm. These parameters should be manipulated by the consulting radiologist. Ensure that he or she understands what the objective of the examination is so that the required images can be provided.

Any disturbance of tissue structure will lead to local expansion of the extracellular space. Pharmaceuticals known to function as tracers for the extracellular space are used to demonstrate these changes. Intravenous gadolinium-DTPA is used as a contrast medium. Following intravenous injection, well vascularized areas normally have greater signal intensity than avascular tissue. The intervertebral disk is normally avascular and has low signal intensity. Gadolinium-DTPA can be used to demonstrate secondary capillarization in a chronically prolapsed disk.

Normal Findings

Normal findings will depend on the selected excitation sequence. The following section briefly discusses the standard findings for T1 and T2-weighted images. The same structures will have different signal inten-

Table 8.**43** Overview of the sequences and imaging planes used in MRI of the spine

Clinical setting	Sequence	Imaging plane
Disk prolapse	Phase-contrast T1-weighted*, for example partial saturation with phase contrast, PS 500/10	Axial, sagittal
Disk prolapse and scar tissue	Phase-contrast T1-weighted, SE T1-weighted (∓Gd-DTPA)**	Axial, sagittal, coronal
Spinal stenosis	SE T1-weighted GRE T2-weighted	Sagittal, coronal
Lateral stenosis	SE T1-weighted GRE T2-weighted Phase-contrast T1-weighted	Axial, coronal oblique
Tumor	SE T1-weighted (∓Gd-DTPA)** Short-time inversion recovery (STIR) GRE T2-weighted	Sagittal, axial, coronal
Spondylitis	Short-time-inversion recovery (STIR) SE T1-weighted (∓Gd-DTPA)**	Sagittal Sagittal, axial, coronal
Intramedullary pathology	SE T1-weighted (∓Gd-DTPA)** GRE T2-weighted	Sagittal, axial, (coronal)

* Gadolinium-DTPA where edema, granulation, or venous stasis should be confirmed or excluded
** (∓Gd-DTPA): first *without* and then *with* gadolinium-DTPA

sity in T1 and T2-weighted images. In general, fat is "bright" on T1-weighted images and hydrated structures are "dark." On T2-weighted images, fat is "dark" and hydrated structures are "bright." In T1-weighted images, the vertebral body and epidural and paravertebral fat are "bright," and the spinal cord and nerve roots are of medium intensity; they are surrounded by hypointense cerebrospinal fluid. Intramedullary hematomas can vary from hyperintense to hypointense, depending on how old they are. Their signal intensity decreases with time. Depending on the T1 weighting, the intervertebral disks will vary in appearance from moderately intense to hypointense. The anterior and posterior longitudinal ligaments usually appear hypointense, whereas the flaval ligament will be of greater signal intensity. In T2-weighted images, fluids usually appear hyperintense. Cerebrospinal fluid and the intact well-hydrated nucleus pulposus are visualized as bright structures. The higher signal intensity of the inner portions of the intervertebral disks makes it possible to distinguish the nucleus pulposus from the anulus fibrosus. Degenerated disks with a low degree of hydration will appear hypointense in contrast. The spinal cord usually is of medium signal intensity in moderately T2-weighted images. This makes intramedullary edema readily discernible. An acute intramedullary hematoma (less than 4 days old) will be "bright" in T2-weighted images, although the finding is not specific. Older hematomas (more than 4 days old) can be visualized as specific findings in both T1-weighted and T2-weighted images. Nerve roots have low signal intensity. The vertebral end-plates and cortical bone appear hypointense in both imaging techniques (Figs. 8.**218a-d**).

Abnormal Findings in the Cervical Spine

Traumatic Changes

Visualization of traumatic changes in the cervical spine exploits the high soft-tissue resolution of MRI to identify intramedullary findings such as edema, hematoma, or ruptures of the spinal cord with high sensitivity. MRI usually provides prognostic information because remission of neurologic symptoms in the presence of intramedullary edema or contusion has been reported, whereas the prognosis for intraspinal hemorrhage is unfavorable (Flanders et al. 1990, Kulkarni et al. 1987). The short-term prognosis for edema is better, although its long-term prognosis is not as favorable due to posttraumatic sequelae such as spinal atrophy, myelomalacia, or syringomyelia. MRI remains the imaging method of choice for visualizing these changes.

MRI also permits precise evaluation of significant injuries to the capsular ligaments and the intervertebral disk. However in the commonly seen acceleration/deceleration injury, whiplash, MRI only identifies findings in the most severe cases. Abnormal changes seen in severe hyperextension trauma to the cervical spine include dissociation of the intervertebral disk from the vertebral end-plates, prevertebral hematoma, or a rupture of the anterior longitudinal ligament (Davis et al. 1991).

Degenerative Changes

Degenerative changes in the cervical spine are frequently discogenic. They often lead to a stenosing process. As in the lumbar spine, the **lower cervical intervertebral disks** are primarily affected by degenerative changes. Since CT is susceptible to artifacts in a   b   c   d

Figs. 8.**218a–d**   MR sagittal sections of the lumbar spine. (**a**) SE 20 300, (**b**) SE 600/40, (**c**) SE 2400/20, (**d**) SE 2400/80. The T1-weighting decreases from (**a**) to (**d**), and the T2-weighting increases. The decrease in T1-weighting causes the cerebrospinal fluid to increase in signal intensity. The normal intervertebral disks at segments L3–L4 increase in signal intensity as T2-weighting increases, whereas the pathologic disks (L1–L2, L2–L3, L4–L5, and L5–S1) do not increase in signal intensity as T2-weighting increases.

this particular region, MRI is the imaging modality of choice for visualizing disk disorders in the lower spine. The ability to distinguish the nucleus pulposus from the anulus fibrosus allows early degenerative changes to be detected in the form of small radial tears in the anulus fibrosus. As the disorder progresses, protrusion of the nucleus pulposus can progress to extrusion if the continuity of the anulus fibrosis is compromised. Clear visualization of the posterior longitudinal ligament in MR images makes it possible to differentiate **subligamentous disk prolapse** from **extraligamentous prolapse.** In **sequestrated prolapse,** MRI has the advantage of providing better images since the sequestrum will not necessarily be located at the same level as the prolapsed disk.

As in all advanced spinal imaging, findings must be carefully correlated to the clinical examination and the history. As an example, consider the following study of clinically normal test subjects. Prolapsed cervical disks were diagnosed in MR images in 10% of test subjects below the age of 40 and in 5% of those over the age of 40 (Boden et al. 1990) (Fig. 8.**219**).

Use of a contrast medium (gadolinium-DTPA) can facilitate the diagnosis of postoperative scarring, which can be identified by typical contrast enhancement and by its location. Recurrent disk prolapse can be difficult to distinguish from scar tissue in CT and myelograms of patients who have undergone previous surgery. In MR images, a prolapsed disk can be distinguished from vascularized postoperative granulation tissue because avascular structures will not enhance.

In advanced degenerative disorders of the cervical spine, **osteophytes** can lead to compression of the spinal cord and nerve roots. Since it provides greater contrast between soft tissue and bone, CT can more

Fig. 8.**219**   MR image of the cervical spine in the sagittal plane (GRE, 500/10, out of phase) showing compression of cord by prolapsed disk tissue. The posterior longitudinal ligament remains intact.

Fig. 8.**220**   MR image of the cervical spine in the sagittal plane (STIR 1900/125). The image shows decreased height of the sixth cervical vertebra with narrowing of the spinal canal due to osteophytes at segment C5–C6. Significant osteophyte bridging is present anteriorly. Disk prolapse at the C6–C7 levels can be identified (image shows the same patient as in Figs. 8.**221**–8.**223**).

Fig. 8.**221**   MR image of the cervical spine in the sagittal plane (GRE 500/10). Osteophytes are seen to narrow the anterior arachnoid space at the level of C4–C5 and C5–C6, and a disk prolapse is readily identifiable at the level of C6–C7.

Fig. 8.**222**   Axial MR image of the cervical spine at the level of C6–C7 (GRE 500/10), showing a left lateral prolapse with a tear of the posterior longitudinal ligament.

Fig. 8.**223**   MR image of the cervical spine in the coronal plane (GRE 500/10), showing osteochondrosis with paramedian stenosis on the left side at the level of C5–C6. A left lateral disk prolapse is visible at the level of C6–C7.

precisely visualize bony structures. However, MRI is regarded as the imaging modality of choice for documenting secondary changes in the spinal cord that involve cervical myelopathy (Figs. 8.**220**–8.**223**).

Stenoses in the intervertebral foramina are well visualized in oblique views on plain radiographs. Here, MRI is used to precisely visualize **stenosis inside and outside the foramina** and the associated secondary changes to the nerve root.

Abnormal Findings in the Thoracic Spine

Traumatic Changes

In addition to plain-film radiography, CT is the imaging modality of choice for injuries to bony structures of the spine. In the thoracic spine, the same considerations apply as in the lumbar spine (Figs. 8.**224a, b** and 8.**225a–c**).

Eighth thoracic vertebra

Figs. 8.**224a, b**   MRI of the thoracic spine.
(**a**) Sagittal plane (GRE 500/10). Fracture of the eight thoracic
vertebra with a significant reduction in height and stenosis of
the spinal canal due to posterior fracture element. The fracture line is visible in this imaging plane.
(**b**) Sagittal plane (SE 500/20). The T1 proton-weighted
images show the fractured thoracic vertebra with generally
reduced signal intensity. The posterior longitudinal ligament
can be identified. It is intact and thickened in this image.

Figs. 8.**225a–c**   MRI of the thoracic spine. (**a**) Sagittal plane
(SE 500/20). (**b**) Sagittal plane (STIR 1900/125). (**c**) Axial plane
(SE 500/20).

The images show destruction of the tenth thoracic vertebra
from a gunshot wound. The posterior fragment is seen to narrow the spinal canal and compress the spinal cord. The axial
image demonstrates displacement of the spinal cord to the
left with significant scarring on the right side and destruction
of the right pedicle.

a

b

Figs. 8.**226a, b** MRI of the thoracic spine. (**a**) Sagittal plane (GRE 500/10). The image shows significant protrusion of disk tissue at the level of T6–T7 and T9–T10. (**b**) Axial plane (GRE 500/10). The slice was obtained at the level of T9–T10, showing a medial disk prolapse with significant compression of the spinal cord.

Degenerative Changes

Degenerative changes in the thoracic spine occur frequently but are rarely symptomatic. If pain from a suspected degenerative disorder is present, plain-film radiography and MRI are the imaging modalities of choice (Figs. 8.**226a, b**).

Abnormal Findings in the Lumbar Spine

Traumatic Changes

Injuries to the lumbar spine generally involve bone. Plain-film radiography and CT are the primary diagnostic imaging methods used. MRI is used in cases where there are **intramedullary changes** or **intraspinal bleeding.** Subarachnoid bleeding in the spinal canal is difficult to diagnose, even in MR images.

MRI is highly sensitive in the identification of **occult fractures** (see p. 444). These can be identified by signal changes in cancellous bone. MRI can also distinguish between **acute** and **chronic fractures** with gadolinium-DTPA contrast enhancement. An acute fracture will normally show changes such as bleeding or edema while such findings will be missing in a chronic fracture (Stoller and Genant 1990).

Degenerative Changes

MRI is regarded as an excellent imaging method for visualizing the intervertebral disks, frequently the site of degenerative changes in the lumbar spine. Disk degeneration begins at an early age and is a part of the natural aging process (Modic and Ross 1991). Degeneration of the disk is closely related to dehydration (Modic et al. 1984), which is seen as a change in signal intensity. However, the mere presence of disk signal change does not by itself signify disk pathology. In the initial phase of dehydration, small spots of altered signal density will be identifiable, which are attributable to fluid-filled fissures in the anulus fibrosis (Stoller and Genant 1990, Yu et al. 1987). Transverse and concentric tears in the anulus fibrosus are frequently encountered and are regarded as normal changes that occur with aging (Modic and Ross 1991). However, radial tears are regarded as a characteristic of a degenerated intervertebral disk (Yu et al. 1989). Immediately adjacent to intervertebral disks with degenerative changes, changes in signal intensity in the bone marrow adjacent to the vertebral end-plates were found in about 30% of all cases. These changes in signal intensity are time related. High signal intensity in T2 or STIR sequences are due to edema of an unspecific inflammatory reaction. In time, red marrow is replaced by yellow marrow in these areas (Assheuer) (Figs. 8.**227** and 8.**228**).

Prolapsed disks are classified as involving **protrusion** and **extrusion,** with or without sequestration (see pp. 391 and 414). The anulus fibrosus and posterior longitudinal ligament play a decisive role in this classification system. MRI makes it possible to clearly distinguish the nucleus pulposus from the anulus fibrosus (Heithoff 1990, Stoller and Genant 1990). A tear of the posterior longitudinal ligament can be reliably identified by the lack of a hypointense halo around the herniation. Distinguishing extrusion from protrusion can be difficult in a CT image, which cannot distinguish between the nucleus pulposus and anulus fibrosus. Even a sequestrated disk extrusion is difficult to diagnose in images because it may lie in a different plane in the spinal canal and may not be included in the slices of the intervertebral spaces. Sagittal imaging planes are best for this indication; the sequestrum will appear as an area of altered signal intensity that will reflect the age of the lesion (Figs. 8.**229a–f**).

Fig.8.**227** MRI of the lumbar spine, sagittal image (STIR 1900/125). The image shows degenerated disks L4 and L5 with low signal intensity. Adjacent to the endplates, areas of high signal intensities are present in the vertebrae L4 and L5 representing non-specific inflammation.

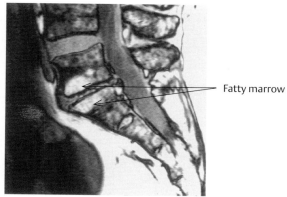

Fig.8.**228** MRI of the lumbar spine, sagittal image (GRE 500/10, out of phase). The image shows reduction in height of the intervertebral disk L4–L5 with high signal intensities in the vertebrae L4 and L5, adjacent to the endplates, representing fatty marrow.

Secondary changes immediately adjacent to disk tissue can be demonstrated with contrast MRI. Such changes include venous stasis and focal edema of the nerve root (Castro et al. 1995) (Figs. 8.**229c, d, f** and 8.**230a, b**).

Epidural fibrosis in the form of postoperative scarring can produce similar symptoms to a prolapsed disk. It is important to precisely document these changes prior to revision surgery. Surgery in the presence of fibrosis often produces poor results ("failed back surgery syndrome"). Scarring can frequently be identified with respect to the nerve root by its location and typical post-contrast enhancement.

Scar tissue is distinguished from recurrent prolapse in contrast MR images with gadolinium-DTPA (Figs. 8.**231a, b**). Usually the vascularized granulation tissue will enhance. The prolapsed disk tissue as a rule does not enhance. Occasionally, chronically prolapsed disks can enhance after application of contrast medium due to secondary capillarization.

The accuracy of contrast MRI using this technique is 96% (Ross et al. 1990) compared to 67–100% for contrast CT (Braun et al. 1985, Teplick and Haskin 1984). CT and MR studies can complement each other. For example, CT with its higher contrast between bone and soft tissue can more precisely differentiate osteophytes from prolapsed disks.

Not every prolapsed disk demonstrated by MRI is clinically significant. Studies on clinically normal test subjects have demonstrated prolapsed lumbar disks in 20% of patients below the age of 60, and in 36% of patients over the age of 60 (Boden et al. 1990). For this reason, extreme care should be taken when attributing clinical symptoms to a morphologic change.

MRI complements CT in the diagnosis of **lateral recess spinal stenosis.** It can image the surrounding soft-tissue structures that define the nerve-root canal such as disk tissue, venous plexuses, the ligamentum flavum, or fibrous tissue and edema (Heithoff 1990) (Figs. 8.**232a, b**). However, CT with its higher contrast between bone and soft tissue can provide a more precise overview of bony structures. This can be helpful because spondylotic osteophytes and facet-joint hypertrophy are significant attributing factors in the cause of spinal stenosis.

Other Abnormal Findings

The atlantoaxial junction can be critically affected by **rheumatoid disease.** Erosion of the dens, alar ligaments, and cruciform ligament of the atlas can result in instability that can cause neurologic deficits. Extensive pannus can also lead to compression of the spinal cord with associated symptoms. MRI with gadolinium-DTPA can visualize the inflammatory tissue and demonstrate the severity of spinal cord involvement (Figs. 8.**233a–d**).

MRI in the cervical spine is also indicated to diagnose **basilar impressions,** which can be reliably evaluated in MR images (Figs. 8.**234a, b**).

Arachnoiditis is a possible cause of radiating low-back pain that can be identified in MR images. These show changes seen as nerve root conglomerates. The examination should be performed as a dynamic study by changing the patient's position to exclude coincidental nerve-root conglomerates due solely to positioning.

◀ Figs. 8.**229a–f**   MR images of the lumbar spine in three planes. (**a**) Sagittal plane (GRE 500/10). (**b**) Sagittal plane (STIR 1900/125). (**c**) Sagittal plane after administration of gadolinium-based contrast medium (SE 1000/30). (**d**) Sagittal plane, subtraction image before and after intravenous gadolinium-based contrast medium (GRE 500/10). (**e**) Axial image at L4–L5 (GRE 500/10) and coronal image (**f**) after intravenous injection of gadolinium-based contrast medium.

The images show a prolapsed disk at L4–L5 with significant contrast enhancement corresponding to (**c**), (**d**), (**e**), and (**f**). The STIR images demonstrate massive disk prolapse with compression of the dural sac. The prolapsed disk itself has relatively high signal intensity, indicative of an acute lesion.

The increase in signal intensity after administration of gadolinium-based contrast medium is more prominent in the coronal slices corresponding to edema and hyperemia. The axial slices show a paramedian prolapse on the left side with displacement of the dural sac. At the level of L5–S1, the STIR image shows the decrease in signal intensity indicative of degeneration. (From Castro, Assheuer, Schulitz 1995 – see references).

a   b

Figs. 8.**230a, b**   MR images of the lumbar spine in two planes after administration of gadolinium-based contrast medium (GRE 500/10). (**a**) Increase in signal intensity surrounding the disk prolapse (focal edema). (**b**) Focal increase in signal intensity extending caudally. Nerve root L5 is enhanced, indicating the presence of a nerve-root edema.

a   b

Figs. 8.**231a, b**   Axial MR images of the lumbar spine after administration of gadolinium-based contrast medium (GRE 500/10). (**a**) Demarcation of the recurrent prolapse. (**b**) Significant enhancement of scar tissue after laminectomy on the left side at L5.

Figs. 8.**232a, b**   MR images of the lumbar spine. (**a**) Coronal plane (GRE 500/10). (**b**) Axial plane (PS 500/10).
Increase in signal intensity is visible in the synovia of facets L3–L4 on both sides and at L4–L5 on the left side. The axial slice also shows significant enhancement in the facet-joint synovia at L4–L5 on the left side. These changes are signs of facet inflammation.

a   b

Figs. 8.**234a, b**   MR images of the cervical spine in the sagittal plane (SE 500/20). (**a**) Vertical dislocation of the dens with relative superior displacement. (**b**) Bulbous deformity of the cervical spinal cord with syringomyelia and basilar impression.

a   b

c

Figs. 8.**235a–c**   MR images of the lumbar spine.
(**a**) Sagittal plane (STIR 1900/125). The image shows a circumscribed structure (posterior longitudinal ligament and epidural tissue) of increased signal intensity extending from the middle of L3 to the level of the distal border of L4 and apparently compressing the dural sac.
(**b**) Axial plane (SE 600/20) after administration of gadolinium-based contrast medium. The image shows increased enhancement in the intraspinal structure with a central hypointense area (abscess).
(**c**) Sagittal plane (GRE 500/10) after administration of gadolinium-based contrast medium. The image shows increased enhancement of vertebrae L4 and L5 and a circular pattern of increased posterior intraspinal enhancement surrounding the abscess at segment L4–L5. The intraspinal nerve roots show increased enhancement.
The diagnosis was vertebral osteomyelitis with an intraspinal abscess.

◀ Figs. 8.**233a–d**   MR images of the cervical spine.
(**a**) Sagittal plane (GRE 500/10). The image shows compression of the spinal cord in the region of the atlanto-occipital joint with anterior dislocation of the atlas. The distance between atlas and dens is increased due to soft tissue of medium signal intensity in the presence of known rheumatoid arthritis.
(**b**) Sagittal plane (SE 500/20). The tissue surrounding the dens is of medium signal intensity.
(**c**) Axial plane (GRE 500/10). The distance between dens and atlas is increased, with destruction of the cruciform ligaments of the atlas and the alar ligaments. The spinal cord is compressed by anterior dislocation of the atlas.
(**d**) CT image of the same patient showing increase in the distance between dens and atlas. Findings show rheumatoid arthritis of the atlantoaxial joint with anterior dislocation of the atlas and compression of the spinal cord.

Figs. 8.**236a–d** MR images of the lumbar spine.
(**a**) Sagittal plane (SE 500/20) shows a band-shaped intraspinal structure with slightly increased signal intensity extending from the middle of the fourth lumbar vertebra to the middle of the fifth lumbar vertebra.
(**b**) Sagittal plane (SE 500/20) after administration of gadolinium-based contrast medium. This study was performed on postoperative day 5 following disk surgery on segment L4–L5 in a patient with intense pain in the lumbar spine, increased erythrocyte sedimentation rate, and low-grade fevers. The band-shaped structure shows a significant increase in signal density. This sign of an intraspinal band-shaped area of increased signal intensity extending across the operative site itself was evalated as an early characteristic sign of retrodiscal infection.
(**c**) Sagittal plane (STIR 1900/125); (**d**) Sagittal plane (GRE 500/10) after administration of gadolinium-based contrast medium. These images demonstrate the complete clinical syndrome of vertebra osteomyelitis developed within 3 weeks after the patient discontinued antibiotic treatment.

MRI is helpful in the diagnosis of **vertebral oste-omyelitis.** It is superior to both conventional radiography and CT for this indication (Modic et al. 1985). Studies cite a sensitivity of 96%, specificity of 92%, and accuracy of 94% in diagnosing purulent **vertebral osteomyelitis.** MRI is more specific than nuclear medicine studies (Stoller and Genant 1990). The infected area appears as the zone of altered signal intensity. Soft-tissue tumors identifiable as areas of aberrant signal intensity are frequently encountered in the advanced stages of the disorder (DeRoss et al. 1986) (Figs. 8.**235a–c** and 8.**236a–d**).

In **spinal tuberculosis** (Pott disease), MRI permits precise anatomic localization of the vertebral and paravertebral abscesses in several planes and evaluation of compression of the spinal cord. How-

a

b

Figs. 8.**237a, b**   MR images of the cervical spine.
(**a**) Sagittal plane (SE 500/20). The image shows an intraspinal mass with a central area of reduced signal intensity posterior to the body of the third cervical vertebra.
(**b**) Sagittal plane (SE 500/20) after administration of

gadolinium-based contrast medium. A halo-shaped pattern of contrast enhancement and a central area of reduced signal intensity are seen in the mass.
Histologic examination revealed a cystic meningeoma with central necrosis.

a

b

Figs. 8.**238a, b**   MR images of the cervical spine.
(**a**) Coronal plane (SE 500/20). The image shows destruction of the left transverse process of the fifth cervical vertebra with stenosis of the cervical spinal canal.
(**b**) Coronal plane (SE 500/20) after administration of

gadolinium-based contrast medium. The image shows increased contrast medium in the mass and destruction of the left transverse process of the fifth cervical vertebra.
The diagnosis for a patient with known prostate cancer was bone metastasis.

ever, CT images the posterior aspect of the vertebral body with greater precision than MRI due to its higher contrast between bone and soft tissue.

MRI permits reliable differentiation between normal bone marrow and marrow with **metastatic infiltration** (Sarpel et al. 1987). In T1-weighted images, normal bone marrow will appear as areas of relatively high signal intensity. Lesions in bone marrow usually reduce signal intensity. Fat-suppressing sequences (STIR) allow higher contrast between normal and

abnormal bone marrow. MRI is generally able to distinguish between **vertebral subsidence due to osteoporosis** and subsidence due to metastatic disease. In osteoporotic subsidence, changes in cancellous bone will be seen to surround the fracture site. However, a metastasis will appear as a focal finding because of its high contrast. Proliferation of neoplastic changes in the paravertebral soft tissue, particularly intraspinal changes, are more readily identifiable in MR images than in CT studies (Figs. 8.**237a, b**–8.**240a-c**).

a   b

Figs. 8.**239a, b**   MR images of the lumbar spine.
(**a**) Sagittal plane (GRE 500/10 out of phase, with Gd-based contrast medium). The image shows enhancement in the posterior portion of the third lumbar vertebra protruding against the spinal canal. The posterior portion is particularly hyperintense. The posterior margin of the vertebral body is no longer distinguishable.

(**b**) Sagittal plane (STIR 1900/125). The entire vertebral body of L3 appears hyperintense with compression of the dural sac. A small fracture of the superior vertebral end-plate is present. This is a metastasis to the body of the third lumbar vertebra. There is instability at this level, and the dural sac is compressed.

References

Algra PR, Bloem JL, Tissing H, et al. Detection of vertebral metastases: comparison between MR imaging and bone scintigraphy. *Radiographics.* 1991; 11: 219

Assheuer J. Personal communication. Cologne 1995

Assheuer J, Lenz G, Lenz W, et al. Fett-Wassertrennung im Kernspintomogramm. Darstellung von Knochenmarkreaktion bei degenerativen Bandscheibenveränderungen. *Fortsch Geb Rontgenstr Nuklearmed.* 1987; 147: 58

Bell G, Stearns K, Bonutti P, Boumphrey F. MRI diagnosis of tuberculous vertebral osteomyelitis. *Spine.* 1990; 15: 462

Boden S, Davis D, Dina T, et al. Abnormal magnetic resonance scans of the lumbar spine in asymptomatic subjects: a prospective investigation. *J Bone Joint Surg.* 1990; 72-A: 403

Braun I, Hoffman J, David P, et al. Contrast enhancement in CT differentiation between recurrent disk herniation and postoperative scar: Prospective study. *AJR.* 1985; 145: 785

Castro WHM, Assheuer J, Schulitz KP. Haemodynamic changes in lumbar nerve root entrapment due to stenosis and/or herniated disk of the lumbar spinal canal — a magnetic resonance imaging study. *Eur Spine J* 1995; 4: 220

Davis S, Teresi L, Bradley W, et al. Cervical spine hyperextension injuries: MR findings. *Radiology.* 1991; 180: 245

DeRoss A, et al. MRI of tuberculous spondylitis. *AJR.* 1986; 146: 79

Flanders A, Schaefer D, Doan H, et al. Acute cervical spine trauma. Correlation of MR imaging findings with degree of neurologic deficit. *Radiology.* 1990; 177: 25

Heithoff K. Computed Tomography and Plain Film Diagnosis of the Lumbar Spine. In: Weinstein J, Wiesel S, eds. *The Lumbar Spine.* Philadelphia: WB Saunders; 1990

Kulkarni M, McArdle C, Kopanicky D, et al. Acute spinal cord injury. MR imaging at 1.5T. *Radiology.* 1987; 164: 837

Link M, Sciuk J, Fründt H, et al. Wirbelsäulenmetastasen — Wertigkeit diagnostischer Verfahren bei der Erstdiagnostik und im Verlauf. *Radiologe.* 1995; 35: 21

Modic M, Pavlicek W, Weinstein M, et al. Magnetic resonance imaging of intervertebral disk disease. Clinical and pulse sequence considerations. *Radiology.* 1984; 152: 103

Modic M, Ross J. Magnetic resonance imaging in the evaluation of low back pain. *Orthop Clin North Am.* 1991; 22: 283

Modic M, et al. Vertebral osteomyelitis: Assessment using MR. *Radiology.* 1985; 157: 157

Ross J, et al. Use of Gd-DTPA in the postoperative lumbar spine. *AJNR.* 1990; 11: 771

Sarpel S, et al. Early diagnosis of spinal-epidural metastasis by magnetic resonance imaging. *Radiology.* 1987; 164: 887

Stoller D, Genant H. Magnetic Resonance Imaging of the Lumbar Spine. In: Weinstein J, Wiesel S, eds. *The Lumbar Spine.* Philadelphia: WB Saunders; 1990

a

b

c

Figs. 8.**240a–c** MR images of the lumbar spine intraspinal metastasis in a patient with known prostate cancer.
(**a**) Sagittal plane (SE 500/20). The image shows a sharply demarcated intraspinal mass resembling a cyst, with erosion of vertebra S1.
(**b**) Axial plane (SE 500/20). The image shows a circumscribed intraspinal mass on the right side with a thickened wall that almost appears lobulated.
(**c**) Axial plane (SE 500/20). The wall of the mass is enhanced and has displaced the dural sac to the left.

Teplick J, Haskin M. Intravenous contrast enhanced CT of the postoperative lumbar spine. *AJR.* 1984; 143: 845

Yu S, Haughton V, et al. Criteria for classifying normal and intervertebral disks. *Radiology.* 1989; 170: 523.

Yu S, Ho P, Sether L, et al. *Nucleus pulposus degeneration: MR imaging.* 73rd scientific assembly and annual meeting of the Radiological Society of North America, Chicago (IL) 1987.

8.9 Discography

Indications, Diagnostic Value, and Clinical Relevance

Discography is an invasive method for visualizing the nucleus pulposus that makes it possible to **provoke and reproduce pain (distension test).** In combina-

tion with subsequent CT imaging (CT discography), discography is regarded as one of the most reliable methods for visualizing **degenerative disk disorders** (Bernard 1990; Grubb et al. 1987; Sachs et al. 1987). CT discography is regarded as more sensitive than MRI for detecting degenerative disk changes in their early stages because it can visualize tears in the anulus fibrosus at their onset (Bernard 1990). However, other authors regard MRI as the more precise and reliable method for visualizing degenerative disk disorders (Gibson et al. 1986). The advantage of discography lies in the combination of imaging and pain-reproduction testing (Table 8.**44**). Other causes of pain such as facet or sacroiliac joint pathology, spinal stenosis, segmental instability, and muscle pain symptoms should be excluded prior to performing discography. As an invasive procedure, discography

Table 8.**44**   Clinical value of discography

Bone structure	–
Facet arthritis	–
Disk prolapse	++
Symptomatic disk without prolapse	+++
Trauma	–
Spondylitis	–
Deformities	–
Tumor	–
Spinal stenosis (central)	–
Lateral stenosis	–

– No information content
(+) Low information content
+ Moderate information content
++ High information content
+++ Very high information content

forms the final link in the diagnostic imaging chain (Bernard 1990; Greenspan 1993; Sachs et al. 1987). The Diagnostic and Therapeutic Committee of the North American Spine Society defines the indication for discography as follows:

— In patients with persistent symptoms in whom discogenic causes are suspected but noninvasive imaging methods are inconclusive.
— In patients in whom spinal fusion is planned to visualize adjacent and possible symptomatic intervertebral disks to determine the extent of fusion necessary.
— In patients with persistent symptoms after spinal surgery.
— In patients in whom minimally invasive disk surgery is planned where it is necessary to determine preoperatively whether a contained disk is present.

Cervical discography provides less diagnostic information than the lumbar method. This is because degenerative changes are encountered far more frequently with increasing age and therefore do not correlate sufficiently with clinical symptoms (Merriam and Stockdale 1983).

Discography as an invasive method can involve complications. These include the risk of infection, which according to the literature ranges from 0.1–4.0% (Jackson and Jacobs 1990; Osti et al. 1990) to 0.1–0.2% (Guyer and Ohnmeiss 1995), and the risk of allergic reaction to the contrast medium. Occasionally a temporary increase in the existing symptoms is observed after injection. This usually completely reverses. Although theoretically possible, there is no evidence that aspiration and injection in the nucleus pulposus provokes disk prolapse. Retrospective studies of patients who have undergone multiple discographies have failed to demonstrate any detrimental effects of this method on the intervertebral disk (Bernard 1990; Johnson 1989; Park 1976).

Technique, Instrumentation, and Examination Procedure

The patient is in a stable lateral position with the legs flexed (Fig. 8.**241**). The examination is performed under sterile conditions via a posterolateral approach to the desired disk after carefully disinfecting the skin, draping the patient, and administering local anesthesia. The examination should include multiple levels. The disks at levels L3–L4, L4–L5, and L5–S1 are often involved in discogenic symptoms (Bernard 1990, Jackson and Jacobs 1990). The segment of interest is visualized using fluoroscopy. The injection is performed using the approach described by McCulloch and Waddell (1978) approximately 8–10 cm lateral to the row of spinous processes parallel to the intervertebral disk compartment of interest. This pro-

Fig. 8.**241**   Patient positioning for lumbar discography (from Castro W. M., Schilgen, M., Kreuzschmerzen, Springer Verlag 1995).

cedure is monitored under fluoroscopy. To examine segment L5–S1, an entry point 1 cm further lateral is selected, which lies slightly proximal to the injection site for L4–L5. The "double-needle" technique is used. This involves advancing a thicker needle to slightly above the facet joint, which represents the actual bony impediment. Then, only the thinner needle contained within the thick needle is advanced to avoid accidental contact with a nerve root, which could cause unnecessary pain. Using the "double-needle" technique is also thought to reduce the risk of diskitis (Guyer and Ohnmeiss 1995).

The needle should be located exactly in the center of the intervertebral space (i.e., nucleus pulposus) to avoid false positive findings from injection into the anulus fibrosus or against an end-plate. The contrast medium is injected under close fluoroscopic control. Injection into a normal disk is not usually painful (Bernard 1990). However, studies by Grubb et al. (1987) reported a painful (positive) distension test in 12% of test subjects despite an intact intervertebral disk. In these cases, either degenerative changes were present in the adjacent disks, or the patients showed psychogenic abnormalities. Patients may frequently report a certain sensation of pressure, which should be regarded as normal. Strong resistance will be felt after injection of 1–4 mL of contrast medium on average. A healthy disk will rarely accept more than 2.5 mL (Jackson and Jacobs 1990). Degenerative or prolapsed disks will hold a large volume.

The provocative test should be performed. This supplements evaluation of the morphologic appearance of the disk and provides important diagnostic information. The **distension test** describes the quality of discomfort during injection of contrast medium into the nucleus pulposus. It is not clear what generates the pain. Possible causes include distension of pain-conducting fibers in the outer layers of the anulus fibrosis (Bernard 1990). During injection, ask the patient to describe whether the pain felt is typical (reproducible pain) or whether it is a new pain not previously experienced (atypical pain). Three different degrees of pain are distinguished: not painful (grade 0), atypical pain (grade 1), and typical pain (grade 2). Other authors expand the gradation and distinguish between no pain/tenderness, atypical pain, similar pain, and identical pain (Sachs et al. 1987).

The distension test will be negative in most intact intervertebral disks, i.e., there will be no significant pain. Other studies (Guyer and Ohnmeiss 1995) report an accuracy of 64% for the distension test in diagnosing a prolapsed disk. The incidence of false negative findings cited is 57%.

Normal Findings

In a normal lateral discogram, the nucleus pulposus will appear as an oval, smoothly demarcated, area of contrast slightly posterior to the center of the intervertebral space. The normal intervertebral disk can appear in one of three physiologic forms. They are referred to according to their appearance as "cotton ball", "pancake," or "cookie sandwich" (Figs. 8.**242a–c** and 8.**244**).

The distension test and the morphologic appearance of the disk will not always coincide. Grubb et al. 1987 reported a negative distension test in 22% of patients with abnormal disk changes. The extent of degenerative damage to the disk does not always correlate with reproducible pain. In multilevel disk degeneration, "typical" pain was not always reported in the segment with the most severe degeneration, but often in segments with less pronounced pathology.

Degenerative changes of the anulus fibrosus can be a problem. They can involve fissures and subtotal rupture up to and including protrusion of the anulus fibrosus tissue (Yasuma et al. 1988). This last form simulates the clinical symptoms of protrusion of nucleus pulposus tissue but is difficult to diagnose in the discogram. Yasuma et al. reported on patients with negative discography findings who underwent discectomy. Histologic examination of these patients

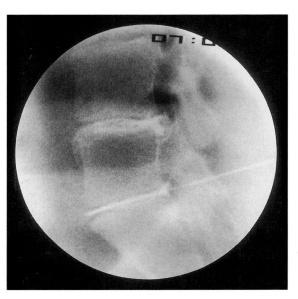

Fig. 8.**243** Discography of the two distal lumbar disks in the sagittal plane. Contrast medium is seen to spread throughout the entire disk, indicative of degeneration. The second disk from the bottom also shows slight posterior protrusion.

a   b   c

Figs. 8.**242a–c** Schematic diagram of normal findings during discography.

Fig. 8.**244** Discography of the two distal lumbar disks in the sagittal plane. The second disk from the bottom is normal and shows a "cookie sandwich" pattern of contrast enhancement. The bottom disk shows degenerative changes. The contrast medium is seen to spread throughout the entire disk.

Fig. 8.**245** Discography of the second to last lumbar disk in the sagittal plane. After injection, contrast medium not only flows into the disk but also extends to an epidural location. The column of contrast medium is clearly visible in the entire spinal canal caudally to the affected disk. This is a sign of a posterior defect in the anulus fibrosus.

revealed protrusion in 32% of the study group and prolapse of anulus fibrosis tissue with an intact nucleus pulposus in 56%. This illustrates that isolated degeneration of the anulus fibrosis without continuity into the nucleus pulposus cannot be excluded in the discogram.

Abnormal Findings

Disk degeneration begins with an initial **decrease in the height of the intervertebral space** with uniform symmetric protrusion of the intervertebral disk (bulging disk). As the disorder progresses, disk degeneration is characterized by increased dehydration and an irregularly bounded nucleus pulposus with radial fissures in the anulus fibrosus (Yu et al. 1989). This appears in the discogram as an irregularly bounded nucleus pulposus with spread of contrast into large portions of the intervertebral space (Figs. 8.**243** and 8.**244**). Advanced degeneration can lead to **protrusion** of the nucleus pulposus with the anulus fibrosis at least partially intact (contained disk). In disk protrusion, the anulus fibrosus is not yet interrupted (subannular displacement of the nucleus). **Extrusion** is when the anulus fibrosis is ruptured, in which case the nucleus tissue is still covered by a thin fibrous layer (see pp. 391 and 402). Extrusion is often referred to as a **subligamentous disk prolapse** since the posterior longitudinal ligament is not yet compromised (Castro et al. 1995). Where the posterior longitudinal ligament is ruptured, one refers to an **extraligamentous disk prolapse.** This can be located in the peridural space as a **free fragment or seques-**

tered disk if the continuity of the disk is interrupted. The classification described is taken from the Düsseldorf Diagnostic Disk Program, which determines whether a minimally invasive or open surgical procedure is indicated, depending on the degree of severity (Castro et al. 1995, Schulitz and Schöppe 1994).

In a sequestrated disk, the distension test may well be negative due to the lack of continuity with the nucleus pulposus (Bernard 1990). Any form of contrast-medium leakage, whether anterior or posterior, is considered abnormal (Fig. 8.**245**).

A **CT scan** performed immediately after discography (CT discography) can be used to further describe the protrusion as broad-based or narrow-based. This is done to evaluate minimally invasive therapeutic interventions (Figs. 8.**207**–8.**210**, p. 392). Diagnosing a sequestrated disk in CT images can be difficult because the free fragment may be at a different level than the disk; depending on the slices selected, it can be easily overlooked. In such cases, MR images in the sagittal plane should be obtained.

The accuracy of discography in diagnosing disk prolapse is cited at 58%, and the incidence of false negative results at 18% (Jackson and Jacobs 1990). Differentiating between contained and noncontained prolapsed disks is crucial to selecting the proper surgical procedure.

References

Bernard T. Lumbar discography followed by computed tomography. 1990; 15: 690

Castro WHM, Bongartz G, Schultz KP. Stellenwert der CT-Diskographie in der differenzierten Therapie des Bandscheibenvorfalles. *Deutsches Ärzteblatt.*1995; 92: 352

Gibson M, Buckley J, Mawhinney R, et al. Magnetic resonance imaging and discography in the diagnosis of disk degeneration. *J Bone Joint Surg.* 1986; 68B: 369

Greenspan A. *Skelettradiologie.* Weinheim–London: Chapman & Hall; 1993

Grubb S, Lipscomb H, Guilford B. The relative value of lumbar roentgenograms, metrizamide myelography, and discography in the assessment of patients with chronic low-back syndrome. *Spine.* 1987; 12: 282

Guyer RD, Ohnmeiss DD. Contemporary concepts in spine care – Lumbar discography. *Spine.* 1995; 20: 2048

Jackson R, Jacobs R. Computed Tomography – Discography. In: Weinstein J, Wiesel S, eds. *The Lumbar Spine.* Philadelphia: WB Saunders; 1990

Johnson R. Does discography injure normal disks? *Spine.* 1989; 14: 424.

McCulloch JA, Waddell G. Lateral lumbar discography. *Brit J Radiol.* 1978; 51: 498

Merriam W, Stockdale H. Is cervical discography of any value? *Eur J Radiol.* 1983; 3: 138

Osti O, Fraser R, Vernon-Roberts B. Discitis after discography. *J Bone Joint Surg.* 1990; 72B: 271

Park W. Lumbar Discography. In: Jayson M, ed. *The Lumbar Spine and Back Pain.* New York: Grune & Stratton; 1976

Sachs B, Vanharanta H, Spivey M, et al. Dallas discogram description. *Spine.* 1987; 12: 287

Schultz KP, Schöppe K. Die neuroradiographische Diagnostik degenerativer Bandscheibendiagnostik – Das Düsseldorfer diagnostische Diskusprogramm (DdD). *Z Orthop.* 1994; 132: 25

Yasuma T, Ohno R, Yamauchi Y. False-negative lumbar discograms. J Bone Joint Surg. 1988; 70A: 1279

Yu S, Haughton V, et al. Criteria for classifying normal and intervertebral disks. *Radiology.* 1989; 170: 523

8.10 Diagnostic Injection Techniques

Facet Infiltration

Indications, Diagnostic Value, and Clinical Relevance

Facet infiltration with a local anesthetic is regarded as a valuable method in diagnosing **facet syndrome** (Jerosch and Castro 1994; Schaerer 1978, Schultz and Lenz 1984). It is used to exclude other causes of pain and to identify the level of the joints causing pain. However, only a brief relief of symptoms can usually be expected from successful facet infiltration (Jerosch et al. 1993).

Experience to date has shown that facet infiltration with subsequent short-term pain relief involves uncertainties regarding the diagnosis of facet syndrome and the prognosis after spinal fusion. Studies have shown that spinal fusion is successful in only 50–80% of patients free of pain after facet infiltration (Jerosch and Castro 1994).

However, studies by Lorenz et al. (1983) and Nachemson (1963) have been able to define various physical factors that correlate with relief of pain after facet infiltration. These include a history of persistent low-back pain without leg pain, pain that does not increase as intrathecal pressure is increased (Valsalva maneuver), and advanced age. Additional factors include normal weight, lack of muscle spasms, and maximum pain upon extension after bending forward.

In addition to an excessively large injection volume (see below), incorrect needle placement can result in periarticular facet injection instead of intra-articular injection. This can lead to a false positive diagnosis of facet syndrome where structures supplied by the sinuvertebral nerve are anesthetized. Additional infiltration methods such as paravertebral or epidural injection, and radiologic provocation methods such as discography, can be used to evaluate a recurrent pain component caused by the sinuvertebral nerve (Jerosch and Castro 1994).

The response to facet joint infiltration must be interpreted carefully. Studies have shown a placebo response rate of up to 32 % and a false positive rate as high as 38 %.

Technique, Instrumentation, and Examination Procedure

The patient is prone with the skin disinfected over a wide radius around the injection site. The injection is performed under sterile conditions. A 22-G spinal needle is inserted in a paravertebral position approximately 2 cm between the spinous processes, and advanced under fluoroscopic control as far as the joint and subsequently through the joint capsule. An oblique projection (45°) achieved by using cushions and tilting the C-arm facilitates identification of the vertebral joints. The needle should be placed in the inferior articular recess to avoid cartilage damage (Jerosch and Castro 1994) (Figs. 8.**246a, b**).

Approximately 0.5 mL of a local anesthetic is then injected into the inferior articular recess. Using a larger volume of local anesthetic increases the risk of cartilage injury and periarticular leakage. This can anesthetize other structures that caused pain and in so doing, reduce the selectivity and diagnostic value of this examination method (Hildenbrandt and Weyland 1987; Jerosch and Castro 1994; Schultz and Lenz 1984). Contrast medium may first be injected to verify proper positioning of the spinal needle. However, arthrography is not routinely performed.

Selective Nerve Root Block

Indications, Diagnostic Value, and Clinical Relevance

In patients with leg pain, a selective nerve root block may be used to diagnose clinically relevant nerve root compression. Castro and Akkerveeken (1991) defined the following five indications in their prospective

a   b

Figs. 8.**246a, b**   Lumbar facet infiltration. Thin aspiration needles are advanced as far as the vertebral joint, 2 cm paravertebral between the spinous processes.

study on the diagnostic value of selective lumbar nerve-root block:

1. Patients with possible radicular pain in one or both legs without a neurologic deficit and nerve root compression sign. Radiographic signs of entrapment of at least one nerve root on the same side as the leg pain must be present.

2. Patients with a classic nerve root compression syndrome with a positive sign of nerve root irritation (positive Lasègue sign) and radiographic signs of entrapment of more than one nerve root.

3. Patients with a classic nerve root compression syndrome with radiographic signs that do not correspond to the clinical picture.

4. Patients with leg pain that increases when walking or standing. Absence of the typical signs of neurogenic intermittent claudication, but radiographic signs of nerve root entrapment, with or without stenosis of the spinal canal.

5. Patients with the typical signs of neurologic claudication syndrome with radiographic signs of nerve root entrapment and stenosis of the spinal canal.

As in facet infiltration, false results can be caused by injecting too large a volume of local anesthetic. Therefore the volume of local anesthetic should be kept as small as possible. This in turn requires accu-

racy in needle positioning, which should be verified by fluoroscopy. Performing the examination under CT control may be necessary in exceptional cases, such as severely deformed spines or in scoliosis.

Technique, Instrumentation, and Examination Procedure

The patient may be positioned either on the unaffected side, supported by a cushion, or prone. An S1 block should always be performed with the patient prone. The examination is performed under fluoroscopy. An 18-G or 21-G spinal needle is advanced under sterile conditions after careful disinfection of the skin. Correct positioning of the needle inferolateral to the pedicle can be verified in the AP plane (Figs. 8.**247a, b**).

To administer a block at L5, the tip of the needle is positioned inferolateral to the pedicle of the fifth lumbar vertebra, anterior to the transverse process. With the patient in a lateral position, the needle is advanced as in discography and aimed at the intervertebral foramen.

Performing a nerve root block with the patient in a lateral position is recommended in patients who have undergone previous spinal fusion in the region of the injection. Here, fused bone could prevent aspi-

a   b

Figs. 8.**247a, b** Placement of the needle for administering a nerve root block as visualized in the AP and sagittal planes.

ration of the nerve root sheath from a medial approach with the patient prone. The patient should always be prone when a block at S1 is administered. Advance the tip of the needle into the foramen of the first sacral vertebra and locate the sheath of the nerve.

Before administering anesthesia, we recommend verifying proper positioning of the aspiration needle by injecting approximately 0.5 mL of contrast medium while evaluating pain provocation (Fig. 8.**248**). The patient should feel a sharp stabbing pain in the leg corresponding to the area supplied by the nerve root. Pain in the back alone or pseudoradicular radiating pain is not sufficient. Next, inject a maximum of 0.5 mL of local anesthetic. Larger volumes of local anesthetic increase the rate of false positive results by anesthetizing adjacent structures (Castro et al. 1994).

A reversible total loss of motor and sensory function of the nerve root can occur after a successful selective nerve root block. In a positive test, the leg pains disappear and gradually return after several hours. The test is negative if the leg pains are not influenced by this procedure. Inconclusive results are also possible (Castro and Akkerveeken 1991).

Fig. 8.**248** The course of nerve root S1 is demonstrated under fluoroscopic control after aspiration of the root pocket and injection of contrast medium.

References

Castro WHM, Akkerveeken PF. Der diagnostische Wert der selektiven lumbalen Nervenwurzelblockade. *Z Orthop.* 1991; 129: 374

Castro WHM, Grönemeyer D, Jerosch J, et al. How reliable is lumber nerve root sheath infiltration? *Europ Spine J.* 1994; 3: 374

Hildebrandt J, Weyland A. Die perkutane lumbale Facettendenervation. *Z Orthop.* 1987; 125: 154

Jerosch J, Castro WHM. *Das Facettensyndrom: Ursachen, Diagnostik, Therapie, Prophylaxe.* (Bücherei des Orthopäden, vol. 62). Stuttgart: Enke; 1994

Jerosch J, Castro WHM, Halm H, Müller-Silvergieter G. Langzeitergebnisse nach perkutaner lumbaler Facettenkoagulation. *Z Orthop.* 1993; 131: 241

Lorenz M, Patwardhan A, Vanderby R. Load-bearing characteristics of lumbar facets in normal and surgically altered spinal segments. *Spine.* 1983; 8: 122

Nachemson AL. The influence of spinal movements on the lumber intradiscal pressure and on the tensile stresses in the annulus fibrosus. *Acta Orthop Scand.* 1963; 33: 183

Schaerer JP. Radiofrequency facet rhizotomy in the treatment of chronic neck and low-back pain. *Int Surg.* 1978; 63: 53

Schulitz KP, Lenz G. Das Facetten-Syndrom, Klinik und Therapie. In: Hohmann et al. eds. *Neuroorthopädie.* 2nd ed. Berlin: Springer; 1984

9 | Pelvis

9.1 Introduction

The pelvis is a closed ring of bone formed by the two innominate bones and the sacrum. The pelvis transmits the forces acting on the spinal column to the lower extremities and protects the pelvic organs. Parts of the proximal pelvic ring provide insertions for the musculature of the trunk, and parts of the hip and thigh musculature insert into its distal parts. Therefore, evaluation of any pelvic pathology should also include examination of the spine and lower extremities.

Degenerative changes lead to chronic irritation of the pubic symphysis and sacroiliac joints. Unbalanced stresses resulting from deficient posture can produce arthritic changes in the sacroiliac joint. Predisposing factors include scoliosis and leg-length difference.

Sacroiliac dysfunction is a disturbance of the motion at the sacroiliac joint.

The sacroiliac joint is also frequently involved in rheumatic disorders. Table 9.1 provides an overview of types of sacroiliac arthritis.

Pelvic trauma can involve soft-tissue damage or bone injuries. Bone injuries include pelvic rim fractures (such as an avulsion fracture of the anterior superior iliac spine), fractures of the pelvic ring, and acetabular fractures.

Pelvic ring fractures are divided into three categories according to the condition of the posterior segment of the ring, which is crucial for the biomechanical stability of the pelvis (Table 9.2):

- stable (type A injuries);
- rotationally unstable (type B injuries);
- rotationally and vertically unstable (type C injuries).

There is no universally accepted classification system for pelvic ring fractures. Table 9.2 shows the 1991 ver-

Table 9.**1**   Arthritis of the sacroiliac joint in rheumatic disorders

Disorder	Characteristics/symptoms	HLA type
Ankylosing spondylitis	Initial manifestation often in the sacroiliac joint	HLA-B27
Reiter syndrome	At least two joints are involved with at least one of the following symptoms: urethritis, cervicitis, conjunctivitis, or Shigella dysentery	HLA-B27 in 80% of all cases
Psoriatic arthritis	Frequently associated with joint and fingernail symptoms (stippling, nail grooves, or nail loosening)	Often HLA-B27 and occasionally HLA-Bw38
Whipple disease	Inflammation of the sacroiliac joints as in ankylosing spondylitis	
Bowel disorders (Crohn disease, ulcerated colitis) with involvement of the sacroiliac joint	Joint involvement is more frequent when the colon is involved	HLA-B27 positive in 70% of all cases
Rheumatic arthritis	Sacroiliac joints are less frequently affected, usually unilaterally	HLA-Dw4 and HLA-DR4
Sjögren syndrome	Triad: dry eyes, dry mouth, HLA-Dw3 and arthritis; primarily (90%) in middle-aged women	HLA-Dw3
Associated arthritis	In infections (bowel or urogenital tract) caused by Yersinia, salmonella, or gonococci	Frequently HLA-B27 positive

Table 9.**2**   AO/ASIF classification of pelvic ring fractures (1991)

Type	Lesion
A	**Stable**
A1	Fractures without involvement of the pelvic ring (avulsion fractures)
A2	Fractures of the iliac wing without involvement of the pelvic ring Pelvic ring fractures without (significant) displacement
A3	Transverse fractures of the sacrum and coccyx without involvement of the pelvic ring
B	**Rotationally unstable, vertically stable**
B1	External rotation injury (open book), i.e., rupture of the pubic symphysis
B2	Compression injury with internal rotation deformity of one half of the pelvis
B2.1	Ipsilateral type
B2.2	Contralateral type
B3	Bilateral type B injuries
C	**Rotationally and vertically unstable (vertical shear)**
C1	Unilateral
C1.1	Fracture of the ilium
C1.2	Rupture or fracture dislocation of the sacroiliac joint
C1.3	Fracture of the sacrum
C2	Bilateral incomplete
C3	Bilateral complete C lesion with additional acetabular fracture

sion of the AO/ASIF classification system as proposed by Pennal et al. (1980). Since then, the AO/ASIF system has undergone further revision. The 1995 version is a combined classification of the anterior and posterior pelvic ring. It is designed as an open system, which enables it to encompass a wide variety of pelvic ring injuries and permit precise scientific documentation. The classification of pelvic fractures is in evolution and the literature should be reviewed for more detailed information.

An example of a rotationally unstable pelvic ring injury (i.e., unstable in the horizontal plane) is an isolated rupture of the pubic symphysis caused by an anteroposterior (AP) force in which the anterior ligaments of one or both sacroiliac joints are also torn. Vertical stability of the pelvis is not compromised because the crucial biomechanical posterior ligament connections remain intact. However, shear forces will produce a rotationally and vertically unstable injury (the classic Malgaigne fracture), such as can occur when landing on one leg after a fall from a height.

The system developed by Letournel and Judet (1993) has become the standard for classifying **acetabular fractures.** The acetabulum is divided into anterior (iliopubic) and posterior (ilioischial) columns. For each of these locally, basic forms of fractures (fracture of the acetabular rim, column fracture, and transverse fracture) are distinguished from combined fracture forms, such as a fracture of both col-

umns. This classification was modified by the AO/ASIF according to Table 9.**3**.

The incidence of **pelvic fractures** varies between 3% and 10%, depending on the author and patient group. Automobile accidents are cited as the most frequent cause, accounting for 80–90% of all injuries. This is followed by falls from a great height and crush injuries. Injuries to the pelvis and hip represent a relatively insignificant number of athletic injuries, accounting for 2–3% of these injuries. Fatigue fractures in the hip and pelvis are also relatively rare; only about 3% of all fatigue fractures occur as the result of athletic activity.

Pelvic injuries can be categorized according to their cause as **extrinsic** (externally caused) and **intrinsic injuries.** The latter are due to forces acting within the body itself and include such injuries as avulsion fractures or muscle tears. In addition to the classic cases of sudden trauma, stress in the form of chronic improper use or overuse can also cause injuries. Examples of this are the rare stress fractures of the pubic bone that can occur in joggers.

Extrinsic soft-tissue injuries include skin abrasions (frequently superficial) and crush injuries at structures such as the iliac crest where the bone is only covered by a thin layer of soft tissue. Blunt trauma in the lateral and posterior pelvis can result in extensive compression of the surrounding muscle layers. These injuries may present as broad hematomas (Table 9.**4**).

Table 9.**3**   AO/ASIF classification of acetabular fractures (1991)

Type A	**Involvement of only one column of the acetabulum while the second column is intact**
A1	Fractures of the posterior acetabular rim with variants
A2	Fractures of the posterior column with variants
A3	Fractures of the anterior acetabular rim and the anterior column
Type B	**Characterized by a transverse fracture component whereby at least a portion of the acetabular roof is intact and must remain in contact with the ilium**
B1	Transverse fractures through the acetabulum with or without a fracture of the posterior rim of the acetabulum
B2	T-shaped fractures with variants
B3	Fractures of the anterior column of acetabular rim associated with a posterior "hemi-transverse" fracture
Type C	**Fractures of both columns: the fracture lines course through both the anterior and posterior columns. In contrast to type B fractures, all articular fragments including the acetabular roof are separated from the rest of the ilium**
C1	Fracture of the anterior column coursing as far as the iliac crest
C2	Fracture of the anterior column coursing into the anterior margin of the ilium
C3	Transverse fractures extending into the sacroiliac joint

Table 9.**4**   Soft-tissue injuries in the pelvis

Extrinsic	**Intrinsic**
Contusions, crush injuries, skin abrasions (for example at the iliac crest), hematomas in the gluteal region	Muscle pulls and small tears in the muscles inserting into the pelvis, such as the adductors, rectus femoris, iliopsoas, abdominal oblique muscles, and rectus abdominis

Intrinsic soft-tissue injuries include the numerous types of muscle pulls and tears. Injuries to the adductors are common. Injuries to the proximal portion of the rectus femoris are also observed. In rare cases, tears in the insertions of the iliopsoas can also occur. Minor tears can also occur in the abdominal oblique muscles at the iliac crest, and in the rectus abdominis in the region of the pubic bone (Table 9.**4**).

The group of **extrinsic bone injuries** includes traumatic damage to the pubic bone, ischium, sacrum, or coccyx. Extreme trauma can also disrupt the pelvic ring. These injuries are often complicated by associated injuries to neurovascular structures, the urethra, or the bowels (complex pelvic trauma). Less severe injuries of this type include fractures of the coccyx (Table 9.**5**).

Intrinsic bone injuries (avulsion fractures) are caused by muscular traction on the origin of the apophysis. They frequently occur in teenagers and young adults and primarily involve the anterior superior and anterior inferior iliac spines, the pubic bone, and, rarely, the iliac crest and ischial tuberosity (Table 9.**5**).

Overuse fractures can also be included among the intrinsic bone injuries. Sites include the pubic bone and, rarely, the ischium and sacrum.

The pelvis may be involved in systemic disorders. These include disturbed calcium and phosphate metabolism that may result from vitamin D deficiency, primary hyperparathyroidism, or renal dysfunction, which itself can lead to secondary hyperparathyroidism. Sequelae of these metabolic changes

Table 9.**5**   Bone injuries in the pelvis

Extrinsic	**Intrinsic**
Fractures These may be caused by direct external trauma, for example fractures of the pelvic ring due to extreme trauma such as a riding or motorcycle accident	Avulsion fractures The cause is uncoordinated powerful muscular traction on the origin of the apophysis, usually in the second decade of life. Predisposed sites include the anterior superior and anterior inferior iliac spines, pubic bone, and (rarely) the iliac crest and ischial tuberosity
	Stress fractures The cause is chronic overuse. Predisposed sites: pubic bone, less frequently the coccyx and sacrum
	Other overuse injuries Arthritis in the sacroiliac joints

observed in the pelvic bones include osteomalacia with softening of the bone and structural insufficiency. In children for example, chronic vitamin D deficiency leads to flattening of the pelvis typical of rickets.

Another systemic skeletal disorder primarily affecting the pelvis in older patients is Paget disease (osteitis deformans). The cause of this disorder is unclear. Symptoms include "rheumatic" symptoms, spontaneous fractures, and skeletal deformations.

Finally, there are inflammatory disorders (such as osteomyelitis) and tumors. Tumors are often metastatic in origin. Osteoblastic metastases proceed from prostate and breast carcinomas. Osteolytic metastases generally stem from bronchial, thyroid, and kidney carcinomas, occasionally from breast carcinomas. Primary tumors in the pelvic region include chondrosarcomas and Ewing sarcomas.

9.2 Clinical Standard Examination

Since the pelvis is the bridge between the spine and the lower extremities, the history and examination of pelvic symptoms should also include the history and examination of the spine and lower extremities, particularly the hip.

Physical examination of the pelvis begins with inspection. In addition to observation of the morphology of the pelvis, include evaluation of gait. Palpation includes the muscular insertions and important bony structures such as the anterior and posterior iliac spines, the pubic symphysis, and the joints. Always examine pelvic version, and document any pathologic anterior movement of the posterior iliac spines indicative of limited motion in the sacroiliac joints when the patient bends over. This is followed by examination of the sacroiliac joints in particular, and by functional testing of the muscles of the pelvic girdle.

The final phase of the pelvic examination consists of neurovascular examination of the lower extremities and of the genitals where pelvic trauma is present.

The tentative diagnosis reached on the basis of clinical examination can be verified or modified by subsequent diagnostic imaging studies (Table 9.**6**).

Table 9.**6** Standard examination procedure

- History
- Inspection
- Palpation
- Neurovascular examination
- Diagnostic imaging studies

Patient History

Interpreting information from the history is difficult in the presence of pelvic symptoms, particularly where there are atypical **chronic symptoms** such as groin pain or "diffuse" pelvic pain. The patient should be routinely asked the following questions:

- **How long have the symptoms been present and under what conditions did they first occur?**

Sudden symptoms in the sacroiliac region that occur with body motion are a sign of sacroiliac joint dysfunction.

- **Does the pain occur at rest or during exercise? What stresses is the patient subjected to?**

Irritation of the adductors and iliopsoas in particular can decrease or disappear during exercise. Frequently it can reappear with increased intensity after exercise. Persistent groin pain radiating into the buttocks or thigh can occur following strenuous exertion, for example in distance runners. Groin pain can be a sign of a stress fracture of the ischium, pubic bone, or proximal femur. These fractures are most often encountered in female runners; the history should always include sports activities.

- **Does the pain occur independently of exercise? Does it disturb the patient's sleep?**

Pain occurring independently of exercise or which disturbs the patient's sleep always suggest a disorder other than trauma or overuse, such as appendicitis, prostatitis, urinary tract infection, kidney disorders, gynecologic disorders, osteomyelitis, or tumors in the pelvis or groin region.

- **What is the nature of the pain?**

Intermittent episodes of dull pain in the sacrum or lower lumbar region occurring primarily in the morning suggest rheumatic disorders, primarily ankylosing spondylitis. If the patient reports these symptoms, you should inquire about pain in other parts of the body, particularly in the joints.

- **Where is the pain localized? To where does it radiate?**

It is important to determine whether referred pain can be linked to a certain dermatome or area of distribution of a peripheral nerve. The differential diagnosis should consider pathology in the lumbar spine. Nerve roots L1 through S5 are responsible for the sensory supply of the lower extremities, buttocks, and genitals (see Fig. 8.**40b**, p. 311).

Obtaining a history with **acute injuries** to the pelvis is usually easier. Pelvic injury in an accident usually requires trauma involving significant kinetic energy. The patient will often have multiple trauma so that reconstructing the mechanism of injury will require information from other sources. The patient's age is significant because the same pelvic injuries may require far less trauma in older patients than in younger patients because of osteoporosis. The risk of associated pelvic and extrapelvic injuries in older patients is higher. Ask patients who are conscious and responsive about blood in the urine or perianal bleeding. These can be important signs of associated injuries to the urogenital system or the bowel. Always inquire about disturbed sensation and/or paralysis in the lower extremities. This can be a sign of injury to the femoral, sciatic, or obturator nerves, or the lumbosacral nerve plexus.

Describing the mechanism of injury (crush injury, fall, or automobile accident) including the direction of forces acting on the pelvis is important for diagnosing acute injuries of soft tissue and bone. In **adductor tears** or avulsions in the region of the pubic bone, the patient will feel a stabbing pain in the groin at the moment of injury. Adducting the legs will be painful. Adductor tears typically occur with abrupt excessive abduction. Sports such as soccer, ice hockey, skiing, and hurdle events entail an increased risk of these injuries. Such injuries can occur in everyday situations where the patient attempts to avoid a fall. Less frequent causes of avulsion fractures include electrical accidents and tetanus.

The **abdominal muscles** that insert into the pelvis on the pubic bone (especially the rectus abdominis) are especially prone to tear in overuse injuries from weight lifting, gymnastics, crew, and wrestling.

Physical examination

Observation

Observation of the pelvis begins when the patient enters the examining room. Gait irregularities may be due to:

— pain (Duchenne gait);
— muscular weakness (Trendelenburg sign);
— leg shortening (compensatory limp);
— arthrodesis of the hip (compensation for a fused joint).

In the **antalgic gait** (Duchenne's gait), the patient attempts to reduce stress on the painful hip by reducing the stance phase of the affected leg in a typically truncated gait, or by shifting the upper body, and thus the body's center of gravity, over the affected joint in the stance phase.

In the **Trendelenburg gait,** weakness of the hip abductors causes the pelvis to dip toward the unaffected side in the stance phase, and the patient shifts the upper body over the affected side (see Figs. 8.**19a, b**, p. 302). The stance phase is not as sharply truncated as in an antalgic gait. Bilateral insufficiency of the gluteal musculature produces a typical waddling gait.

In a **compensatory limp with leg shortening,** the upper body is shifted slightly over the leg in the stance phase. Otherwise, the gait is relatively smooth.

In a gait that attempts to **compensate for hip fusion,** the increased tilt of the pelvis in the sagittal plane, as it moves from hyperlordosis into lumbar kyphosis, produces femoral anteversion in the swing phase.

For a complete examination, the patient should **undress** completely (seriously injured patients should be undressed). You should observe the undressing as closely as possible because it can provide important information about possible limited motion in the lumbar and sacral spine and/or painful motion, for example in hip flexion. Evaluate the gait again after the patient has undressed.

Document any **skin changes** such as external signs of injury (scrapes, contusions, or hematomas), discoloration (for example erythema as a sign of inflammation), congenital skin changes, swelling, penetration, and the position of skin folds. The patient's underwear may contain residual **secretions** indicative of associated injuries with pelvic fractures, such is bleeding from the anus and/or urethra.

When inspecting the patient **from the front,** note the position of the anterior iliac spines. Normally they should be at the same level. Deviation can be a sign of pelvic obliquity or a difference in leg length.

Observing the pelvis **from the side** will give you an impression of the inclination of the pelvis. Lack of normal lumbar lordosis can be a sign of a spasm in the paravertebral musculature. Hyperlordosis or increased anterior pelvic version can be a sign of insufficiency of the abdominal musculature, of a weakness in the extensors, or of a flexion contracture in the hips.

Observe the contour of the musculature of the buttocks on the **posterior aspect** of the pelvis. Asymmetry in the marginal skin folds can be due to diseases of the hip (developmentally dislocated hip), neuromuscular diseases, or leg-length differences. Patients who are not excessively obese will have two small depressions ("sacral dimples") superior to the posterior iliac spines (Fig. 8.7, p. 297). Deviation of one of these depressions from horizontal is a sign of pelvic obliquity.

A leg-length difference in trauma patients can be a sign of an unstable injury of the pelvic ring with superior displacement of one hemipelvis, or an acetabular fracture with central dislocation of the hip.

Palpation and Examination

Palpation may be performed with the patient standing or supine. This will depend on the pattern of injury and the degree to which the patient is impaired.

Both sides should be palpated simultaneously if possible. This provides information about differences in skin temperature or unilateral swelling.

• **Examination with the patient standing**
When examining the patient **from the front,** rest

Fig. 9.**1**   Observation and palpation of the position of the anterior pelvis with the patient standing.

Fig. 9.**2**   Observation and palpation of the position of the posterior pelvis with the patient standing.

both hands on the patient's waist with your thumbs on the patient's iliac spines. Place your fingers on the anterior iliac crest. Compare both sides, and note any pelvic obliquity (Fig. 9.**1**).

To evaluate the position of the pelvis from **behind** with the patient standing, place your thumbs on the patient's posterior superior iliac spines. Move your index finger from lateral across the iliac crests (see p. 301). This may be difficult in obese patients. Normally the anterior and posterior iliac spines and the iliac crests will be at the same level (Fig. 9.**2**).

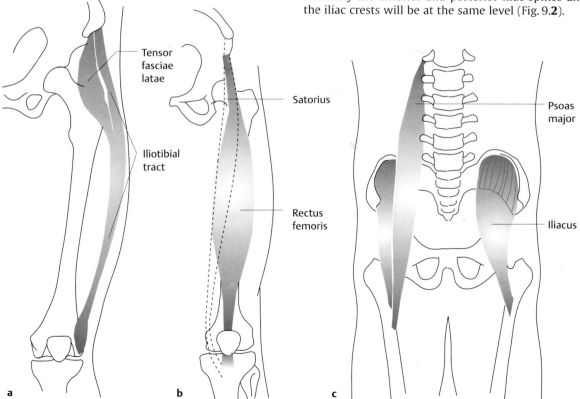

Figs. 9.**3a–c**
(**a**) Tensor fasciae latae and iliotibial tract.
(**b**) Sartorius in relation to the rectus femoris.
(**c**) Psoas major and iliacus, which together form the iliopsoas.

Painful neuromas may be found in the region of the iliac crests following removal of bone graft since the cluneal nerves can be injured in this procedure.

● **Examination with the patient supine**
Muscular insertions can be palpated with the patient **supine.** The tensor fasciae latae is located lateral to the **anterior superior iliac spine** (Fig. 9.3a). The origin of the sartorius is palpable anteriorly (Fig. 9.**3b**). Tenderness to palpation in these regions suggests tenosynovitis at the muscular insertions or an avulsion fracture. The iliopsoas, consisting of the iliacus and psoas, is located medially (Fig. 9.**3c**). The iliacus is palpable in the lateral inguinal canal; the psoas can be palpated through the abdominal wall next to the rectus abdominis. Have the patient flex his or her legs to relax the abdominal wall. This will make it easier to palpate the psoas. Overexertion from lifting weights with simultaneous deep knee bends or intensive kicking practice in football or soccer can produce irritation of the psoas that presents as tenderness to palpation. A tear or bursitis of the insertion of the iliopsoas produces tenderness to palpation at its insertion on the lesser trochanter. The **anterior inferior iliac spine** lies inferior to the anterior superior iliac spine. This is where the rectus femoris has its origin (Fig. 9.**3b**). It can also be irritated by overuse (for example in kicking practice, frequent sprinter starts, or weight training), torn, or even injured in an apophyseal fracture or avulsion fracture. Apophyseal fractures most frequently occur in adolescent athletes. An unrecognized fracture or malunion can result in thickened callus that can simulate a tumor. In relatively rare cases, this in turn can produce local pain or compressive neuropathy in what is referred to as entrapment syndrome.

Fig. 9.**4** Position of the hip in relation to the most important neurovascular structures in the groin.

The **hip** lies at the intersection of the inguinal ligament and the femoral artery (Fig. 9.4). It is not directly accessible to palpation. Tenderness in this region may be regarded as a sign of hip pathology. Swelling proximal to the inguinal ligament suggests an inguinal hernia; swelling distal to it may be a sign of a femoral hernia. Examination of the **hernial orifices** (Fig. 9.5a) and palpation of the inguinal canal (Fig. 9.**5b**) with the patient standing or supine is indi-

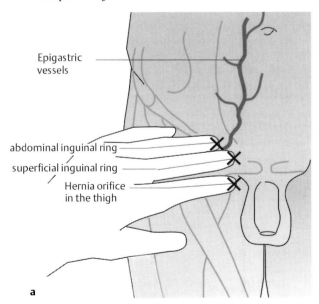

Figs. 9.**5a, b**
(**a**) Location of the three different hernial orifices in the right groin.

(**b**) Palpation of the inguinal canal with the patient standing or supine. Instruct the patient to bear down or cough after you insert your finger.

Fig. 9.**6** Palpation of the pubic symphysis and the pubic tubercle with the patient standing.

Fig. 9.**7** Positions of the various hip adductors relative to each other.

Pectineus

Adductor longus

Adductor magnus

Gracilis

cated whenever swelling is present. The differential diagnosis should exclude swelling of an **inguinal lymph node.** Exploration of the inguinal region includes palpation of the **femoral artery.** Its pulse is normally palpable midway between the anterior superior iliac spine and the pubic tubercle. A weakened pulse in trauma patients can be a sign of vascular injury.

The **pubic symphysis** or the **pubic tubercle** can be palpated anteriorly at the level of the trochanters with the patient supine or standing (Fig. 9.**6**). Note whether the two pubic tubercles are level with each other. Displacement can occur in a rupture of the pubic symphysis. Physiologic painful loosening occurs during pregnancy. Since the rectus abdominis also inserts here, the area will be tender to palpation when the muscle is irritated. Another cause of pain can be inflammation of the pubic symphysis. This is most often due to overuse, but can also be caused by infection. The pectineus inserts lateral to the pubic tubercle; the adductor longus and brevis insert inferior to it (Fig. 9.**7**). Tears in these muscles produce significant swelling inferior to the pubic bone from the contracted muscle belly and often a hematoma; they also leave a depression at the pubic bone.

Important examination sites on the posterior pelvis in the **lateral position** and **prone position** include the ischial tuberosity, sacroiliac joint, posterior hip musculature, sacrum, and coccyx.

The **ischial tuberosity** is located approximately at the level of the gluteal folds. It is the origin of the hamstrings, which include the semitendinosus, semi-membranosus, and long head of the biceps femoris (Fig. 9.**8**). Since it is difficult to palpate with the hip in extension when the patient is standing, this part of the examination is best performed with the patient in a lateral position with the hip flexed (Fig. 9.**9**). Here too, tenderness to palpation suggests a tendon disorder, bursitis, or an apophyseal avulsion fracture.

The **sciatic nerve** lies midway between the ischial tuberosity and the greater trochanter. It is palpable with the patient prone or in the lateral position. It may also be palpable when the hip is flexed since this moves the gluteal musculature superiorly (Fig. 9.**10**). Irritation of the nerve such as can occur with a prolapsed intervertebral disk or as a direct sequela of trauma can produce extreme tenderness to palpation at **Valleix's points** (see p. 306). It is important to differentiate the sciatic nerve from the ischial tuberosity, since bursitis there can produce similar pain which can lead to misdiagnosis.

Arthritic, inflammatory, or traumatic changes in the **sacroiliac joints** can manifest themselves in local tenderness to palpation. Palpate the prone patient with both hands. Move your thumbs from lateral across the posterior iliac spine to the midline in the depression between the iliac spine and the median sacral crest. Palpate the entire length of the joint on both sides for comparison.

There are a number of tests to further evaluate sacroiliac joint dysfunction (see section 8.3). These can be performed with the patient standing, supine, or prone and include:

- Standing:
  Test for pathologic anterior movement of the posterior iliac spines when the patient bends over
  Spine test
- Prone:
  Mennell's first sign
  Three-step test
  Shaking test
- Supine:
  Patrick's four-point sign
  Mennell's second sign
  Elasticity test
  Leg-length changes.

The greater part of the outer contour of the posterior pelvis is defined by the **gluteus maximus** (Fig. 9.**8**). This is best palpated with the patient prone. Instruct the patient to press the buttocks together. Palpate with both hands, noting tone, size, and form. Palpating the muscles while they are tensed and relaxed will reveal hematomas or abscesses (for example from intramuscular injections). These pathologic changes are often not visible in their initial stages.

- **Examination of the injured patient**

Some of the examination procedures described above are very specific and time consuming. The preliminary examination following severe trauma with suspected pelvic fracture must be performed quickly. The purpose of this examination is to establish the severity of **pelvic instability** (Figs. 9.**11a, b**). Examine the patient with both hands, applying lateral compression to the iliac wings and anterolateral or AP compression to reveal any abnormal mobility of the two halves of the pelvis. Palpate the injured hemipelvis while carefully applying traction or compression to the ipsilateral leg to determine vertical instability. Comparative palpation of the posterior iliac spines will reveal posterior instability of one hemipelvis. A palpable gap in the pubic synthesis may be seen if it is ruptured and the patient is not overly obese. Pain to compression of the hip can be a sign of an acetabular fracture. Avoid abrupt manipulation, particularly if the patient is conscious.

Fig. 9.**8**   Diagram of the hamstrings in relation to the gluteus maximus.

Rectal and **vaginal examination** must be performed. This can reveal injuries of the rectum or urogenital system. Perforation of the vaginal or rectal wall is a sign of an open fracture of the pelvic ring. Lack of blood on the palpating finger means that injury to the lower rectum or vagina can be largely excluded. Vaginal injury must not be confused with menstrual bleeding. Evaluate sphincter tone during the rectal examination. Sphincter dysfunction or caudal symptoms suggest a sacrum fracture. Rectal examination should also be performed for direct

Fig. 9.**9**   Palpation of the right ischial tuberosity with the patient in a left lateral position with the ipsilateral hip flexed.

Fig. 9.**10**   Palpation of the sciatic nerve with the patient in a left lateral position. The sciatic nerve can occasionally be palpated midway between the ischial tuberosity and the greater trochanter when the hip is flexed.

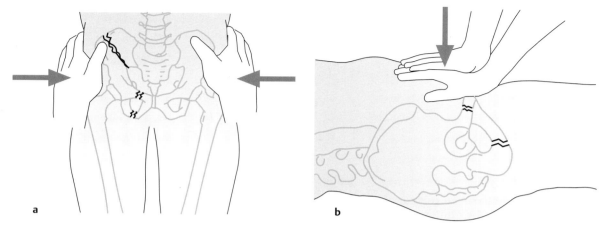

Figs. 9.**11a, b**   Lateral (**a**) and anterior to posterior (**b**) compression is applied to provoke pain in the supine patient with a pelvic fracture.

Fig. 9.**12**   Rectal examination of the coccyx and sacrococcygeal joint with the patient in a lateral position.

trauma such as a fall on the buttocks to exclude deformities in the coccygeal region (Fig. 9.**12**).

Urethral tears in males are characterized by abnormal mobility or superior displacement of the prostate. In the examination, the prostate or its tip will be palpable in the middle of a "rubbery" hematoma displaced toward the abdominal cavity. Frequently cited in the literature, this sign of a **superiorly displaced prostate** may be difficult to ascertain, especially in young patients due to the small size of the prostate. Often the nature of the injury will prevent optimum positioning for rectal palpation with the hip flexed. Blood at the urethral meatus or an abnormal prostate examination dictate that a retrograde urethrogram has to be performed before the urethra is instrumented with a catheter.

Functional Examination

Aside from the hips, there are no true joints in the pelvis. The sacroiliac joints and the pubic symphysis are articulations with limited motion.

However, there are a few functional tests that provide information about injuries to the pelvis and the musculature inserting into it.

Painful limitation of adduction against resistance with the legs extended or complete loss of adduction are signs of irritation or a tear in the muscles responsible for this motion. Flexing the hip against resistance is painful if the iliopsoas or the adjacent bursa is injured. If extending the knee also produces groin pain, this can be a sign of a proximal injury to the rectus femoris. Pain or limited motion experienced when raising the upper body from a supine position with the hips in 90° flexion combined with pain in the pubic bone suggests an abdominal muscle tear.

The nature and diagnosis of sacroiliac joint dysfunction has been discussed in the section Palpation and Examination.

Neurovascular Examination

As already mentioned, pelvic injuries, tumors, and inflammation can cause nerve irritation or injury. For this reason, examination of the pelvis should also include preliminary neurologic examination as discussed in Chapter 8, p. 309. This examination is of little use in patients with an endotracheal tube in place.

Always **palpate the peripheral pulses.** Lack of a peripheral pulse in the legs can be a sign of vascular injury as a result of pelvic trauma, for example injury to the iliac or femoral artery.

9.3 Radiology

Indications, Diagnostic Value, and Clinical Relevance

Radiographs of the pelvis are mandatory diagnostic imaging studies. The plain pelvic radiograph is the starting point for diagnostic evaluation. It provides an

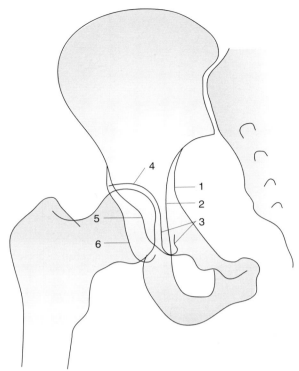

Fig. 9.**14**   Schematic diagram of the bony structures in the region of the acetabulum in the plain AP pelvic radiograph. 1 Iliopectinal line, 2 ilioischial line, 3 Köhler's teardrop figure, 4 acetabular roof, 5 anterior rim of the acetabulum, 6 posterior rim of the acetabulum.

Figs. 9.**13a, b**   Plain pelvic radiograph with the patient standing (**a**) and supine (**b**). When positioned supine, the patient is disrobed with the knees extended and the feet internally rotated about 15°. The central ray is aimed directly at the center of the pelvis.

Standard Views

AP plain pelvic radiograph: The patient is undressed and stands with his or her back to the film cassette. The knees are extended, and the feet are internally rotated about 15°. Any leg-length difference should be compensated. The central ray is aimed at the middle of the pelvis; gonad protection should be used if possible (Fig. 9.**13a**). This examination may also be performed with the patient supine (Fig. 9.**13b**); this will often be necessary in trauma patients. The plain pelvis radiograph visualizes both ilia, the sacrum, pubic bone, coccyx, and the proximal femur. It provides information on fractures of the pelvis, proximal femur, femoral neck, and trochanteric region. It also reveals signs of inflammatory processes and osteolytic or osteoplastic changes. The AP pelvic radiograph is not always sufficient for evaluating the entire sacrum, sacroiliac joints, and acetabulum (Fig. 9.**14**). Often either a PA view (with or without tilting of the X-ray to 30°–35° caudally) or a Ferguson view will be required.

Ferguson view: For this view, the patient is positioned supine as for the plain AP radiograph of the pelvis. The difference is that the X-ray tube is inclined cranially 30°–35°. The central ray is aimed at the center of the pelvis (Fig. 9.**15**). This technique provides

Fig. 9.**15**   Ferguson view of the pelvis. The patient is positioned supine and disrobed with the knees extended and the feet internally rotated 15°. The central ray is aimed directly at the center of the pelvis, and the X-ray tube is tilted cranially 30°–35°.

overview of the entire pelvis and provides a basis for any subsequent special views that may be required.

Fig. 9.**16**   Plain pelvis radiograph showing bilateral anterior fractures of the pelvic ring and a sacroiliac fracture dislocation on the left.

Fig. 9.**17**   Plain pelvic radiograph showing a left acetabular fracture (central hip dislocation).

Fig. 9.**18**   Plain pelvic radiograph showing rupture of the pubic symphysis and the right sacroiliac joint (Type C1.2 according to the AO/ASIF classification, corresponding to the CT scan in Fig. 9.**48**, p. 442).

Fig. 9.**19**   Plain pelvic radiograph. The fracture of the anterior roof of the acetabulum is only clearly discernible in the CT scan (Fig. 9.**47**), but not in the plain pelvic radiograph, the iliac wing view (Fig. 9.**36a**), or the obturator view (Fig. 9.**34a**).

the examiner with a tangential view of the sacroiliac joints and the sacrum, and it visualizes the pubic bone and coccyx.

The goal of this technique is to provide better information on possible injuries to the sacrum, pubic bone, and coccyx.

Abnormal Findings

• Changes due to trauma

The plain pelvis radiograph provides a good overview where there are multiple fractures of the pelvis (Fig. 9.**16**). However, it does not reliably image injuries of the acetabular region (Fig. 9.**17**) or the sacroiliac joint (Fig. 9.**18**). With acetabular fractures (Fig. 9.**19**),

one is often surprised by the extent of the injury. Special views, and CT scans in particular, are mandatory in such cases (see section Special Views and Computed Tomography).

• Tumors

A **chondrosarcoma** is defined as a malignant neoplasm derived from cartilage cells. It can develop on an existing endochondroma or a cartilaginous exostosis. A primary form also exists. When the tumor develops from the center of a bone, it is known as a central chondrosarcoma. Tumors that spread from the surface of a bone are referred to as periosteal chondrosarcomas. These must be distinguished from periosteal osteosarcomas. Fifty percent of chondro-

Fig. 9.**20** Partial plain pelvic radiograph. The lateral aspect of the left iliac wing shows an irregularly demarcated dense bony deposit. A calcified structure is also discernible lateral to the acetabular convexity, which at least in the plain film is not in direct contact with the pelvic bone. This was diagnosed as a chondrosarcoma.

Fig. 9.**22** Partial plain pelvic radiograph. The bone structure of the right acetabulum and the ilium largely shows pathologic changes; the normal bone structure is no longer present. "Cloudy" areas of sclerosis are present. This was diagnosed as an osteosarcoma.

sarcomas discovered are found in the pelvis and proximal femur. Men are affected by the primary form twice as often as women. The disorder most often occurs above the age of 30.

In the radiograph, the chondrosarcoma typically

Fig. 9.**21** Plain pelvic radiograph showing bone destruction with a moth-eaten appearance at the sacroiliac joint involving the adjacent portion of the sacrum. This was diagnosed as a Ewing sarcoma.

appears as an osteolytic tumor with cortical destruction and varying degrees of matrix ossification (Fig. 9.**20**).

Ewing sarcoma occurs primarily in children and adolescents. It is highly malignant. Ewing's sarcoma is thought to proceed from bone marrow cells. One of the most frequent sites is the pelvis. In radiographs, it can appear as moth-eaten destruction of bone with an associated periosteal reaction and a large soft-tissue mass. This soft-tissue mass may be the main characteristic (Fig. 9.**21**).

Osteosarcoma represents one of the most frequently encountered primary bone tumors. All types are characterized by malignant cells that form osteoid and bone matrix. This tumor most frequently develops between the ages of 10 and 20 (as a primary osteosarcoma). Men are affected slightly more often than women. This tumor can occur in different forms: as an osteolytic osteosarcoma, an osteoblastic osteosarcoma, or as a combined form. Its radiographic appearance varies. The classic appearance is moth-eaten areas of osteolysis with islands of osteosclerotic foci. The demarcation of tumor from healthy surrounding tissue is ill-defined. Periosteal reactions such as formation of spicules or layered bone remodeling are frequent associated findings (Fig. 9.**22**).

Giant-cell tumors are locally aggressive bony changes containing histologic osteoclastic giant cells. Occurrence in the pelvis is atypical. Women between the ages of 20 and 40 are most frequently affected; the ratio of women to men is 2 : 1. These tumors appear in radiographs as purely osteolytic areas without a sclerotic halo (Fig. 9.**23**).

An aneurysmatic bone cyst in the pelvis is rare. It can develop on a chondroblastoma, osteoblastoma, giant-cell tumor, or in fibrous dysplasia, or it can appear in the absence of existing changes. Most often these cysts occur before the age of 20. Usually several cysts will be found together. The tumor tends to expand (Fig. 9.**24**).

There are many tumors that can metastasize into the skeleton. These include lung, breast, prostate, and kidney cancer. Several of these tumors produce both osteoblastic and osteolytic **metastases** (Figs. 9.**25**–9.**28**).

Fig. 9.**23**   Partial plain pelvic radiograph. A typical sharply delineated area of osteolysis without a sclerotic halo in the right ilium adjacent to the sacroiliac joint. This was diagnosed as giant-cell tumor.

Fig. 9.**24**   Partial plain pelvic radiograph. Extensive polycystic lesions with destruction of the right iliac wing. Secondary findings include multiple vascular clips in situ following a kidney transplant. This was diagnosed as aneurysmatic bone cysts (corresponds to Figs. 9.**51a, b**, p. 443).

Fig. 9.**25**   Plain pelvic radiograph showing diffuse bony metastases of a breast carcinoma of mixed osteolytic-osteoblastic type (corresponds to Figs. 8.**139a, b**, p. 353).

Fig. 9.**26**   Plain pelvic radiograph showing multiple irregular areas of increased bone density, some extensive, throughout the entire visualized portion of the pelvic including both proximal femurs and the sacrum. This was diagnosed as osteoblastic metastases of a breast carcinoma.

Fig. 9.**27**   Plain pelvic radiograph showing decreased bone density superior to the left acetabulum in the lateral ilium without sharp demarcation. This was diagnosed as osteolytic metastases of an adenocarcinoma (prior to chemotherapy).

Fig. 9.**28**   Plain pelvic radiograph. In contrast to the image in Fig. 9.**27**, the previously osteolytic areas appear as sclerotic areas of dense bone after chemotherapy.

Fig. 9.**29**   Plain pelvic radiograph in a 26-year-old female patient. Extensive dense or sclerotic area extending to the acetabulum is visible in the left iliac wing. This was diagnosed as chronic osteomyelitis, although neoplasms can have the same radiographic appearance.

Fig. 9.**30**   Plain pelvic radiograph showing ankylosis of both sacroiliac joints, traction osteophytes at muscle insertions, and osteoarthritis of the right hip. This was diagnosed as ankylosing spondylitis.

● **Other changes**

Osteomyelitis. The signs of acute osteomyelitis in plain radiographs include destruction of cortical bone and bone marrow, periosteal reactions, and the presence of bone sequestrae. Chronic osteomyelitis is discernible as an area of dense bone (Fig. 9.**29**).

Ankylosing spondylitis. Typical changes in the pelvis in ankylosing spondylitis (Bechterew disease) include ankylosis of both sacroiliac joints and traction osteophytes at the muscular insertions. Chronic osteoarthritis of the hip can develop when the large joints are involved (Fig. 9.**30**).

Fibrous dysplasia. This disorder involves fibrotic changes in bone that belong to the group of developmental dysplasia disorders. The **monostotic form** most frequently occurs in the femur, followed by the tibia and ribs. It develops in the center of the bone and then spreads to the marrow. The higher the proportion of fiber in the bony changes, the more radiolucent they will appear. In contrast to the polyostotic form, this form of the disorder is often an incidental finding.

The **polyostotic form** is a significantly more aggressive disorder. It primarily involves the pelvis, followed by the long cortical bones, skull, and ribs. The disease is progressive until the skeleton matures. Foci usually increase in size and number. In 95% of all cases, these foci do not change after growth has ceased. The typical complication is a pathologic fracture. It is often combined with skin changes, particu-

Fig. 9.**32**   Plain pelvic radiograph showing diffuse increase in bone density in the right hip. This was diagnosed as Paget disease. Incidental findings included a radiodense metallic structure projected on the right sacrum, consistent with a projectile (such as a pistol bullet).

Fig. 9.**31**   Partial plain pelvic radiograph showing areas with loss of trabecular structure in the cancellous bone. The lesions have a "ground glass" appearance. Areas of increased sclerosis are also seen. This was diagnosed as fibrous dysplasia.

larly café-au-lait spots. The radiographic appearance of fibrous dysplastic foci depends on the relationship and distribution between the connective-tissue and bony components. Bubble-like honeycomb cystic patterns can appear. These are usually sharply demarcated from the surrounding bone by a sclerotic halo. The bone can be greatly distended with thinning of the cortex, particularly in the polyostotic form of the disorder (Fig. 9.**31**).

Paget disease. This is a chronic progressive dysfunction of bone homeostasis where osteoclastic and osteoblastic functions become uncoupled. Its precise cause is not known. Usually the disease occurs between the ages of 45 and 55. Men are most often affected; the ratio of men to women is 3 : 2. The pelvis is most frequently involved, followed by the femur, skull, tibia, vertebrae, clavicle, humerus, and ribs. Three radiographic phases are differentiated (Fig. 9.**32**):

1. Osteolytic or hot phase: This involves bone resorption in the form of a radiolucent wedge, which is also referred to as a "candle flame" because of its shape.

2. Intermediate phase: In addition to bone destruction, the onset of bone remodeling is also discernible. This appears on the radiograph as a widening of the cortex. The cancellous bone shows a course trabecular pattern.
3. Cold phase: The bone now shows a diffuse increase in density. It also appears widened and enlarged; the cortex and the border between cortex and cancellous bone is indistinct.

Deformation of the bone can also occur. Complications of Paget disease include secondary osteosarcomas and high-output cardiac failure.

Special Views

These studies provide imaging of those areas that are not well visualized on standard views. The advent of CT scanning has lessened the utility of some of these studies.

Judet Views (Obturator and Iliac Wing Views)

The extent of an acetabulum fracture is often underestimated on the plain pelvis radiograph. Overlapping shadows of bone structures make it very difficult to imagine the three-dimensional structure of a fracture. These two perpendicular oblique views of the hip permit better orientation in determining the course of a fracture.

Anterior (internally rotated) view or obturator view. The patient is positioned supine with the body rotated 45° toward the contralateral side. A wedge-shaped cushion is usually placed under the side of interest to stabilize the patient in this position. The central ray is aimed at the affected hip (Figs. 9.**33a–c**).

This exposes the obturator foramen. Fractures of the anterior (iliopubic) column of the hip and the

Figs. 9.**33a–c**   Judet view (anterior oblique view or obturator view). Patient positioning:
(**a**) oblique supine position.
(**b**) The patient is turned 45° to the contralateral (unaffected) side. A wedge-shaped cushion is usually placed under the affected side to stabilize the patient in this position.
(**a, c**) The central ray is aimed at the affected hip.

posterior rim of the acetabulum can be demonstrated in this view (Figs. 9.**34a, b**).

Posterior (externally rotated) view or iliac wing view. In contrast to the anterior view, the patient is rotated 45° toward the affected side, and the contralateral side is supported with a wedge-shaped cushion. The central ray is again aimed at the affected hip (Figs. 9.**35a–c**).

The full width of the iliac wing is visualized. The posterior (ilioischial) column of the hip and the anterior acetabular margin, projected far laterally, are clearly visible (Figs. 9.**36a, b**).

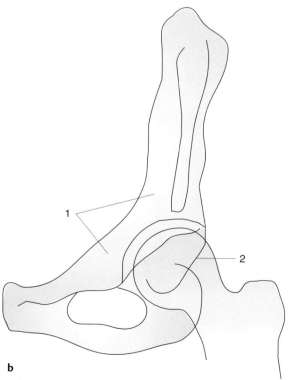

Figs. 9.**34a, b**   Judet view (anterior oblique view or obturator view). Patient positioning:
(**a**) Plain radiograph corresponding to Figs. 9.**19**, 9.**36a**, and 9.**47**.
(**b**) Schematic diagram of the obturator view: 1 anterior column, 2 posterior column.

a   b   c

Figs. 9.**35a–c**   Judet view (posterior oblique view or iliac wing view). Patient positioning:
(**a**) Oblique supine position.
(**b**) The patient is turned 45° onto the affected side. A wedge-shaped cushion is usually placed under the affected side to stabilize the patient in this position.
(**a, c**) The central ray is aimed at the affected hip.

Inlet and Outlet Views According to Pennal and Tile

Inlet and outlet views of the pelvis described by Pennal and Tile provide information in injuries to the pel-

vic ring. These two projections are approximately perpendicular to each other.

Inlet view. The patient is supine with the central ray aimed caudad at the middle of the pelvis at an angle

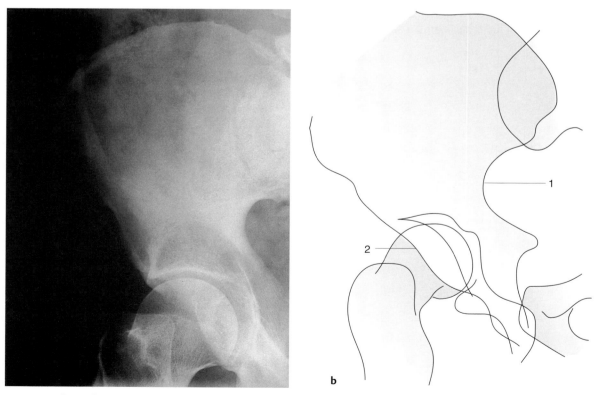

a   b

Figs. 9.**36a, b**   Judet view (posterior oblique view or iliac wing view).
(**a**) Plain radiograph corresponding to Figs. 9.**19**, 9.**34a**, and 9.**47**.
(**b**) Schematic diagram of the iliac wing view: 1 posterior column, 2 anterior acetabular rim.

of approximately 45° to the film cassette. In this position, the central ray is approximately perpendicular to the pelvic inlet and parallel to the plane of the sacrum (Fig. 9.**37**). This view best demonstrates the ring configuration of the pelvis; any narrowing or widening of the diameter of the pelvic ring will immediately be apparent. The inlet projection is also the best projection for visualizing posterior dislocation of one hemipelvis (Figs. 9.**38a, b**). Internal or external rotation of one hemipelvis will be readily visible.

Outlet view. With the patient positioned supine, the central ray is angled cephalad 45° to the film cassette and aimed at the pubic symphysis, perpendicular to the plane of the sacrum (Fig. 9.**39**). The full length of the sacrum is visible, as are the sacral foramina. The anterior pelvic ring is superimposed over the posterior pelvic ring in this tangential view. This projection demonstrates superior or inferior dislocations (Figs. 9.**40a, b**).

Fig. 9.**37**   Inlet view of the pelvis. The patient is supine with the central ray aimed caudad at the pelvis at an angle of approximately 45° to horizontal.

b

Figs. 9.**38a, b**   Inlet view of the pelvis.
(**a**) Dislocation fracture through the left ilium (sacroiliac fracture dislocation). The posterior displacement of the left hemipelvis is readily visible.
(**b**) Schematic diagram of an inlet view of the pelvis in a fracture of the left sacrum.

a

Fig. 9.**39**   Outlet view of the pelvis. The patient is supine with the central ray aimed cephalad at the pelvis (pubic symphysis) at an angle of approximately 45° to horizontal.

a

b

Figs. 9.**40a, b**   Outlet view of the pelvis.
(**a**) Dislocation fracture through the left ilium sacroiliac fracture dislocation
(**b**) Schematic diagram of an outlet view of the pelvis in a disruption of the left sacroiliac joint demonstrating the superior displacement of the left hemipelvis.

Risser View

This view is used to visualize the iliac crests to determine skeletal age (Fig. 8.**165** [see p. 368] and Table 9.**7**). The patient is supine with the hips and knees flexed to reduce the lumbar lordosis. Gonad protection should be used. The cassette is placed beneath the iliac crests, and the ray is aimed at them (Figs. 9.**41**).

Figs. 9.**41**   Risser view of the pelvis. The patient is supine with the hips and knees flexed. The central ray is aimed at the iliac crests.

Fig. 9.**42**   PA symphysis view. The patient stands facing the film cassette with the pubic symphysis against its surface. The central ray is aimed at the pubic symphysis.

Table 9.**7**   Risser stages (see Fig. 8.**165**, p. 368)

Development of the iliac crest apophysis	
Stage I	25%
Stage II	50%
Stage III	75%
Stage IV	100%
Stage V	Completely closed

Symphysis Views

PA symphysis view. The patient stands facing the film cassette with the symphysis against its surface. The symphysis is palpated and marked posteriorly. The ray is aimed at the pubic symphysis (Fig. 9.**42**).

Craniocaudal symphysis view. The patient leans back from a sitting position on the table and with the legs extended and the arms supporting the upper body. The film cassette is beneath the symphysis, and the central ray is aimed at the palpable aspect of the symphysis. The patient exhales and holds his or her breath as the image is taken (Fig. 9.**43**).

Symphysis stress view. The patient stands on one leg facing the film cassette with the pubic symphysis in contact with the film cassette. Instability will create a step-off in this view that must be compared with the normal PA view (Figs. 9.**44**, 9.**45a, b**).

Similarly, chronic posttraumatic pelvic instability can be revealed in plain pelvic radiographs as abnormal mobility of one hemipelvis as the patient stands alternately on each leg.

Tomography

Tomographic images are helpful in evaluating the extent of the fracture line and the position of the fragments in a trauma setting. They are also suitable for demonstrating the size and proliferation of masses or inflammatory processes. The projection used depends on the region of interest.

Conventional tomography has largely been replaced by the use of CT scans.

Angiography

Conventional angiography or digital subtraction angiography (DSA) can be useful, particularly in the evaluation of tumors. The main vessel supplying the region of interest is catheterized, and the catheter is advanced under fluoroscopic control. Contrast medium is injected when it reaches the affected area. This permits precise evaluation of the vascular regions supplying the area. DSA uses special algorithms to remove superfluous visual information from digital images to obtain more precise or isolated visualization of the vascular structures. In orthope-

Fig. 9.**43**   Craniocaudal symphysis view. The patient sits on the table and leans back with the legs extended and the arms supporting the upper body. The image is obtained after the patient exhales. The central ray is aimed at the pubic symphysis.

Fig. 9.**44**   Stress view of the pubic symphysis. The patient stands alternately on the left and right leg while facing the film cassette with the pubic symphysis against the surface of the cassette. The central ray is aimed at the pubic symphysis.

a   b

Figs. 9.**45a, b**   Stress view of the pubic symphysis in a 51-year-old female patient with osteomyelitis of the left sacroiliac joint. Instability in the left sacroiliac joint resulted after extensive surgical excision. This is demonstrated in the stress views (left and right single-leg stance), which show motion at the symphysis.

Fig. 9.**46**   An angiogram demonstrating the vascular supply to an osteosarcoma in the right iliac wing. Notable findings include an extensive irregular vascular network with abrupt changes in vascular diameter.

dics, this technique is used primarily in tumor surgery (Fig. 9.**46**). In a trauma setting, it can provide important information about possible associated vascular injuries. In pelvis fractures, it can also be used for selective embolization of injured vascular structures, such as the branches of the internal iliac artery.

Retrograde Urethrocystography

In pelvic trauma, the urethra and bladder can be visualized with a water-soluble contrast medium in retrograde urethrocystography, permitting diagnosis and evaluation of injuries to the urethra and/or bladder. Contrast-medium leakage will be seen in injuries. A bladder tear will appear as a more or less diffuse leakage of contrast medium into the peritoneum or preperitoneal space depending on the severity of the injury. In an extraperitoneal tear, this will typically appear as a "teardrop bladder." In a pelvic fracture, the teardrop form of the bladder in a cystogram can also be due to extravasated blood and/or urine (urinoma) and is not necessarily a characteristic sign of an extraperitoneal tear. In a tear, contrast medium will also leak from the bladder; otherwise the teardrop shape will be formed by the surrounding hematoma. A complete periprostatic tear of the intrapelvic urethra with superior displacement of the bladder will produce a high-riding bladder syndrome.

9.4 Ultrasound

Indications, Diagnostic Value, and Clinical Relevance

Ultrasonography of the pelvis is of limited importance. Soft-tissue injuries can be diagnosed. These include hematomas or inflammatory masses, such as an abscess from an injection. Ultrasound may conceivably be used to diagnose muscle tears in the adductors, or for diagnosing instability of the pubic symphysis.

Ultrasound studies of the abdomen can be performed on trauma patients with pelvic fractures to diagnose associated injuries, particularly ruptures of the spleen or liver (abdominal and pelvic trauma).

9.5 Nuclear Medicine Studies

Nuclear medicine studies of the pelvis are discussed in conjunction with nuclear medicine studies of the spine in Chapter 8, p. 380.

9.6 Computed Tomography

Indications, Diagnostic Value, and Clinical Relevance

Computed tomography (CT) is the preferred diagnostic imaging modality after plain radiography in the diagnosis of fractures or tumors. Compared to conventional radiographs, CT permits detailed, unobstructed visualization of deeper-lying bone structures such as the sacrum or sacroiliac joints. Superimposed intestinal gas, which can greatly complicate the interpretation of conventional radiographs, does not influence CT imaging. Physicians can obtain three-dimensional reconstruction from the CT images. This representation of the fracture or tumor may then be used for preoperative planning. These reconstructions allow the surgeon to verify the involvement of acetabulum and femoral head, the position of the fragments, or the presence of intra-articular loose bodies or fragments following acetabular fractures or hip dislocations. CT is especially useful after trauma to the sacrum or sacroiliac joints. The **sensitivity** of CT lies between 85% and 100% for evaluating the sacrum and sacroiliac joint, ilium, roof of the acetabulum, posterior rim of the acetabulum, pubic rami, or intra-articular loose bodies, depending on slice thickness. Its **specificity** is 100% in all of these cases.

Technique, Instrumentation, and Examination Procedure

The patient is symmetrically positioned on the CT examining table to permit accurate comparison of both sides in the slice images. A preliminary scan is obtained to aid in selecting the area of interest. Next the CT slice images are obtained. A **slice thickness** of 5–10 mm is adequate for many tumors or fractures. Acetabular fractures are an exception since they may involve intra-articular loose bodies. In this case and with smaller bone or soft-tissue tumors, one should select a slice thickness not greater than 3–5 mm. If two-dimensional or three-dimensional reconstruction is planned, the slices should be 1–2 mm thick. Slice thicknesses of 2 mm are preferred in these cases to protect the patient against excessive radiation exposure.

Intravenous **contrast medium** can be used to obtain information about the vascularization of neoplasms. Decisions about slice thickness, reconstructions, and contrast must be discussed with the consulting radiologist.

Abnormal Findings

Changes Due to Trauma

CT of the pelvis provides more precise information about the presence, location, and relationship of fragments to each other than can conventional radiography (Fig. 9.**47**). Injuries of the sacroiliac joints are often difficult to determine on plain radiographs. CT permits detection of even minor injuries or diastasis. Contralateral comparison in axial images is especially helpful (Fig. 9.**48**). Plaster casts do not degrade images. A further advantage is that CT examinations require only minimal movement of trauma patients.

Three-dimensional reconstruction permits precise visualization of fracture fragments. This is important for proper treatment of the fracture (Figs. 9.**49a–c**).

Even chronic injuries to the pelvis can be visualized in CT scans. The additional information provided by the CT examination can be clearly seen in an avulsion fracture of the anterior superior iliac spine (Figs. 9.**50a, b**). A plain pelvis radiograph would not have been sufficient to evaluate the shape and extent of bony structures at the anterior superior iliac spine following an avulsion fracture.

Tumors

The advantages of CT apply to diagnosing tumors. In addition to providing unobstructed visualization, CT scans also make it easier to diagnose discrete cortical destruction, endosteal changes, and minor matrix calcifications. This provides more information about the size of the tumor, and it also helps to identify the type of tumor. The use of intravenous contrast permits limited evaluation of tumor components extending

Fig. 9.**47**   CT of the pelvis in the transverse plane. The fracture fragment is only clearly identifiable in the CT scan (corresponding to Figs. 9.**19**, 9.**34a**, 9.**36a**).

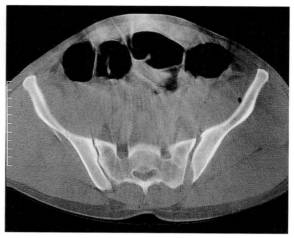

Fig. 9.**48**   Axial CT of the pelvis showing disruption of the right sacroiliac joint (corresponding to Fig. 9.**18**, p. 430).

a

b

Figs. 9.**49a–c**   Plain pelvic radiograph and CT reconstruction.
(**a**) Radiograph showing fracture of the left pelvis involving the acetabulum.
(**b, c**) Three-dimensional CT reconstruction of the same fracture.

c

beyond the bone, and it can demonstrate the size of necrotic areas and the relationship of the tumor to vascular structures.

The advantages of CT over conventional radiography in diagnosing are seen in Figures 9.**51a** and **b**, which show an aneurysmal bone cyst. The CT slices of the pelvis were obtained from the same patient as the plain pelvic radiographs in Figure 9.**24**. This patient had received a renal transplant 8 years prior to the occurrence of the tumor. In addition to showing the topographic relationship of the tumor to the organs, the CT demonstrates the typical tumor structure (i.e., polycystic and proliferative).

b

Figs. 9.50a, b
(**a**) Partial plain pelvic radiograph.
(**b**) Axial CT scan of the pelvis in a 16-year-old patient showing a chronic avulsion of the anterior superior iliac spine. Bone remodeling has produced a mass that could be confused with a tumor if the history or initial films were unknown. This can produce symptoms by irritating adjacent neurovascular structures. In contrast to plain radiography, the CT image precisely demonstrates the shape and size of the mass.

a

a   b

Figs. 9.51a, b Axial CT scan of the pelvis. The images show an extensive, relatively sharply demarcated mass in the left ilium that anteriorly displaces the pelvic organs and soft tissue. The slices show the relationship of the tumor to adjacent structures and demonstrate its polycystic structure. This was diagnosed as an aneurysmal bone cyst (corresponding to Fig. 9.24, p. 432).

9.7 Magnetic Resonance Imaging

Indications, Diagnostic Value, and Clinical Relevance

Magnetic resonance imaging (MRI) has become an important modality for the evaluation of soft-tissue and bony structures in the pelvis in recent years. Its particular advantage lies in its ability to detect inflammatory changes and tumors at an early stage. It is the only method aside from nuclear medicine studies that can detect occult fractures.

Technique, Instrumentation, and Examination Procedure

Since the pelvis is a large region of the body, a **body coil** is frequently used. However, surface coils may be used under certain circumstances to image smaller areas. The coil images major vascular structures including the aorta, common iliac artery, internal and external iliac arteries, inguinal artery, and femoral artery. Pulsatile motion of these vascular structures can produce **ghosting.** Other **motion artifacts** may be caused by breathing or intestinal motion and can interfere with the image similarly to pulsatile ghosting.

Enteral administration of contrast media is helpful for distinguishing the bowel from other soft-tissue structures. **Intravenous administration of gadolinium-DTPA** is particularly useful in demonstrating and identifying tumors as benign or malignant, but it can also be helpful in evaluating infiltrative processes such as the spread of a prostate carcinoma to the wall of the bladder.

The **slice thickness** depends on the required degree of detail. Differentiating postoperative conditions, residual tumor tissue, and recurrent tumors is a particular problem. As with other diagnostic imaging modalities, regular follow-up examinations are frequently necessary. The **imaging plane** should also be chosen according to the pathology and anatomy. Coronal oblique imaging planes in addition to oblique transverse planes are needed for evaluating sacral processes. Processes in the inguinal canal frequently require an oblique sagittal imaging plane.

Abnormal Findings

Occult Fractures and Changes Due to Trauma

Common pelvic fractures are easily visualized using radiographic methods, i.e., plain radiography or CT. With the introduction of MRI, bone changes that escape detection in radiographic studies were described. These are referred to as occult fractures (Figs. 9.**52a, b**). In addition to cancellous fractures due to metabolic dysfunction, these findings can theoretically include changes in bone metabolism resulting from impaired perfusion or remodeling processes due

to biomechanical dysfunction. These changes are visible especially in fat-suppressing pulse sequences. These findings may be diffuse. There is never a visible cortical lesion with these changes.

Tumors

Differentiating between benign and malignant bone tumors is difficult in MR images. Characteristics such as sharp demarcation, a purely tissue-displacing pattern of growth, and homogeneous signal behavior suggest a benign tumor, although some malignant tumors such as the chondrosarcoma behave similarly (Figs. 9.**53a–c**). Biopsy is indicated to evaluate any bone tumors in the pelvis. Depending on the type of the tumor, T1 or T2-weighted images will provide the best contrast between the tumor and adjacent tissue. A fat-suppressing sequence (Figs. 9.**54a, b**) has the highest sensitivity in detecting tumors since the pathophysiologic changes always include a locally enlarged extracellular space. T1-weighted images with gadolinium-DTPA are indicated to demonstrate the tumor borders and help identify the type of tumor.

Specificity depends on the morphology, behavior after application of contrast medium, and, to a lesser extent, the T1 and T2 relaxation times.

Differentiating tumor from surrounding tissue in MR images is possible with a high degree of accuracy using fat-suppressing sequences (to distinguish it from healthy marrow) and T1 sequences before and after application of gadolinium-DTPA.

a   b

Figs. 9.**52a, b**   MR images of the pelvis.
(**a**) SE 500/20 in the coronal plane showing reduced signal intensity in the right side of the sacrum.
(**b**) STIR 1900/125 in the coronal plane showing increased signal intensity in the sacrum. The change does not extend beyond the margins of the bone. Signal intensity is also slightly increased lateral to the right foramen between S1 and S2. This was diagnosed as a contusion of the right side of the sacrum following a fall. The corresponding plain pelvic radiograph was normal.

Figs. 9.**53a–c**   MR images of the sacral region.
(**a**) GRE (500/10, out of phase) in the sagittal plane showing a well-demarcated tumor mass that includes the sacrum and extends into the pelvis and the spine. It is relatively homogeneous with slightly increased signal intensity.
(**b**) GRE (500/10, out of phase) in the sagittal plane after administration of gadolinium-based contrast medium. Contrast-medium enhancement is seen in the tumor masses, which continue to be well demarcated.
(**c**) GRE (500/10, out of phase) in the coronal plane. The tumor is still well demarcated and includes the entire sacrum except for the lateral mass adjacent to the joint. This was diagnosed as a recurrent chondrosarcoma.

a   b

Figs. 9.**54a, b**   MR images of the pelvis.
(**a**) STIR 1900/125 in the coronal plane showing a mass of high signal intensity that includes the iliac spine but also extends into the pelvis and into gluteal musculature.
(**b**) STIR 3000/100 in the transverse plane showing destruction of the iliac spine by tumor tissue of median signal density. The far posterior portions of the tumor again appear with high intensity and surround the iliac wing. This was diagnosed as a largely necrotic metastasis to the iliac wing.

MRI can demonstrate whether a tumor respects bone borders or has passed through them, particularly in the sacroiliac joints and the facet joints (Figs. 9.**55a–e**).

Lipomas are easily identified and distinguished from non-fatty tissue because of their high fat content. However, intracutaneous lipomas without a discernible mass can avoid detection. Differentiating intracutaneous lipomas and **liposarcomas** can also be difficult. Septation in sarcomas is one criterion for differentiation.

Inflammatory Changes

In **osteomyelitis** the physician will only be able to document pathologic findings about 10 days to 2 weeks after the onset of clinical symptoms using conventional radiography or CT. MRI can detect changes in bone as early as 3 days after infection. Nuclear medicine studies are similarly sensitive but less specific. Inflammation produces hyperemia and edema in the marrow. The increased fluid content extends the T1 relaxation time, which reduces the signal in a T1-weighted sequence. At the same time, hyperemia and edema will extend the T2 relaxation time and increase the signal in T2-weighted sequences. Since marrow has a high content of fatty tissue, these findings are often difficult to discern in

T2-weighted sequences because fat also has a long T2 relaxation time. For this reason, **fat-suppressing pulse sequences** are preferred. These sequences visualize the free water content of tissue with high signal intensity according to its relaxation time (Figs. 9.**56a–c**). The criterion for differentiating **chronic** from **acute osteomyelitis** is the periosteal zone of irritation, which can be readily demonstrated in the T1-weighted images after administration of gadolinium-DTPA. **Chronic osteomyelitis** can be recognized by the reactive thickening of the cortex. The reactive periosteal halo is also missing in chronic osteomyelitis except when it is reactivated. However, the early **acute process** is not sharply demarcated. The change extends over a wide area of the marrow. A **sequestrum** resulting from osteomyelitic changes will be discernible in all sequences as a zone of low signal intensity within the inflamed area.

Soft-tissue infections appear in T2-weighted images as areas of high signal intensity, showing significant diffuse boundary disruption visible as contrast enhancement. If an **abscess** develops, the abscess itself will appear as a homogeneous structure of high signal intensity in T2-weighted and fat-suppressing pulse sequences. The abscess membrane is usually hyperemic and will show circumscribed halo-like enhancement after administration of gadolinium-DTPA (Figs. 9.**57a–c**, 9.**58a, b**).

Figs. 9.**55a–e**   MR images of the pelvis.
(**a**) STIR 1900/125 in the coronal plane showing a mass of high signal intensity in the left inferior pubic ramus that disrupts the boundary of the bone and extends into soft tissue.
(**b, c**) GRE (500/10, out of phase) in the transverse plane. No lesion is discernible.
(**d, e**) GRE (500/10, out of phase) in the transverse plane after administration of gadolinium-based contrast medium. A circumscribed area of increase signal intensity in the superior and inferior pubic rami with significant boundary destruction. The mass is seen to extend into the adductors that insert here.
This was diagnosed as a metastasis of an adenocarcinoma to the left superior and inferior pubic rami.

a

b

c

Figs. 9.**56a–c**   MR images of the pelvis.
(**a**) STIR 1900/125 in the coronal plane showing an area of increased signal intensity in the body of the right ilium that also involves the lateral mass of the sacrum. There is an increase in signal intensity around the bone in the gluteal musculature of the right side.
(**b**) GRE (500/10, out of phase) in the coronal plane. Signal intensity is increased in the body of the right ilium compared with the contralateral side.
(**c**) GRE (500/10, out of phase) in the coronal plane after administration of gadolinium-based contrast medium. Significant signal enhancement is seen in the body of the ilium and in the tissue surrounding the bone.
This was diagnosed as osteomyelitis of the right ilium extending to the right lateral mass of the sacrum.

a

b

c

Figs. 9.**57a–c**   MR images of the pelvis.
(**a**) STIR 1900/125 in the coronal plane showing strips of increased signal intensity in the right gluteal musculature extending into the sheath of the biceps femoris. At the level of the trochanter there is a relatively circumscribed subcutaneous area with a halo of increased signal intensity. Increased signal intensity is also seen in the skin.
(**b**) GRE (500/10, out of phase) in the coronal plane after administration of gadolinium-based contrast medium. The infiltrated area appears enhanced, and the decrease in signal intensity in the fatty tissue is apparent.
(**c**) GRE (500/10, out of phase) in the sagittal plane. A circumscribed area of increased signal intensity is visible at the level of the greater trochanter.
This was diagnosed as an abscess of the gluteal musculature at the level of the greater trochanter with infiltration into the biceps femoris.

a   b

Figs. 9.**58a, b**   MR images of the pelvis.
(**a**) STIR 1900/125 in the coronal plane showing a large infiltrative process of high signal intensity extending from the psoas and iliopsoas through the inguinal region into the adductors and vastus medialis. There is a zone of increased signal intensity in the femoral head and the right acetabulum. A moderate effusion into the hip is present.
(**b**) PS 500/10 in the coronal plane after administration of gadolinium-based contrast medium showing significantly increased signal intensity in the iliopsoas. The process shows reduced signal intensity with increased marginal signal intensity in the adductors and vastus medialis.
This was diagnosed as an abscess proceeding from the psoas with a large abscess cavity in the adductors and vastus medialis. The image shows accompanying inflammation of the hip and the onset of osteomyelitis of the right femoral head and acetabulum.

References

Bernau A, Berquist TH. *Orthopaedic Positioning in Diagnostic Radiology.* Munich–Vienna–Baltimore: Urban & Schwarzenberg; 1983

Biedert R. Sportverletzungen und Sportschäden. *Therapeutische Umschau.* 1987; 44: 855

Dalton SE. Overuse injuries in adolescent athletes. *Sports Med.* 1992; 13: 58

Dunn EL. Berry PH, Connally JD. Computed tomography of the pelvis in patients with multiple injuries. *J Trauma.* 1983; 5: 378

Frisch H. *Programmierte Untersuchung des Bewegungsapparates.* Chirodiagnostik. Berlin–Heidelberg: Springer; 1995

Greenspan A. *Skelettradiologie.* Weinheim–London: Chapman & Hall; 1993

Häring R, Zilch H. *Diagnose und Differentialdiagnose in der Chirurgie.* Vol 2. Weinheim–London: Chapman & Hall; 1995

Hegglin J. *Chirurgische Untersuchung.* Stuttgart–New York: Thieme; 1988

Jend HH, Tödt HC. *Wegweiser Bildgebende Diagnostik.* Stuttgart: Hippokrates; 1992

Hoppenfeld S. *Klinische Untersuchung der Wirbelsäule und der Extremitäten.* Stuttgart–Jena–New York: Fischer; 1992

Klose HH, Schuchardt E. Die beckennahen Apophysenausrisse. *Orthopäde.* 1980; 9: 229

Letournel E, Judet R. *Fractures of the Acetabulum.* Berlin–Heidelberg–New York: Springer; 1993

Lissner J, Fink U (ed). *Radiologie I.* Stuttgart: Enke; 1990

Matta JM, Cockin J, Letournel E, Rüedi T. Acetabulum. In: Müller ME, Allgöwer M, Schneider R, Willenegger H, eds. *Manual of Internal Fixation. Techniques Recommended by the AO-ASIF-Group.* Berlin–Heidelberg–New York: Springer; 1991: 501

McRae R. *Klinisch-orthopädische Untersuchung.* Stuttgart–New York: Fischer; 1989

Metzmaker JN, Pappas AM. Avulsion fractures of the pelvis. *Am J Sports Med.* 1985; 13: 349

Neumann HD. *Manuelle Medizin.* Berlin–Heidelberg–New York: Springer; 1989

Nutton RW, Pinder IM, Williams D. Detection of sacroiliac injury by bone scanning in fractures of the pelvis and its clinical significance. *Injury.* 1982; 13: 473

Pennal GF, Tile M, Waddell JP, Garside H. Pelvic disruption: assessment and classification. *Clin Orthop.* 1980; 151: 12

Peters PE, Matthias HH, Reiser M. *Magnetresonanztomographie in der Orthopädie* (Bücherei des Orthopäden, Vol 56). Stuttgart: Enke; 1990

Pitt MJ, Lund PJ, Speer DP. Imaging of the pelvis and hip. Radiographic imaging in orthopedics. *Orthop Clin North Am.* 1990; 21: 545

Renström P. Swedish research in sports traumatology. *Clin Orthop.* 1984; 191: 144

Rieger H. *Das instabile Becken – Diagnostik, Therapie und Prognose der Beckenringfraktur.* Munich–Bern–Vienna–New York: Zuckschwerdt; 1996

Schils J, Hauzeur JP. Stress fracture of the sacrum. *Am J Sports Med.* 1992; 20: 769

Tscherne H, Pohlemann T. Tscherne Unfallchirurgie, Becken und Acetabulum. Berlin–Heidelberg–New York: Springer; 1998

Tile M, Burri C, Poigenfürst J. Pelvis. In: Müller ME, Allgöwer M, Schneider R, Willenegger H, eds. *Manual of Internal Fixation. Techniques Recommended by the AO-ASIF-Group.* Berlin–Heidelberg–New York: Springer; 1991: 485

Wenz W, Laubenberger J. Sportverletzungen als Herausforderung für die moderne Bildgebung. *Radiologe.* 1989; 29: 537

Index